Psychiatric Nursing Care Plans

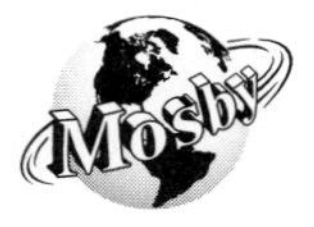

Visit our website at **www.mosby.com**

Psychiatric Nursing Care Plans

Katherine M. Fortinash, RN, MSN, CS
Certified Clinical Specialist
Adult Psychiatric–Mental Health Nursing
Clinical Nurse Specialist/Clinical Educator
Mesa Vista Hospital
Sharp Hospital Behavioral Health Services
San Diego, California

Consultant
San Diego, California

Patricia A. Holoday-Worret, RN, MSN, CS
Certified Clinical Specialist
Adult Psychiatric–Mental Health Nursing
Associate Professor, Psychiatric Mental Health Nursing
Palomar College
San Marcos, California

Consultant
San Diego, California

Third Edition

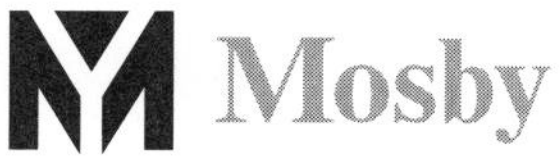

St. Louis Baltimore Boston Carlsbad Chicago Minneapolis New York Philadelphia Portland
London Milan Sydney Tokyo Toronto

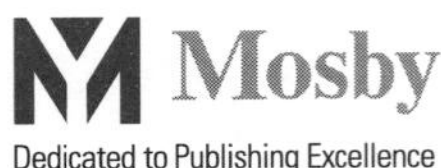

Mosby
Dedicated to Publishing Excellence

A Times Mirror Company

Publisher: Sally Schrefer
Editor: Jeanne Allison
Associate Developmental Editor: Jeff Downing
Project Manager: John Rogers
Designer: Yael Kats
Cover Design: John Ritland, Ritland Publishing Services
Cover Illustration: Diana Ong/SuperStock
Manufacturing Supervisor: Debbie LaRocca
Editing and Production: Graphic World Publishing Services

Third Edition

Composition by Graphic World, Inc.
Printing/binding by World Color Press-Taunton

Mosby, Inc.
11830 Westline Industrial Drive
St. Louis, Missouri 63146

Library of Congress Cataloging in Publication Data
Fortinash, Katherine M.
Psychiatric nursing care plans / Katherine M. Fortinash, Patricia A. Holoday-Worret.—3rd ed.
p. cm.
Includes bibliographical references and index.
ISBN 0-323-00403-2
1. Psychiatric nursing. 2. Nursing care plans. I. Holoday-Worret, Patricia A. II. Title.
[DNLM: 1. Psychiatric Nursing—methods. 2. Nursing Care—methods. 3. Patient Care Planning. WY 160 F742p 1999]
RC440.F57 1999
610.73'68—dc21
DNLM/DLC
for Library of Congress 98-29832
CIP

98 99 00 01 02 / 9 8 7 6 5 4 3 2 1

Preface

Psychiatric Nursing Care Plans, third edition, continues with the quality of the previous work. Focus is placed on the client's psychosocial needs and the responses of the nurse and other health care providers in achieving, maintaining, and promoting the psychosocial integrity related to those needs. We continue to believe that the text's clear language and "real life" examples help to distinguish it as a unique and powerful clinical tool and are largely responsible for its positive impact on students and instructors.

INTENDED USE

The primary intention of this text is to help nurses deliver professional, quality care in the psychiatric mental health environment. The text has also proven useful for other clinicians who interact with persons experiencing mental or emotional problems, in a variety of settings.

To maintain the structural integrity of this text, we continue to use the North American Nursing Diagnosis Association's (NANDA) Taxonomy I Revised, 1994, and the American Psychiatric Association's Diagnostic and Statistical Manual, fourth edition (DSM-IV), 1994.

NEW ADDITIONS TO TEXT

- New clinical pathways (mania and psychosis) in Chapter 1 (see Figures 1-4 and 1-5)
- New appendixes:
  - — Grief and Loss
  - — Spirituality
  - — Crisis Intervention
- New second color to emphasize and enhance content and readability
- Four universal principles in the general principles section preceding care plans. The authors believe that these are essential for promoting mental health and treating mental disorders.

  Four Universal Principles:
  1. Continue to monitor assessment parameters listed under *Defining Characteristics* section
  2. Continue to consider the etiologic factors listed under *Etiologic/Related Factors* section
  3. Utilize principles of the *Therapeutic Nurse–Client Relationship* (Appendix G)
  4. Address clients' spiritual and cultural needs

The collaborative, time-proven efforts of nursing and medicine provide the organizational framework for effectively managing client problems in both a practical and scientific manner. As in previous editions, this text emphasizes the dynamic progress of nursing and the interdisciplinary health care team in achieving quality client care. Future editions will continue to reflect the trends in NANDA and DSM-IV as they are revised, expanded, and refined; to meet the changes in health care delivery systems and standards of care. Terminology used in this text reflect the most current information found in professional nursing and medical publications.

CHAPTER 1 THE NURSING PROCESS

Chapter 1 presents a comprehensive narrative description of the nursing process. It explains why the process is cyclic and continuous, not linear or episodic, and includes a newly refined diagram reflecting these concepts. Each of the six phases of the nursing process (assessment, nursing diagnosis, outcome identification, planning, implementation, and evaluation) is discussed with emphasis on the nursing diagnosis, its historical development, and evolvement in relation to NANDA.

NANDA's Taxonomy I Revised, 1994, which is NANDA's conceptual framework and classification system for ordering nursing diagnoses, is described in the narrative and illustrated in tables for clarity. The framework comprises nine human response patterns (exchanging, communicating, relating, valuing, choosing, moving, perceiving, knowing, and feeling). Chapter 1 also includes:

- Two clinical pathways used in clinical settings, entitled *Mania* and *Psychosis* (Figures 1-4 and 1-5). The pathways include variances and are accompanied by a narrative description of each component, such as client outcomes, processes (interventions), intervals (days depicting length of stay), and other critical elements. Clinical Pathways, also known as *Caremaps* or *Critical Pathways,* are currently used in both hospital and home care and other community settings and are continuously revised and refined for greater efficacy. They are not intended to replace critical narrative documentation.
- A comprehensive client history and assessment tool designed to help the learner develop care plans from the content throughout this textbook. It includes a client case study with relevant assessment data, client physiologic and psychologic problem lists, client learning needs, nursing diagnoses, client outcomes, and nursing interventions with rationale.
- A community home health narrative illustrating case management concepts for the psychiatric client outside the hospital setting. The authors believe this to be essential information pertinent to the ongoing changes in health care delivery systems. Community and home health nurses have constantly expanded roles in mental health

as they manage interdisciplinary home care teams with the goal of delivering cost-effective, quality care while meeting both client and family needs.

CHAPTERS 2 THROUGH 11

Each of these chapters begins with a comprehensive narrative description of the mental disorders categorized in the DSM-IV (e.g., Anxiety Disorders, Mood Disorders, Schizophrenia, Personality Disorders). These discussions are organized by headings, such as etiology, epidemiology, and diagnostic categories related to the disorder. The authors believe this format is essential in providing the learner with a basic understanding of psychopathology and its manifestations, treatment, and management. A sample outline of the format follows:

Sample Outline

- Concise, comprehensive narrative of the disorder
- Etiology (accompanied with box)
- Epidemiology
- Assessment (phases and symptoms)
- Diagnostic types, according to DSM-IV
- Prognosis box (favorable and unfavorable course)
- Interventions that include the following descriptions:
  - — Hospitalization
  - — Pharmacotherapy
  - — Psychosocial therapy
  - — Therapeutic nurse–client relationship
  - — Group therapy
  - — Family therapy
  - — Cognitive-behavioral therapy
- Discharge criteria

The organization of this content provides information that is readily accessible and understood by the reader and remains constant throughout. The reader is effectively acquainted with the content in a timely manner, which enhances meaning of the material that is subsequently presented in the care plans. Preceding the care plans, nursing management strategies are detailed in boxed summaries entitled *General Principles for Interacting and Assisting Clients to Manage (the mental disorder presented in that chapter).* It is here that the authors include four universal principles, newly added to this area of the text. These principles appear in each disorder chapter as the authors believe they are significant for every disorder. The four principles are followed by general principles that are relevant to each specific disorder.

Following these interventions (principles) are the titles of the care plans that pertain to each chapter. For the convenience of the reader, we have included a list of the medical diagnoses and nursing diagnoses. Note that there may be more than one nursing diagnosis for each medical diagnosis, since nursing diagnoses are defined as "clinical judgment about individual, family, or community responses to actual or potential health problems/life processes. Nursing diagnoses provide the basis for selection of interventions to achieve outcomes for which the nurse is accountable" (NANDA, 1990). Therefore, although medical and nursing diagnoses may complement each other, they remain separate entities.

NURSING CARE PLANS

Nursing care plans throughout the text reflect the following client needs:

- Biologic
- Psychologic
- Spiritual
- Cultural
- Age-specificity
- Sexual
- Family/significant others
- Community involvement
- School/work/activities
- Social/relational

Each care plan is preceded by the identifying medical diagnosis from which it emerges, such as anxiety, depression, or mania. The care plan begins with a selected nursing diagnosis. Many of the nursing diagnoses are followed by definitions that more clearly describe or explain the health problem or nursing diagnosis statement. For example: *Nursing Diagnosis: Impaired Social Interaction. The state in which an individual participates in an insufficient or excessive quantity or quality of social exchange.*

Under this statement are two headings: One is *Focus,* which briefly describes the client's behaviors to which the care plan is directed. The second column, *NANDA Taxonomy,* lists the appropriate *Human Response Pattern* under which the nursing diagnosis is categorized and the definition of the pattern.

The care plans are then developed according to the remaining nursing process steps: outcome identification and evaluation (combined) and planning and implementation (combined). Nursing interventions and rationales are listed in the Planning and Implementation section. Assessment criteria can be found in the narrative discussions of each disorder chapter.

In some instances, especially in the care plans listed in the chapter on personality disorders (Chapter 6), we have assisted the reader by identifying client responses and behaviors commonly noted in each of the nursing diagnoses we identified. These responses and behaviors, such as anger, mistrust, jealousy, or passive/aggression, are listed sequentially, directly under each main heading. In this way the reader is able to track each behavior until it is treated or resolved by nursing in the intervention section. Special care has been taken to include client responses and behaviors as well as the nursing diagnosis statements in the index, to help the reader quickly locate relevant information.

The nursing diagnoses selected reflect a wide range of problems, most of which are commonly encountered in psychiatric–mental health settings, as noted in our chapters on anxiety, depression, schizophrenia, personality disorders, substance-related disorders, disorders of childhood and adolescence, and eating disorders. We have also included care plans that pertain to such interesting, challenging topics as dissociative disorders (more specifically, dissociative identity disorder formerly called *multiple personality disorder*), sexual dysfunction, and posttraumatic stress syndrome. Gerontologic issues are extensively discussed in the chapter pertaining to delirium, dementia (all types), and amnestic and other cognitive disorders. The family and community are addressed along with the individual, because we believe that the problems of one individual affect the family and society as a whole. **Cultural** and **Spiritual** considerations are interspersed throughout the care plans, as well as being placed in a special section in the appendixes.

Finally, the last sections include a bibliography with both current and classic sources, a thorough and extensive glossary, and appendixes, containing information and strategies (e.g., a medication section, age-specific growth and development stages, psychosocial therapies) that are timely and useful in the care of clients with mental or emotional disorders.

SUMMARY

Psychiatric Nursing Care Plans, third edition, represents our efforts to continue to present the reader with the most illuminating information that a psychiatric care plan text can offer. It consists of the most currently researched information in areas of both psychiatric–mental health nursing and the psychiatric medical profession, with a strong scientific basis in both its content and organizational structure.

It is our continued belief that the first step in theory-building within a profession is to name what it is we do. The next step is to use the language to make it easier for nurses everywhere to communicate and relate to each other, as well as to other health care professionals. We believe that the vast accumulation of information in the area of psychiatric–mental health nursing, and in the nursing profession in general, mandates the use of a commonly shared language to help practitioners of nursing formulate complex clinical decisions for clients whose mental and physical health changes day by day.

We have thus elected to persist in using the language of our profession in the development of the nursing care plans throughout this text. We have endeavored to clarify meanings through frequent examples and descriptive use of words and phrases.

We believe strongly that this text serves two purposes: (1) to educate and inform the reader with new and current knowledge relevant to the practice and profession of nursing, and (2) to use the language of nursing to enhance and distinguish it as a discipline. We believe this goal has been accomplished. We wish you success and enrichment as you use this comprehensive, research-based care plan text in your area of practice, whether you are a new graduate or seasoned practitioner.

ACKNOWLEDGMENTS

The writing of any text involves an intricate mingling of ideas, concepts, artistry, and talent of special persons other than just the authors. We wish to thank the following people who share our goal, which is to transform ideas and concepts into a finished product and state-of-the-art text.

- Phillip R. Deming, MA, MDiv, Chaplain, Pastoral Care and Education, Sharp HealthCare Behavioral Health Services, San Diego, Calif., for the spirituality content in Appendix F.
- The people at Mosby Nursing Editorial Division:
  — Jeanne Allison, Managing Editor
  — Jeff Downing, Associate Developmental Editor
  — Leslie Mosby, Editorial Assistant
- Carol O'Connell at Graphic World Publishing Services.

Thanks to All!

Kathi Fortinash and Pat Worret

Contents in Brief

Contents

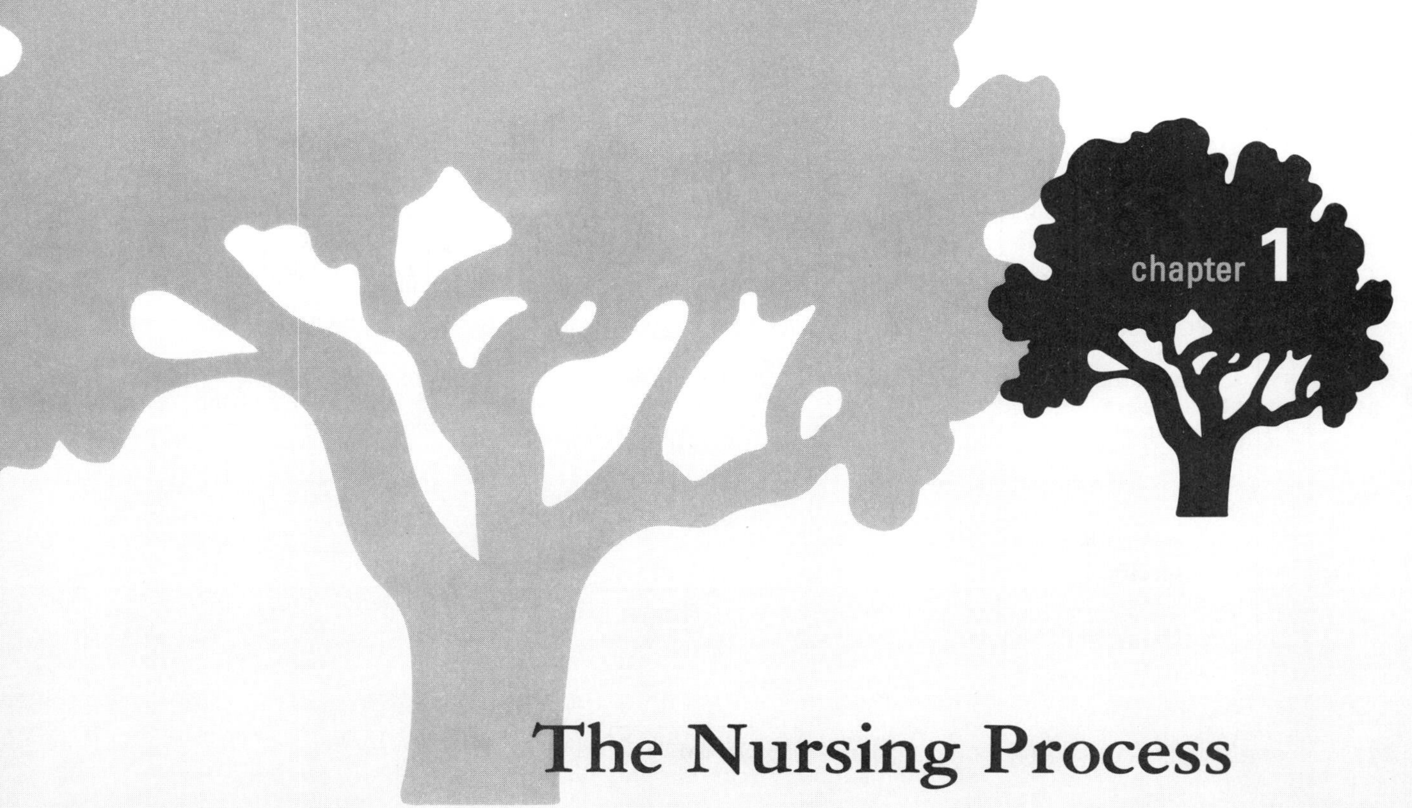

The Nursing Process

The nursing process is more than just an organized, systematic, six-step approach to a client's clinical problems. Unlike episodic or linear problem-solving methods in which a problem is identified, diagnosed, and resolved (hence the process ends with the resolution), the nursing process is an ongoing, multidimensional, cyclic approach in which data are collected, critically analyzed, and incorporated into the client's treatment plan in accordance with the client's fluctuating responses to health and illness (Fig. 1-1). Thus, as the client's health state is dynamic rather than static, so too is the nursing process—challenging the seasoned nurse to make sound clinical judgments and decisions and guiding the novice toward practicing and eventually mastering clear, analytic, critical thinking and keen organizational skills.

Psychiatric–mental health nursing practice presents a unique and exciting challenge for the application of the nursing process. Clients responses to mental and emotional illness are manifested through cognitive, affective, and behavioral domains—all dynamic forces constantly subject to change. Thus assessment of clients' responses depends on the nurse's ongoing planned observations of the client's behavior and the client's reports of perceptions, thoughts, and feelings.

The six phases or steps of the nursing process are assessment, nursing diagnosis, outcome identification, planning, implementation, and evaluation (see Box 1-1). Figure 1-2 details the nursing process of actual and risk problems.

ASSESSMENT

Assessment, the initial step of the nursing process, is its most essential, integral component because it provides the nurse with relevant data from which nursing diagnoses, the crux of treatment planning, are developed. Throughout the assessment phase, the psychiatric–mental health nurse collects data through learned interactive and interviewing skills and through observations of verbal and nonverbal behaviors, based on a broad biopsychosocial background and knowledge of normal and dysfunctional behaviors. In the discipline of psychiatric–mental health nursing, assessment takes place in a number of settings within the milieu, so the nurse has many opportunities to observe the client and modify assessment data in accordance with the client's continued adjustment to the milieu, as well as progress made throughout hospitalization.

Ideally, the client is the major source of information during the assessment phase, although data may be obtained via client records, other staff, and physicians as well. Occasionally, the client may be unable to offer a complete or accurate health history. In such instances, a reliable source may be interviewed on the client's behalf, with the understanding that such information will be evaluated in terms of that person's relationship with the client.

Assessment of the individual includes the following criteria: physical, psychiatric/psychosocial, developmental, family dynamics, cultural, spiritual, and sexual. The method of assessment includes the client's subjective report of symptoms and problems and the nurse's objective findings.

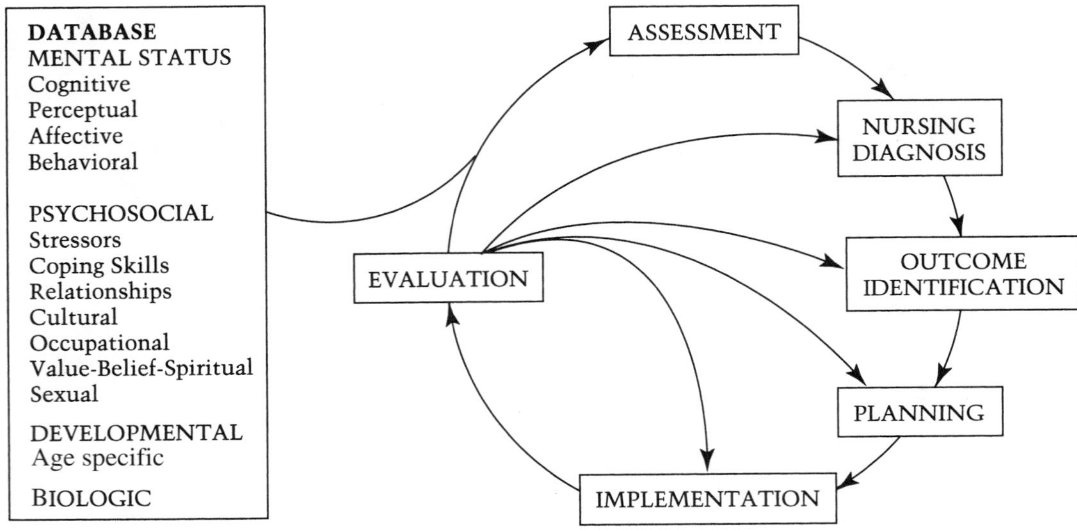

Fig. 1-1 Cyclic nature of the nursing process.

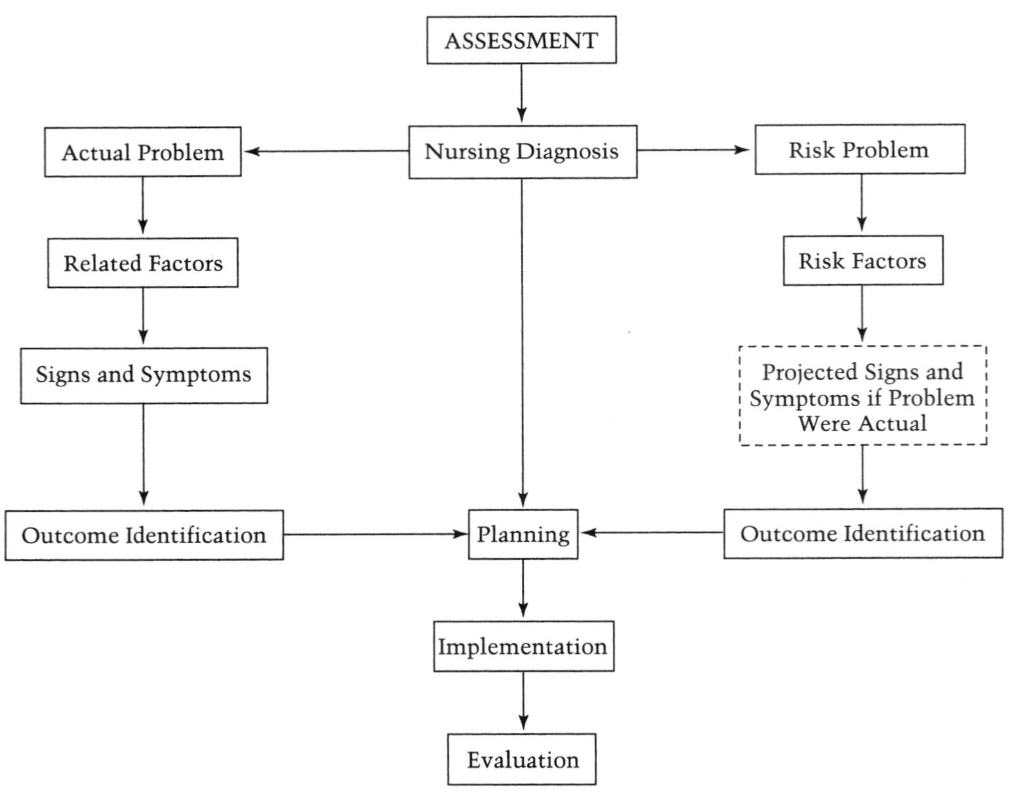

Fig. 1-2 Nursing process of actual and risk problems.

Assessment of Mental Status

The psychiatric–mental health component of total client assessment is called the *Mental Status Examination.* It is a basis for subsequent medical and nursing diagnoses and management of care. The *Mental Status Examination* is an organized collection of data that reflects an individual's level of functioning at the time of the interview. See Figure 1-3.

A major focus of the Mental Status Examination is identification of the individual's strengths and capabilities for interaction with the environment, such as the

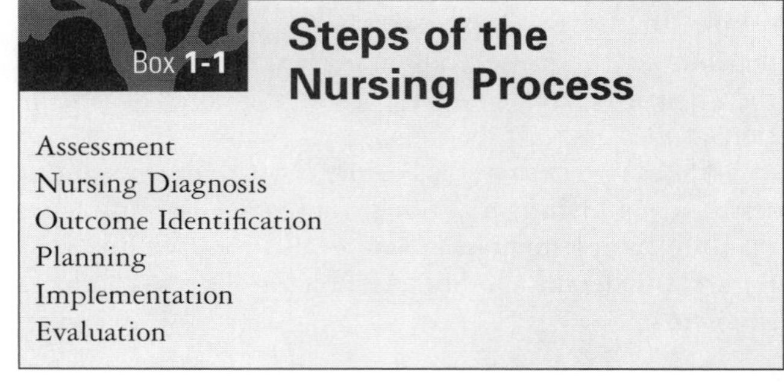
Box 1-1 **Steps of the Nursing Process**

Assessment
Nursing Diagnosis
Outcome Identification
Planning
Implementation
Evaluation

Psychiatric Nursing History and Assessment

GENERAL ADMISSION INFORMATION

Client Name ______________________ Age/Sex __________ Marital Status __________
Medical Record Number ______________________ Room Number ______________________
Insurance Company ______________________ Admission Date ______________________
Address ______________________ Telephone ______________________
Significant Other ______________________ Telephone ______________________
Company/School ______________________ Telephone ______________________

CONDITIONS OF ADMISSION

Voluntary ______________________ Involuntary ______________________
Accompanied to Facility by: (family, friend, police, other) ______________________
Route of Admission: (ambulatory, wheelchair, gurney) ______________________
Admitted from: (home, other facility, street, place of destination) ______________________

OTHER

Vital Signs: P __________ B/P __________ Resp __________ Temp __________
Level of Consciousness __________ Orientation (person, place, time, situation) __________
Allergies __________ Diet __________ Height/Weight __________
Culture ______________________ Value/Belief System ______________________
Place/City of Residence ______________________ Dominant Language ______________________
Special Needs ______________________ Strengths/Coping Skills ______________________
Discharge to: (home, facility, other) ______________________ Estimated Length of Stay __________
Chief Complaint (client's own words) ______________________

PREDISPOSING FACTORS

Genetic/Biologic Influences
Family of Origin (Use Genogram if applicable)
Present Family/Significant Persons
Family Dynamics (Describe significant interpersonal relationships among family members) ______________________

MEDICAL/PSYCHIATRIC HISTORY

Client: ______________________

Family Members: ______________________

Recent Stressors: (physical, emotional, psychosocial, psychiatric disorder) ______________________

Other physical, psychosocial, cultural, sexual, financial, environmental factors, relevant to current problem: (physical disability, cultural change, loss of income or bankruptcy, trauma from living in high-crime neighborhood, homelessness, abuse, domestic violence) ______________________

Health Beliefs and Practices: (personal responsibility for health, wellness, special practices) ______________________

Religious/Spiritual Beliefs and Practices ______________________

Educational Background/Interests: ______________________

Fig. 1-3 A psychiatric nursing history and assessment form.

Psychiatric Nursing History and Assessment—cont'd

MEDICAL/PSYCHIATRIC HISTORY—cont'd

Significant Losses/Changes/Grief Responses: ____________________

Support System: (peers/friends/others) ____________________

Occupational/Academic History ____________________

Previous Patterns of Coping with Grief/Stress (adaptive) ____________________

(maladaptive) ____________________

Growth and Development Resources (Erikson)

Stages of Development ____________________

Tasks/Skills Mastered ____________________

Tasks/Skills Not Met ____________________

Contributions/Areas of Productivity ____________________

Precipitating Event: Describe Situation or Events That Influenced This Hospitalization/Illness/Exacerbation ____

Client's Perception of Stressor/Stressor Event ____________________

LEVELS OF ANXIETY (check one)

__________ Mild __________ Moderate __________ Severe __________ Panic

MEDICATION/DRUG HISTORY (including alcohol)

Use of Prescribed Drugs:

Name	Dose	Reason Prescribed	Results/Effects

Use of Over-the-Counter Drugs

Name	Dose	Reason Taken	Results/Effects

Use of Street/Illicit Drugs/Alcohol

Name	Amount Used	Frequency	When Last Used	Effects Produced

Fig. 1-3—cont'd A psychiatric nursing history and assessment form.

ability to initiate and sustain meaningful relationships and attain satisfaction congruent with one's sociocultural life-style. Knowledge of the psychodynamics and psychopathology of human behavior is essential for assessment of the individual's adjustment or maladjustment to internal and external life stressors.

The Interview

The client interview is the most important process in gathering critical information about overall health status. It is a more meaningful, flexible method of collecting data than questionnaires or computers, and it allows the examiner to use all the senses to explore specific topics and concerns the person identifies through verbal and nonverbal responses.

In the mental status assessment, the primary instrument of evaluation is the nurse interviewer. The success of the interview depends on the development of trust, rapport, and respect between the nurse and the client. Keen therapeutic communication skills such as active listening and reflective questioning are used throughout the interview. (See Appendixes F and G.)

Components of Assessment

Total assessment of the individual in the psychiatric–mental health setting includes the components listed in Box 1-2.

NURSING DIAGNOSIS

Nursing diagnosis is a process whereby nurses interpret data collected during the assessment phase of the nursing process and apply standardized labels to clients' health problems and responses to illness. Nursing diagnoses are statements that describe an individual's health state or an actual or potential alteration in a person's life processes. The statement may reflect biologic, psychologic, sociocultural, developmental, spiritual, or sexual processes (Table 1-1).

The National Task Force for the Classification of Nursing Diagnoses was organized in 1973 by a group of nurses and is now called the *North American Nursing Diagnosis Association (NANDA).* At NANDA's ninth conference in March 1990, nursing diagnosis was defined as "a clinical judgment about individual, family, or community responses to actual or potential health problems/life processes. Nursing diagnoses provide the basis for selection of nursing interventions to achieve outcomes for which the nurse is accountable."

NANDA is in the process of collecting, defining, describing, and refining nursing diagnoses submitted by practicing nurse colleagues and categorizing them within the constructs of an organizational conceptual framework known as *Taxonomy I Revised* (see inside back cover and Table 1-2). This classification system for ordering nursing diagnoses is divided into several broad patterns known as *human response patterns.* Each pattern has an accompanying definition that describes its nature in relation to the human condition (Table 1-2).

Taxonomy and Nursing Diagnosis Systems Defined

A taxonomy is a classification system that organizes known phenomena (nursing diagnoses) under a hierarchic structure (taxonomy), whereas an alphabetical list of nursing diagnoses is a nomenclature, or system of names. The first step in science-building is naming, and the second step is organization of names. Both the taxonomy and the diagnostic nomenclature assist and guide nurses toward building a solid scientific foundation for the profession, which additionally serves as a standardized communication system.

The authors of this text remain true to NANDA's continuing efforts to refine and standardize nursing diagnoses, and each nursing diagnosis statement throughout this book is accompanied by the pattern under which it is ordered in the NANDA Taxonomy I Revised.

Nursing diagnosis as a standard vocabulary. Nursing diagnosis provides nursing with a vocabulary that is distinctive to its own discipline and that serves to enhance communication among nurses in regard to the health problems that they assess and treat. The concept of nursing using its own language to describe or name the conditions and responses that it treats reflects significant growth and credibility in a profession once dependent on the medical profession for labeling of diseases and disorders. Thus the evolution of nursing diagnosis fosters nursing's theory- and science-building efforts and its ability as a profession to stand on its own merit by clarifying its distinct service to society.

Nursing diagnoses and medical diagnoses. Nursing diagnoses and medical diagnoses may complement each other, but they remain separate entities. Nursing diagnoses can be formulated based on the client's maladaptive responses, whether or not a medical diagnosis exists. In the medical model of psychiatry, the health problems are the mental disorders as defined in the *Diagnostic and Statistical Manual of Mental Disorders,* 4th edition (DSM-IV), from which many nursing diagnoses emerge. See Table 1-3 for some sample comparisons of DSM-IV and NANDA diagnoses.

Components of the Nursing Diagnosis Statement

The three distinct components to an actual nursing diagnosis statement are (1) problem, (2) etiology, and (3) signs and symptoms. The format for documentation of these components is known as the *PES format.*

P = Problem. A problem is a concise statement of the client's actual or potential response to health problems/life processes, also known as its *diagnostic label.* Problem statements come from the list of approved nursing diagnoses (NANDA). *Example:* Ineffective Individual Coping.

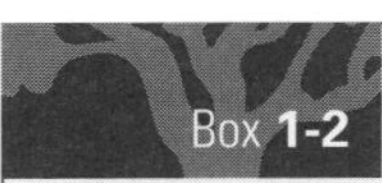

Components of Assessment

Mental Status Examination

Appearance

Dress, grooming, hygiene, cosmetics, apparent age, posture, facial expression

Behavior/activity

Hypoactivity or hyperactivity, rigid, relaxed, restless or agitated motor movements, gait and coordination, facial grimacing, gestures, mannerisms, passive, combative, bizarre

Attitude

Interactions with the interviewer: cooperative, resistive, friendly, hostile, ingratiating

Speech

Quantity: poverty of speech, poverty of content, voluminous
Quality: articulate, congruent, monotonous, talkative, repetitious, spontaneous, circumlocutory confabulating, tangenital, pressured, stereotypical
Rate: slowed, rapid

Mood and affect

Mood (intensity, depth, duration): sad, fearful, depressed, angry, anxious, ambivalent, happy, ecstatic, grandiose
Affect (intensity, depth, duration): appropriate, apathetic, constricted, blunted flat, labile, euphoric, bizarre

Perceptions

Hallucinations, illusions, depersonalization, derealization, distortions

Thoughts

Form and content: logical vs. illogical, loose associations, flight of ideas, autistic, blocking, broadcasting, neologisms, word salad, obsessions, ruminations, delusions, abstract vs. concrete

Sensorium/cognition

Levels of consciousness, orientation, attention span, recent and remote memory, concentration; ability to comprehend and process information; intelligence

Judgment

Ability to assess and evaluate situations, make rational decisions, understand consequences of behavior, and take responsibility for actions

Insight

Ability to perceive and understand the cause and nature of own and others' situations

Psychosocial Criteria

Stressors

Internal: psychiatric or medical illness, perceived loss, such as loss of self-concept/self-esteem
External: actual loss, e.g., death of a loved one, divorce, lack of support systems, job or financial loss, retirement, dysfunctional family system

Coping skills

Adaptation to internal and external stressors, use of functional, adaptive coping mechanisms and techniques, management of activities of daily living

Relationships

Attainment and maintenance of satisfying interpersonal relationships congruent with developmental stage; includes sexual relationship as appropriate for age and status

Reliability

Interviewer's impression that individual reported information accurately and completely

Cultural

Ability to adapt and conform to prescribed norms, rules, ethics, and mores of an identified group

Spiritual (value-belief)

Presence of a self-satisfying value-belief system that the individual regards as right, desirable, worthwhile, and comforting

Occupational

Engagement in useful, rewarding activity, congruent with developmental stage and societal standards (work, school, recreation)

Many diagnoses are accompanied by definitions that more clearly describe or explain the health problem, a feature useful to students who may need more specific clarification of the problem than the label conveys. *Examples:*

1. The definition that accompanies the diagnosis Social Isolation stipulates it is a condition of aloneness perceived by the individual as a negative state and imposed on him or her by others. It distinguishes social isolation from the situation in which the individual prefers to be alone and thus becomes isolative.
2. The definition that accompanies the diagnosis Powerlessness explains that it is a state in which the individual perceives that her or his own actions will not significantly affect an outcome—that nothing he or she could do would make a difference. Without this definition, the reader may interpret the diagnostic label by itself to mean that the person has no power or control in a given situation.

For additional clarity, some nursing diagnoses require qualifying statements based on the nature of the health problems as it is manifested in each particular client response or situation (Table 1-4).

Table 1-1

Nursing Diagnosis Statements in Relation to Life Processes

Nursing Diagnosis	Life Process
Altered nutrition	Biologic
Self-esteem disturbance	Psychologic
Impaired social interaction	Sociocultural
Altered growth and development	Developmental
Spiritual distress	Spiritual
Altered sexuality patterns	Sexual

Table 1-2

NANDA Taxonomy I Revised

Human Response Patterns	Definitions
1. Exchanging	Mutual giving and receiving
2. Communicating	Sending messages
3. Relating	Establishing bonds
4. Valuing	Assigning of relative worth
5. Choosing	Selection of alternatives
6. Moving	Activity
7. Perceiving	Reception of information
8. Knowing	Meaning associated with information
9. Feeling	Subjective awareness of information

Table 1-3

Comparisons of DSM-IV and NANDA Diagnoses

DSM-IV Diagnosis	NANDA Diagnosis
Generalized Anxiety Disorder	Anxiety; Coping, ineffective individual
Bipolar Disorder (Mania)	Violence, risk for; Coping, defensive
Schizophrenia	Thought processes, altered; Sensory/perceptual alterations
Major Depression	Hopelessness; powerlessness
Obsessive Compulsive Disorder	Social interaction, impaired
Posttraumatic Stress Disorder	Rape–trauma syndrome

Table 1-4

Examples of NANDA Diagnoses and Qualifying Statements

NANDA Diagnosis	Qualifying Statement
Nutrition, altered	Less than body requirements
Self-care deficit	Bathing, grooming, feeding, total
Noncompliance	Medication, milieu activities
Knowledge deficit	Medication, treatments

Table 1-5

Examples of NANDA Diagnosis and Etiologies

NANDA Diagnosis	Etiologies (Related To)
Anxiety	Threat to biologic, psychologic, and/or social integrity Ineffective use of coping mechanisms Depletion of coping strategies

E = Etiology. The etiology is the second part of the PES format and is considered the source from which the nursing diagnosis emerges. Etiologies are also known as *related or contributing factors* and are considered to be the cause of the problem to the extent that cause can be determined. Nursing diagnoses are often accompanied by several etiologic factors that serve to interact to produce the health problem. They may be of psychologic, biologic, relational, environmental, situational, developmental, or sociocultural origins—yet all are in some manner associated with the problem. Examples of nursing diagnosis and etiologies are presented in Table 1-5.

As previously noted, many etiologic factors are broad categories or examples that require more specific information based on the nature of the problem and the client who is the focus of treatment. For example, the first etiology listed in Table 1-5 is a threat to biologic, psychologic, or social integrity. Considering the source of anxiety in a particular client, the nurse needs to be more precise in delineating which aspects of biologic, psychologic, or social integrity are threatened: recent illness, injury (biologic); loss of job or status, either actual or a perceived feeling of abandonment or isolation (psychologic); divorce, separation, dysfunctional relationship (social).

Etiologies: the focus of treatment. Etiologies may be treated by nurses independently or in collaboration with other health care professionals, as determined by the client's needs. The nurse, however, is primarily responsible for constructing the client's treatment plan and formulating etiologies that are both specific to the client's identified problem and managed and treated largely by nurses. Thus the treatment plan for any given nursing diagnosis must include interventions aimed at managing or resolving etiologic factors, as well as the health problem. The authors believe that the etiologies listed throughout this text illustrate the need for nurses to explore multicausal factors that are both specific to the identified nursing diagnoses and treated by nurses who, "by virtue of their education and experience, are capable and licensed to treat" (Gordon, 1994).

Nursing diagnoses as etiologies. Nursing diagnoses can also be appropriately used as etiologies for other nursing diagnoses. Some examples are the following:

1. Anxiety—related to powerlessness
2. Impaired social interactions—related to self-esteem disturbance
3. Ineffective individual coping—related to anxiety when nursing interventions are focused exclusively on etiologic (causative) factors, which in turn will reduce or resolve the health problem (nursing diagnosis), it is most advantageous when the etiology is another nursing diagnosis.

Medical diagnoses as etiologies. It is considered inadvisable to cite medical diagnoses as etiologies for nursing problems, for the following reasons:

1. The health problem is reduced and resolved through interventions that are primarily nursing therapies.
2. The problem statement should retain its identity as a health state that is treated and resolved by nurses.
3. The etiologies that accompany nursing diagnoses become the focus of nursing interventions in the treatment of the overall problem.

However, many symptoms and behaviors consequent to mental disorders and medical conditions are of great concern to nurses and highly amenable to management and treatment by nurses. Some examples are the following:

1. Altered thought processes as a result of the schizophrenic process
2. Altered nutrition: less than body requirements as a result of anorexia nervosa

In such situations, the nurse should isolate those aspects contributing to the symptoms or pathology that can be modified or treated by nursing interventions and cite those as etiologic factors. Some examples are the following:

1. Altered thought processes related to:
   — increased internal and external stressors
   — impaired ability to process internal and external stimuli
2. Altered nutrition: less than body requirements related to:
   — inadequate intake and hypermetabolic need
   — loss of appetite secondary to constipation

These etiologic factors that accompany the problem statements more clearly specify the focus for nursing interventions and are examples of the etiologies used throughout this text.

S = Signs and symptoms. The signs and symptoms, also known as *defining characteristics,* are the observable, measurable manifestations of clients' responses to the identified health problem. Defining characteristics are listed for every nursing diagnosis and, like the problem statement and etiologies, they often require more specific descriptions to better represent the needs of the client being diagnosed. For example, the diagnosis Ineffective Individual Coping has as one of its critical defining characteristics ineffective problem solving. As the nurse constructs this diagnostic statement for the benefit of clinical use, specific examples that describe the client's impaired problem solving should be cited. Often, the nurse can clarify the defining characteristic statements by quoting the client. Examples of ineffective problem solving:

- "I can't decide if I should stay with my family or move to a board and care home."
- "I can't decide what to do first—get a job or begin day treatment."

Therefore, major characteristics, when applicable, must be present in the nurse's assessment criteria to give some validity to the health problem that is being diagnosed. *Examples:* Major characteristics of the diagnosis (e.g., chronic low self-esteem) are those that are persistent and long-standing. They are listed as follows:

Self-negating verbalization
Expression of shame or guilt
Evaluates self as unable to deal with events
Rationalizes away or rejects positive feedback
Exaggerates negative feedback about self
Hesitant to try new things or situations

Other noncritical, or "minor," characteristics may be added as defining characteristics. Major defining characteristics have been tested for reliability as predictors of the diagnosis based on research or extensive clinical experience.

Risk nursing diagnoses

Risk factors. Risk factors are used in assessing potential health problems to describe existing risk states that may contribute to the potential problem becoming actual. Thus in a risk nursing diagnosis there are no defining characteristics because the actual problem has not been manifested. Also, there is no etiologic factor in a potential (risk) problem because cause cannot exist without effect. Therefore a risk nursing diagnosis carries a two-part statement, whereas an actual nursing diagnosis consists of a three-part statement. Some examples follow:

Risk problem (two-part statement)

Part 1 Nursing diagnosis:
  Violence, risk for, directed at others

Part 2 Risk factors (predictors of risk problem):
  History of violence
  Panic state
  Hyperactivity, secondary to manic state
  Low impulse control

Actual problem (three-part statement)

Part 1 Nursing diagnosis:
  Post-trauma response

Part 2 Etiologic factors (related to):
  Overwhelming anxiety secondary to
    Rape or other assault
    Catastrophic illness
    Disasters
    War

Part 3 Defining characteristics:
  Reexperience of traumatic events (flashbacks)
  Repetitive dreams or nightmares
  Intrusive thoughts about traumatic event
  Excess verbalization about traumatic event

Risk factors as predictors of risk problems. The prediction of a risk health problem in a particular client requires an estimation of probability of occurrence. Risk problems can be ascribed to almost any individual in a compromised health state. For example, a client taking a tricyclic antidepressant medication may be at risk for several potential problems or conditions as a result of the actions of these drugs on many of the body systems, such as risk for injury (hypotension, dizziness, blurred vision), risk for constipation, risk for urinary retention, and risk for altered oral mucous membranes (dry mouth). For the nurse to construct a treatment plan that lists all these diagnoses with outcome criteria and interventions, without considering the probabilities, would be time-wasting. The nurse should first appraise the client's overall health state and identify those factors that place the individual at a higher risk for the health problem than the general population. For example, a client on tricyclic antidepressant medications who is poorly hydrated, refuses to drink juice or water, and doesn't eat fibrous foods is at a higher risk for constipation than the general population. Therefore, the risk nursing diagnosis of constipation must be stated on the client's individualized treatment plan. The two-part nursing diagnosis would be the following:

Nursing diagnosis:	Constipation, risk for
Risk factors:	Effects of tricyclic antidepressant medications
	Refusal to drink water, juice, etc.
	Noncompliance to high-fiber foods

This risk diagnosis was specifically selected to remind the psychiatric nurse that although the focus of this text is psychiatric nursing, all body systems are considered during management of client care.

This client's remaining problems would not need to be stated on an individual treatment plan but should instead be part of a Standard of Care Record, which would require the monitoring and interventions necessary to avoid the problems. The diagnosis of risk for constipation, with its greater risk factors, should be stated so that additional and/or more intensified interventions can be prescribed.

OUTCOME IDENTIFICATION

In the outcome identification phase of the nursing process, the nurse identifies outcomes, which are specific indicators derived from the nursing diagnoses. The nurse identifies expected client outcomes and individualizes them to the client and the client situation. In the evaluation phase, outcomes are examined by nurses to determine whether the actual problem was resolved or reduced, or if the risk problem ever occurred.

Outcomes are measurable and mutually formulated with the nurse, client, and other caregivers. Whenever possible, they are realistic and achievable in relation to the client's current and potential capabilities and available sources and support system (see Box 1-3).

Outcomes serve to provide direction for continued, effective management of care and can include a predicted time estimate for attainment based on the nurse's accumulated knowledge and experience as to when specific outcomes are typically achieved. An outcome statement, then, is a projected influence that nursing interventions will have on the client in relation to the identified problem. Outcomes are not considered client goals or nursing goals and should not describe nursing interventions.

As previously noted, problems can either be actual or risk. An example of a risk problem is risk for violence, self-directed. When problems are risk, actual signs and symptoms are absent; therefore, risk problem statements are accompanied by risk factors that may be precursors to the signs and symptoms, should the problem become actual. Outcome criteria are then developed from what would be the signs and symptoms if the risk problem were to become actual (see Fig. 1-2).

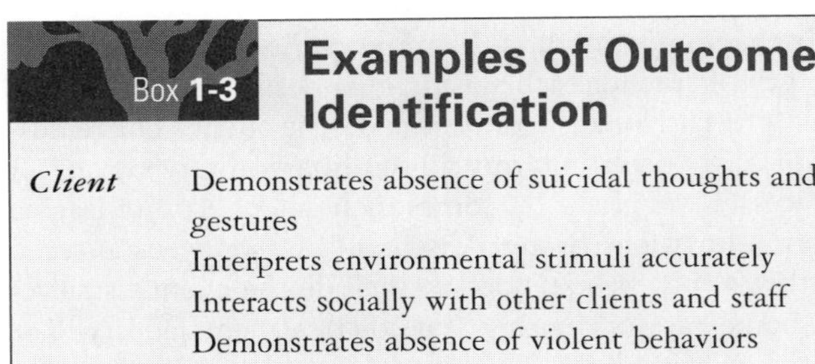

Box 1-3 **Examples of Outcome Identification**

Client	Demonstrates absence of suicidal thoughts and gestures
	Interprets environmental stimuli accurately
	Interacts socially with other clients and staff
	Demonstrates absence of violent behaviors

PLANNING

In the planning phase of the nursing process, the nurse develops a plan of care that prescribes interventions with accompanying rationale to achieve expected client outcomes. Nurses individualize care plans to accommodate the client's condition, needs, and situation, based on actual problems or risk factors. The process of planning includes the following:

1. Collaboration by the nurse with the client, family, significant others, and treatment team members
2. Identification of signs, symptoms, risk factors, and priorities of care
3. Decisions regarding use of psychotherapeutic principles and practices
4. Coordination and delegation of responsibilities according to the treatment team's expertise as it relates to client needs

Plans reflect current nursing practices and may include input from other disciplines involved in the treatment when the approach to client care is multidisciplinary. Nursing care plans, no matter what the format, should provide for continuity and efficiency of client care management and progress.

Clinical Pathways

A *clinical pathway* (also referred to as *a critical pathway, care path,* or *Care Map*) is a standardized format used to provide and monitor client care and progress via the case management interdisciplinary health care delivery system. Although nursing is a primary proponent of the critical pathway method, other disciplines responsible for client care in the psychiatric setting are strongly involved in the planning and developing of each individualized critical pathway. Such disciplines include social services, occupational therapy, therapeutic recreation, and dietary services, with strong collaborative input from psychiatrists. Consultations may be provided by psychologists, family practice physicians, or other professionals, depending on the special needs of the client.

A clinical pathway refers primarily to a written clinical process that identifies projected caregiver behaviors and interventions and expected client outcomes, based on the client's mental disorder as defined in the *Diagnostic Statistical Manual,* edition 4, which is in line with the *International Classification of Diseases,* edition 10. The pathway is mapped out along a continuum that depicts chronologic milestones or timelines that are generally the number of days that reflects the client's estimated length of stay for each specific diagnosis.

The pathway is a projection of the client's entire hospital stay, detailing multidisciplinary interventions or processes and client outcomes each day of hospitalization from admission through discharge. In some instances, a pathway may be extended to include the client's transfer to home care or another type of treatment facility. The pathway would then continue for as long as necessary. Clinical pathways may also originate for clients in a home care situation and would then be developed by the interdisciplinary home care team.

Key client outcomes. Pathways may identify key outcomes to be achieved by the client that are considered critical to the client's recovery or prognosis. These outcomes generally require several interventions specifically intended to assist the client to achieve the identified key outcome. For example, in a client experiencing mania, a phase of bipolar disorder, key client outcomes would be identified as: "Demonstrates reduction in movement, racing thoughts, grandiosity, euphoria, and irritability; sleeps 4-6 hours a night; lithium level within therapeutic range (generally 1.0 mEq/L, the usual level at which a client safely functions in a nonmanic and nontoxic state). Lithium is also the primary treatment for patients in the manic phase of bipolar disorder. Because a major focus in pathway implementation is linking key processes (interventions) with key client outcomes, some critical interventions necessary for the client to achieve these outcomes that should be progressively documented along the pathway are:

1. Initiate lithium level (to determine baseline admission level)
2. Administer lithium (and/or other relevant medications) according to protocol
3. Teach client and/or family about lithium and symptom recognition and link symptoms to precipitating events
4. Check lithium levels for therapeutic range; titrate doses accordingly
5. Assess/reassess for lithium toxicity
6. Continue to check lithium levels until desired level and stable mood are achieved

Noncritical outcomes may be considered those related to the client's secondary levels of treatment, such as attending special occupational or recreational groups or facilitating grooming skills. Although such tasks are important in the client's overall treatment regimen and reflect a general functional level, they may not be considered key or critical outcomes for the client's diagnosis and prognosis.

Variances. Variances (also known as *outliers*) occur when a client's response to interventions is different than what is typically expected. A variance may therefore be considered an unexpected or aberrant client response that "falls off" the pathway, requiring separate documentation and further investigation by the interdisciplinary team. Causes of pathway variances may be related to client/family, caregivers, hospital, community, and payer (including insurance companies, health maintenance organizations, or managed care organizations). A variance may be positive or negative and affect the client's length of stay and/or outcomes. An example of a positive variance would be a client who responds more rapidly to medication or other forms of treatment than expected and leaves the hospital before the estimated length of stay. An example of a negative variance would be a client who fails to achieve the desired nonmanic state or therapeutic lithium level in accordance with the time line designated on the clinical pathway continuum (generally by date of discharge), and whose length of stay is therefore prolonged.

The clinical pathways of case management help ensure timely lengths of stay, prevention of complications, cost effectiveness, and continued quality improvement. Also, overall coordinated management of each client's care and progress by the RN case manager and the interdisciplinary team is assured.

Figure 1-4 is a clinical pathway describing a client who is experiencing mania; the clinical pathway in Figure 1-5 describes a client who is experiencing psychosis. Each has a length of stay of 8 days, the average length of stay for the designated related groups of these categories of mental disorders, according to a recent search. In reviewing the pathway format, note that the elements are separated into two parts, outcomes and processes. *Outcomes* are the expected client outcomes that are predicted along the 8-day continuum that is noted in the interval row across the top of the pathway. Outcomes have four distinct client categories: physiologic, psychologic, functional status/role, and family/community reintegration. Processes, also known as interventions, comprise the bottom section of the clinical pathway. They consist of several categories, which are listed along the left column. Processes reflect the client's needs and the pathway's interdisciplinary focus. Processes are expected to promote/affect the client's identified outcomes in a progressive, timely manner along the pathway continuum. The pathway is, in effect, the client's care plan, the outcome of which is used to evaluate the client's progress on a daily basis. Variances, described previously, are categorized by either letters or numbers along the bottom of each pathway. In the pathways depicted in this text, two types of variances have been developed: Pathway Variances, which the staff would indicate by writing the codes (P1, P2, etc.) in the Interval (Days) section across the top of the pathway, and Element Variances, which the staff would indicate by writing the codes (1.1, 2.2, etc.) in the body of the pathway itself, according to where they occur. Clinical pathways continue to be developed, improved, and implemented in a variety of health care settings and are expected to reflect the changing trends and complexities of current health care delivery systems.

IMPLEMENTATION

In this phase of the nursing process, the nurse implements the interventions that have been prescribed in the planning phase. Nursing interventions, also termed *nursing orders* or *prescriptions,* are the most powerful components of the nursing process. They comprise the management and treatment approach to an identified health problem. Interventions are selected to achieve or attain outcomes and prevent or reduce problems. Some shortcomings noted in nursing interventions, both in the literature and in clinical practice, are that they are weak, vague, and nonspecific. The interventions listed throughout this text reflect both actual and typical nursing responses and behaviors derived from educational preparation and clinical experience. They are substantive, expressive, and inclusive. In the psychiatric–mental health setting, treatment or therapies frequently constitute verbal communication skills, a major source of psychosocial intervention. Such treatments are intended to effect a change in the client's present condition or circumstance, not merely maintain the problem in its present state. Prescriptions or orders serve to recommend a course of action, not simply support an existing regimen.

Nursing interventions for nursing diagnoses should explicitly describe a plan of therapeutic activity that will help mobilize the client toward a healthier or more functional state.

Examples (therapeutic):

1. Gradually engage client in interactions with other clients, beginning with one-to-one contacts and progressing toward informal gatherings and eventually structured group activities, occupational therapy first, then recreational therapy.
2. Teach client and family that therapeutic effects of antidepressant medications may take up to 2 weeks but that uncomfortable effects may begin immediately.

Examples: (nontherapeutic):

1. Assist the client to interact with others.
2. Teach client and family about medications.

The correct examples demonstrate clarity and substance, as opposed to the weaker, vaguer, incorrect statements. Nursing interventions that simply regurgitate doctors' orders are not substantive enough to treat or manage the health problem effectively. *Example* (nontherapeutic):

1. Monitor the client's progress, check lithium levels; notify social services; obtain client's consent form; report change in mood and affect.

Effective nursing interventions should have the capability of moving the client from a less functional to a more functional health state by virtue of their clarity, substance, and direction.

In the psychiatric–mental health setting, clients' health states are constantly assessed, diagnosed, and treated by nurses. Thus the challenge for nurses today is to formulate strong, effective nursing interventions that address and modify the client's health problem, based on researched, independent nursing therapies.

Interventions' Impact on Etiologies

Interventions have the greatest impact when they are directed toward the etiologies (related factors) that accompany the nursing diagnosis or, if the problem is a risk nursing diagnosis, are aimed at the risk factors. This suggests that the etiologies of a problem can be modified by

Text continued on p. 18.

Mania

	Interval	Day of Admit	Day 2	Day 3	Day 4	Day 5	Day 6	Day 7	Day 8
	Location								
OUTCOMES	Physiologic	*Takes adequate nutrition, fluids with assistance *Complies with lithium level evaluation	*Demonstrates increased sleep/ rest time *Demonstrates adequate elimination	*Takes adequate nutrition/fluid with reminders *Demonstrates adequate elimination	*Sleeps 4-6 hours *Demonstrates adequate elimination	*Takes adequate nutrition/fluid *Sleeps 4-6 hours *Lithium level in therapeutic range *Other drug level in therapeutic range	*Sleeps 5-8 hours *Absence of drug toxicity	*Sleep 5-8 hours	*Sleeps 5-8 hours *Able to manage food and activity requirements independently
OUTCOMES	Psychologic	*Involved in stimulation-reducing activities with staff supervision	*Oriented to person and place	*Demonstrates reduction in: movement racing thoughts grandiosity/euphoria irritability	*Demonstrates increased attention span *Reality tests with staff *Oriented to person, place, time, and situation	*Demonstrates more reality-based thoughts *Able to focus on one topic ×5-10 minutes	*Demonstrates euthymic mood *Able to focus on one topic ×5-10 minutes	*Able to complete activities and unit assignments	*Able to complete activities and unit assignments independently *Able to plan and structure day
OUTCOMES	Functional Status/Role	*Tolerate orientation to the unit *Refrains from harming self/others with assistance	*Interacting with staff as tolerated *Attends to hygiene/grooming needs with assistance *Refrains from harming self/others with assistance	*Engages in unit activities with staff supervision	*Maintains impulses with reminders *Complies with meds with reminders	*Demonstrates less intrusive behaviors	*Able to interact with peers *Able to make simple decisions	*Demonstrates safe, appropriate activities/behaviors *Independently complies with medical regimen	*Verbalizes need for ongoing med compliance
OUTCOMES	Family/Community Reintegration	*Family/significant other aware of treatment program/goals *Family/significant other provide history including meds	*Identifies family/significant other to staff	*Attends community meetings with staff supervision *Communicates with SW for increased understanding of treatment goals/DC plans	*Family/significant other involved in treatment/discharge planning	*Identifies discharge needs	*Identifies discharge needs	*Identifies discharge needs *Able to identify supports and their appropriate use	*Able to utilize supports and lists ways to access them *States specific plans to manage symptoms, comply with meds, and aftercare

Note: This Clinical Pathway is a tool to assist health care providers in achieving quality patient outcomes by providing appropriate and timely patient care. It is not intended to establish a community standard of care, replace a clinician's medical judgment, establish a protocol for all patients, or exclude alternative therapies. (See Variances at end of figure.)

Abbreviations: *CBC,* complete blood chemistry; *DC,* discharge; *ELOS,* estimated length of stay; *eval,* evaluation; *H/O,* history of; *I&O,* intake and output; *milieu,* therapeutic patient environment; *OT,* occupational therapist; *Reise writ,* hearing to determine if patient is cognitively able to make a decision to refuse psychotropic medication; *S&R,* seclusion and restraint; *SW,* social worker; *UR,* utilization review.

Fig. 1-4 Clinical pathways design sheet: Mania.

	Interval	Day of Admit	Day 2	Day 3	Day 4	Day 5	Day 6	Day 7	Day 8
	Location								
PROCESSES	Discharge Planning	*SW assessment *Identify DC placement *ELOS, contact family/significant other *Nursing assessment *Identify H/O chronicity *Med compliance, strengths, needs, knowledge deficit	*Team: Involved in DC planning discuss with MD *UR notify managed care ( )	*SW eval completed *Treatment team meeting #1 ( ) *Specific DC plans, placement facility identified ( )	*Involve family/significant other in DC plans *Review DC plans with patient	*Assist patient/family/significant other discharge needs *UR contact managed care as needed ( )	*Continue to problem solve discharge needs with patient, family/significant other	*Transition to day treatment if indicated *Assist patient, family/significant other in finalizing discharge plans *Treatment team meeting #2 ( )	*Discharge to least restrictive environment completed *UR inform managed care as needed ( )
	Education	*Orient to unit *Inform of patient's rights *Assess patient's and family's/significant other knowledge of disorder/meds	*Assist with symptom recognition and importance of compliance *Teach family/significant other as needed	*Continue with symptom recognition *Continue teaching patient and family/significant other learning needs	*Assist in linking symptoms with precipitating events	*Teach patient/family/significant other about med effects on symptom management *Instruct in med, diet, exercise regimen	*Emphasize importance of compliance with meds after discharge *Teach about drug-to-drug effects on symptom management	*Develop aftercare plan to manage symptoms and contact supports	*Reinforce aftercare teaching plan with patient, family/significant other as needed
	Psychosocial/Spiritual/Legal	*Assess: Safety ( ) *Mental status ( ) Spiritually ( ) *Legal status: Voluntary ( ) 72 hour hold ( ) *Reise writ () Payer ( ) Conservator ( )	*Continue to assess: Safety issues Mental status Spiritual needs Legal status	*Continue to assess: Safety issues Mental status (e.g., racing thoughts, grandiosity, euphoria, irritability) Spiritual/legal needs	*Continue to assess: Safety issues Mental status (e.g., racing thoughts, grandiosity, euphoria, irritability) Spiritual/legal needs	*Continue to assess: Safety issues Mental status Spirituality Voluntary status	*Continue to assess: Safety issues Mental status Spirituality Voluntary status	*Continue to assess: Safety issues Mental status Spirituality Voluntary status	*Complete assessments and confirm: Safety Mental status Spirituality Legal status
	Consults	*Physical exam within 24 hours *Other consults	*Other consults as needed	*Other consults as needed	*Other consults as needed	*Complete consults as ordered	*Complete consults as ordered	*Complete consults as ordered *Arrange for aftercare consults as ordered	*Complete all consults as ordered
	Tests/Procedures	*Lithium level ( ) *Tegretol level ( ) *Drug screen ( ) *Thyroid function ( ) *CBC/SMAC ( ) *Other ( )	*Tests/procedures as ordered	*Tests/procedures as ordered	*Tests/procedures as ordered	*Check lithium level for therapeutic range *Check other drug levels for therapeutic range as needed *Test procedures as needed	*Check lithium level for therapeutic range *Check other drug levels within therapeutic range as needed *Tests procedures as needed	*Check lithium level for therapeutic range *Check other levels within therapeutic range as needed *Test procedures as needed	*Confirm lithium level for therapeutic range *Confirm other levels within therapeutic range as needed *Test procedures as ordered aftercare

Fig. 1-4—Mania, cont'd For legend see page 12.

Continued

	Interval	Day of Admit	Day 2	Day 3	Day 4	Day 5	Day 6	Day 7	Day 8
	Location								
PROCESSES	Treatment	*Monitor: I&O *Sleep/rest patterns *Level of observation 1:1 ( ); every 15 min ( ); every 30 min ( ) *Reduce milieus stimulation *S&R yes ( ) or no ( ) *Other	*Monitor: I&O *Sleep/rest patterns *Level of observation 1:1 ( ); every 15 min ( ); every 30 min ( ) *Reduce milieu stimulation *S&R yes ( ) no ( ) *Other	*Level of observation 1:1 ( ); every 15 min ( ); every 30 min ( ) *Continue with treatment plan: Monitor: I&O Sleep/rest Other	*Continue with treatment plan: Monitor: I&O Sleep/rest Other	*Level of observation 1:1 ( ); every 15 min ( ); every 30 min ( ) *Continue with treatment plan I&O Sleep/rest Other	*Level of observation 1:1 ( ); every 15 min ( ); every 30 min ( ) *Continue with treatment plan I&O Sleep/rest Other	*Level of observation 1:1 ( ); every 15 min ( ); every 30 min ( ) *Aftercare treatment instructions reviewed with patient, family/significant other as needed	*DC with aftercare treatment instructions
	Medications (IV & Others)	*Meds as ordered *See relevant protocols: *Lithium *Other *Monitor side effects *Toxicity	*Meds as ordered *Continue to monitor side effects/toxicity	*Meds as ordered *Continue to monitor side effects/toxicity	*Meds as ordered *Continue to monitor side effects/toxicity	*Meds as ordered *Contact managed care if any change in med regimen	*Meds as ordered *Contact managed care if any change in med regimen	*Meds as ordered *Review of meds with patient, family/significant other as needed	*DC with meds and instructions as ordered
	Activity	*OT assessment *1:1 brief contacts *Reality orientation *Intervene to manage impulses: prevent harm to self/others	*Engage in stimulation-reducing activities as tol *Assist with hygiene, grooming, ADLs *Prevent harm to self/others during activities	*OT eval completed *Encourage hygiene, grooming, ADLs with reminders *Prevent harm to self/others during activities	*Engage in 2 groups per day *Increase group stimulation as tolerated *Prevent harm to self/others during activities	*Encourage: Independent hygiene and grooming Independent ADLs Increased participation in groups	*Engage in all unit activities and groups *Encourage independent decision making	*Reinforce active participation in all unit activities and groups; independent decision making	*Confirm ability to complete activity assignments independently, ability to make decisions independently
	Diet/Nutrition	*Nutritional screening *Elicit food preference *Offer adequate nutrition and fluids; normal salt intake *Baseline weight (weekly unless otherwise ordered)	*Provide simple meals Finger foods Easy to carry drinks	*Encourage meals in patient community as tolerated with staff supervision	*Encourage meals in patient community as tolerated with staff supervision	*Teach family/significant other importance of adequate foods/fluids/salt intake	*Teach family/significant other importance of adequate foods/fluids/salt intake	*Reinforce adequate nutrition/fluids and normal salt intake *Weekly weight	*Confirm patient/significant other/family knowledge of adequate foods/fluids/salt intake

Pathway Variances: P1. CP completed early P2. Patient off CP P3. Pathway Completed & Patient Not Discharged P4. Initial Interval Not Appropriate

Element Variances:

1. Patient/Family:
   1. Patient physiologic status
   2. Patient psychologic status
   3. Patient/family refusal
   4. Patient/family unavailable
   5. Patient/family other
   6. Patient/family communication barrier
   7. Element met early
2. Clinician:
   1. Order differs from CP
   2. Action differs from CP
   3. Response time
   4. Clinician other
   5. Court/guardianship
3. Operating Unit
   1. Bed/appointment not available
   2. Lack of data
   3. Supplies/equipment not available
   4. Department overbooked/closed
   5. Court/guardianship
   6. Operating unit other
4. Community
   1. Placement not available
   2. Home care not available
   3. Ambulance delay
   4. Transportation not available
   5. Community other
5. Payer
   1. Delayed giving authorization number
   2. Payer limitations
   3. Payer other

Fig. 1-4—Mania, cont'd For legend see page 12.

Psychosis

	Interval	Day of Admit	Day 2	Day 3	Day 4	Day 5	Day 6	Day 7	Day 8
	Location								
OUTCOMES	Physiologic	*Takes adequate fluid/nutrition with assistance *Tolerates meds	*Takes adequate fluid/ nutrition with assistance *Increased sleep/rest time *Adequate elimination	*Adequate nutrition with reminders *Adequate elimination	*Sleeps 3-6 hours *Adequate elimination	*Takes adequate nutrition/fluids *Drug levels therapeutic range	*Sleeps 5-8 hours *Absence drug toxicity side effects	*Sleeps 5-8 hours	*Sleeps 5-8 hours *Able to manage food/activity requirements independently
	Psychologic	*Tolerates orientation to unit within capacity	*Oriented ×2	*Oriented ×3 *Demonstrates reduction in hallucinations and delusions	*Oriented ×4 *Reality testing with staff *Increased trust demonstrated	*Demonstrates more reality-based thoughts	*Able to focus on one topic 5-10 minutes	*Able to complete unit assignments and activities	*Able to complete unit assignment and activities independently *Able to plan/ structure day
	Functional Status/Role	*Refrains from harming self or others with assistance	*Refrains from harming self *Attends to basic ADLs *Seeks staff when anxious	*Refrains from harming self *Increased trust demonstrated *Increased ADLs *Complies with meds with reminders	*Increased ADLs *Controls impulses with assistance *Utilizing basic stress management techniques with assistance	*Demonstrates less psychosis and intrusive behavior	*Interacts with peers *Able to make decisions	*Able to maintain safety *Demonstrates safe behaviors	*Able to maintain safety *Independently complies with medical regime
	Family/Community Reintegration	*Family/significant other aware of treatment program goals *Family/significant other provide history including meds	*Identifies family/significant other to staff	*Attends community meetings/milieu activities with staff supervision. *Identify family/ significant other *Communicates with SW for increased understanding of Treatment goals/DC plans	*Family/significant other included in treatment/DC plans	*Identifies DC needs	*Identifies DC needs	*Identifies DC needs *Able to identify supports and how to use them	*Able to utilize supports and list ways to access them *State specific plans to manage symptoms, comply with meds and aftercare

Note: This Clinical Pathway is a tool to assist health care providers in achieving quality patient outcomes by providing appropriate and timely patient care. It is not intended to establish a community standard of care, replace a clinician's medical judgment, establish a protocol for all patients, or exclude alternative therapies. (See Variances at end of figure.)

Abbreviations: *CBC,* complete blood chemistry; *DC,* discharge; *ELOS,* estimated length of stay; *eval,* evaluation; *H/O,* history of; *I&O,* intake and output; *milieu,* therapeutic patient environment; *OT,* occupational therapist; *Reise writ,* hearing to determine if patient is cognitively able to make a decision to refuse psychotropic medication; *S&R,* seclusion and restraint; *SW,* social worker; *UR,* utilization review.

Fig. 1-5 Clinical pathways design sheet: psychosis.

Continued

	Interval	Day of Admit	Day 2	Day 3	Day 4	Day 5	Day 6	Day 7	Day 8
	Location								
PROCESSES	Discharge Planning	*(SW) initiate assessment *Identify DC placement ELOS contact family/significant other (nursing) initiates assessment *Identify H/O med compliance knowledge deficit and chronicity	*Team involved in DC planning *Discussed with MD *UR notify managed care	*SW evaluation completed *Specific DC plan identified *Treatment team meeting #1	*Involve family/significant other in DC plan *Review with patient	*Patient, family/significant other communicate understanding DC plan and follow-up *UR contact manage care	*Reinforce patient, family/significant other understanding DC plan and follow-up	*Transition to day treatment if indicated *Continue to identify/reinforce support system	*DC to least restrictive environment
	Education	*Orient to unit *Patient's rights *Assess patient/significant other *Assess knowledge of meds and chronicity	*Assist with symptom recognition and importance of compliance *Include family/significant other as necessary	*Continue with symptom recognition *Continue to assess level of knowledge re: disorder and meds	*Assist in linking symptoms with precipitating event	*Assist in linking symptoms with precipitating events (noncompliance, drug abuse)	*Reinforce med education *Importance of compliance	*Develop aftercare plan to manage symptoms *Contact supports	*Develop aftercare plan to manage symptoms and contact supports
	Psychosocial/ Spiritual/Legal	*Assess: Safety issues Mental status Spirituality Voluntary status	*Continue to assess: Safety issues Mental status Spirituality Voluntary status	*Continue to assess: Safety issues Mental status Spirituality Voluntary status	*Complete assessments and confirm: Safety Mental status Spirituality Legal status	*Continue to assess: Safety issues Mental status Spiritual Voluntary status	*Continue to assess: Safety issues Mental status Spiritual Voluntary status	*Continue to assess: Safety issues Mental status Spirituality Voluntary status	*Legal, psychosocial, spiritual eval completed
	Consults	*Physical exam within 24 hours ( )	*Other consults as needed	*Other consults as needed	*Other consults as needed	*Other consults as needed	*Other consults as needed	*Arrange aftercare consults as ordered	*Complete all consults
	Tests/Procedures	*Med levels ( ) *Drug screen ( ) *CBC ( ) *Thyroid function ( ) *SMAC ( )	*Other test/procedures as ordered	*Other test/procedures as ordered	*Other test/procedures as ordered	*Other test/procedures as ordered	*Other test/procedures as ordered *Check drug levels in therapeutic range	*Other test/procedures as ordered	*Test procedures as ordered outpatient
	Treatment	*Monitor I&O *Monitor sleep/rest patterns *Level of observation 1:1 ( ); every 15 min ( ); every 30 min ( ) *Reduce milieu stimulation *Treatment as ordered *S&R ( ) yes ( ) no ( )	*Monitor I&O *Monitor sleep/rest patterns *Level of observation 1:1 ( ); every 15 min ( ); every 30 min ( ) *Treatment as ordered	*Monitor I&O *Monitor sleep/rest patterns *Level of observation 1:1 ( ); every 15 min ( ); every 30 min ( ) *Treatment as ordered	*Monitor I&O *Monitor sleep/rest patterns *Level of observation 1:1 ( ); every 15 min ( ); every 30 min ( ) *Continue treatment plan as ordered	*Level of observation: 1:1 ( ); every 15 min ( ); every 30 min ( ) *Treatment plan as ordered *Monitor sleep/rest pattern	*Level of observation: 1:1 ( ); every 15 min ( ); every 30 min ( ) *Treatment plan as ordered *Monitor sleep/rest pattern	*Level of observation: 1:1 ( ); every 15 min ( ); every 30 min ( ) *Treatment plan as ordered *Monitor sleep/rest pattern	*Discharge with specified treatment confirmed for aftercare

Fig. 1-5—Psychosis, cont'd For legend see page 15.

	Interval	Day of Admit	Day 2	Day 3	Day 4	Day 5	Day 6	Day 7	Day 8
	Location								
PROCESSES	Medications (IV & Others)	*Meds as ordered *Protocols for anti-psychotic med management *Monitor side effects *Toxicity	*Meds as ordered *Protocols for anti-psychotic med management *Monitor side effects *Toxicity	*Meds as ordered *Protocols for anti-psychotic med management *Monitor side effects *Toxicity	*Meds as ordered *Protocols for anti-psychotic med management *Monitor side effects *Toxicity	*Meds as ordered *Contact managed care with med changes *Protocols for anti-psychotic med management *Monitor side effects *Toxicity	*Meds as ordered *Protocols for anti-psychotic med management *Monitor side effects *Toxicity *Review meds with family/significant other	*Meds as ordered *Protocols for anti-psychotic med management *Monitor side effects *Toxicity	*Discharge with meds and instructions as ordered
	Activity	*OT assessment *1:1 reality orient/brief contact *Assist with ADLs *Interventions to control self/other harm/impulses	*Continue OT eval *Engage in groups as tolerated *Assist with ADLs *Interventions to control self/other harm/impulses	*OT eval *Engage in groups as tolerated *ADLs with reminders *Interventions to control self/other harm/impulses	*Engage in 2 groups as tolerated *Interventions to control self/other harm/impulses	*Independent ADLs *Engage in 2 groups per day *Provide opportunity for simple decision making	*Independent ADLs *Engage in all unit activities *Provide opportunity for simple decision making	*Independent ADLs *Engage in all unit activities *Encourage independent decision making	*Independent ADLs *Engage in all unit activities *Confirm decision making *Confirm safety
	Diet/Nutrition	*Nutritional screening *Elicit food preference *Offer adequate nutrition/fluids *Baseline weight (weekly unless otherwise ordered)	*Offer adequate nutrition/fluids *Provide simple meals: Finger foods Room-temperature drinks	*Offer adequate nutrition/fluids *Encourage meals in milieu as tolerated with staff supervision	*Offer adequate nutrition/fluids *Encourage meals in milieu as tolerated with staff supervision	*Offer adequate nutrition/fluids *Teach family /significant other importance of adequate nutrition/ fluids	*Offer adequate nutrition/fluids *Teach family/ significant other importance of adequate nutrition/ fluids	*Reinforce adequate nutrition/fluids *Weekly weight	*Confirm patient family/significant other knowledge adequate nutrition/ fluids *Confirm adequate nutrition/fluids

Pathway Variances: P1. CP completed early P2. Patient off CP P3. Pathway Completed & Patient Not Discharged P4. Initial Interval Not Appropriate

Element Variances:

1. Patient/Family:
   1. Patient physiologic status
   2. Patient psychologic status
   3. Patient/family refusal
   4. Patient/family unavailable
   5. Patient/family other
   6. Patient/family communication barrier
   7. Element met early
2. Clinician:
   1. Order differs from CP
   2. Action differs from CP
   3. Response time
   4. Clinician other
   5. Court/guardianship
3. Operating Unit
   1. Bed/appointment not available
   2. Lack of data
   3. Supplies/equipment not available
   4. Department overbooked/closed
   5. Court/guardianship
   6. Operating unit other
4. Community
   1. Placement not available
   2. Home care not available
   3. Ambulance delay
   4. Transportation not available
   5. Community other
5. Payer
   1. Delayed giving authorization number
   2. Payer limitations
   3. Payer other

Fig. 1-5—Psychosis, cont'd For legend see page 15.

nursing. Therefore, to achieve or attain the most successful client outcomes, the nurse should carefully examine each of the etiologic factors and select interventions that would effectively modify each one.

Interventions and Medical Actions

Interventions can include medically focused actions, such as the administration of medications, but the major focus of the intervention should emphasize nursing actions, judgments, treatments, and directives. *Examples* (nontherapeutic):

1. Administer antipsychotic medications as ordered.
2. Observe for extrapyramidal effects.

Note in these examples the absence of any prescribed nursing actions that would influence the client's health state.

Rationale Statements

In many instances, a rationale statement (the reason for the nursing intervention or why it was prescribed) is included next to the intervention statement. This practice enhances the understanding of the nurse's action or treatment. We have liberally used clear and descriptive rationale statements throughout this text (in italics following interventions) to foster the reader's overall understanding of the selected interventions. *Examples:*

Actively listen, observe, and respond to client's verbal and nonverbal expressions. *Lets the client know he or she is worthwhile and respected.*

Initiate brief, frequent contacts with the client throughout the day. *Lets the client know he or she is an important part of the community.*

EVALUATION

Evaluation of achieved or attained expected client outcomes must occur at various intervals as designated in the outcome criteria, with the capability and health state of each client as a primary consideration. There are two steps in the evaluation phase:

1. The nurse compares the client's current mental health state or condition with that described in the outcome criteria: Is the client's anxiety reduced to a tolerable level? (For example, can the client sit calmly for 10 minutes, attend a simple recreational activity for 10 minutes, and engage in one-to-one interaction with staff for 5 minutes without distractions? Is there a significant reduction in pacing, fidgeting, scanning? Were these outcomes attained within the times originally projected?) The degree to which client outcomes are attained or not attained is also an evaluation of the effectiveness of nursing.
2. The nurse considers all the possible reasons why nursing outcomes were not attained, if this is the case. For example, perhaps it is too soon to evaluate and the plan of action needs further implementation (the client needed another 2 days of one-to-one interactions before attending client group activities); or maybe the interventions were too forceful and frequent or too weak and infrequent. It may be that the outcomes were unattainable, impractical, or just not feasible for this client, or perhaps they were not within the client's scope and capabilities on a developmental or sociocultural level. What about the validity of the nursing diagnosis? Was it developed with a questionable or faulty data base? Are more data required: What were the conditions during the assessment phase? Was it too hurried? Were conclusions drawn too quickly? Were there any language or other communication barriers?

Based on conclusions drawn from these queries, specific recommendations are then made, which include either continuing implementation of the plan of action or reviewing the previous phases of the nursing process (data collection, nursing diagnosis, planning, or implementation).

The evaluation of a client's progress and the nursing activities involved in the process are critical because they require—even demand—that nursing be accountable for its own standards of care.

Informal evaluation of client's progress, much like the nursing process, takes place continuously. (Refer to Fig. 1-1.)

THE NURSING PROCESS IN COMMUNITY AND HOME SETTINGS

In the past the nursing process and its multistep format have been most associated with the care of hospitalized clients. Current trends in health care delivery systems have shifted from inpatient facilities to community and home-based settings and provide yet another vital avenue for use of the nursing process. Home health care is a primary alternative to hospitalization, and the nursing process continues to be a major factor in the effective management of home client care.

Psychiatric Home Health Care Case Management System

The changes and demands in today's health care delivery system have resulted in several trends in health care reform designed to bring about cost-effective quality care. Although the case management concept has been around for years in acute care settings and public health arenas, only recently has the private home health model subscribed to total case management, and only more recently has psychiatric home care been incorporated under the case management umbrella.

Psychiatric home care case management is a method by which a client is identified as a candidate for home care and treated on a health care continuum in the familiar surroundings of the home. The interdisciplinary home care team, facilitated by a registered nurse, coordinates all available resources to meet their goals for treatment and to achieve the client's expected outcomes in a quality and cost-effective manner. At one end of the continuum is the highest degree of independent wellness within the client's capacity, and at the other end of the continuum is death, with varying levels of wellness-illness in between.

Critical to successful utilization of case management is the accurate placement of the client at the entry point on the continuum and a clear understanding of the team's best estimate for the date of cessation of home care services.

Nursing-Sensitive Outcomes Classification

Current nursing research in the expansion of patient outcomes was developed by the nursing-sensitive outcomes classification (NOC) research team, formed in August 1991 at the University of Iowa (Iowa Intervention Project, 1996). Its purpose was to conceptualize, label, and classify nursing-sensitive patient outcomes. NOC is complementary to the work of NANDA; both reflect the creation and testing of a professional, standardized language that defines the nursing profession, and they both strive to develop patient outcomes that are responsive to nursing interventions. NOC developed the first comprehensive list of standardized outcomes, definitions, and measures to describe patient outcomes that are influenced by nursing practice.

According to the NOC, patient outcomes are considered to be neutral rather than static, and they reflect patients' ongoing states, such as mobility and hydration (physiologic), or coping and grieving (psychologic). Such fluid states can be measured on a continuum of care, rather than as singular, discrete goals that are either met or not met. Since outcomes are presented by the NOC as neutral concepts, they can be identified and measured in a variety of ways and for different population groups. This is useful in assisting nurses to develop realistic standards that reflect currently achieved outcomes, if the outcomes are satisfactory, or desired, higher standards or achievement.

Identifying outcomes responsive to nursing versus depending on the use of interdisciplinary outcomes developed mostly for physician practice is critical for controlling quality patient care and the further development of nursing knowledge, language, and the profession. Agreement on standardizing nursing-sensitive patient outcomes allows nurses to analyze the effects of nursing interventions along a patient care continuum and across health care settings.

Nursing Interventions Classification

Nursing Interventions Classification (NIC) is the first comprehensive, standardized classification of treatments performed by nurses. NIC works in conjunction with NOC in that patient outcomes need to be identified before an intervention is selected. The classification includes interventions that nurses facilitate for patients both independently and with other disciplines, for direct and indirect care. NIC interventions include both physiologic types (airway suctioning) and psychologic or psychosocial types (anxiety reduction). As with NANDA and NOC, NIC interventions include a variety of patient populations, settings, groups, and cultures. Although most are geared toward the individual, they also apply to families and entire communities. They can be used for illness prevention, health maintenance, education, environmental management, and health promotion. Although NIC interventions are linked to NANDA diagnoses, there are more possibilities with NIC in that nurses need to know the patient and the patient's condition before selecting the appropriate intervention; therefore, the decision-making process is more complex. Principal investigators/editors Bulechek and McCloskey (1992) have outlined three areas in which the nurse must be competent in order to carry out an intervention.

1. Knowledge of scientific rationale
2. Possession of the necessary psychomotor and interpersonal skills
3. Ability to function within the setting to effectively use health care resources

For more information on NIC and NOC and their relationships to NANDA, refer to current literature on these classification systems.

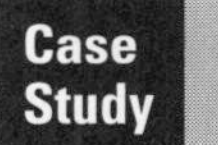

Case Study: Application of the Nursing Process

The assessment tool (Fig. 1-3) and the following case study and plan of care are examples of how the care plans in this book can be adapted to an individual client.

CASE STUDY: CLIENT WITH ANXIETY

John, a 15-year-old high school student, is admitted for the first time to the mental health facility. He is accompanied to the facility voluntarily by his parents, who are noted to be supportive and concerned about their only child. John's chief complaint is quoted as: "I suddenly feel I can't cope with schoolwork, friends, or sports; I feel tense, sweaty, and uncomfortable and find it hard to concentrate on my assignments. My heart pounds and I breathe fast even when I'm not moving around, and I find myself wanting to run out of the classroom." He noted that his symptoms have occurred for 10 days and have been increasing in severity and frequency until he now feels they are interfering with his ability to function in school and perform the activities and sports that he loves.

ASSESSMENT

Problem List

(Based on Psychiatric Nursing History and Assessment; Fig. 1-3)

Physiologic

1. Shortness of breath at rest
2. Rapid heart rate (greater than 120 beats/min) at rest

3. Sweaty palms when performing schoolwork or sports or talking with peers
4. Feelings of generalized discomfort and tension

Psychologic

1. Cannot concentrate or focus on schoolwork/assignments
2. Unable to perform sports or other activities
3. Feels like running away from classroom or peers
4. Unable to cope with current responsibilities, role, and life circumstances

Behaviors observed by RN during assessment and interview

1. Paced back and forth (could not remain seated for more than 1 minute)
2. Burst into tears 3 times during 45-minute interview
3. Difficulty in attending interview questions (Interviewer had to repeat each question at least once.)
4. Spoke in hurried, tense manner (rarely completed a sentence or thought)
5. Stated "I am worried" at least 3 times during the interview

Learning Needs Identified

Client needs to learn the following:

- Stressors/stressor events that are precursors to ineffective coping
- Methods/strategies to increase effective coping skills and decrease or minimize anxiety
- Use of healthy, adaptive defense mechanisms
- Cognitive, reframing, and desensitization skills
- Effective ways to cope with stress
- Problem-solving strategies
- Value of support systems and community resources
- Dose, therapeutic, and adverse effects of anxiolytic medications
- Importance of follow-up care/preventive measures

Medical Diagnosis (Based on DSM-IV Multiaxial Criteria)

Axis I: Generalized Anxiety Disorder
Axis II: No Noted Personality Disorder
Axis III: No Noted Medical Condition
Axis IV: Psychosocial/Environmental Stressors (moderate to severe educational and social stressors noted)
Axis V: Global Assessment of Functioning GAF = 55 (current); GAF = 85 (past year)

Nursing Diagnosis: Coping, ineffective individual

The state in which an individual demonstrates impaired adaptive behaviors and problem-solving abilities in meeting life's demands and roles

Etiologic/Related Factors (Related to):

Anxiety (refer to symptoms/behaviors described previously)
Depletion of usual adaptive/coping methods
Conflicts/stressors that may be associated with current role, relationships, responsibilities
Perceived threat to physical/psychosocial integrity
Possible feelings of powerlessness or helplessness
Expectations for success exceed actual abilities
Knowledge deficit regarding adaptive coping methods

Defining Characteristics (As Evidenced by):

Unable to perform schoolwork, sports, or other activities
Cries easily for no apparent reason or provocation
Experiences urge to leave classroom or run away from peers for no apparent reason
Cannot cope with age-related responsibilities, role, or life circumstances (schoolwork, sports, activities, etc.)
Experiences physiologic symptoms (e.g., rapid heart rate, shortness of breath, sweaty palms) when faced with routine tasks, activities, schoolwork, peers, sports, etc.
Unable to attend or concentrate on age-appropriate tasks/roles, e.g., school assignments, activities, sports, friendships

Outcome Identification and Evaluation

By Day 4 of admission, demonstrates ability to focus/concentrate on assigned unit task/activity
By Day 4, remains seated throughout individual interactions with staff for 15 minutes
By Day 4, performs slow deep breathing techniques and muscle tension-relaxation exercises (See Appendix J.)
By Day 5, practices learned cognitive skills, reframing, and desensitization exercises (See Appendix J.)
By Day 5, completes unit task, activities with minimal or absent anxiety symptoms
By Day 6, communicates and relates effectively with peers/ staff without hesitation or anxiety responses
By Day 7, adaptively and effectively utilizes (with help of staff) defense mechanisms (See Appendix H.), e.g.:

a. Introjection (Role models calm behavior of staff)
b. Suppression (Consciously attempts to forget anxiety-producing stimuli)
c. Compensation (Practices pleasurable, rewarding activities)
d. Displacement (Transfers energy of anxiety to physical exercises, e.g., jogging, walking, bicycling, volleyball, etc.)

Verbalizes ability to effectively perform schoolwork, sports, and other activities without anxiety on Day 8 (Discharge)
By Day 8, exhibits adaptive, healthy coping methods and strategies without supervision.
By Day 8, prioritizes and problem-solves appropriate to age, role, and status with absence of anxiety, e.g.:

a. Places schoolwork first on priority list
b. Makes an effort to interact with peers and support system
c. Participates in sports and other activities
d. Attends school functions with peers
e. Engages in meaningful relationships inside and outside school environment

f. Takes prescribed anxiolytic medication as needed
g. Utilizes resources, supports, and strengths effectively
h. Adheres to follow-up treatment plan and prevention

Verbalizes signs/symptoms of escalating anxiety

Demonstrates learned skills for interrupting progression of anxiety to panic level

Functions effectively with level of anxiety that promotes productivity and creativity

PLANNING AND IMPLEMENTATION

Nursing Interventions and Rationale

Maintain a calm, nonthreatening demeanor while interacting with the client. *Anxiety is transferable, and client will feel more trusting and secure with a calm, controlled staff member.*

Demonstrate active listening, empathy, and understanding as client verbalizes painful feelings. *Client is more likely to vent feelings in a safe, nurturing environment.*

Assure client of his safety and security by remaining with him and not leaving him alone when he is experiencing symptoms of anxiety; dread, or fear. *Client's anxious symptoms worsen when left alone during such times and may escalate to a panic state.*

Use brief, simple messages in a calm, direct manner when speaking with client, especially during initial stages of hospitalization. *Clients who are highly anxious may be unable to tolerate or comprehend complex, stimulating explanations.*

Offer client simple directives vs. asking open-ended questions that require him to respond with lengthy statements, especially in initial hospitalization phase. *The client experiencing anxiety may become even more anxious when asked to come up with too many answers. He needs direction to help focus on relevant matters from staff who anticipate his needs.*

Decrease environmental stimuli as much as possible (e.g., keep lights low, reduce volume on radio or television, disperse people so they do not all congregate in one area). *A stimulating milieu may increase the client's level of anxiety.*

Administer prescribed anxiolytic medication and continue to assess its therapeutic and nontherapeutic effects. *Antianxiety medications may, at times, be the most beneficial therapeutic modality and should always be closely monitored for effectiveness throughout the client's hospitalization. Medications do not take the place of safe, nurturing milieu, but could enhance it when necessary.*

When client's anxiety level has been reduced, engage him in a discussion about his identified stressors (school, sports, peers) and their possible connection to his anxiety. *Identification of possible precipitating factors, even if not the actual underlying cause of anxiety, is the initial step in teaching the client to interrupt further escalation of anxiety and to begin to exercise some control over it.*

Encourage the client to verbalize the extent to which his anxiety has disrupted his role as a student, son, peer, etc., and how this has affected his day-to-day functions. *Ventilation of feelings in a safe, therapeutic environment helps the client confront painful issues and eventually take steps, with staff assistance, to resolve them.*

Teach client to identify signs and symptoms of escalating anxiety and methods to interrupt its progression, such as deep-breathing exercises, relaxation techniques, physical activities such as walking, jogging (if not contraindicated), meditation, reframing, visualization, etc. (See Appendix J.) *Knowledge of impending anxiety and its escalation gives the client the opportunity to utilize learned physical and cognitive methods to interrupt the negative effects of increasing anxiety and prevent its rise to a panic state.*

Anxiety and Related Disorders

Anxiety is a vague, subjective, nonspecific feeling of uneasiness, apprehension, tension, insecurity, and sometimes dread or impending doom. It is a normal alerting and protective response to threats to a person's biologic, psychologic, or social integrity, esteem, identity, or status. The experience of anxiety is universal and an integral part of human existence—everyone becomes anxious at some time. Some anxiety is necessary for the scholar to learn, the artist to create, the builder to construct, and, in general, for all of us to contend with the challenges of living.

RESPONSES TO ANXIETY

Certain physiologic, cognitive, perceptual, emotional, and behavioral responses occur in response to mild, moderate, severe, and panic levels of anxiety (Table 2-1). Nurses must develop skill in recognizing the early stages of anxiety in clients so that calm, immediate interventions aimed at alleviation of symptoms may begin before the client's behavior escalates beyond control.

Early recognition of anxiety is necessary for two other reasons. First, anxiety is contagious. Because it is readily communicated between people, one highly anxious client may quickly upset an entire unit. Second, nurses must be aware of their own anxiety, which can be communicated to clients. The therapeutic effectiveness of an interaction can be greatly reduced or even cease when the nurse fails to recognize and manage self-anxiety.

ETIOLOGY

Specific etiologic factors related to anxiety are listed in Box 2-1.

EPIDEMIOLOGY

Although many individuals report experiencing high levels of anxiety in our fast-paced, demanding times, actual anxiety disorders occur in approximately 1% to 5% of the total population. Post-traumatic stress disorders may occur in 50% to 80% of individuals after a devastating experience. Hypochondriac disorders occur in higher numbers in general client populations than do other anxiety disorders. Some anxiety disorders are more prevalent in women. Age at onset for all anxiety disorders is usually before 30 years.

ADAPTIVE VERSUS MALADAPTIVE RESPONSES

When a threat is perceived, anxiety occurs and evokes automatic responses that may be adaptive or maladaptive. In a general sense, all responses could be considered adaptive because each alleviates tension and discomfort brought on by anxiety. Over time, individuals develop characteristic patterns of responding to anxiety, which become a strong influence in their lives, and these patterns affect the way people view themselves, others, and the world around

Table 2-1

Responses to Anxiety

Anxiety Level	Physiologic	Cognitive/Perceptual	Emotional/Behavioral
Mild	Vital signs normal. Minimal muscle tension. Pupils normal, constricted.	Perceptual field is broad. Awareness of multiple environmental and internal stimuli. Thoughts may be random but controlled.	Feelings of relative comfort and safety. Relaxed, calm appearance and voice. Performance is automatic; habitual behaviors occur here.
Moderate	Vital signs normal or slightly elevated. Tension experienced; may be uncomfortable or pleasurable (labeled as "tense" or "excited").	Alert; perception narrowed, focused. Optimum state for problem solving and learning. Attentive.	Feelings of readiness and challenge, energized. Engage in competitive activity and learn new skills. Voice, facial expression interested or concerned.
Severe	Fight or flight response. Autonomic nervous system excessively stimulated (vital signs increased, diaphoresis increased, urinary urgency and frequency, diarrhea, dry mouth, appetite decreased, pupils dilated). Muscles rigid, tense. Senses affected; hearing decreased, pain sensation decreased.	Perceptual field greatly narrowed. Problem solving difficult. Selective attention (focus on one detail). Selective inattention (block out threatening stimuli). Distortion of time (things seem faster or slower than actual). Dissociative tendencies; vigilambulism (automatic behavior).	Feels threatened; startles with new stimuli; feels on "overload." Activity may increase or decrease (may pace, run away, wring hands, moan, shake, stutter, become very disorganized, or withdrawn, freeze in position/unable to move). May seem and feel depressed. Demonstrates denial; may complain of aches or pains; may be agitated or irritable. Need for space increased. Eyes may dart around room, or gaze may be fixed. May close eyes to shut out environment.
Panic	Above symptoms escalate until sympathetic nervous system release occurs. Person may become pale, blood pressure decreases, hypotension. Muscle coordination poor. Pain, hearing sensations minimal.	Perception totally scattered or closed. Unable to take in stimuli. Problem solving and logical thinking highly improbable. Perception of unreality about self, environment, or event. Dissociation may occur.	Feels helpless with total loss of control. May be angry, terrified; may become combative or totally withdrawn, cry, run. Completely disorganized. Behavior is usually extremely active or inactive.

them. These patterns influence interpersonal interactions and, eventually, help shape personalities.

Adaptive Responses

If anxiety occurs and the individual is able to contain and manage it, positive outcomes are possible. All anxiety is not detrimental; it can be a challenging, powerful motivating factor toward problem solving, conflict resolution, and achievement of higher levels of functioning. For example, a person faced with job obsolescence and the inevitable resultant hardships experiences anxiety that may move him or her to return to school to learn new job skills. A student faced with failure on a major exam because of inadequate study may experience the threat of loss of status, self-esteem, identity, and support, and anxiety occurs. This motivator may help the student seek tutoring and make a focused, concentrated effort to pass the exam.

Other adaptive strategies people commonly use to manage anxiety are talking, crying, sleeping, exercising, and relaxation strategies. These and many other coping methods are used to relieve tension and contend with stress.

Maladaptive Responses

Automatic relief behaviors that protect the individual from anxiety, defend against threats, and provide alleviation and comfort may also lead to maladaptive response patterns that can result in physical or psychologic symptoms, as well as personal, social, and occupational dysfunction. For example, the ego defense mechanisms that serve to protect the person from anxiety may also prevent realistic appraisal of self, other people, situations, or events. (See Appendix I.)

When anxiety is not manageable, the individual may resort to coping mechanisms and strategies that are exaggerated and labeled dysfunctional or abnormal by others. Maladaptive patterns of coping with anxiety include aggressive acting out; withdrawal and isolation; excessive overeating, drinking, gambling, or spending; and drug use or sexual overactivity. Behavior in response to anxiety may become severe enough to be formally labeled an anxiety disorder.

Note that the state of uncontrollable anxiety is not restricted to anxiety disorders—clients with other mental or emotional disorders can experience various levels of anxiety. For example, a client with schizophrenia may experience an increase of symptoms because of overstimulation or environmental stressors that exceed his ability to cope. The symptoms occur in response to anxiety and may not necessarily indicate a worsening of the schizophrenic process.

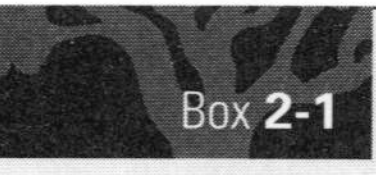

Specific Etiologic Factors Related to Anxiety*

Psychodynamic
Unconscious conflict resulting from guilt, shame; repressed wishes, drives, desires, impulses threaten to invade consciousness, resulting in anxiety

Biologic
Genetic predisposition; inherited vulnerability; CNS and endocrine system interaction

Neurophysiologic
Excessively responsive autonomic nervous system; neurotransmitter disruption (GABA, serotonin, norepinephrine)

Interpersonal
Early interactions with parental figure result in low self-esteem and poor self-concept and are genesis of anxiety

Behavioral
Anxiety is a conditioned response to certain internal or environmental stimuli; learned behavior

Existential
Loss of meaning in life is cause of anxiety

Environmental
Disasters, rape, assault, continual traumas/stressors produce anxiety

*Although a specific etiology for anxiety is still uncertain, a combination of biologic, psychosocial, and environmental factors seem likely; current research is directed toward biologic studies

DIAGNOSIS OF ANXIETY AND RELATED DISORDERS

Generalized Anxiety Disorder

The defining feature of Generalized Anxiety Disorder is persistent, chronic (duration of 6 months or more), excessive, unrealistic worry and anxiety over two or more circumstances or situations in the individual's life. For example, a man who makes a generous salary may be anxious and unnecessarily worried about paying his bills each month and worries that his daughter, who consistently gets high grades, is going to fail college.

Individuals with this disorder are likely to be anxious about things in general. Symptoms of anxiety include the following:

Apprehensive expectation (worry or fear that something awful will happen)
Motor tension (restless, tense, sore muscles, easily fatigued)
Autonomic hyperactivity (shortness of breath, heart palpitations, dizziness, diaphoresis, nausea, frequent urination)
Vigilance and scanning (feeling on edge, easily startled, irritable, trouble falling asleep, continually looking for something negative to happen)

Panic Disorder without Agoraphobia

The defining feature of panic disorder is unexpected recurrence of panic attacks without demonstrable organic etiology or actual life-threatening stimuli. Usually several attacks occur in a week. Symptoms of panic attacks include the following:

- Heart palpitations
- Shortness of breath
- Dizziness
- Trembling

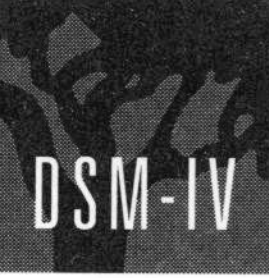

Anxiety Disorders

The essential characteristics of these disorders are anxiety symptoms and avoidance behaviors.

DSM-IV Categories
Generalized Anxiety Disorder
Panic Disorder without Agoraphobia
Panic Disorder with Agoraphobia
Agoraphobia without History of Panic Disorder
Social Phobia
Specific Phobia
Obsessive-Compulsive Disorder
Posttraumatic Stress Disorder
Acute Stress Disorder

- Numbness and tingling
- Hot flashes or chills
- Sweating
- Chest pains
- Derealization/depersonalization
- Fear of dying
- Fear of "going crazy"
- Fear of losing control

At least four of these symptoms occur abruptly and cause extreme fear or discomfort. The individual is usually nervous and apprehensive between attacks and fears the next attack (see Table 2-1).

Panic Disorder with Agoraphobia

Agoraphobia without History of Panic Disorder

Agoraphobia is commonly called fear of the marketplace but really means the unfounded fears that the "marketplace," or life itself, represents—loss of safety or control. The defining feature is fear of being in places or situations from which escape might be difficult or embarrassing, or fear that no help will be available in case of incapacitating symptoms.

This disorder can severely restrict travel or necessitate a constant travel companion. Affected individuals frequently will not leave home because of their extreme discomfort while out of the house alone, in a crowd, or traveling. Most cases of agoraphobia appear to be related to panic disorder; when the latter is treated, agoraphobia usually improves. Avoidance behaviors can greatly interfere with daily functioning. Inability to leave the house to get groceries, go to a job, or transport children to school can be severely incapacitating to individuals with agoraphobia.

Social Phobia

The defining feature of Social Phobia is continual fear that while in public and social situations the individual will do something humiliating or embarrassing. Common examples are fear of choking while eating food with others, fear of saying something foolish in the company of others, and inability to urinate in public rest rooms. These people avoid social phobic situations and usually acknowledge the fear as irrational but seem helpless to eliminate the fear.

Specific Phobia

The defining feature of Specific Phobia is strong fear and avoidance of a specific object or situation, such as an animal (dogs, snakes, insects), enclosed places, heights, or the sight of blood. The person usually acknowledges the intense anxiety that results from exposure to the object or situation as excessive and unreasonable, but the avoidance continues (Table 2-2).

Obsessive-Compulsive Disorder

The defining features of Obsessive-Compulsive Disorder are recurrent thoughts and behaviors that are extremely distressing to the individual or that interfere with a normal life pattern.

Obsessions: Persistent, intrusive thoughts, ideas, images, or impulses that the person knows are irrational or senseless and that cause excessive anxiety. The most common obsessions are thoughts of violence (killing a loved one), contamination (touching doorknobs), and doubt (worry about having done something wrong).

Compulsions: Repetitive, intentional behaviors performed in a stereotypical, routine way. The act may be carried out in direct response to an obsession. Tension and anxiety are relieved by the act. The most common compulsions are hand washing, counting, checking, and touching.

Obsessions and compulsions can be extremely incapacitating. Sometimes individuals get into complex, involved patterns of ritualistic behavior that interfere with normal living. For example, a multistep morning ritual must be completed before leaving the house, but it takes the entire day to perform and prevents the person from getting to work.

Affected individuals usually recognize that the obsessions and compulsions are absurd and irrational, but they continue to persist incessantly. More than half of these persons experience acute onset, usually following a stressful event, and depressive symptoms are not uncommon. Suicide is a special risk in this disorder.

Posttraumatic Stress Disorder

The defining feature of Posttraumatic Stress Disorder is development of anxiety symptoms after an excessively distressing life event that is experienced with terror, fear, and helplessness. The event is serious (seeing a child

Table 2-2 Common Specific Phobias

Feared Situation/Object	Phobia
Heights	Acrophobia
Water	Hydrophobia
Enclosed places	Claustrophobia
Leaving familiar place (home)	Agoraphobia
Animals	Zoophobia
Death	Thanatophobia
Darkness	Nyctophobia
Dirt	Mysophobia
Sex	Genophobia
Venereal disease	Cypridophobia
Being evaluated by others	Social phobia
Women	Gynophobia
Failure	Kakorrhaphiophobia
Homosexual/Homosexuality	Homophobia
Pain	Algophobia

killed, involvement in a major earthquake, fire, plane crash, war, rape, abuse). Symptoms include the following:

Reexperiencing the traumatic event (recurrent recollections, flashbacks, dreams of the event, or intense distress with events that resemble or represent the event)

Avoidance of stimuli, thoughts, or feelings associated with trauma (inability to recall aspects of the event, refusal to go to places that are reminders of the event)

Restricted responsiveness (general numbing, decreased affect, diminished interest, withdrawal from others). This disorder may occur directly after the event or may not be diagnosed until several months or even years later.

Acute Stress Disorder

Symptoms for an Acute Stress Disorder diagnosis are similar to Posttraumatic Stress Disorder, but they develop within the first month after the individual experiences an extremely threatening event or situation. In addition, dissociative symptoms occur in the form of emotional detachment, dazed appearance, depersonalization, derealization, or amnesia in which the person cannot recall part of the traumatic incident. If symptoms extend past 1 month, the diagnosis of Posttraumatic Stress Disorder is considered.

SOMATOFORM DISORDERS

The defining feature of somatoform disorders is the occurrence of physical symptoms that compare with medical disorders but have no identifiable organic pathology or psychopathology. Etiology varies.

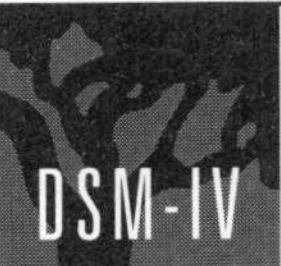

DSM-IV **Somatoform Disorders**

The essential characteristics of these disorders are the occurrence of physical symptoms with no evident organic or physiologic findings and evidence or presumptions that the symptoms are psychologic in origin and not consciously intentional.

DSM-IV Categories

Body Dysmorphic Disorder
Conversion Disorder
Hypochondriasis
Somatization Disorder
Pain Disorder

Body Dysmorphic Disorder

The defining feature of Body Dysmorphic Disorder is preoccupation by a normal-appearing person with perceived bodily flaws or defects or excessive concern over actual minor defects. For example, a woman may constantly look at her nose in the mirror and complain of its shape, although it appears normal to all other observers. Anxiety is always present, and the person may avoid social or occupational situations as a result.

Conversion Disorder

The defining feature of Conversion Disorder is loss or alteration of physical function *not* because of pathophysiology. The symptom usually appears suddenly, at or near the time of a severe psychosocial stressor (e.g., a soldier poised to shoot the enemy suddenly experiences paralysis of his arm; a child listening to her parents fighting aggressively is suddenly unable to hear).

Primary and secondary gains play a part in this disorder. In primary gain, the symptoms keep the actual origin of anxiety out of the person's awareness; in secondary gain the person receives support or is relieved of responsibility or duty as a result of the symptoms.

A lack of concern about the seriousness of the symptoms that is incongruent with the problem may be present *(la belle indifference).*

Hypochondriasis

The defining feature of Hypochondriasis is preoccupation with a belief or fear that the individual has a serious illness or disease when no actual physical problem exists. The belief is based on the patient's interpretations of physical signs and sensations as abnormal. It may involve one or a variety of body parts or functions. These individuals usually seek several doctors in an attempt to gain agreement about the existence of the problem (e.g., a woman believes she has bowel cancer and goes from doctor to doctor to substantiate her belief, which is not supported by medical and technologic exam results).

Somatization Disorder

The defining feature of Somatization Disorder is chronic recurrence of multiple physical complaints of many years' duration with no apparent physical explanation. Presentation of symptoms is frequently exaggerated, dramatic, vague, and very involved. The symptom list is extensive and involves various systems. For example, a client consistently describes a stabbing pain that occurs when she swallows, but all examinations are negative.

Pain Disorder

The defining feature of Pain Disorder is preoccupation with pain that cannot be accounted for through diagnostic evaluation, or, if there is related organic pathology, the complaints or dysfunctions are grossly excessive. Psychologic factors influence pain maintenance, severity, and recurrence.

FACTITIOUS DISORDERS

The defining features of factitious disorders are intentionally produced symptoms of psychologic or physical nature that the individual feigns for the purpose of assuming the "sick role." The person's behavior is voluntary but presumed to be out of his or her control (similar to repetitive compulsive disorder). For example, a hospital laboratory technician repeatedly injected himself with low doses of contaminated normal saline, became ill, and had to be hospitalized. He received much attention from coworkers and family for his "unusual fevers." These disorders are not to be confused with malingering, in which the person fakes symptoms but does so to control the environment, situation, or circumstance. Behavior is voluntary and fully within the control of the individual. For example, a client about to be transferred from the psychiatric unit of a hospital to the less favorable surroundings of a jail suddenly and intentionally develops an acute exacerbation of symptoms of a previously diagnosed mental disorder.

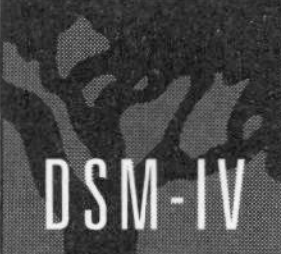

DSM-IV Dissociative Disorders

The essential characteristics of these disorders are disturbance of consciousness, memory, or identity. Onset may be sudden or gradual, and the alteration may be transient or chronic.

DSM-IV Categories

Dissociative Identity Disorder
Dissociative Fugue
Dissociative Amnesia
Depersonalization Disorder

DISSOCIATIVE DISORDERS

Dissociative Identity Disorder

Formerly named multiple personality disorder, the Dissociative Identity Disorder diagnosis reflects the lack of integration of an individual's consciousness, memory, and identity. The defining feature of this disorder is the occurrence of two or more separate and distinct personalities within one individual, with transition from one personality to another (several personalities may exist together). Each personality separately takes full control over the person's behavior. Transitions are usually sudden and occur around psychosocial stressors or conflicts, and the person may or may not have knowledge of all or part of the other personality(ies). Most cases may have been preceded by abuse (frequently sexual abuse) or other severe trauma. This disorder is no longer thought to be as rare as it once was.

Dissociative Fugue

The defining feature of Dissociative Fugue is that the individual suddenly and unexpectedly leaves the usual home or workplace, travels a distance, assumes a new identity, and is unable to recall the previous identity. When the person recovers there is no recollection of events leading to the fugue. The disturbance usually occurs at times of severe psychosocial stress; it is usually brief but may last several months.

Dissociative Amnesia

The defining feature of Dissociative Amnesia is sudden inability to recall information that exceeds mere forgetfulness. Types of amnesia include the following:

1. *Circumscribed or localized:* Most common; inability to recall events surrounding a specific traumatic or distressful event. *Example:* The survivor of a house fire cannot remember any of the details until several months later.
2. *Selected:* Inability to recall parts of a specific event. *Example:* The survivor remembers calling family and friends about the fire but cannot recall any content of the conversation.
3. *Generalized:* Complete inability to recall entire life.
4. *Continuous:* Inability to recall events from a specific time to the present.

Depersonalization Disorder

The defining feature of Depersonalization Disorder is depersonalization that is recurrent or persistent. Symptoms include the sense that one's reality is changed or lost and feelings of detachment from self as if "robotlike" or viewing self from the outside or in a dream. Reality testing remains intact.

PROGNOSIS

In general, the prognosis for most anxiety and related disorders is fair. Frequently the onset of the disorder is near the time of a traumatic event; therefore, if the individual seeks help soon after initial onset, the prognosis is often improved.

Somatization disorders tend to be chronic, and clients rarely go a year without seeking medical attention. Major depression may occur in several of the anxiety and related disorders.

One diagnosis more resistant to treatment is Obsessive-Compulsive Disorder. Approximately 20% to 40% of these individuals remain ill or have worsening of symptoms. Depressive symptoms occur in approximately one third of these clients, and they are at high risk for suicide.

For all anxiety disorders, good premorbid functioning, strong social supports, and the absence of other disorders influence more favorable prognoses.

INTERVENTIONS

Hospitalization

Hospitalization usually is not necessary for anxiety and related disorders in the absence of severe depression or suicidal risk. These individuals have intact reality-testing ability, and if symptoms become intolerable to them or to significant others, they usually seek treatment on an outpatient basis. Occasionally, obsessive rituals reach intolerable levels, and clients require hospitalization to help reduce external environmental stressors, provide a safe environment, and, in some cases, begin a medication regimen.

Pharmacotherapy

Antianxiety medications are often prescribed for persons who experience anxiety; they are among the most widely prescribed drugs. The major problems with antianxiety medications are increased tolerance and resultant overuse, abuse, and substance dependence. Antidepressants and beta-adrenergic antagonists have been successfully used for anxiety disorders. Medications are generally avoided in somatoform disorders unless anxiety or depression is present. Dissociative disorders usually do not require medication intervention unless direct treatment of anxiety is necessary. Clomipramine hydrochloride is sometimes dramatically helpful for some individuals in controlling compulsive rituals. Other antidepressants, particularly the serotonin selective reuptake inhibitors, have been useful in treating obsessive or compulsive symptoms and other anxiety disorders.

Cognitive and Behavior Therapies

Among the most successful interventions for anxiety disorders are the cognitive and behavior therapies. The behavior therapies (systematic desensitization, thought stopping, behavior substitution, reciprocal inhibition, flooding, aversive conditioning, and exposure-response prevention) have all been used to improve behaviors. Client commitment is essential for a successful outcome.

During cognitive therapies for anxiety, clients are assisted in refuting irrational ideas that trigger anxiety. These two therapies are frequently used in conjunction.

Psychotherapies

Insight-oriented therapy may be effective in treating some anxiety disorders, but it is not governed by symptoms alone. Assessment of the client's personality, life circumstances, events, and relationships is also necessary. Psychotherapy is usually refused by clients with somatoform disorders. Group therapies are effective, particularly for clients with posttraumatic stress disorder.

Family Therapy

Family therapy is used to reassure and support the family, help reduce environmental stressors, and educate family members about symptoms, interventions, and expected outcomes. (See Appendix K.)

DISCHARGE CRITERIA FOR ANXIETY AND RELATED DISORDERS

The client:

Identifies situations and events that trigger anxiety and ways to prevent or manage them

Identifies anxiety symptoms and levels of anxiety

Discusses connection between anxiety-provoking situation or event and anxiety symptoms

Discusses relief behaviors openly

Identifies adaptive, positive techniques and strategies that relieve anxiety

Demonstrates behaviors that represent reduced anxiety symptoms

Utilizes learned anxiety-reducing strategies

Demonstrates ability to problem solve, concentrate, and make decisions

Verbalizes feeling relaxed

Sleep through the night

Utilizes appropriate supports from nursing and medical community, family, and friends

Acknowledges inevitability of occurrence of anxiety

Discusses ability to tolerate manageable levels of anxiety

Seeks help when anxiety is not manageable

Continues postdischarge anxiety management, including medication and therapy

Nursing Process for

Anxiety and Related Disorders

Universal Principles for Interactions and Interventions with Clients Who Are Managing Anxiety

- Continue to monitor assessment parameters listed under *Defining Characteristics.*
- Continue to consider the etiologic factors listed under *Etiologic/Related Factors.*
- Use principles of the *Therapeutic Nurse-Client Relationship.* (See Appendix G.)
- Address clients' spiritual and cultural needs.

General Principles

- Recognize early stages of anxiety in clients to prevent escalation and loss of control. Immediate intervention is imperative.
- Recognize and monitor anxiety in the nurse to ensure effectiveness of therapeutic interventions.
- Assist clients to reduce anxiety by using techniques outlined in this chapter and in Appendix K.
- Teach clients strategies to reduce their anxiety.
- Help clients to identify sources of anxiety and connect the sources to relief behaviors.
- Identify coping mechanisms and techniques that are adaptive and maladaptive.
- Assist clients to learn new adaptive coping methods and skills.
- Help client to understand that mild anxiety is inevitable and that it can be tolerated through learned strategies.
- Discuss with clients the role of anxiety as a motivating force for productive behavior.
- Support and monitor the client's medical and psychosocial treatment plans.

Care Plans for Anxiety and Related Disorders

DSM-IV Diagnoses

Anxiety
Phobias (all types)
Obsessive-Compulsive Disorder
Posttraumatic Stress Disorder
Acute Stress Disorder
Somatoform Disorders (all types)
Dissociative Disorders (all types)

NANDA Diagnoses

Anxiety
Coping, ineffective individual
Social interaction, impaired
Post-trauma response
Coping, ineffective individual
Coping, ineffective individual
Violence, risk for: self-directed; violence, risk for: directed at others

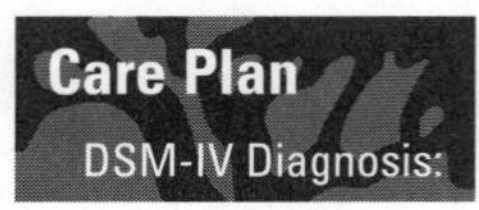

Anxiety (All Types)

Care Plan
DSM-IV Diagnosis:

NANDA Diagnosis: Anxiety

The state in which an individual experiences a vague uneasy feeling, the source of which is often nonspecific or unknown to the individual

Focus:
For the client who experiences mild, moderate, severe, or panic levels of anxiety that may impede growth potential or exceed the person's ability to cope in a functional manner

NANDA Taxonomy
Pattern 9—Feeling: A human response pattern involving the subjective awareness of information

ETIOLOGIC/RELATED FACTORS (RELATED TO)

Threat to biologic, psychologic, and/or social integrity (illness, injury, loss—actual or perceived)
Ineffective use of coping mechanisms/resources
Depletion of coping strategies
Level of stress that exceeds coping abilities
Hopelessness
Powerlessness
Unmet needs/expectations that may be unrealistic or unattainable
Response to long-term illness, hospitalization
Threat to self-esteem
Biologic/psychosocial/environmental factors

DEFINING CHARACTERISTICS (AS EVIDENCED BY)

Subjective (Refer to Table 2-1)

The client verbalizes:
- Trouble breathing
- Increased muscle tension
- Frequent sensation of tingling in hands and feet
- Continuous feeling of apprehension
- Preoccupation with a sense of impending doom
- Inability to identify source/stimulus responsible for emotional/feeling state
- Difficulty falling asleep
- Concerns about change in health status, outcome of illness and hospitalization
- Difficulty concentrating on the task at hand
- Gastrointestinal disturbances (decreased appetite, nausea, vomiting, diarrhea, dry mouth)
- Urinary symptoms (urgency, frequency, hesitancy)
- Narrowed range of perceptions (sight, hearing, pain)
- Selective inattention (removal of threatening stimuli from conscious awareness)
- Selective enhancement (concentrates on one or few details)
- Distortion of environment (objects seem out of proportion to reality)
- Need for increased space:
  - "Everything is closing in on me."
  - "I need to get out of here; I feel trapped."
  - "This room is like a closet."
- Dissociation (feelings of numbness, separateness, or distancing from the environment)

Objective (Refer to Table 2-1)

The client demonstrates:
- Psychomotor agitation (fidgeting, jitters, restlessness, shaking leg or foot, pacing back and forth)
- Tightened, wrinkled brow
- Strained (worried) facial expression
- Hypervigilance (scans environment)
- Startle response
- Distractibility
- Fragmented sleep patterns
- Sweaty palms
- Diaphoresis
- Hyperreflexia
- Tachypnea
- Tachycardia
- Regressive behaviors (crying, biting, curled up in fetal position)
- Voice change to loud, high pitch
- Rapid speech (may be unintelligible)
- Inability to move (frozen to spot) or attempts to flee from immediate area
- Wringing of hands
- Decreased cognitive skills (insight, judgment, problem solving)
- Maladaptive use of ego defense mechanisms (projection, displacement, denial)
- Avoidance behaviors (withdraws from milieu)
- Relief behaviors (pacing, wringing hands)

OUTCOME IDENTIFICATION AND EVALUATION

Expresses feeling calm, relaxed with absence of muscle tension and breathing problems
Demonstrates significant decrease in physiologic, cognitive, behavioral, and emotional symptoms of anxiety
Describes early warning signs of anxiety (increased irritability, gastrointestinal upset, increased heart rate)
Identifies levels of anxiety (mild, moderate, severe, panic)
Effectively employs learned relaxation techniques
Identifies anxiety-producing situations when possible
Utilizes functional coping strategies to assuage anxiety
Demonstrates decreased use of dysfunctional coping mechanisms
Demonstrates absence of avoidance behaviors (withdrawal from milieu, lack of contact with others)
Demonstrates absence of relief behaviors (pacing, wringing of hands)
Exhibits ability to make decisions and problem solve
Expresses hopeful, futuristic plans
Verbalizes control over illness, outcome, and management of care
Seeks support from family, friends, and therapists when necessary

Complies with treatment and medication regimen as needed
Conveys understanding of need to live with mild levels of anxiety
States importance of refraining from caffeine, nicotine, and other central nervous system stimulants

PLANNING AND IMPLEMENTATION

Nursing Interventions and Rationale

Recognize the client's use of relief behaviors (pacing, wringing of hands) as indicators of anxiety. *Early recognition of anxiety is critical to prevent escalation of symptoms and loss of control.*

Observe avoidance behaviors (withdrawal from milieu). *Withdrawal indicates that the milieu is stress-producing to a degree that exceeds the client's ability to cope.*

Assess your own level of anxiety and make a conscious effort to remain calm. *Anxiety is contagious and easily transferred from person to person.*

Approach the client calmly and help him or her to recognize the anxiety:

"Mr. Jones, I see you pacing back and forth. What are you feeling?"

Asking the client to describe the feeling helps the client to identify it as anxiety.

For the Client Who Is Unable to Describe the Feeling as Anxiety:

Assist the client to label the anxiety:

"Mr. Jones, are you feeling anxious?"

Specific labeling helps the client to isolate anxiety as a feeling that the client can begin to understand and manage.

For the Client with Mild to Moderate Levels of Anxiety:

Assist client to slow breathing rate and depth. Role-model as necessary. *Hyperventilation decreases* CO_2*, which increases anxiety.*

Help the client identify the event or situation that preceded the symptoms of anxiety:

"What happened just before you had these anxious feelings and began to pace the halls?"

This assists the client to connect the feeling of anxiety with a stimulus or stressor that may have provoked it.

Encourage the client to determine the level of anxiety according to client's perception (refer to Table 2-1). *The client's knowledge of his or her typical responses to anxiety-producing stimuli assists the client to begin to manage them.*

Inform the client that pacing releases the tension caused by anxiety. *The client is calmed by the knowledge that relief behaviors reduce anxiety and that the nurse understands and does not criticize or ridicule the behaviors.*

Walk with the client as you and the client discuss the anxiety. *The physical exercise of walking tends to reduce the tension associated with anxiety. A low-key discussion may calm the client by allowing ventilation. Remaining with the client is critical, because persons who are anxious feel out of control and the presence of a confident, therapeutic nurse offers control and safety.*

Help the client associate feelings of anxiety with possible unmet needs or expectations that may represent a threat to the self-system:

"So you're saying you expected to be discharged by 5 o'clock and it's 7 o'clock and you're feeling anxious."

The client's knowledge that unmet needs and expectations can precipitate anxiety may also bring relief.

Help the client recognize that desired outcomes may differ from actual outcomes, especially if the client does not consider all the facts:

"I know you hoped to be discharged by 5 o'clock, but the exact time of your discharge has not been established yet."

The client's understanding that expectations may not always be fulfilled and that occasionally it may be due to a misperception rather than punitive action may decrease the anxiety that often stems from anger, frustration, low self-esteem, and unmet needs.

Suggest to the client alternate steps that may achieve desired outcomes (if feasible):

"Let's telephone your doctor to find out if you can get a tentative discharge time."

Helping the client to meet needs when possible builds trust, acknowledges the client's worth, and reduces anxiety.

Assist the client to accept delayed need gratification while acknowledging his or her anxiety:

"I realize you are anxious about not going home when you planned, but it may be a few more days before you will be ready for discharge."

Offering the client factual information while recognizing feelings helps to promote trust and decreases the anxiety that generally accompanies uncertainty and disappointment.

Discuss with the client activities that may be initiated to help ease the tension until desired outcomes can be achieved:

"What kinds of activities will best help you pass the time until your doctor can give you a firm discharge date?"

Demonstrating that staff are willing to help ease the client's disappointment by problem solving with the client is in itself anxiety-reducing. Engaging in meaningful activities will redirect anxiety-producing energy and occupy the client so that less time will be spent on concerns about discharge.

Help the client bear the burden of anxiety that stems from unmet needs by pointing out alternative outcomes that can be realistically achieved:

"It's difficult for you to accept the fact that you will be living in a residential treatment center instead of your parents' home, but you can visit your parents every week as planned."

Softening disappointing facts with some positive information offers the client hope and decreases the impact of anxiety.

For the Client Whose Anxiety Escalates or Who Suddenly Experiences Severe to Panic Levels of Anxiety:

Accompany the client to a smaller, quieter area away from others, using direct, gentle reassurance:

"I'll go with you to a quieter place where we can talk if you like."

A quiet, stimulating environment with just the client and a reassuring nurse assists the client to gain control over anxiety that threatens to be overwhelming.

Remain with the client, continuing with a calm approach. *Persons who demonstrate high levels of anxiety tend to experience feelings of fright, dread, awe, or terror. The nurse's calm presence offers safety, support, and control at a time when the client's self-system is threatened and coping mechanisms are depleted. A client who is left alone during such times may experience serious physical or psychologic complications.*

Reduce all environmental stimulation (noise from radio or television, bright lights, people moving and talking). *Increased stimulation tends to increase anxiety; decreased stimulation tends to decrease anxiety.*

Consider administration of prescribed anxiolytic or other appropriate medication as needed. *Medication may be the most therapeutic and least restrictive measure to decrease severe or panic levels of anxiety.*

Consider seclusion and/or restraint for clients who may be a danger to self or others as a result of high anxiety. (See Appendix L.) *Seclusion and restraint may be the method of choice for the client's and others' immediate safety if all other interventions fail.*

For the Client Who Is Able to Focus and Discuss the Experience of Anxiety and Problem Solve Strategies to Prevent or Reduce It:

Actively listen to and accept the client's concerns regarding subjective feelings of anxiety and the threat it poses to that patient's self-system. *Active listening and unconditional acceptance of the client's experience of anxiety convey respect, validate the client's self-worth, assure the client that concerns will be addressed, and provide an avenue for ventilation, all of which reduce anxiety.*

Assist the client to build on previously successful coping methods to manage anxiety symptoms, illness, and treatment and to integrate them with newly learned strategies. Sample statements:

"What methods have helped you get through difficult times like this in the past?"

"How can we help you to use those methods now?"

"Let's discuss some new alternative strategies that may fit into your particular situation."

Use of previously successful coping methods in conjunction with newly learned techniques equips the client with multiple skills to manage anxiety.

Help the client identify support persons who can help the client take care of personal and/or business details while the client is hospitalized. *Significant supportive individuals can help to reduce the client's anxiety by reassuring the client that matters of concern will be attended to in a safe, reliable manner.*

Inform the client frequently of status and progress made during hospitalization:

"You were able to sit calmly through the meeting today, Bob."

Clients who are well informed of their condition are better able to control illness, outcome, and treatment regimen, which tends to reduce anxiety generated from helplessness and loss of control.

Encourage the client to use coping mechanisms such as **suppression and displacement** to manage anxiety effectively when the client is unable to do so through more direct methods.

Suppression:

"It's perfectly OK to think about those things at a time when you feel less anxious."

"Let's talk about a less-troubling topic for a while; we can discuss this subject later."

Displacement:

"Some exercise or activity may help you feel more relaxed."

"Perhaps a game of Ping-Pong will help expend your energy."

When client is not ready to face troubling issues, use of adaptive coping mechanisms may successfully assuage anxiety that cannot be averted through confronting techniques.

Instruct the client in the following anxiety-reducing strategies (individualize according to the client's preference and ability):

- Progressive relaxation (tense and relax all muscles progressively from toes to head)
  Progressive relaxation relieves stress-related muscular tension and reduces the physiologic effects of anxiety.
- Slow, deep-breathing exercises
  Breathing exercises provide slow, rhythmic, controlled breathing patterns that relax and distract the client while slowing the heart rate, thus decreasing feelings of anxiety.
- Focusing on a single object or person in the room
  Focusing on one object or person helps the client to disengage from all other visual stimuli and promotes control and relaxation.
- Listening to soothing music or relaxation tapes (clients may prefer to close eyes)
  Soothing music or tapes reduce anxiety by providing relaxing effects and an overall tranquil environment.
- Visual imagery (visualization of an image that evokes a soothing, peaceful sensation such as an ocean, a waterfall, or a field of flowers)
  Visual imagery provides the client with a mental representation that inhibits anxiety by invoking an opposing, peaceful image.

  Note: Visual imagery employs the concept of reciprocal inhibition, a behavioral approach used for clients with phobic disorder who experience panic when exposed to a feared object or situation. With this method, anxiety-producing stimuli are paired with stimuli associated with an opposite feeling strong enough to diminish the anxiety. Other behavioral techniques such as systematic desensitization, flooding, aversive methods, hypnosis, biofeedback, and yoga are also used to treat anxiety and related disorders. (See Appendix K for additional description of psychiatric therapies.)

Provide simple clarification of environmental events or stimuli that are not related to the client's illness and management of care but may still elicit anxiety. Sample statements:

"The nurse is preparing medication for another client."

"That client is concerned because visitors are late."

"Staff are not upset with you; they're busy giving report."

Clarification of events or stimuli that are unrelated to the client helps the client to disengage from external anxiety-provoking situations; thus apprehension and anxiety are decreased.

Teach the client to distinguish between anxiety that can be connected to identifiable objects or sources (illness, prognosis, hospitalization) and anxiety for which there is no immediate identifiable object or source:

"The shortness of breath you're experiencing is not unusual during times of anxiety."

"Frequently it is difficult to determine exact causes of anxious symptoms."

"It's OK to feel upset when people you expect don't visit you."

"It's understandable to feel anxious about being in a hospital with people you hardly know."

A client who is informed and reassured about expected symptoms of anxiety emanating from a recognizable stressor is better able to control anxiety and maintain a realistic perspective of illness, prognosis, and hospitalization. Awareness that anxiety cannot always be traced to a specific source or object reduces the threat of anxiety and allows the client to concentrate on anxiety-reducing strategies.

Inform the client of the importance of abstaining from caffeine, nicotine, and other central nervous system stimulants *to reduce anxiety.*

Teach the client to tolerate mild levels of anxiety and to channel anxiety toward constructive behaviors and activities. *Anxiety is an integral part of human existence that can be accepted and tolerated in its mild to moderate states and may be used to motivate productive, satisfying behaviors.*

Continue to support and monitor prescribed medical and psychosocial treatment plans *to prevent escalating symptoms and subsequent anxiety.*

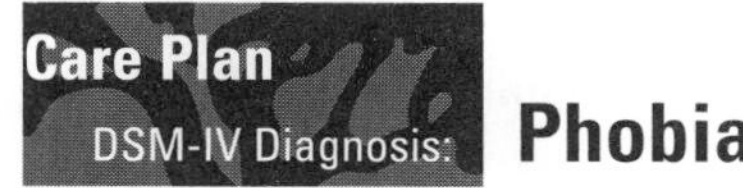

Phobia

NANDA Diagnosis: Coping, ineffective individual

The state in which an individual demonstrates impaired adaptive behaviors and problem-solving abilities in meeting life's demands and roles

Focus:
For the client with a persistent, irrational, or excessive fear* of a specific object, situation, or event, which may induce a panic anxiety state when the client is exposed to such stimuli. The client may fear being harmed or out of control, and resultant avoidant behaviors often interfere with personal growth, adaptive coping, and social and occupational functioning

NANDA Taxonomy
Pattern 5—Choosing: A human response pattern involving the selection of alternatives

ETIOLOGIC/RELATED FACTORS (RELATED TO)

Phobic response (see Table 2-1)
Fear of subsequent phobic response (anticipatory state)
Life-style of avoidant behaviors secondary to fear of phobic stimulus
Perceived threat of feared object, situation, or event
Powerlessness secondary to phobic disorder
Knowledge deficit regarding adaptive methods of coping
Depletion of adaptive coping mechanisms/strategies
Unidentified conflicts/stressors
Biologic/psychologic/environmental factors

DEFINING CHARACTERISTICS (AS EVIDENCED BY)

Persistently avoids such things as other clients, eating in the dining room, and group activities or outings
Continuously avoids public places such as shopping malls, movie theaters, restaurants, bathrooms, open spaces
Refuses to use elevators or to be enclosed in small areas
Demonstrates increased anxiety or panic symptoms when exposed to specific feared object or situation (e.g., animals, heights, freeways, restaurants) (see Table 2-1)
Verbalizes dread of eating in public places for fear of uncontrolled episodes of choking, urination, defecation, or other such embarrassing occurrences
Expresses excessive fear of speaking in public or of giving a prepared speech
Remains housebound for an excessive length of time (months or years)
States fear of being out of control when outside an enclosed building or house
Repeatedly avoids driving on busy freeways, even when late for work or appointments

*Psychoanalytic theory differentiates fear from anxiety in that fear emanates from a known source and anxiety evolves from an unknown, unresolved conflict.

Enlists family or friends to run errands such as grocery shopping and transporting children to school, appointments, and activities

Verbalizes inability to meet the demands of everyday life

"I need my prescription, but I can't cope with the crowds in the drugstore."

"My kids missed their bus and I'm afraid to drive them to school."

"I can't go to Jane's house; she has cats."

"I can't accept that job; it means I'll have to use the elevator every day."

"I won't go on the client outing; there are bugs and animals in the woods."

"I can't attend group; I could get germs or others will laugh at me."

"I won't eat in the dining room; I might choke or wet my pants."

"I'm afraid to go to sleep tonight; I might die."

OUTCOME IDENTIFICATION AND EVALUATION

Verbalizes significant decrease in phobic response during progressive exposure to feared objects, events, or situations (decreased physiologic and emotional symptoms of severe to panic anxiety states)

Demonstrates significant reduction in avoidance behaviors when threatened with exposure to feared stimuli (remains in dining room despite fear of crowds and/or eating in public, remains in area with small pets, refrains from going to room during visiting hours or other peak times)

Tolerates feared objects, events, or situations commensurate with level of progress (attends outings, visits shopping malls, eats in the dining room or public restaurants, verbalizes in groups, confronts small animals)

Relates increase in understanding of phobic disorder and behaviors needed to manage phobic response

Limits intake of caffeine, nicotine, and other central nervous system stimulants that produce physiologic symptoms of anxiety

Participates actively in prescribed treatment plan and learned therapeutic strategies to reduce phobic responses (deep breathing, relaxation exercises, visual imagery, reframing, desensitization) (See Appendix M.)

PLANNING AND IMPLEMENTATION

Nursing Interventions and Rationale

The nurse must be aware of own level of anxiety (see Table 2-1) and use appropriate strategies (deep breathing, relaxation, cognitive techniques, etc.) to decrease anxiety to a tolerable level prior to approaching client. *Anxiety is readily transferred from person to person.*

Approach the client in a calm, direct, nonauthoritarian manner using soft voice tone. *A calm, direct approach helps the client gain control, decreases apprehension and anxiety, and fosters security. A nonauthoritarian manner decreases powerlessness.*

In early stages of the relationship, to establish trust:

Listen actively to the client's fears and concerns no matter how irrational they may seem. *Active listening signifies unconditional respect and acceptance for the client as a worthwhile individual. It builds trust and rapport, guides the nurse toward problem areas, encourages the client to vent concerns without fear of ridicule or reproach, and sets the stage for management of phobic responses.*

Acknowledge the client's feelings, concerns, and limitations in a simple, matter-of-fact manner:

"It sounds as if you're frustrated with your responses."

"It is difficult to avoid certain situations and objects."

"It's OK right now to do only those things you *can* handle."

Acknowledgment of the client's feelings and concerns regarding the limitations induced by the phobic disorder illustrates that staff understands and will be supportive.

Refrain from exposing the client to identified feared object or situation (e.g., if the client adamantly refuses to attend an outing with the rest of the clients for fear of exposure to small animals, snakes, or bugs, it is best not to insist that the client comply at this time; if the client is afraid to eat in the dining room with others, allow him or her to eat in an uncrowded area). *Exposure to feared stimuli without adaptive coping strategies could escalate the client's anxiety to a panic state. Forced compliance increases powerlessness and loss of control and decreases the client's trust in staff and treatment regimen.*

Schedule an alternative, less-threatening activity for the client while the group attends the outing, such as chess, checkers, or occupational or recreational activities. *Participation in milieu activities increases the client's confidence, self-esteem, and control.*

Inform the client that staff understands that refusal to attend the group outing is not attributable to resistance to treatment but rather to the phobic disorder for which the client is seeking management. *Acknowledgment of the client's diagnosis minimizes a sense of failure and conveys hope.*

When the nurse assesses that the client is able to discuss phobic responses without experiencing incapacitating anxiety:

Assist the client to describe physiologic responses to identified feared objects, situations, or events (see Table 2-1). *Teaching the client to identify autonomic nervous system responses to anxiety in the early stages helps the client to acknowledge the feelings rather than to deny or avoid them. This sets the stage for symptom management.*

Assist the client to identify factors that increase or decrease phobic responses, such as size of object (small or large bug or animal), texture of object (perceived "sliminess" of a snake, furry or hairy bugs or animals), and movement (wiggling worms, crawling spiders, flying bugs or birds). *Helping the client to differentiate between most and least feared objects gives the client some control and decreases feelings of powerlessness. It also sets the stage for therapeutic strategies such as desensitization techniques. (See Appendix K.)*

Assist the client to determine other factors associated with feared stimuli that may precipitate a phobic response:

"What else bothers you about this situation?"

"You were able to eat with the group yesterday. What is different about today?"

The client's recognition that factors such as increased noise or fatigue may contribute to his or her vulnerability may encourage the client to modify those situations or elements that can be controlled.

Teach the client about the effects of caffeine, nicotine, and other central nervous system stimulants. *Caffeine and nicotine stimulate the central nervous system to produce physiologic effects of anxiety (increased heart rate, jitteriness, etc.).*

Explore with the client previously successful coping methods:

"What methods have helped you handle your reactions in the past, and how can we help you use those methods now?"

Use of previously successful coping strategies, in conjunction with newly learned skills, better prepares the client to deal with the anxiety of the phobic disorder and promotes more control over the feared situation, object, or event.

Discuss with the client why usual coping methods no longer seem to work. (Perhaps usual support systems, persons, or situations are no longer available, new stressors have emerged, or the client can no longer avoid feared stimuli.) *Identification of possible reasons why usual coping methods have failed is the first step toward helping the client manage the phobic response.*

Help the client identify alternative adaptive coping techniques to manage the anxiety that emanates from excessive or irrational fears rather than use avoidance behaviors. *The client may need help in activating adaptive coping strategies because energy and motivation are depleted in times of anxiety. (See Appendix K for the following therapies: relaxation exercises, deep breathing, visual imagery, and cognitive techniques.)*

Practice with the client alternative adaptive coping strategies commensurate with the client's lifestyle and capabilities. *Role playing useful therapeutic techniques when the client is in a calm state enables the client to more readily activate such strategies in times of anxiety.*

For the Client Who Is Able to Use Cognitive-Perceptual Skills:

Utilize relabeling or reframing techniques to change the client's perceptions of feared objects, situations, or events:

Client: "I feel so nervous when I think about going into that crowded activity room."

Nurse: "When you feel that way, relabel the word 'nervous' with a less-threatening word like 'excited' and note the change in symptoms."

Reframing or relabeling volatile words with less-threatening terms helps the client place thoughts and feelings in a different perspective and tends to decrease anxiety. (Refer to Appendix K for reframing/relabeling techniques.)

Teach the client to combine reframing techniques with another learned strategy when necessary:

Client: "I feel so anxious and begin to breathe very fast whenever I go off the unit to a store or on a pass."

Nurse: "When you get that feeling, relabel the word 'anxious' with 'overactive' and begin the deep-breathing exercises we practiced."

Combining a newly learned skill with a previously learned strategy provides the client with more than one technique to cope adaptively with anxiety, each strategy reinforcing the other.

Teach the client thought substitution and behavioral substitution strategies:

Client: "I'm afraid to go for a walk; a snake might crawl out of the bushes."

Nurse: "When you think about snakes crawling out of the bushes, focus your thoughts on the bush, on the color of the foliage or flowers on the bush. Then, use your learned relaxation technique."

Replacing the fearful thought or image with a pleasant one and performing concomitant relaxation techniques tends to diminish anxiety. (Refer to Appendix K for thought and behavioral substitution therapies.)

For the Client Who Has Successfully Practiced the Preceding Strategies:

Assist the client to confront the feared object under safe conditions, if the client is willing and able:

Client: "I'd like to go to Jane's party, but when I'm in her house I'm preoccupied with avoiding her cat and I can't enjoy myself."

Nurse: "It sounds like you're using a lot of energy with your concern about the cat. Would you be willing to locate the cat as soon as you enter Jane's house and perhaps even stroke it once?"

Confronting the feared object in a familiar setting diminishes the phobic response and the anticipatory anxiety that precedes it. (Refer to Appendix K for desensitization technique.)

Expose the client progressively to feared stimuli. Example for the client who fears dining with crowds:

The nurse can initially dine alone with client; then, one or two familiar persons may be added. Next, the client can progress to a secluded or quiet area of the dining room. Finally, the client can sit in a more populated area of the dining room with significant reduction in phobic responses.

For the Client Who Refuses to Go on Outings Because of a Fear of Small Animals:

The nurse can go with the client on a short group outing where small animals will be seen and stay with the client throughout. Next, take the client on a longer outing, leaving him or her with familiar persons. Continue exposing the client to longer outings with more frequency until the client can tolerate exposure to small animals with a significant reduction in phobic responses.

Clients who are gradually and serially exposed to anxiety-provoking situations (predetermined by the client's treatment planning team) and graded from least to most anxiety-provoking are eventually desensitized to the feared stimulus. (Refer to Appendix K for desensitization technique.)

Offer positive reinforcement whenever the client demonstrates a decrease in avoidance behaviors or an increase in socialization skills and other milieu activities:

"It showed strength to stay in the dining room, John."

"It was a sign of real progress to stroke the cat, Sara."

"Attending the group outing was a fine effort, Sam."

Positive statements convey confidence and hope and reinforce the client's adaptive coping skills.

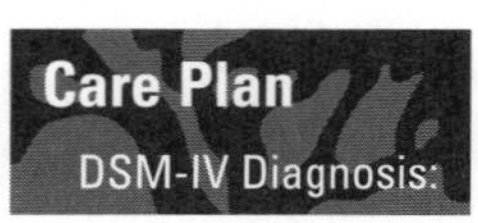

Obsessive-Compulsive Disorder

NANDA Diagnosis: Social interaction, impaired

The state in which an individual participates in an insufficient or excess quantity or ineffective quality of social exchange

Focus:

For the client with *obsessions* (thoughts, images, impulses), involuntarily produced, persistent, and recurring, that invade consciousness and are generally perceived as intrusive, repetitive, senseless, and anxiety-producing AND *compulsions* (repetitive, seemingly purposeful actions or behaviors) performed in a stereotypical, ritualistic fashion in an attempt to ignore, suppress, negate, or neutralize anxiety. Obsessive-compulsive behaviors occur together and inhibit the client's interpersonal social interactions and relationships.

NANDA Taxonomy

Pattern 3—Relating: A human response pattern involving established bonds

ETIOLOGIC/RELATED FACTORS (RELATED TO)

Overwhelming anxiety (exceeds ability to cope adaptively)

Altered thought processes (intrusive and recurrent)

Inability to control thoughts, images, or impulses in a purposeful, voluntary manner

Repetitive, ritualistic behavior patterns that interfere with social interactions

Ambivalence, indecisiveness

Inflexible thought and behavior patterns

Guilt, shame, or doubt

Depletion of effective coping mechanisms/strategies

Knowledge deficit regarding adaptive measures to manage anxiety

Impaired judgment and insight

Perceptual/cognitive impairment

Unidentified early life conflicts/stressors

Unresolved/misdirected anger

Powerlessness

Decreased psychologic and physical energy/endurance secondary to obsessive-compulsive behaviors

Biologic/psychologic/environmental factors

DEFINING CHARACTERISTICS (AS EVIDENCED BY)

Verbalizes irrational, recurrent thoughts of violence, contamination, or doubt:

"I keep thinking and worrying that I'm going to kill my baby."

"I can't even go into my best friend's bathroom; I'm afraid the toilet is contaminated."

"After I stop driving, I constantly worry that I've caused an accident."

Expresses awareness that thoughts, images, or impulses are alien to self-perception and self-concept.

"I know my thoughts are foolish and absurd and have nothing to do with my life."

States inability to prevent intrusion of repetitive thoughts, images, or impulses:

"I can't stop these thoughts from occurring and I can't stop them once they begin."

Demonstrates repetitive, stereotypical rituals (compulsive acts) in response to anxiety produced by the obsessions that may or may not be related to the obsessions (e.g., cleans room several times a day; checks doors and windows throughout the night; dresses and undresses many times during the day and evening; washes hands continuously until skin is red, cracked, or bleeding).

Repeats same story or belief automatically, generally related to doubt, violence, or contamination:

"I know it's foolish, but I keep thinking I won't wake up tomorrow."

"I continually think about making love to our parish priest."

"I never go to the movies because the theater is full of germs."

Demonstrates difficulty completing routine activities of daily life. (Much of client's time is spent in compulsive ritualistic behaviors.)

Reports diminished satisfactory interpersonal relationships.

OUTCOME IDENTIFICATION AND EVALUATION

Verbalizes understanding that thoughts, impulses, or images are involuntary and may worsen with stress

Expresses understanding that involuntary, automatic obsessions may be related to biochemical factors and/or repressed conflicts

Relates knowledge that ritualistic behaviors may be an attempt to decrease the anxiety produced by the obsessions

Verbalizes awareness that early conflicts may remain repressed, but obsessions and compulsions can be reduced or eliminated by more adaptive management of anxiety and stress.

Participates actively in learned therapeutic strategies to manage anxiety and decrease obsessive-compulsive behaviors

States significant reduction in obsessive thoughts, images, or impulses

Verbalizes reduction of intrusive, involuntary thoughts

Demonstrates significant reduction in compulsive ritualistic acts and behaviors (e.g., pacing, cleaning, checking, hand washing)

Demonstrates absence of suicidal ideation, gestures, or attempts

Verbalizes significant increase in control over involuntary thoughts and repetitive behaviors

Uses majority of time to complete basic tasks and activities of daily life (e.g., nutrition, hygiene, grooming, socialization, occupation)

Participates in milieu activities without being interrupted by compulsive acts and rituals

Continues to participate in planned psychosocial and medical treatment regimens

PLANNING AND IMPLEMENTATION

Nursing Interventions and Rationale

The nurse must be aware of own level of anxiety (see Table 2-1) and use appropriate strategies (deep breathing, relaxation exercises, cognitive techniques, etc.) to decrease it to a tolerable level prior to approaching the client. *Anxiety is readily transferred from person to person.* (See Appendix K.)

Approach the client in a calm, direct, nonauthoritarian manner, using soft voice tone. *A calm, direct approach decreases anxiety and allows the client to regain some control. A nonauthoritarian manner decreases powerlessness and agitation. These clients are generally proud and knowledgeable, and an autocratic approach may be demeaning.*

Actively listen to the client's obsessive themes no matter how absurd or incongruent they seem, without focusing too intently on the rituals. *Active listening signifies respect for the client as a worthwhile person and helps the nurse elicit the client's feelings and intent (violence, guilt, powerlessness, ambivalence) in order to individualize care. The less focus placed on the rituals, the less anxiety will occur, with a possible decreased need for the compulsive act.*

Acknowledge the effects that automatic thoughts and ritualistic acts have on the client by demonstrating empathy rather than disapproval.

Therapeutic responses:

"I know these thoughts and behaviors are troubling; staff notices that they are difficult to control."

"I saw you undress several times today; that must be tiring for you."

"I realize that thoughts of death are very troubling. Staff will be available when you want to talk to us about it."

Reflecting the client's feelings in an empathetic manner reduces the intensity of the ritualistic behavior and promotes trust and rapport that encourage compliance with the treatment plan.

Nontherapeutic responses:

"I know these thoughts and behaviors are annoying. They bother me too."

"Try to dress only once a day and you won't be so tired."

Intimating that the client's behaviors are annoying or bothersome to others gives the client a sense of disapproval by staff that may inhibit trust and rapport, increase anxiety, and promote dysfunctional behaviors. Client may become more resistant to the treatment plan.

Assist the client to gain control of overwhelming feelings and impulses through verbal interactions.

Example:

Nurse to client who is pacing the hall and wringing hands with a worried facial expression just prior to an activity:

"You seem upset about going to the activity; let's walk together and you can tell me what's troubling you."

Anxiety is relieved by expressing thoughts and feelings, being understood by another person, and actively walking and talking. The client therefore feels more in control. Concerned staff builds trust and rapport.

For the Client Who May Be a Danger To Self or Others:

Assess the client for suicidal or self-destructive thoughts or impulses regularly. *Clients with obsessive-compulsive disorder may be at risk for suicide.* (Refer to care plans in Chapter 3 for suicide intervention.)

Protect the client who is at risk for suicide or self-destructive acts *to prevent harm, injury, or death to the client.* (See Appendix J.)

Assess the client for homicidal ideation or impulses. *Clients with obsessive-compulsive disorder may harbor violent thoughts toward others.*

Protect others in the environment from a client who is potentially violent *to prevent harm, injury, or death to others.*

Protect the client as much as possible from the curiosity of other clients or visitors. *The client may feel embarrassed or undignified if others seem offended or amused by the compulsive acts. All clients deserve as much privacy as possible when their behavior is out of control.*

For the Client with Excessive Ritualistic Hand-Washing Behaviors that Threaten Skin Integrity and Quality of Life:

Interact verbally with the client to encourage protection of skin until rituals can be better managed via learned strategies:

"I notice that your hands are becoming raw from too many hand washings. There are several things you can do to protect them: apply petroleum jelly to your hands before washing them; apply hand lotion to your hands after washing them; begin to wash your hands once every 15 minutes instead of once very 5 minutes; begin to wash your hands for 10 seconds instead of 30 seconds. Staff will remind you."

Protects the client from pain or damage to skin integrity, while giving the client the opportunity to reduce ritualistic behaviors. The nurse can also assess the client's ability to use problem-solving methods to control the compulsive acts, which can be used as a guide in treatment planning.

For the Client Whose Excessive Rituals Promote Activity Intolerance:

Assist the client in planning rest periods between planned activities and rituals. Rest periods may become progressively longer as the client learns strategies that reduce anxiety and decrease ritualistic behaviors *to conserve energy and strength for leisure activities and activities of daily living (hygiene, grooming, socializing).*

For the Client Who Is in the Midst of a Ritualistic Act:

Allow the client to complete the ritualistic act initially, knowing that it emanates from the anxiety produced by the troubling, automatic thoughts, images, or impulses (unless it poses a threat or danger to the client or others). *The client may not yet possess adaptive means to reduce anxiety, as obsessions are initially beyond his or her control. Anxiety may escalate to a panic state if rituals are abruptly interrupted.*

Assess the client's ability to control the compulsive act, the level of intensity during the rituals, the frequency and duration of the behaviors, and the stage of the client's involvement in the treatment regimen. (Is the client newly admitted? Has trust been established? Which strategies have been taught, if any? Is medication also needed to decrease anxiety?) *The level of the client's progress is a critical factor in determining and structuring psychosocial interventions. A client who is forced to control compulsive acts when anxiety exceeds his or her ability to focus on strategies or a client who has not yet mastered strategies may fail and become discouraged.*

For the Client with Whom Trust Has Been Established:

Work with the client to manipulate the schedule to satisfy both the client's and the facility's routines.

"You have been missing breakfast every morning because it takes an hour to clean your room and get dressed. What do you think about getting up at 6 o'clock instead of 7 o'clock so you can make it to breakfast?"

Setting up directives for the client in a collaborative manner provides the structure and relief the client needs when impulses and functions are out of control. A nonauthoritarian approach preserves the client's dignity. Obsessive-compulsive clients are generally proud, knowledgeable, overly perfectionistic individuals who may feel anger, shame, or guilt if they are reprimanded.

For the Client Who Is Ready and Able to Focus on Strategies:

Suggest activities that will reduce stress or anxiety (e.g., a warm bath, listening to music, taking a walk, performing simple exercises). *Simple, familiar activities can have a calming effect on the client and also interrupt obsessive themes and ritualistic behaviors.*

Assist the client to learn stress-reduction strategies, e.g., deep breathing, relaxation exercises, visual imagery, cognitive techniques, and behavior modification. (See Appendix K.) *Stress-management strategies reduce and channel anxiety in an adaptive, functional manner. They also interrupt automatic thoughts and substitute for ritualistic acts.*

Engage the client in constructive activities when able, e.g., quiet games (chess, checkers, dominoes) and arts and crafts (needlepoint, ceramics, painting, leatherwork). *Planned activities offer the client less time for obsessive thoughts and compulsive behaviors and help the client to focus on adaptive and creative endeavors that offer positive feedback.*

For the Client Who Is Able to Tolerate Limit Setting:

Help the client, for example, to schedule activities at least 1 hour apart to provide a reasonable, but not excessive, amount of time for ritualistic behaviors. *Planned activities offer the client structure and meaning and substitute for ritualistic behaviors. At the same time, the client's anxiety could escalate to a panic state if initially there was not sufficient time for compulsive acts.*

Allow the client eventually to choose the amount and frequency of time needed for ritualistic behaviors, while encouraging the client to perform anxiety-reducing strategies when necessary. *This provides the client with some control over the obsessive-compulsive sequence, supported by learned therapeutic techniques.*

Offer praise and positive reinforcement (e.g., your time, attention, interactions) when the client engages in meaningful activities or attempts to manage ritualistic behaviors through learned strategies *to increase the client's self-esteem and promote continued adaptive behaviors. A behavioral therapy called Exposure and Response Prevention may be effective in reducing anxiety and decreasing obsessive and ritualistic behaviors.* (See Appendix K.)

For the Client Who Is Receptive to Learning about the Disorder:

Teach the client and family about the obsessive-compulsive disorder (the meaning and purpose of the behaviors) in accordance with the treatment plan, their level of understanding, and their readiness to learn. One theory states that a biochemical disruption in the brain has a role in this disorder; another theory states that early conflicts and/or life stressors may have some influence; these troubling behaviors may be the body's way of managing anxiety that comes from the intrusive thoughts. Often a combination of medication and stress-reducing strategies can decrease anxiety, which in turn may reduce the troubling thoughts and behaviors. *Information and knowledge help to uncover the mystery that generally surrounds mental health disorders and decreases the client's powerlessness, while increasing hope for successful symptom management.*

For the Client and Family Who Are Preparing for Discharge:

Summarize with the client and family the meaning and purpose of the behaviors (that they occur to reduce the anxiety that stems from the troubling, automatic thoughts, impulses, and images), the feelings that emerge when the behaviors occur (guilt, shame, anger), and the identifiable stressors that may precipitate the rituals (loss of job, status, persons, finances). *Reinforcing learned knowledge prior to discharge gives the client control over the disorder and the confidence to manage it.*

Review with the client the learned behavioral and cognitive strategies that are used to manage anxiety and reduce the symptoms of the disorder. *Reviewing therapeutic strategies prior to discharge reminds the client that there are successful methods to manage anxiety and reduce obsessive-compulsive behaviors. The client will then approach discharge with confidence and hope.*

Teach the client's family and close friends (with the client's permission) about obsessive-compulsive disorder and how they can assist the client to manage anxiety and ritualistic acts. *Significant others add support and understanding and are critical adjuncts to the success of the client's overall treatment plan.*

Support and monitor the client's prescribed psychosocial and medical treatment plans.

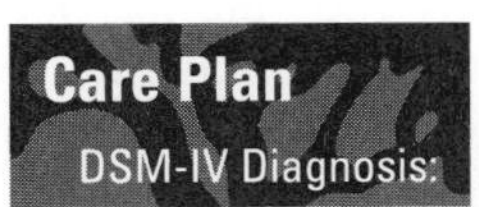

Posttraumatic Stress Disorder and Acute Stress Disorder

NANDA Diagnosis: Post-trauma response

The state in which an individual experiences a sustained painful response to an unexpected extraordinary life event(s)

Focus:

For the client who develops fear, terror, dread, or helplessness following exposure to a traumatic event (e.g., rape, war, natural disaster, abuse, experiencing or witnessing serious trauma or violence). Symptoms range from emotional "numbness" to vivid nightmares in which the traumatic event is recalled.

NANDA Taxonomy

Pattern 9—Feeling: A human response pattern involving the subjective awareness of information

ETIOLOGIC/RELATED FACTORS (RELATED TO)

Overwhelming anxiety secondary to:

War experiences/military combat

Natural disasters (earthquake, hurricane, tornado, flood)

Personal assaults (rape, incest, molestation, beatings, abuse)

Kidnap of self or significant others

Catastrophic illness or accident

Prisoner of war, death camp, or hostage experiences

Learning of a loved one's serious accident, injury, or maiming

Destruction of home or valued resources

Witnessing a serious accident or act(s) of violence (e.g., car crash, building collapse, mother being beaten, killing of family member)

Viewing a scene in which there are dead and/or maimed bodies (e.g., the aftermath of war, plane or train crash, earthquake)

Threat to physical and emotional integrity (all of the above)

DEFINING CHARACTERISTICS (AS EVIDENCED BY)

Relates frequent intrusive recollections of past traumatic experience

States that recollections are accompanied by feelings of dread, terror, helplessness, powerlessness, cardiac palpitations, shortness of breath, and other symptoms of emotional physical reactivity: "I feel out of control and terrified when I recall the event; I get out of breath and my heart beats faster and faster; I have a sense of doom, as if something terrible is going to happen." (See Table 2-1.)

Describes recurrent dreams or nightmares in which vivid details of traumatic event are relived or reenacted: "I had another horrible nightmare last night and went through the same trauma and anxiety all over again."

Expresses feelings of "numbness," detachment, or loss of interest toward people and the environment (generally occurs immediately after the traumatic event)

Demonstrates avoidance or lack of responsiveness toward stimuli associated with the traumatic event (in rare instances, may experience psychogenic amnesia)

- A war veteran may avoid hospitals, injured persons, bandages, blood
- An accident victim may demonstrate flat affect while listening to a news report describing a traumatic event

Demonstrates symptoms of physiologic reactivity (anxiety symptoms) when exposed to events that resemble or symbolize the original trauma

- A young woman develops fear, dread, terror when she attempts sexual intimacy with her partner because it reminds her of the time she was raped
- A prison camp victim experiences sympathetic nervous system stimulation (e.g., rapid heart rate, shortness of breath, nausea, diarrhea) while sitting in a cell-sized room

- A war veteran who fought in a hot, humid climate experiences dread and terror when exposed to similar weather many years later

Demonstrates symptoms of increased arousal, e.g., inability to fall asleep or remain asleep, hypervigilance, exaggerated startle response

Manifests unpredictable episodes of explosive anger or aggression

Verbalizes inability to concentrate or complete tasks: "I'm too distracted to make my bed or go to an activity; I can't concentrate on my crafts; I can barely shower and groom myself."

Relates inability to express angry feelings: "I feel as if I might explode, but I can't let it out; I can't begin to express my anger."

Expresses thoughts of self-blame and guilt regarding a traumatic event: "If only I had locked the door, it wouldn't have happened; if I had been there on time, it wouldn't have happened."

Verbalizes anger at others for perceived role in traumatic event: "If they had helped more, he would have lived; if they had called for help right away, I wouldn't be so badly injured."

OUTCOME IDENTIFICATION AND EVALUATION

Verbalizes awareness of psychologic and physiologic symptoms of anxiety that accompany recollections of a past traumatic event

Identifies situations/events/images that trigger recollections and accompanying responses of a past traumatic experience (e.g., small or enclosed spaces, hot or cold climate, arguments or fights, sexual intimacy)

Communicates and interacts within the milieu to control and manage anger and relieve thoughts of self-blame and guilt

- Communicates thoughts/feelings to a trusted person
- Problem solves source of thoughts/feelings
- Participates in group activities
- Engages in physical activities/exercise
- Attends process groups (see Appendix K) for group therapy

Utilizes learned adaptive cognitive and behavioral therapeutic strategies to manage symptoms of emotional and physical reactivity

- Slow, deep breathing techniques
- Progressive relaxation exercises
- Thought, image, and memory substitution
- Cognitive restructuring
- Systematic desensitization
- Behavior modification
- Assertive behaviors (See Appendix K for assertiveness training.)

Relates understanding that anger, self-blame, and guilt are common in persons who have experienced or witnessed traumatic events in which others were injured, assaulted, or threatened: "I realize others who have gone through this have had similar reactions."

Verbalizes ability to control or manage symptoms of emotional and physical reactivity that tend to occur during recollections of the traumatic event:

"I can deal with my anxiety much better now."
"My symptoms are much less troubling now."
"I feel more in control of my reactions."

Demonstrates ability to remain significantly calmer when exposed to situations or events that symbolize or are similar to the original traumatic event (displays relaxed affect and facial expression; smooth, nonagitated psychomotor movements)

Expresses relief from anger, self-blame, or guilt related to the traumatic event:

"I'm not so hard on myself anymore; I realize things happen that we can't control or change."
"I'm not overcome with anger anymore."

Verbalizes realistic hopes and plans for the future with absence of suicidal thoughts:

"I'm going back to my old job; I have a lot of reasons to live; my family needs me."

Identifies significant support systems, e.g., family, friends, community groups

Identifies the normal progression of grief symptoms that may be a part of the traumatic event (shock, denial, awareness, anger, restitution, acceptance)

Verbalizes self-forgiveness and forgiveness of others for actions or nonactions perceived by the client to have influenced the traumatic event:

"I can finally forgive myself for being human."
"They did what they could to help at the time."
"It's time to forgive and get on with my life."

PLANNING AND IMPLEMENTATION

Nursing Interventions and Rationale

Listen actively to the client's details and ruminations about the recollections surrounding the traumatic event. *Active listening builds trust, allows the client to vent, decreases feelings of isolation, and guides the nurse toward significant problem areas (e.g., guilt, self-blame, anger).*

Encourage the client to identify and describe specific areas surrounding the traumatic event that are most troubling and that elicit powerlessness or loss of control. *Talking it out with a trusted person helps the client bring the details of the event out into the open during a safe, nonthreatening time. It gives the client an opportunity to gain some influence over the traumatic event and decreases apprehension about intrusive recollections.*

Assist the client in structuring time for basic needs (hygiene, grooming, rest, nutrition) *to increase self-esteem, promote health and safety, and provide fewer opportunities for painful recollections of the traumatic event.*

Conduct a suicide assessment *to provide for the client's safety.* (See Appendix J.)

Assess the client's anxiety level *to prevent escalation of symptoms through early interventions.* (See Table 2-1.)

Encourage the client to communicate and interact within the milieu in accordance with level of tolerance. Have the client:

- Engage in frequent one-to-one interactions with assigned staff
- Eat all meals in the clients' dining room
- Participate in recreational activities
- Attend community meetings

This is to prevent and decrease feelings of isolation and detachment from others and the environment, enhance socialization, use energy in rewarding here-and-now activities, and decrease opportunities for painful recollections of the traumatic event.

Avoid statements that dictate to the client what to feel, think, and do. *Client's behaviors and decisions are best influenced by the client's needs, desires, and life-style, not by the singular opinions of others. Preaching to the client will elicit resistance and delay the therapeutic process.*

Nontherapeutic responses:

"You really have to stop blaming yourself and get on with your life."

"Don't feel that way; it's self-destructive."

"If I were you, I would break off with your old war buddies."

Teach the client adaptive, cognitive, and behavioral strategies to manage symptoms of emotional and physical reactivity (dread, terror, helplessness, sense of doom, cardiac palpitations, shortness of breath, etc.) that accompany intrusive recollections of the traumatic event.

- Slow, deep breathing techniques
- Relaxation exercises
- Cognitive therapy
- Desensitization
- Assertive behaviors

Breathing and relaxation exercises provide slow, rhythmic, controlled patterns that decrease physical and emotional tension, which reduces the effects of anxiety and the threat of painful recollections. Cognitive therapy helps the client to substitute irrational thoughts, beliefs, or images for more realistic ones and thus promotes a greater understanding of one's actual role in the traumatic event, which may decrease the client's guilt and self-blame. Systematic desensitization helps the client gain mastery and control over the past traumatic event by progressive exposures to situations and experiences that resemble the original event, which eventually desensitizes the client and reduces the painful effects. Assertive behaviors enable the client to manage anger and self-doubt by choosing to respond to painful recollections through use of adaptive strategies rather than being controlled by painful consequences. (See Appendix K.)

Assist the client to develop objectivity in perceptions of the traumatic event by providing a fresh perspective, *to promote a greater understanding of the client's actual versus perceived role in the event and assuage feelings of self-blame and guilt:*

"Rape is not a mutual sexual act; it is an act of violence that cannot be anticipated or prevented."

"No one could have predicted the accident; it just happened."

Problem solve with the client those areas in which some control is possible versus those that are beyond control:

"No one can control who lives and who dies in a war, but the survivors can be helped to deal with the memories."

"It's hard to know if the robbery would have occurred if your door was locked, but anyone can forget to lock a door."

"The past can't be changed, but the impact can be reduced in time."

This is to help the client begin to "let go" of aspects that are impossible to resolve (death, loss, injury) and begin to focus on areas that can be influenced (attitudes, coping methods).

Assist the client to develop an internal locus of control rather than feeling externally influenced by the effects of the traumatic event by involving the client in decisions about care and treatment *to foster feelings of power and control:*

"What are some of the behaviors and coping methods you prefer to decrease anxiety and control intrusive recollections?"

"I notice the methods you've been using seem to reduce your symptoms effectively; what is your perspective?"

Engage the client in group therapy sessions with other clients with posttraumatic stress disorder (when the client is ready for the group process) *to obtain additional support and understanding through the concept of universality.* (Refer to Appendix K for group therapy.)

Promote the client's awareness of own avoidance of experiences similar to the traumatic event *to give the client the opportunity to integrate the past traumatic event into present and future life experiences without fear or apprehension.*

Provide realistic feedback and praise whenever the client attempts to use learned strategies to manage anxiety and reduce posttraumatic stress response *to increase self-esteem and promote compliance with treatment plan:*

"The staff has noticed you practicing the relaxation exercises."

"You handled your anger well in the assertiveness training class today."

"Your thoughts about yourself have become more realistic."

Assist the client and family to develop realistic life goals (school, work, community, and leisure activities) *to prepare for a hopeful future that will absorb and alleviate the posttraumatic stress response.*

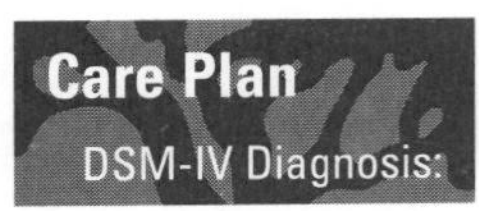

Somatoform Disorders

NANDA Diagnosis: Coping, ineffective individual

The state in which an individual demonstrates impaired adaptive behaviors and problem-solving abilities in meeting life's demands and roles

Focus:

For the client who manifests physical symptoms or loss of physical functions as a means of coping with anxiety. The anxiety generally arises from unresolved conflicts/stressors that are too painful to be exposed to the conscious mind.

NANDA Taxonomy

Pattern 5—Choosing: A human response pattern involving the selection of alternatives

ETIOLOGIC/RELATED FACTORS (RELATED TO)

Psychologic conflicts/stressors
Severe anxiety, repressed
Fear of responsibility, failure, or loss
Value–belief system
Psychosocial stressors
Past experience with true organic disease (self or others)
Exposure to persons with actual physical symptoms
Ineffective use of adaptive coping mechanisms/strategies
Dependent personality traits/disorder
Histrionic personality traits/disorder
Narcissistic personality traits/disorder
Obsessive-compulsive personality traits
Depressed mood state (secondary to dysthymic or major depressive disorder)
Negative self-concept (low self-esteem)

DEFINING CHARACTERISTICS (AS EVIDENCED BY)

Preoccupation with body functions such as heartbeat, sweating, or peristalsis, or with minor problems such as mild cough or sore throat:
"I can't seem to stop concentrating on my heartbeat."
"I can't get my mind off my physical problems."
Interprets body functions or sensations as evidence of a serious disease:
"I'm sure I have cancer somewhere in my body; I can feel it."
"I just know I'm going to have a heart attack soon."
Verbalizes continued need to seek medical assistance for perceived physical symptom(s) in spite of physician's reassurance of no demonstrable organic pathology ("doctor-shopping"):
"If I don't get any satisfaction, I'll just see another doctor."
"I'll keep going for checkups until they find out what's wrong with me."
Relates history of excessive visits to physicians, clinics, emergency departments, and possibly multiple surgeries
Presents elaborate or detailed lengthy history of perceived physical symptomatology
Demonstrates anger and frustration toward physicians when perceived physical symptoms are not diagnosed or treated:
"I'm frustrated and upset at those doctors who refuse to give my symptoms a name."
"How can they treat me if they can't figure out what I have?"
Promotes anger and frustration in health care providers who cannot find a physiologic basis for client's perceived symptoms
Denies correlation between physical symptoms and psychologic conflicts/stressors:
"I'm so fed up with everyone who thinks it's all in my head."
Experiences continuing deterioration of health care provider relationships as a result of mutual anger and frustration:
"I'm very upset that I can't find a doctor who will stay with me."
"My doctor is avoiding me like all the others did after a while.
Relates family's frustration regarding inability of medical profession to diagnose and treat perceived symptomatology:
"My family is so upset about this; sometimes I think they blame me."
"My husband says we may need counseling to get through this."
Relates history of family members with similar symptoms as client, some of whom are deceased:
"My greataunt died and she suffered from the same symptoms that I have."
"My dad had trouble swallowing before he died, and I always feel as if I have a lump in my throat."
Demonstrates excessive dramatic or histrionic behavior when describing perceived physical signs and symptoms
Demonstrates intermittent symptoms of anxiety that rapidly decrease as physical symptoms emerge
Focuses on self and physical symptoms during interactions and group activities with clients and staff
Examples:
Persistently discusses physical symptoms in all conversations, no matter what the original topic
Demonstrates exaggerated physical dysfunctions or alterations during group meetings and activities
Refuses to attend recreational activities because of perceived limitations rendered by physical symptoms or dysfunctions:
"You know I can't play Ping-Pong; I can't stand or walk."
"How can I play bingo? I can't see the numbers with my double vision."
Relates history of dependency on significant family members:

"My father always protected me when I was a young girl."

"I don't know what I'd do without my husband; he does everything for me."

"I have wonderful kids; they take care of the house and do all the cooking."

Manifests depressed mood states that have occasionally required hospitalization:

"I've been treated for depression, but they still couldn't find the cause of my physical symptoms."

Relates history of prescription drug use for perceived physical pain, dysfunction, or other symptomatology

Verbalizes progressive reduction in social activities that client directly attributes to perceived physical deterioration:

"I hardly see my friends anymore; I'm too sick to socialize."

"My physical problems have really limited my social life."

Relates prolonged history of job absences directly related to long-standing symptoms or problems for which there are no demonstrable organic findings or pathology (e.g., back pain, nausea and vomiting, muscle weakness or paralysis, painful menstruation, fainting, dizziness, blurred vision)

OR

Relates work history that began early in life and involved strenuous work with rare breaks or vacations (workaholic):

"I never missed a day of work in my life; now my back hurts so much, I can't work."

"I used to work overtime for years, but since my head injury I have blurred vision."

Attributes present perceived physical symptoms to an old injury:

"My back pain is due to bending over the wrong way many years ago; this hip pain is due to an old auto accident; these headaches are the result of bumping into an open door during childhood."

Refuses persistently to attribute perceived physical symptoms to possible psychologic or emotional factors or influences:

"They're trying to tell me that psychotherapy might help my pain; I can't believe it!"

"My problems are physical, so how could they be caused by anything emotional or psychologic?"

"How could some emotional problem that happened long ago have anything to do with these physical symptoms?"

Demonstrates a loss of or alteration in physical functioning of a body part or system that generally suggests, but is not limited to, a neurologic disease (e.g., paralysis, aphonia, seizures, blindness, anesthesia, coordination disturbance), which is an expression of a psychologic conflict or need. *Examples:*

A man who is dependent on his wife claims he cannot stand or walk when she threatens to divorce him to prevent her from deserting him.

A woman is unable to speak after becoming enraged during an argument (rather than expressing anger outwardly), but no organic pathology exists.

Demonstrates markedly decreased anxiety concomitant with the manifestations of perceived physical symptoms, dysfunctions, or alterations. (Primary gain: conflict is kept out of conscious awareness as anxiety is converted to a physical symptom.)

Avoids particular activities or behaviors as a result of physical dysfunction or alteration. (Secondary gain: support is obtained from the environment that may not be forthcoming if the client functions normally.) *Examples:*

A man who thinks he is unable to stand or walk can relinquish responsibility and remain dependent on the environment.

A woman who believes she cannot see gains support and sympathy from others.

OUTCOME IDENTIFICATION AND EVALUATION

Verbalizes absence or significant reduction of physical symptoms, dysfunctions, or alterations. *Examples:*

Able to feel normal sensations in previously "numbed" arm

Stands and walks on legs that were once "paralyzed"

Experiences significant decrease in duration and frequency of "gastrointestinal distress"

Demonstrates a significant decrease in anxiety in the absence of physical symptoms, dysfunctions, or alterations (indicates that anxiety is being managed via adaptive coping mechanisms/methods rather than being converted to a physical symptom, dysfunction, or alteration)

Verbalizes awareness of correlation between physical symptoms and psychologic conflicts/stressors:

"Perhaps my early troubled childhood did influence my physical problems."

"I can see how my combat experience may have played a part in my physical symptoms."

"I was always afraid I would get sick and die like my brother did; maybe that did affect my body."

Explains body structure and functions in realistic terms:

"I can tell the difference between a normal heartbeat and a racing one."

"I know it's OK for my stomach to feel fluttery when I'm excited or nervous."

Communicates and interacts with others in the milieu:

- Seeks out staff for one-on-one interactions
- Discusses thoughts and feelings with concerned clients
- Problem solves source of thoughts and feelings
- Participates in community and didactic groups
- Engages in physical activities/exercises
- Shares information in process groups

Uses learned adaptive cognitive and behavioral therapeutic strategies to manage and reduce anxiety:

- Slow, deep breathing techniques

- Relaxation exercises
- Thought, image, and memory substitution
- Cognitive restructuring
- Desensitization
- Behavior modification
- Assertive behaviors (See Appendix K.)

Recognizes the need to grieve normally for actual loss/impairment of body structure, function, or integrity:

"It's OK to feel bad that my arm will never be totally normal, as long as I don't dwell on it."

"I want to be able to get angry about all those surgeries I've had and then get on with my life."

"I need to have a good cry about my back injury and then try to make the best of it."

Accepts laboratory tests and clinical diagnostic results as valid criteria for health status:

"I realize that repeated laboratory tests indicate accurate results of my condition."

"Several doctors have examined me, and all of them agree that they could find nothing significantly wrong."

Refrains from discussing perceived physical symptoms, dysfunction, or alterations with clients, staff, and family

Functions independently and assertively in social and personal situations:

- Takes care of basic needs without asking for help
- Interacts as mature role model in milieu
- Facilitates adult role with spouse and children
- Initiates work or school role with positive attitude

Demonstrates absence of physical symptoms, dysfunctions, or alterations (unless there is actual residual impairment)

Verbalizes absence of physical pain or discomfort (unless there is actual residual discomfort)

PLANNING AND IMPLEMENTATION

Nursing Interventions and Rationale

Review all current laboratory and diagnostic results with the client in clear terms, in accordance with the client's level of comprehension:

"Mrs. Jones, your test results are all normal."

Mr. Smith, your test results indicate no physical disorder."

The client has the right to knowledge about health status. Anxiety may inhibit learning, so clear, concise terms are helpful. It's also important to offer information that will assist the client to accept facts regarding health status.

Ensure that the client's treatment team members are equally informed of the latest relevant test results. *It is imperative that the client be given consistent, accurate information to decrease anxiety about health status and promote trust.*

Convey your understanding that, although the symptom is real to the client, no organic pathology has been found:

"Mrs. Jones, I know you feel the pain in your arm. Exams and tests have been taken and no physical cause has been found."

"Mr. Brown, I realize you still have trouble standing and walking. X-rays and lab studies have shown no physical cause."

"Ms. Smith, I understand you feel no sensation in your hand. Test results did not show any physical cause."

Denial of the client's feeling could inhibit trust and decrease the client's self-esteem. Reassurance that no organic pathology has been found presents facts that are incongruent with the client's symptom(s) and difficult to challenge.

Assist the client in basic needs, routines, and activities in the initial stages of the therapeutic relationship with the realization that prolonged help may result in secondary gains (e.g., the client may use the physical symptom(s) to preserve dependency and relinquish milieu responsibilities):

"Miss Day, staff will help you organize your daily routine for the first two days."

"Mr. Brown, staff will show you the shower and laundry rooms so you'll be able to bathe and wash your clothes tomorrow."

"Mrs. Jones, I'll let you know when activities are today and I'll give you a written schedule for the rest of the week."

The client needs some assistance during times of vulnerability, and to deny it at a time when trust is being established could result in increased anxiety and intensification of physical symptoms and other maladaptive behaviors.

Decrease gradually the time and assistance given to the client according to the client's level of progress and establishment of trust:

"Mr. Brown, if you get to the dining room early, you can finish dinner and still have time to wash and dry your shirt before visiting hours."

"Miss Day, your clothes and makeup looked nice today. It looks like you can manage those things well now."

"Mrs. Jones, I didn't call you for group because yesterday I gave you a schedule for all activities. You were on time for everything else, so I know you can do it."

Fostering the client's independence at the right time enhances self-esteem, promotes adaptive coping and continuity of independent behaviors (organizational and problem-solving skills), and distracts the client from dwelling on physical symptoms and impairment.

Listen actively to the client's verbalizations of fears and anxieties without encouraging or focusing on physical symptom(s) or dysfunctions. *Expression of feelings with a trusted person enables the client to vent pent-up emotions, which in itself decreases anxiety. It also helps the client clarify unresolved issues or conflicts and guides the nurse toward problem areas. Not drawing attention to the client's physical symptoms discourages repetition of maladaptive behaviors.*

Redirect the focus of communication whenever the client begins to ruminate about physical symptom(s) and impairments:

"Bob, you were talking about baseball a few minutes ago and then you got off track to talk about your behavior; let's talk more about baseball. What is your favorite team?"

"Sue, let's go back and continue our talk about your relationship with your sister."

"Steve, I'd like to hear more about what happened on the group outing."

This helps the client to dwell on topics that are more therapeutic and beneficial to recovery.

Inform the client (when trust has been established) whenever physical abilities and behaviors are incongruent with the client's verbal statements regarding physical symptoms and impairments:

"Joe, I noticed you moving your legs and crossing them more often today; you may be able to stand and walk too."

"Jackie, that was a good game of Ping-Pong; your arm seems to be much stronger today."

Assist the client to associate onset of physical symptom(s) with stressful events through exploration of past experiences (those that can be recalled) *to help the client correlate stressful situations with onset of physical symptoms, eliminate maladaptive denial, and stop relying on physical symptoms to manage anxiety.*

Discuss with the client alternative coping strategies to reduce anxiety in accordance with client's capabilities and life-style:

- Deep-breathing techniques
- Relaxation exercises (See Appendix K.)
- Physical activities (walking, running, exercising, sexual activities)
- Milieu activities (checkers, chess, cards, Ping-Pong, bingo)

As client's denial decreases and the client no longer relies on physical symptoms to manage anxiety, adaptive coping techniques become meaningful ways to reduce anxiety and to prevent anxiety from escalating. (See Appendix K.)

Teach the client therapeutic cognitive and behavioral strategies to manage anxiety and reduce the need to rely on physical symptoms:

- Cognitive therapy
- Desensitization
- Reframing-relabeling
- Assertive behaviors

As the client becomes more aware that physical symptoms may be influenced by psychologic and emotional stressors, cognitive-behavioral skills can be used to effect a more positive change in attitude and to reduce or eliminate ineffective coping behaviors. (Refer to Appendix K.)

Praise the client realistically for using adaptive coping behaviors to manage anxiety rather than resorting to physical symptoms, dysfunctions, or impairments to reduce anxiety:

"Jane, your use of deep breathing has helped slow down your heartbeat."

"John, you have made a real effort to concentrate on your thoughts and not on your physical problem."

"Jim, I've noticed that you can be calm now without focusing on your leg pain."

"Sue, it seems the relaxation techniques have helped reduce your anxiety; you haven't discussed your stomachache in three days."

Positive feedback increases the client's self-esteem, offers hope for recovery, and encourages repetition of functional behavior.

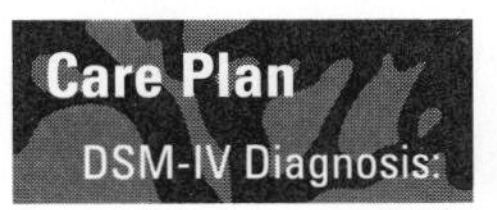

Dissociative Disorders

NANDA Diagnosis: Coping, ineffective individual

The state in which an individual demonstrates impaired adaptive behaviors and problem-solving abilities in meeting life's demands and roles

Focus:
For the client whose disturbances or alterations in normally integrative functions of identity, memory, or consciousness (e.g., Dissociative Identity Disorder, Dissociative Amnesia or Fugue Disorders, Depersonalization Disorder) are a result of ineffective coping (e.g., denial) related to painful, unresolved conflicts and can lead to inability to cope with subsequent stressors, as noted by impaired problem-solving/decision-making skills, relationships, and independent functioning

NANDA Taxonomy
Pattern 5—Choosing: A human response pattern involving the selection of alternatives

ETIOLOGIC/RELATED FACTORS (RELATED TO)

Personal or psychosocial vulnerability

Overwhelming stressors that exceed the ability to cope

- Childhood: sexual abuse, trauma
- Adulthood: accident, trauma, military combat

Inadequate or ineffective support systems (family, early role models)

Anxiety, fear, doubt

Anger, guilt, shame

Threat to self-concept or physical integrity

Ineffective denial

Depressed mood

DEFINING CHARACTERISTICS (AS EVIDENCED BY)

Dissociative behavior in general

Demonstrates inappropriate use of defense mechanisms (e.g., maladaptive denial) evidenced by

- Amnesic episodes
- Presence of alternate personalities
- Loss of perception and experience of self
- Loss of sense of external reality

Verbalizes inability to recall selected events or experience related to dissociative states

Expresses confusion/disorientation about sense of self and purpose or direction in life

Relates altered perception or experience of self, ego boundaries, and sense of external reality

Reports lost or distorted periods of time with episodes of confabulation in an attempt to "fill in" the memory gaps (common in alcoholic amnesic states)

Verbalizes history of ineffective coping since childhood, with specific symptoms emerging at various stages of growth and development

Demonstrates inability to meet role expectations in stages of growth and development subsequent to traumatic events

Dissociative identity disorder

Experiences two or more distinct personalities or personality states that interfere with goal-directed activities (personalities may or may not be aware of one another)

Demonstrates changes in physiologic and/or psychologic characteristics from one personality to another. *Examples:*

- One personality may experience physical symptoms (generally allergic in nature), and another personality may be asymptomatic
- Different personalities may have different eyeglass prescriptions
- Different personalities may respond differently to psychologic tests or intelligence (IQ) tests
- One or more of the personalities may report being of the opposite sex or a different age or race

Manifests discrepancies in attitude, behavior, self-image, and/or problem-solving abilities from one personality to another. *Examples:*

- A person may alternate between one personality that is shy, quiet, and retiring and another personality that is flamboyant and promiscuous.
- A person may have one personality that responds to aggression with childlike fright, a second personality that responds with submission, and a third personality that responds with counterattack.
- A person may have one personality that is reasonably functional or adaptive (e.g., be gainfully employed) and another personality that is clearly dysfunctional or appears to have a specific mental disorder.

Relates history of destructive behavior directed at self or others, alcohol/drug abuse, sex-related crimes

Demonstrates anger, fear, confusion, guilt, shame, or frustration associated with inability to cope with unresolved early conflicts and subsequent stressors (may also be a symptom of other dissociative states)

Addresses each identified personality by its own proper name or symbolic meaning, which usually differs from the person's birth name. *Examples:*

- "Melody" may be a personality that expresses itself through music
- The "Protector" may present a function given to a personality whose role is to protect the individual or group of alternate personalities

Psychogenic fugue

Experiences episodes of sudden, unexpected travel away from home or work with assumption of a new identity

Demonstrates inability to recall previous identity when questioned, with concomitant episodes of confusion and disorientation (rule out mental disorder)

Exhibits completely different behavioral characteristics during fugue periods than those manifested in the original identity. *Examples:*

- An individual who is usually quiet and passive may become more gregarious and uninhibited during a fugue period
- A person may change names or residences and engage in functional, complex social activities that do not reflect the existence of a mental disorder

(The travel and behavior noted in psychogenic fugue are generally more purposeful than the confused wandering observed in clients with psychogenic amnesia.)

Psychogenic amnesia

Exhibits sudden inability to recall important personal information to a greater extent than ordinary forgetfulness, generally associated with a circumscribed period of time, e.g., the first few hours after a profoundly traumatic event or accident

Demonstrates perplexity, disorientation, and purposeless wandering during amnesic experience (generally reported by others)

Displays an indifferent attitude toward memory impairment during amnesic period (See Glossary for definition of *la belle indifference.)*

Depersonalization

Demonstrates persistent, recurrent episodes of altered perception or experience of the self in which the usual sense of reality is lost or changed

Expresses feelings of detachment or of being an "outside observer" of own body or mental processes or as if in a dream

Verbalizes feelings like an "automated" robot or as if out of control of actions and speech, with various types of sensory "numbness" (experiences are ego-dystonic and the client maintains intact reality testing)

Perceives bizarre alterations in surroundings so that sense of external reality is lost (derealization). *Examples:*

- Objects may appear to have altered sizes or shapes
- People may seem mechanical or "dead"
- Sense of time may be distorted
- Anxiety
- Depression
- Obsessive-compulsive ruminations
- Fear of going insane
- Somatic concerns

OUTCOME IDENTIFICATION AND EVALUATION

Identifies ineffective coping behaviors, e.g., fugue states, depersonalization, or alternative personalities, and their negative effects on life functions, relationships, and activities

Expresses feelings appropriately in an attempt to cope with and more effectively manage anxiety, fear, anger, confusion, guilt, or shame

Identifies stressful situations that may trigger fugue states, depersonalization, transition from one personality to another, and other dissociative states, and develops methods to avoid them. *Examples:*

- Seeks out staff for support, interaction, medication
- Alters stress-producing environment
- Leaves stressful area or situation

Demonstrates use of effective coping methods. *Examples:*

- Verbally expresses fear, anger, confusion, guilt, embarrassment, with trusted staff person
- Writes thoughts and feelings in a diary or log
- Engages in milieu activities and exercises

Engages in ongoing, insight-oriented therapy with specialist in dissociative disorders

Exhibits significant reduction in or absence of fugue states, amnesic episodes, and depersonalization

Demonstrates progress toward integration of identified personalities or personality states

Identifies helpful resources and support systems available upon discharge. *Examples:*

- Relatives or friends who replace dysfunctional family
- Employer who is willing to learn about the problem and work with the client
- Day-treatment team (nurses and health care personnel)
- Psychotherapist
- Social services
- Community services

PLANNING AND IMPLEMENTATION

Nursing Interventions and Rationale

Be aware of your own feelings, thoughts, doubts, and beliefs regarding dissociative disorders (especially multiple personality disorder) prior to coming in contact with patients. *The diagnosis must be accepted and understood by staff because any doubts or misinterpretations will be transferred to the client as anxiety or fear and pose a barrier to treatment.*

Discuss concerns with qualified staff or therapist *to gain knowledge about these disorders and assuage own doubts and confusion because these clients generally fear being doubted or questioned about the validity of their disorder.*

Assure the client that he or she is not to blame for behaviors that occur during dissociative states, *to reduce the client's fears, guilt, and embarrassment during times when the client is vulnerable and unable to cope effectively with internal conflict.*

Assure the client that staff will remain with him or her during times of overwhelming anxiety, dissociation, or transition from one personality to another, *to promote feelings of trust, support, and psychologic safety during stressful times when the client is too frightened and confused to cope effectively.*

Demonstrate to the client that staff will intervene to help the client cope more effectively during times of dissociation, depersonalization, or personality transition, *to assure the client that someone is in control when he or she is unable to cope and may fear "going insane" or "falling apart."* Examples:

- Remain calm and accepting of the client's behavior
- Assess the type of dissociative behavior being experienced
- Listen actively to the client and try to identify which personality is currently dominant (if dissociative identity disorder)
- Arrange protection if a violent personality dominates
- Direct primary personality to monitor and control the behaviors of the potentially violent personality. (Usually one primary personality can be called on to prevent violence.)

Verbalize to the client the importance of discussing stressful situation(s) and exploring feelings associated with those times. *Ventilation of feelings in a nonthreatening environment may help the client come to terms with serious issues that may be associated with the dissociative process (treatment team should consult and agree on intervention strategies).*

Help the client understand that confusion, fear, and disequilibrium are normal during disclosure of painful experiences and resolve when integration occurs and adaptive coping methods return. *The client who is aware of what to expect during disclosure of feelings and resolution of dissociative state is more apt to engage in treatment with less apprehension and a greater sense of trust.*

Demonstrate acceptance of whatever experiences are disclosed by the client, making certain that your nonverbal behavior does not reveal disapproval, shock, or surprise. *Because of fear of criticism, clients with dissociative disorders find it difficult to disclose experiences, even in a trusting relationship. Care should be taken to let the client know that the experience will be treated tactfully.*

Structure the environment to reduce stimulation such as loud noises, bright lights, or extraneous movement, *to create a less stressful external environment that may help calm the client's internal state and prevent or minimize dissociative symptoms.*

Protect the client from harm or injury during dissociative episodes (e.g., amnesic states, loss of external reality, altered self-perception, poorly defined ego boundaries, distorted sense of time, emergence of alternate personality). *Client may become confused, disoriented, or frightened during dissociative episodes and may require safety measures by an alert staff. Examples:*

- Accompany client to assigned areas in the milieu
- Move furniture against the wall
- Distinguish boundaries through explanation and touch

- Prevent others from injury owing to client's confused state
- Initiate seclusion and restraint, if necessary (see Appendix J)

Help the client identify effective coping methods used in the past during stressful situations or experiences, *so that the client can recall prior successful coping strategies whenever anxiety is overwhelming.*

Assist the client to utilize new alternative coping methods *to deal with painful feelings, thoughts, and conflicts in a healthy, effective manner rather than using maladaptive denial.* Examples:

- Provide opportunities for the client to vent anger, fears, frustration, shame, or doubt in a trusted environment
- Engage the client in physical activities that require energy and concentration
- Encourage the client to write thoughts, feelings, and fears in a diary or log

Assist the client to evaluate the benefits of each coping strategy and its consequence, *to help the client problem solve and develop a plan of action for future anxiety-provoking incidents and to promote autonomy.*

Praise the client for the use of effective coping strategies *to reinforce repetition of adaptive behaviors.*

Assess the client for the possibility of substance use because *a significant number of clients with dissociative identity disorder and other dissociative behaviors use alcohol or drugs as a means of coping, masking symptoms, or interfering with treatment and progress.*

Assess the client for the presence and degree of depression, depletion of coping methods, and suicidal ideation (e.g., threats, gestures, plans), especially clients with multiple personality disorders in whom one or more personalities may be suicidal. *Clients with dissociative disorders may become discouraged and depressed because treatment is a long-term process (may be 10 years or more), and the client needs protection against self-destructive acts.*

Engage the client in appropriate therapies (e.g., insight-oriented therapy) *to promote expression of anxieties, fear, guilt, anger, or shame. Dissociative symptoms arise from internal conflicts and serve to protect the client from psychic pain. Subsequent stressors can produce similar reactions. Insight-oriented therapy with a knowledgeable therapist in a supportive setting allows the client to explore past and painful conflicts and eventually resolve them.*

Discuss with the client feelings and problems related to lengthy treatment. *Feelings of frustration and discouragement are bound to occur owing to the long-term treatment regimen, and the client may resort to old, ineffective coping methods and/or destructive behaviors.*

Help the clients identify support systems that will assist in coping with early conflicts that cannot be completely resolved (childhood incidents of sexual abuse or trauma), *to provide a network of support to strengthen the client's coping abilities and ease the pain that stems from old memories that continue to interfere with the client's life functions.* Examples:

- Trusted therapist
- Treatment team (inpatient and day treatment)
- Identified significant persons (may have to give up dysfunctional family members for newer, healthier friends)
- Social services
- Community resources

Educate the client and significant others about available information regarding dissociative disorders, particularly multiple personality disorder. *Obtaining current knowledge from professionals helps to dispel confusion and fear surrounding these disorders, reinforces continued treatment, and offers hope.*

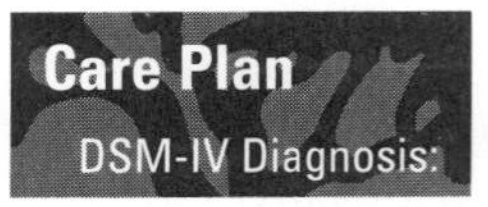

Dissociative Disorders

NANDA Diagnosis: Violence, risk for: self-directed; Violence, risk for: directed at others

The state in which an individual experiences behaviors that can be physically harmful to the self or others

Focus:
For the client whose normally integrative functions of identity, memory, or consciousness (e.g., Dissociative Identity Disorder, Dissociative Amnesia or Fugue Disorders, Depersonalization Disorder) are a result of ineffective coping related to early life conflicts, can lead to inability to manage subsequent stressors, resulting in destructive acts toward self or others

NANDA Taxonomy
Pattern 9—Feeling: A human response pattern involving the subjective awareness of information

RISK FACTORS

Anger, frustration, rage related to amnesic episodes
Anger, frustration, rage reaction of one or more personalities (Dissociative Identity Disorder)
Perceived threat to self-concept or physical integrity
Panic anxiety state
Overwhelming stressors that exceed the ability to cope in a reasonable manner
Conflicts between personalities (Dissociative Identity Disorder)
Depressed mood
History of suicidal threats/behaviors
History of loss of control/violence toward others
Low self-esteem

OUTCOME IDENTIFICATION AND EVALUATION

Demonstrates nonviolent behavior:

- Absence of suicidal threats/gestures

- Absence of aggressive acts toward others

Absence of panic/rage reactions

Uses assertive behaviors to meet needs:

- Maintains relaxed, nonthreatening posture
- Uses calm, matter-of-fact manner

Uses resources and support systems effectively to help maintain self-control and prevent violence:

- Releases anger through verbal expression
- Write volatile feelings in diary or log
- Seeks out trusted individuals for help when overwhelmed with anger
- Engages in physical activities to release angry feelings

Verbalizes understanding that disorder requires long-term treatment and that strategies to reduce anger and eliminate violence are continuous

Engages in appropriate insight-oriented therapies in the hospital and after discharge to reduce the risk of suicide and violence toward others

Demonstrates self-confidence and increased self-esteem as integration of personalities takes place, minimizing risk of violence

PLANNING AND IMPLEMENTATION

Nursing Interventions and Rationale

Assure the client that staff will protect him or her and others from harm or injury during dissociative episodes (e.g., amnesic state, loss of eternal reality, altered self-perception, poorly defined ego boundaries, distorted sense of time, emergence of alternate personalities). *Clients may demonstrate fear, anger, panic, anxiety, or rage during dissociative episodes and need help to control behaviors they cannot yet manage alone. Knowing that qualified staff will be there to prevent violent episodes is in itself anxiety-reducing.*

Be aware of behavioral changes that are clues to destructive acts. Clients with dissociative disorders, especially Dissociative Identity Disorder, can switch behaviors dramatically from calm to violent, as different personalities have different behaviors. *Examples of behavioral changes that are clues to a risk for violence:*

- Voice tone changes from calm and passive to loud and harsh
- Facial expressions change from blunted or smiling to troubled or scowling
- Movements change from smooth and relaxed to erratic with possible pacing
- Verbal expressions change from benign or friendly to hostile and threatening

Take immediate and decisive action when violence to client or others is imminent, according to severity of threat and history of previous violence, *to protect the client and others from harm or injury.*

- Seclude and/or restrain if necessary
- If the client has Dissociative Identity Disorder, direct the primary personality to monitor and control the behaviors of the potentially violent personality (e.g., tell the personality to "stop" until the personality calms down). (There is usually one primary personality or "protector" that can be called on to prevent violence.)
- Offer appropriate prn medication

Refrain from passing judgment on the client; instead, let the client know he or she is a worthwhile individual with strengths and is not responsible for early childhood trauma and sexual abuse, *to relieve client from blame, decrease guilt and shame, and build self-esteem.*

Structure the environment to reduce external stimulation. *Calm surroundings precipitate a less stressful internal state within the client and reduce the risk for violence.* Examples:

- Reduce noise, lights, extraneous movement
- Assist the client to avoid stressful environment when practical

Assess presence and degree of depression and evidence of suicidal ideation in any of the personalities that emerge. *Clients may become discouraged and depressed because treatment is a long-term process (may be 10 years or more), and the client needs protection against self-destructive behavior.* (See Appendix J.)

Examine the client's behaviors closely for abrupt changes that may signal a risk for suicide, e.g., threats, gestures, or plans, *to be able to intervene early and interrupt self-destructive act.*

Assist the client to identify alternatives to aggression or violence, e.g., verbalize feelings in a safe setting, engage in physical activities, write thoughts and feelings in a diary, *to divert overwhelming impulses of anger and hostility toward constructive behaviors.*

Engage the client in appropriate, insight-oriented therapy with a specialist in dissociative disorders, specifically Dissociative Identity Disorder, *to bring painful conflicts and feelings into the consciousness and reduce the risk for dysfunctional coping, suicide, and violence toward self or others.*

Educate the client and family about the most current information regarding dissociative disorders, especially Dissociative Identity Disorder, *to dispel the myths surrounding these disorders, reduce fear and confusion, and reinforce continued treatment with a specialized therapist.*

Praise the client for attempts to control anger and rage and for participation in ongoing therapeutic regimen, *to increase self-esteem and reinforce continued treatment. Because treatment for dissociative disorders is a long-term process (may be 10 years or more), positive reinforcement is necessary.*

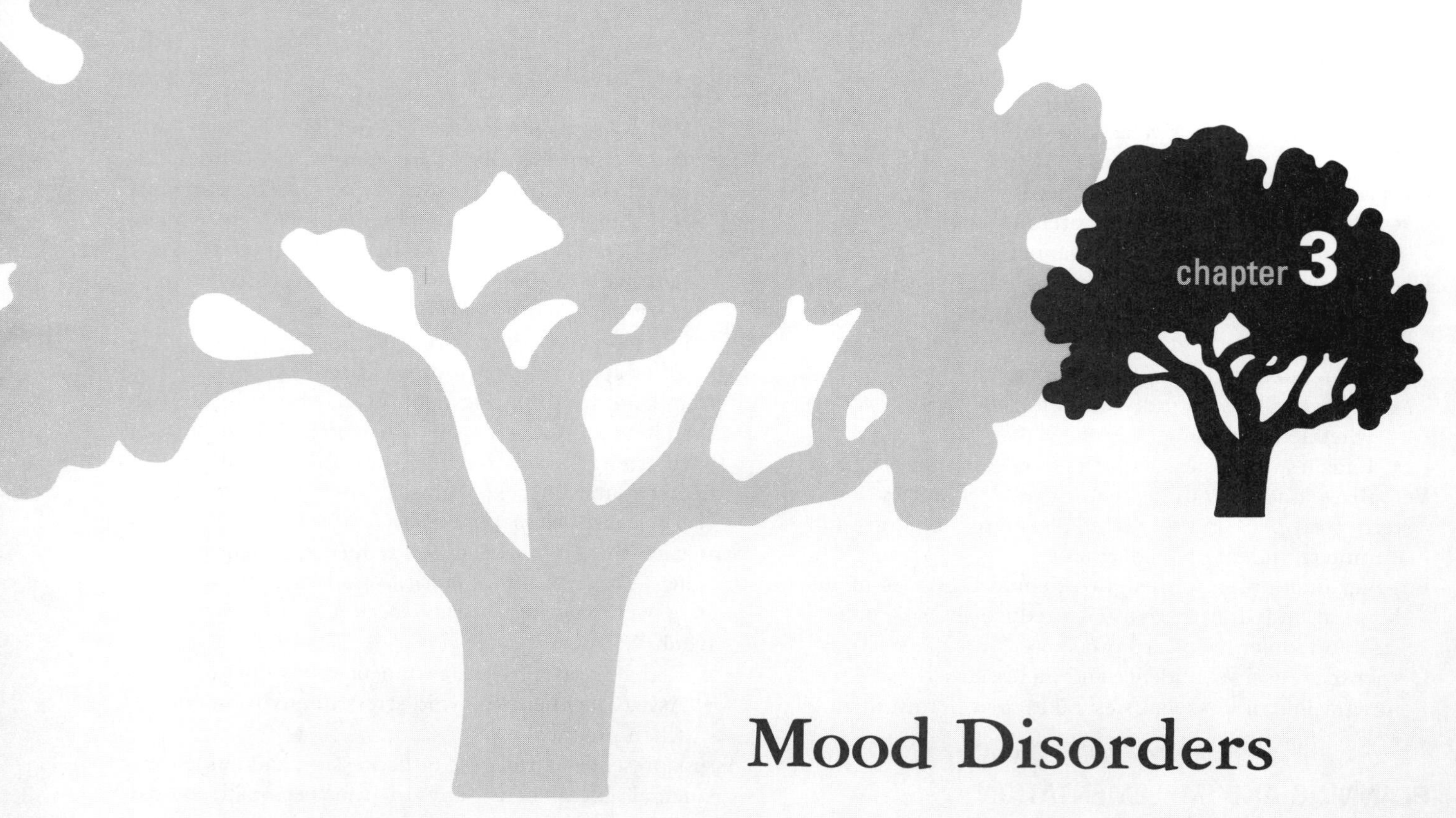

Mood Disorders

The term *mood disorders* represents a group of diagnostic categories that describe a range of emotional disturbances. *Mood* is the internal, subjectively experienced emotion that is pervasive and sustained and colors all the person's psychic life. The client may report a mood as a feeling (sad, depressed, happy, angry). *Affect* is the external, observable manifestation of emotion (flat, blunted, constricted, expansive, labile).

Individuals normally experience a wide range of mood and expressions of affect but are usually in control of both. Mood disturbances severe enough to be named *mood disorders* bring a substantial decrease in, or an entire loss of, control over mood. Mood is either significantly elevated or depressed, with consequences of impairment of interpersonal, social, and occupational functioning and subjective feelings of distress.

People who experience only depressive episodes are said to have major depressive disorder, or unipolar depression; those who experience episodes of exaggerated, expansive, or elevated mood (mania) *or* have both depressed and manic episodes are said to have bipolar disorder. Two distinct symptom patterns exist in mood disorders: one for depression, the other for mania.

Clients who have recurrent depressive episodes and who have relatives with bipolar disorder may at some time during their lives demonstrate mania. Mania and depression represent opposite poles of the same entity, "two sides of the same coin."

ETIOLOGY

Specific etiologic factors related to mood disorders are listed in Box 3-1.

EPIDEMIOLOGY

Mood disorders, particularly unipolar depression, are among the most common psychiatric disturbances in adults. Twice as many women as men have unipolar depression, and the prevalence of bipolar disorder is slightly higher in women. Although major depression can occur at any age, even during infancy, most clients have onset between ages 20 and 50, with a mean age of onset of about 40 years; onset of bipolar disorder usually occurs in early adulthood. The occurrence of mood disorders is not race-specific, but bias in diagnosis may underdiagnose mood disorders and overdiagnose schizophrenia in nonwhites. Incidence is higher in individuals who lack close interpersonal contacts (widowed, single, divorced, or separated).

DIAGNOSIS OF MOOD DISORDERS

Major Depression

The most distinguishing features of clinical depression are depressed mood and loss of interest or pleasure in life (anhedonia). Other symptoms of major depression include the following:

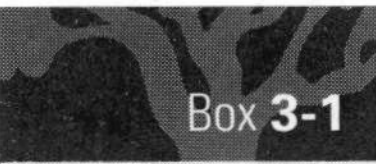

Box 3-1

Specific Etiologic Factors Related to Mood Disorders*

Biologic

Genetic

High incidence of mood disorders in families with history of mania or depression

Biochemical

Dysregulation of neurotransmitters (GABA, norepinephrine, serotonin) at brain synapses
Acetylcholine dysregulation
Abnormalities of biogenic amine metabolites
Neuroendocrine dysfunction (hypersecretion of cortisol; hormonal dysregulation)

Psychodynamic

Loss of libidinal object
Introjection of an ambivalently loved object

Psychosocial

Stressful life events (major losses, disappointments, deaths, divorces)
Premorbid personality types that use internalizing (rather than externalizing) defense mechanisms
Negative cognitive distortions about the self, environment, and life experiences
Learned helplessness

*Although a specific etiology for mood disorders has not been established, a combination of biologic, psychosocial, and environmental factors is implicated. Current research emphasizes biologic studies.

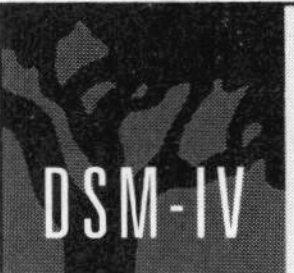

DSM-IV

Mood Disorders

The essential characteristic of these disorders is a disturbance of mood accompanied by a full or partial manic or depressive syndrome.

DSM-IV Categories

Major Depression, Single Episode
Major Depression, Recurrent Episode
Dysthymic Disorder
Bipolar I Disorder
Bipolar II Disorder
Cyclothymic Disorder
Mood Disorder due to Medical Condition
Substance-Induced Mood Disorder

Marked change in appetite
Significant weight loss or gain
Insomnia or hypersomnia
Psychomotor retardation or agitation
Fatigue, lack of energy
Lack of libido
Feelings of hopelessness, worthlessness, guilt
Decreased ability to think or concentrate
Recurrent thoughts of death or suicide

Severely depressed clients may appear extremely despondent, a mood that is distinctly different from the normal mood of sadness or "the blues." These clients express loss of capacity to enjoy life, family, friends, activities, or events that previously brought pleasure; complain of low energy; often resist or refuse others' efforts to help them or to get them to help themselves; and they describe themselves or their situation as hopeless.

Clients may cry often, or they may be unable to cry or express feelings of sadness but continue to withdraw and isolate themselves. It is often painfully difficult for them to engage with others, even concerned staff. They feel worthless and are unable to accept praise and approval. Other manifestations of major depression are guilt, helplessness, and indecisiveness. Ruminations of negative feelings and experiences may be prevalent. Low self-esteem, negative self-concept, and poor self-image seem pervasive.

Physiologic systems are slowed down, and neurovegetative symptoms may occur. Most clients lose their appetite with resultant weight loss, but some clients overeat and gain weight, often with the explanation that eating fills the "emptiness." The sleep-wake cycle is disturbed, and patients may experience hypersomnia (sleeping most of the day and night) or hyposomnia (decreased ability to sleep), difficulty falling asleep, or multiple awakenings. Constipation is common and is worsened by antidepressant medications. There is a loss of libido (frigidity in women, impotence in men), and amenorrhea is not unusual in depressed women.

Depressed clients often describe persistent thoughts of death or suicide, and staff must always be aware of their potential for self-harm. Suicide gestures and attempts are sometimes made when the client appears to be "better" and staff thinks the depression is lifting. Brighter affect may signify the client's relief from ambivalent feelings because of having finally made the decision to end his or her life, and this relief brings energy to commit the act. See Box 3-2.

Psychotic features may be present in depression. Severely depressed clients may have hallucinations, which usually take the form of hearing voices that self-degrade. Delusions are generally mood-congruent and follow themes of poverty, nihilism, guilt, death, personal inadequacy, or disease (somatic). *Examples:*

A man refuses to eat, saying that there is no need to eat because the world has ended (nihilistic type).

A woman believes her body is rotting away, her heart is made of stone, and she doesn't deserve to live (somatic type).

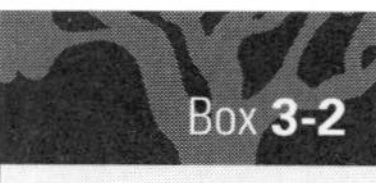

Box 3-2

Risk Factors for Suicide

Male, adolescent or over 40 years old
Divorced, widowed, or separated
Elderly, infirm
Impulsive or seclusive style
History of previous attempt, with or without injury
Attempts that have been unsuccessful in changing the behavior of others
Lack or perceived lack of support systems
Giving away possessions
When mood begins to lift following depression
Major illness
Alcoholism or drug abuse
Bipolar disorder
Major depression

Occasionally clients experience hallucinations and delusions at the same time, as in the following example:

A woman hears her dead husband's voice, sees his image, and tells him she caused his cancer and resultant death.

This symptomatology is sometimes referred to as *primary depression* when it occurs in a client without a history of a recent psychiatric or medical illness. When depression follows another disease or disorder (e.g., cancer, AIDS, schizophrenia), it is called *secondary depression.* Depression is sometimes called *exogenous* when it follows clearly defined external psychosocial stressors (death of a loved one, divorce); the term *endogenous* is used when no obvious psychosocial stressors exist (etiology is biologic).

Major depression with melancholia is a severe form of depression. Diagnostic criteria are similar to those listed previously, with a defining feature of marked anhedonia. The following symptoms may also be noted: psychomotor agitation, early morning awakening, diurnal variation (client feels worse in the morning and may experience some relief as the day progresses).

Seasonal type depression recurs and remits at or about the same time over successive months or years. For example, a person may become depressed every winter. Another indication for this diagnosis is when full remission or a change from depression to mania occurs at specific, rather predictable time periods.

Postpartum Depression

Up to 80% of women experience postpartum "blues" after having a baby because of hormonal and other physiologic and psychologic changes. It is a transient condition characterized by sadness, mood swings, and fatigue and is *not* to be confused with the longer-lasting symptoms of major depression. Pregnancy is not a cause of psychiatric disorders, but physical, psychologic, and environmental stressors may exacerbate a preexisting disorder or trigger a latent disorder. Symptoms of postpartum depression are similar to those of major depression.

Dysthymic Disorder

Dysthymia is a chronic (rather than episodic) disorder with an absence of psychotic features. Symptoms may be almost as severe as major depression and include overeating or poor appetite, sleep changes (insomnia or hypersomnia), fatigue, low self-esteem, difficulty concentrating, and hopelessness. Clients with dysthymia may be introverted, brooding, demanding, and self-degrading. Diagnosis is made after 2 years of chronic symptoms (1 year for children and adolescents).

Bipolar Disorders

Bipolar I Disorder. The defining feature of Bipolar I Disorder is one or more manic episodes or mixed episodes (both manic and major depressive episodes occur every day for at least 1 week). Often the person has had one or more major depressive episodes.

Bipolar II Disorder. Defining characteristics of Bipolar II Disorder are one or more major depressive episodes and at least one hypomanic episode.

Manic Episode

The most distinguishing feature of mania is elevated, expansive, or irritable mood. Other symptoms include the following:

Inflated self-esteem
Grandiosity
Decreased need for sleep
Pressured or excessive speech
Flight of ideas
Distractibility
Increased activity, with decreased purposefulness
Excessive involvement in activities that have high potential for painful consequences

Insight and judgment are poor in the manic phase, and before hospital admission the client may have been engaged in excessive activities such as gambling or spending sprees, wild and/or excessive sexual activity, phoning family and friends in the middle of the night to "party," and engaging in ill-fated business ventures that the individual is not prepared to handle. When admitted to the hospital, the manic client may be hyperactive, pacing or running up and down the halls, intruding in others' activities, sleeping and eating little, and changing clothing several times a day. Clothing, jewelry, and makeup may be excessive, with unusually bright, garish combinations. During this acute phase, the manic client is hyperverbal, demonstrates pressured speech, and talks constantly and rapidly to anyone who will listen. The client says whatever comes to mind and rapidly changes topics (flight of ideas), described by the client as "racing" thoughts. He or she may frequently insult staff and clients, often with foul or sexually explicit language. The client tests unit rules and limits, insists on having his or her own way, is often

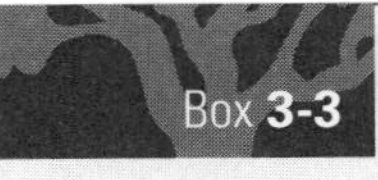

Box 3-3

Depressive Symptoms May Also Be Noted in the Following Conditions

Substance use/abuse
Organic disorders (Alzheimer's disease and multiinfarct dementia)
Prescription/over-the-counter drug use/abuse
Dysfunctional grief
Personality disorders
Anxiety disorders
Schizoaffective disorder
Schizophrenia (all types)

manipulative, and may become hostile and combative when thwarted, exploding in an angry tirade. Some manic patients exploit the weaknesses of other clients and staff, dividing staff and causing management problems. The client may be seductive, flaunt sexuality, or invite other clients and staff to engage in sexual acts.

Sometimes the client with mania describes the euphoric mood as feeling "high" and may elect to stop taking lithium to achieve this state. Manic clients are frequently preoccupied with religious, political, sexual, or financial ideas that may reach delusional proportions. The most common delusions of mania are of *grandeur* or *persecution.* Delusions of grandeur represent the client's attempt to compensate for feelings of low self-esteem (e.g., a woman believes she is the queen of England and is charged with gathering all nations to form a peace treaty; a man believes that he is the son of God and has omnipotent powers), and delusions of persecution represent the client's projected fears and threats to the self-system (e.g., a man working in an office thinks his coworkers are plotting to get him fired from his job and fears retaliation from the opposition, which is "out to get him"; a woman believes all her neighbors belong to a cult and are planning to kill her and her children).

The essential feature of bipolar disorder is one or more manic episodes that may or may not be accompanied by depressive episodes. Diagnosis depends on the symptoms of the *current* episode. Clients sometimes cycle between manic and depressed states in what is termed "rapid cycling," or moods may fluctuate between manic and depressed states with periods of normal mood in between. Episodes of mania in bipolar disorder have a more rapid onset and are of shorter duration than depressed episodes in major depressive disorder.

Hypomanic Episode

Hypomania (not a diagnostic category) is characterized by a predominant mood that is elevated, expansive, or irritable, with associated symptoms as described for manic episodes. However, the symptoms are less severe and may not impair social or occupational functioning or necessitate hospitalization. Psychotic features are absent.

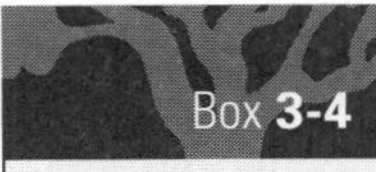

Box 3-4

Manic Symptoms May Also Be Noted in the Following Conditions

Substance use/abuse
Prescription/over-the-counter use/abuse
Attention deficit hyperactivity disorder (ADHD)
Anxiety disorders
Physiologic impairment of the central nervous system
Schizophrenia
Schizoaffective disorder

Cyclothymic Disorder

The essential features of *cyclothymia* are a disturbance in mood for at least 2 years (1 year for children and adolescents) involving numerous hypomanic episodes and numerous periods of depressed mood or loss of interest or pleasure. The severity and duration are less than in major depression or bipolar disorder. Hospitalization is seldom required for this disorder, which is chronic and fluctuating in nature.

Mood disorder due to medical condition. This condition is diagnosed when there is a persistent and prominent mood disturbance as the result of an already existing medical diagnosis.

Substance-induced mood disorder. Mood disturbance that is prominent and enduring as a result of the physiologic effects of chemical substances is called a Substance-Induced Mood Disorder.

INTERVENTIONS FOR MOOD DISORDERS

Hospitalization

Persons with severe depression or mania often require hospitalization. Suicide or homicide risk or an inability to meet the needs for food, clothing, and shelter is direct indication for hospitalization. Other indications for hospitalization of clients with depression or mania include severity of symptoms, rapid escalation of symptoms, and lack of availability or capability of an individual's support systems. Frequently persons with mood disorders resist suggestions for hospitalization because of the very nature of the disorders. Severely depressed people are unable to make decisions because of slowed and impaired cognitive functions, their hopeless, bleak outlook on life, or feelings of unworthiness; manic clients may believe that hospitalization is absurd because of delusional systems that significantly impair their perception, judgment, and insight.

Biologic Therapy

Most studies reveal a higher rate of treatment success for clients with mood disorders when psychopharmacologic and other psychotherapeutic interventions are combined. Medications given for depressed episodes are broadly categorized as antidepressants. Selective serotonin reuptake inhibitors (SSRIs) such as Prozac, Paxil, and Zoloft are more recent (third generation) antidepressants. Effexor (venlafaxine HCl) is another newer antidepressant medication that inhibits reuptake of both serotonin and norepinephrine. Luvox, another recent SSRI, has shown promise in treatment for depression and obsessive-compulsive disorder.

Lithium, a naturally occurring salt, is the drug of choice for mania; however, other medications have been used when clients are unable to take lithium or when it is ineffective. Two such medications are Depakote (valproate) and Tegretol (carbamazepine), which are categorized as anticonvulsants. Antipsychotic medications may be prescribed in the initial stages of mania to slow down clients' activities or reduce psychotic symptoms. Refer to Appendix M for more information on these drugs.

Electroconvulsive therapy (ECT), sometimes referred to as *electroshock therapy* (EST), is an effective biologic intervention for major depression, the disorder for which it is most frequently administered. ECT remains a subject of much controversy. Some data indicate that ECT may be beneficial for acute manic states and some cases of schizophrenia, particularly Schizoaffective Disorder, in which mood is disrupted.

Psychosocial Therapies

Nurse-client relationship therapy. (See Appendix G.)

Cognitive therapy. Cognitive theorists believe that depression is the consequence of a person's negative thoughts about self and circumstances. Cognitive therapy involves helping the individual identify, modify, and eventually change negative thought patterns by practicing thinking realistically about self and situation. Emphasis is on immediate issues and interpersonal relationships, not on intrapsychic phenomena. The care plans in this chapter provide several practical cognitive and behavioral techniques nurses may utilize. (See Appendix K.)

Behavior therapy. Behavioral theory proponents state that the most effective way to alleviate depression is to change the behavior. Reinforcement of negative behaviors is seen as the principal element of depression. Behavioral therapies vary in focus and specific techniques that identify goals, methods for attaining the goals, and reinforcers for goal attainment. (See Appendix K.)

Family therapy. Family therapy can be an effective treatment modality for clients with mood disorders; the focus is on the family unit and the role it plays in perpetuating depression. Family therapy also evaluates the effect depression has on the family as a whole. Marriages and family functions are frequently imperiled, and divorce rates are high in families of mood-disordered clients. Symptoms result in impaired relationships in families of clients with mood disorders. This often leads to psychosocial dysfunction. *Secondary gain* (attention from others as a result of negative behaviors) reinforces dysfunctional behavior. (See Appendix K.)

Group therapy. Group therapy represents a microcosm of a larger society in which clients can interact and express themselves safely. If clients are able to tolerate the interpersonal process, groups are therapeutic for mood-disordered clients. Groups enhance communication and socialization, both of which are essential goals for manic and depressed clients. (See Appendix K.)

DISCHARGE CRITERIA FOR MOOD DISORDERS

Verbalizes plans for future, with absence of suicidal thoughts or behavior
Verbalizes realistic perceptions of self and abilities
Relates realistic expectations for self and others
Sets realistic attainable goals
Identifies psychosocial stressors that may have negative influences
Describes methods for minimizing stressors
States positive methods to cope with threats and stressors
Identifies signs and symptoms of disorder
Contacts appropriate sources for validation and/or intervention when necessary
Utilizes learned techniques and strategies to prevent or minimize symptoms
Verbalizes knowledge of food-drug and drug-drug interactions and potential problems
States therapeutic effects, dose, frequency, untoward effects, and contraindications of medications
Makes and keeps follow-up appointments
Expresses guilt and anger openly, directly, and appropriately
Engages family or significant others as sources of support
Structures life to include appropriate activities

Nursing Process for

Depression

Universal Principles for Interactions and Interventions with Clients Who Are Managing Mood Disorders

- Continue to monitor assessment parameters listed under *Defining Characteristics.*
- Continue to consider the etiologic factors listed under *Etiologic/Related Factors.*
- Use principles of the *Therapeutic Nurse-Client Relationship* (Appendix G).
- Address clients' spiritual and cultural needs.

General Principles

- Protect the client from self-destructive behavior.
- Maintain adequate nutrition, rest, and hygiene.
- Modify an environment that is impoverished or unfavorable.
- Increase activity and involvement.
- Reestablish or teach adaptive coping methods.
- Promote support systems.
- Maintain physiologic and psychologic integrity.
- Teach the client how to identify psychosocial stressors and how to recognize, manage, and prevent symptoms.
- Educate the client about medication effects.

Care Plans for Depression

DSM-IV Diagnoses

Major Depression, Single Episode
Major Depression, Recurrent Episode
Dysthymic Disorder

NANDA Diagnoses

Violence, risk for: self-directed
Social interactions, impaired
Self-esteem, chronic low
Coping, ineffective individual
Hopelessness
Powerlessness
Self-care deficit

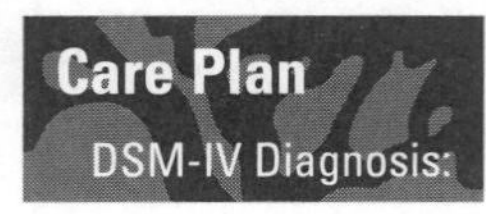

Care Plan

DSM-IV Diagnosis: **Depression (All Types)**

NANDA Diagnosis: Violence, risk for: self-directed

The state in which an individual experiences behaviors that can be physically harmful to the self

Focus:

For the client who is severely depressed, with suicidal ideation, and who threatens suicide and demonstrates suicidal gestures and attempts

NANDA Taxonomy

Pattern 9—Feeling: A human response pattern involving the subjective awareness of information

RISK FACTORS

History of attempts to harm self during depressed episodes

Overt attempts to harm self (cheeks and hoards medications; self-mutilates; attempts to hang self)

Verbalizes suicidal ideation or plan:

"I don't want to live anymore. I'm going to take an overdose of medication."

Expresses sadness, dejection, hopelessness, or loss of pleasure or purpose in life:

"Nothing gives me any joy. Life just isn't worth living anymore."

"Everything is hopeless."

Refusal to eat

Resists or refuses medication and treatments

Relates inability to see any future for self

Suddenly gives or wills away possessions

Frequently tearful, agitated, or morose

Progressive withdrawal from milieu

Affect does not brighten as day goes on

Potentially positive situations, events, or interactions fail to change client's ideation

Refusal to sign a "no self-harm" contract

Loss of self-esteem (*Subjective:* "I'm just not worth anything. I don't deserve to live." *Objective:* self-care deficit, e.g., impaired grooming, hygiene, and appearance, isolation and withdrawal)

Ambivalence (experiencing two opposing feelings, thoughts, drives, or intentions at the same time, e.g., wanting to live and not wanting to live)

Displays *sudden* mood elevation or calmer, more peaceful manner, with more energy (may indicate relief from ambivalent thoughts and feelings about killing self, which is a signal to staff that suicide attempt may be imminent)

OUTCOME IDENTIFICATION AND EVALUATION

Verbalizes absence of suicidal ideation or plans:

"I want to live."

"I no longer think about dying."

Expresses desire to live and lists several reasons for wanting to live:

"I want to get on with my life."

"My kids need me and count on me."

"I have lots of things I want to do for me and my family."

Displays consistent, optimistic, hopeful attitude. Affect appears brighter. Client may smile appropriately. Conversation focuses on present activities or future-oriented plans of positive nature.

Makes plans for the future that include follow-up care and medication compliance.

"My first priority is to go back to work part-time."

"I'll definitely keep my appointments and take my medications without fail."

PLANNING AND IMPLEMENTATION

Nursing Interventions and Rationale

Client safety is the nurse's first priority.

Check client and room for potentially destructive implements (sharp objects, belts, shoelaces, socks, chemicals, hoarded medications) *to protect the client from self-destructive acts.*

Begin "close watch" protocol (every 15 minutes at irregular intervals).

Evaluate the seriousness of the suicidal ideation (ask for intent and plans) *because there is always a chance that the client will act on his or her thoughts, and the more concrete the plans, the greater the risk of completion.* (See Appendix J.)

Refrain from judgment, preaching, and shocked facial expression, *so the client does not feel embarrassed, threatened, or "wrong" and will continue to communicate.*

Listen actively to the client *because verbalization helps relieve pent-up thoughts and feelings.*

Accept and validate the client's thoughts and feelings *because invalidation may block further communication by the client and promote the risk of self-harm.*

Observe for behaviors that are precursors to self-destructive acts (threats, gestures, giving away possessions, making a will, self-deprecating and command hallucinations, delusions of persecution) *because such behaviors may be signposts of suicidal thoughts and feelings.*

Help the client move from an unrealistic to a realistic belief system by contrasting myths with *facts to decrease guilt and helplessness and increase control and self-esteem.* (See Appendix K, Cognitive Therapy; Rational-Emotive Therapy.)

Determine the client's strengths and coping abilities to *reinforce the strengths and prior successful coping strategies and to encourage the client to utilize positive aspects of self.*

Help the client learn new coping methods and problem-solving techniques *to manage internal and external stressors.* (See Appendix K, Psychosocial Therapies; Assertive Training.)

Identify the client's available support systems. *Additional support, care, and concern will increase the client's feelings of self-worth and decrease feelings of alienation, which may be a precursor to suicide.*

Assist the client in formulating attainable goals, *because attainable goals are more likely to be met and will bring quicker rewards.*

Assist the client in maintaining nutritional needs, hygiene, grooming, and appearance *to promote health, safety, dignity, and self-esteem.*

Reassure client that there is hope *as clients in the throes of active suicidal ideation believe that there is no way out:*

"I know you feel bad now, but you will not always feel this way and we're here to help you through it."

Praise the client for attempts at positive self-evaluation, self-control, and realistic goal-setting *to promote self-esteem and provide continued hope for change:*

"Staff agrees with those positive qualities you listed about yourself."

"Your statements in group today were appreciated."

Seclude and restrain, if necessary, *to protect client from self-harm.* (See Appendix L.)

Educate the client and family about the importance of medication and treatment and elicit their feedback *to ensure client compliance, follow-up care, and safety.*

Continue to support and monitor prescribed medical and psychosocial treatment plans.

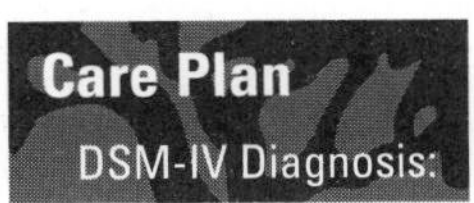

Depression (All Types)

NANDA Diagnosis: Social interaction, impaired

The state in which an individual participates in an insufficient or excessive quantity or ineffective quality of social exchange

Focus:
For the client who is severely depressed who often finds it difficult to communicate, to attain and maintain relationships, or to engage in a therapeutic alliance.

NANDA Taxonomy
Pattern 3—Relating: A human response pattern involving establishing bonds

ETIOLOGIC/RELATED FACTORS (RELATED TO)

Self-concept disturbance (low self-esteem and self-image)
Depletion of coping skills
Hopelessness
Powerlessness
Negative cognitive patterns (mistrust, ambivalence, delusions of persecution)
Knowledge deficit regarding social skills
History of traumatic or unsatisfactory relationships
Insufficient energy to initiate social skills (secondary to depression)
Actual or perceived losses or stressors (breakup of a relationship, change or loss of job/status, death of significant other, altered body image/integrity, financial loss)
Recent traumatic event (life-threatening illness)
Absence of significant other or peers
Dissatisfaction or change in role or relationship
Social isolation

DEFINING CHARACTERISTICS (AS EVIDENCED BY)

Decreased or no participation in activities
Failure to engage other clients or staff in conversation
Unresponsive to others' attempts to initiate communication or to engage client in activities
Remains in room most of the day and evening
Expresses discomfort in social interactions:
"I'd rather stay in my room than go to group."
"Don't bother me; I want to be alone."
Observed discomfort in social situations (slumped posture, head down, avoids eye contact, fidgety, restless)
Refuses/resists visits from significant others
Failure of other patients to seek client's company
Rejection by other clients
States he or she is unworthy of anyone else's time and company
Cites lack of energy as reason for nonparticipation
Claims that attempts at social interactions bring unsatisfactory results:
"I didn't enjoy the activities at all."
"The community meeting was a waste of time."
"I shouldn't have gone bowling in the first place."
Verbalizes inability to achieve a mutual sense of acceptance, caring, or understanding through social interactions:
"We just didn't get along at all."
"There was no understanding between us."
"Our talk was a waste of time."
Resists engaging in a therapeutic alliance with staff
Demonstrates discomfort and resistance when interacting with staff

OUTCOME IDENTIFICATION AND EVALUATION

Engages in therapeutic alliance with staff
Initiates social interactions with peers and staff
Participates actively in all milieu and group activities
Verbalizes satisfaction with social interactions:
"I really enjoyed our talk."
"The activity was fun and everyone got along OK."
Demonstrates comfort and enjoyment during interactions (eye contact, brighter affect, alert responses)
Expresses awareness of some of the problems that precipitated impaired social interactions:
"I do so much better in group once my medication begins to take effect."
"I should do my one-to-one talks with my nurse later in the day, when I feel better."

PLANNING AND IMPLEMENTATION

Nursing Interventions With Rationale

Continue to initiate engaging client in interactions. *Depressed clients resist becoming involved in a therapeutic alliance, so acceptance and persistence are necessary.*

Actively listen, observe, and respond to client's verbal and nonverbal expressions. *Active listening lets the client know he or she is worthwhile and respected. The client will be encouraged to continue seeking out others.*

Initiate brief, frequent contacts with client throughout the day. *This lets the client know he or she is an important part of the community and encourages the client to participate, no matter how minimally.*

Remain with the client even if he or she does not engage in conversation, and offer brief, accepting comments:

"Good morning. I see you are unable to participate today."

"I'll just sit here with you for 15 minutes."

When severely depressed and energy-depleted, the client may be unable to engage in conversation. The presence of a concerned caregiver offers the client comfort and security and increases self-worth.

Use a low-key matter-of-fat approach when offering the client simple choices.

Therapeutic response:

"Good morning. It's 8 o'clock, and breakfast stops being served in the dining room at 8:30."

The nondemanding approach avoids threatening the client with expectations he or she cannot meet, and the choices give the client a sense of having some control.

Nontherapeutic response:

"It's 8 o'clock. You should be up and dressed by now. Everyone in the dining room is waiting for you."

These statements can promote feelings of failure and inadequacy in the client by blaming the client for his or her inability to exercise control over his or her behavior.

Encourage the client to ask for assistance when necessary. *The client must interact to get needs met.*

Refrain from overzealous behaviors (lifting up shades to "let the sunshine in"; excessively cheerful greetings). *The client becomes overwhelmed and feels more despondent when he or she cannot meet or match the nurse's affect and demeanor.*

Initially comment on neutral topics or subjects of common interest (e.g., items in the room, daily news topics, the menu). *Usually, social conversation initially helps establish rapport and aids the client in making the transition toward therapeutic communication.*

Gradually engage client in interactions with other clients, beginning with one-to-one contacts, progressing toward informal gatherings, and eventually taking part in structured group activities; occupational therapy first, then recreational therapy. *Clients experience success when social interactions are pursued in relation to their level of tolerance (simple to complex).* See glossary for descriptions of *therapeutic recreation* and *occupational therapy*.

Suggest journal writing as a means to write about successful social interactions when they occur and feelings provoked by various social experiences. *Writing about social and interactive experiences in a log or journal reinforces repetition of successful behaviors, promotes awareness of feelings, and gives the client more opportunity to better manage social encounters because responses will be expected and less traumatic.*

Encourage phone calls and visits with supportive significant persons. *Reinforce rewarding, supportive relationships.*

Help the client identify the value of his or her attendance at meals, activities, group outings, and so on. *Efforts toward human contact are important, even though enjoyment cannot yet be attained.*

Make available those activities that the client finds rewarding and satisfying. *Activities that interest the client are more apt to provide enjoyment that will act as a catalyst for future social interactions.*

Explore with the client alternative social interactions that may be more appropriate and effective. *Often clients continue to utilize ineffective methods of interacting because change is difficult and results are uncertain.*

Practice with the client alternative interactive techniques in a safe setting, while offering tactful but honest feedback. *Role-playing and constructive criticism, in a safe setting, provide the client with the confidence needed to try out learned skills with others in the environment.*

Discuss with the client the responses of other clients to his or her interactions. *Provides the client with an opportunity to evaluate realistically and accept the effects of his or her behaviors on others, whether negative or positive.*

Help the client set realistic goals and limits in interactions with others *to foster realistic expectations.*

Inform the client that all of his or her needs will not always be met through interactions, *to promote realistic expectations.*

Encourage the client to set specific times for interactions with staff *to ensure positive self-generated interactions.*

Encourage the client to give and accept appropriate praise and compliments during social exchanges *to ensure mutually satisfying social interactions.*

Teach the client to challenge irrational beliefs about self and/or capabilities. *A more realistic view of self may give the client more confidence in social interactions.* (See Appendix K, Cognitive and Rational-Emotive Therapies.)

Develop a written or verbal contract with the client *as a reminder of basic expectations for interacting in the milieu.*

Emphasize the importance of group involvement (e.g., psychosocial therapies, outings, activities). *The client will gain support from others, learn social skills vicariously, and see that his or her problems and concerns are similar to those of others.* (See Appendix K, Psychosocial and Group Therapies.)

Conduct a suicide assessment to prevent harm, injury or death. (See Appendix J.)

Teach the client and family that the therapeutic effects of antidepressant medications may take up to 2 weeks but that uncomfortable effects may begin immediately. *Client and family need to know that the mood will not lift immediately and that adverse effects may initially be troublesome for the client.*

Continue to support and monitor prescribed medical and psychosocial treatment plans.

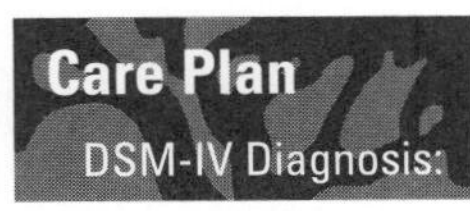

Depression (All Types)

NANDA Diagnosis: Self-esteem, chronic low

The state in which an individual has long-standing negative self-evaluation/feelings about self or self-capabilities

Focus:
For the client with pervasive low self-esteem derived from negative, unrealistic values that the individual ascribes to his or her self-concept (idea, belief, or mental image a person has of self, based on perceived strengths, weaknesses, and status). The person with low self-esteem thinks, feels, and behaves as if unworthy and incapable of achieving or performing at a level consistent with his or her own expectations or the expectations of others.

NANDA Taxonomy
Pattern 7—Perceiving: A human response pattern involving the reception of information

ETIOLOGIC/RELATED FACTORS (RELATED TO)

Long-standing unrealistic perceptions and irrational assumptions about self or situations
Neglectful, abusive, domineering, overprotective relationships
Identity problems (self, sexual)
Negative body image, actual or perceived
Doubt concerning self-worth and abilities
Consistent rejection by others
Unresolved losses, actual or perceived
Role dissatisfaction
Situational crises
Goal obstacles
Psychosocial stressors
Biologic factors (neurophysiologic, genetic, structural)

DEFINING CHARACTERISTICS (AS EVIDENCED BY)

Failure to attend to appearance, hygiene
Weight problems
Difficulty communicating or interacting with others (poor eye contact, reticent, paucity of speech, soft or inaudible voice)
Ruminations and repetitious statements about negative thoughts, situations, experiences
Expressions of incompetence, inadequacy, failure, or inability to deal with situations.
"I'm a flop at everything I try to do."
"I can't do anything right."
"I'm a failure at life."
"I can't handle anything."
Expresses shame or guilt:
"I'm so ashamed of myself for being such a failure."
"I'm responsible for all this misfortune."
Excessive shyness
Rejects positive comments and attention from others
Exaggerates negative feedback about self
Inability to make decisions
Fears trying new things or situations
Demonstrates anxious behaviors
Overly sensitive to critical appraisal
Continually asks for approval from others concerning self or capabilities

OR

Completely avoids interactions regarding self-context
Delusional thinking and expressions (See Glossary for delusion examples.)
Suicidal ideation

OUTCOME IDENTIFICATION AND EVALUATION

Demonstrates self-care (appearance, hygiene) appropriate for age and status
Initiates conversation with staff and others
Demonstrates absence of self-deprecating statements
Verbalizes realistic positive statements about self and others. ("I've always gotten along well with people." "Everyone here is nice to me.")
Stands and walks with a self-assured demeanor
Begins projects and activities without encouragement
Discusses negative mind-set, irrational beliefs, and values with staff
Utilizes techniques to decrease anxiety (See Appendix K, Deep-breathing and Relaxation Exercises.)
Acknowledges encouragement from others
Accepts suggestions for strategies to increase esteem and assertiveness. (Attends assertiveness training and cognitive therapy sessions.)
Practices techniques for increasing esteem and assertiveness. (Asks for assistance when necessary; asserts self to get needs met; speaks in clear, audible tones; replaces negative, self-deprecating thoughts with realistic ones.)
Demonstrates absence of delusions
Verbalizes will to live, reasons for living, plans for future

PLANNING AND IMPLEMENTATION

Nursing Interventions and Rationale

Encourage the client to wash, dress, comb hair, and use appropriate toiletries. *The act of attending to grooming and the results often increase confidence and esteem.*

Praise the client for all attempts at engaging staff appropriately. *Positively rewarded behavior tends to be perpetuated, and this helps the client to distinguish between self-defeating and self-enhancing socialization.*

Engage the family in plans to give genuine praise to the client when warranted. *Some families need reminders to support one another. Positive strokes from significant others go a long way to increase the client's self-worth and esteem.*

Keep all appointments with the client. *Increases client's sense of importance, worth, and esteem.*

Teach the client assertiveness skills. *Becoming assertive helps the client to get his or her needs met, gives the client a sense of control over his or her life, and brings respectful regard from others.* (See Assertiveness Training, Appendix K.)

Encourage the client to identify positive aspects of self by any methods (verbalize, write, draw):

"You have talked about some of the things you like about yourself today. Sometimes making lists helps in thinking of more positive qualities. If you make a list or write about your good qualities in a daily journal or log, we can discuss it during our meeting tomorrow."

The more the client expresses positive aspects of self, the less likely he or she is to focus on negative aspects.

Regarding Irrational Belief System:

Listen to the client's expressions of beliefs and allow the client to vent feelings.

Accept the client's feelings without judging or shutting him or her off because of your discomfort.

Encourage the client to explore alternatives and other perspectives about self.

Respectfully confront persistent irrational convictions.

Encourage thought-stopping and thought-substituting techniques. (Replace irrational thoughts with realistic ones.) *The client will let go of irrational beliefs and behaviors when a more realistic awareness is established. That develops by talking with a therapeutic listener.* (See Thought Substitution/Thought Stopping, Appendix K.)

When the Client Is Delusional:

State your reality, giving accurate information.

Do not ask for detailed explanations regarding the delusion. Focus on feelings engendered by the delusion and not the content.

Do not argue with the delusion regardless of its absurdity.

Discuss realistic interpretations or possible alternatives to perceptions. *This helps correct distorted perceptions.*

Present realistic activities and projects in which the client can succeed. *Graded activities that allow success raise confidence and esteem.*

Recognize the client's anxiety and encourage techniques to control anxiety. (See Appendix K, Deep Breathing and Relaxation Exercises.)

Genuinely praise the client's acceptance of compliments and encouragement from others. *This reinforces self-esteem.*

Encourage participation in group activities and therapies. *The client will experience curative factors of groups (learning that he or she is not alone with his or her problem, altruism, unconditional acceptance, catharsis, etc.).* (See Group Principles, Appendix K.)

Regarding Statements of Suicide:

Encourage the client to discuss thoughts and feelings about wanting to die.

Discuss the client's plan, if any.

Explore alternatives.

Reinforce statements regarding will to live and plans for future. *This helps the client get in touch with feelings, come to self-acceptance, and increase esteem.* (See Appendix J.)

Continue to support and monitor prescribed medical and psychosocial treatment plans.

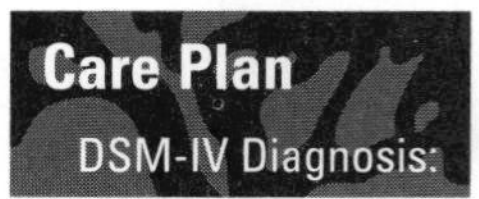

Depression (All Types)

NANDA Diagnosis: Coping, ineffective individual

The state in which an individual demonstrates impairment in adaptive behaviors and problem-solving abilities in meeting life's demands and roles

Focus:

For the client who is depressed and has decreased energy, for whom the tasks of coping with his or her disorder and meeting the requirements of daily living exceed his or her capabilities. Therefore, the individual may resort to coping methods that are maladaptive.

NANDA Taxonomy

Pattern 5—Choosing: A human response pattern involving the selection of alternatives.

ETIOLOGIC/RELATED FACTORS (RELATED TO)

Situational crisis

Personal vulnerability

Ineffective support system (actual or perceived) (e.g., absent, neglectful, or overprotective parents)

Dysfunctional family system (e.g., alcoholic parents or spouse, domineering or abusive role models, history of sexual molestation)

Unresolved grief or anger

Negative cognitive patterns (self-deprecating or self-persecutory thoughts)

Unrealistic or irrational self-perception

Unmet or unrealistic goals

Disturbance in self-concept (feelings of worthlessness or inadequacy)

History of multiple stressors over time (e.g., job or financial loss, breakup of relationship, death of significant other)

Decisional conflict

Hopelessness

Powerlessness

Role dysfunction

DEFINING CHARACTERISTICS (AS EVIDENCED BY)

Expressions of inability to cope or inability to ask for help:

"I don't know how I'll get through this."

"I can't take the stress any more."

"Who can I turn to?"

Frequently cries with no obvious provocation

Demonstrates depletion of coping resources ("I'd be better off dead"; expressions of suicide ideation or actual gestures and attempts)

Problem-grouping (stating several problems together):

"I can't hold a job; my wife and kids have left me; there's nowhere for me to live; my doctor is fed up with me."

Ineffective use of coping methods (unable to express or resolve anger or grief—directs feelings toward self; blames others for illness and hospitalization; regresses to earlier stages of development; seeks help for simple tasks; fails to meet basic grooming and hygiene needs)

Verbalizes delusions:

"I'm going to die soon because I don't deserve to live."

"There's no need to eat because I don't have any insides."

Verbalizes self-deprecating thoughts:

"I'm a failure at everything I do."

"I'm a terrible person."

"I'm a bad parent."

"I'm no good to anyone any more."

Social isolation and withdrawal (spends most of the time in bed or room; resists interacting with staff or clients; refuses to attend meetings and activities)

Fails to assert self to meet own needs

Ineffective problem-solving and decision-making skills

Fails to make decisions regarding care and treatment:

"I can't decide if I should stay with my family or move into a board and care home."

"I can't decide what to do first: get a job or begin day treatment."

Impaired judgment and insight:

"I stopped taking my antidepressants because I felt drowsy."

"I was doing OK before I came in here."

OUTCOME IDENTIFICATION AND EVALUATION

Verbalizes ability to cope in accordance with age and status:

"I think I'll be able to handle my responsibilities when I go back home."

Demonstrates effective problem-solving and decision-making skills:

"I've made up my mind to see my kids once every two weeks instead of every week for now."

"I've decided to walk every morning before breakfast for my daily exercise."

Verbalizes increased insight and judgment:

"I tend to get sick when I do too much, so I'll take one day at a time."

"I know if I continue to take my medicine, I will do better."

Demonstrates effective coping strategies (absence of blaming or accusing others for own problems; absence of angry or hostile remarks; displaces feelings appropriately, e.g, talking, exercising)

Exhibits self-restraint and control in situations that previously invoked crying spells

Demonstrates effective prioritizing of problems:

"I think I'll get back on my feet before I take on parenthood."

Expresses sense of self-worth:

"I deserve the love of my family and friends."

"I'm worth being helped."

Verbalizes realistic thoughts and situations about self:

"Everything hasn't been perfect, but my family is still together and loves one another."

"I didn't get to be supervisor but at least I'll have time to pursue that book I'm writing."

Demonstrates absence of delusions

Verbalizes feelings of hopefulness:

"Things seem to be getting better each day."

"I can't wait to see my new grandchild."

Verbalizes sense of power and control:

"I know now I can do many things to prevent becoming so depressed."

Demonstrates absence of suicidal thoughts and actions

PLANNING AND IMPLEMENTATION

Nursing Interventions and Rationale

Encourage client to focus on strengths rather than weaknesses. *This brings to the client's awareness the fact that he or she has positive qualities and capabilities that have helped him or her cope in the past.*

Help the client identify individuals who help the client to cope and who support his or her strengths.

"I notice you seem more relaxed during your sister's visits; you seem upset each time your friend calls. I'm here if you want to talk about it."

This increases the client's awareness of the positive effect supportive individuals have in his or her life.

Assist the client to learn strategies that will effect more positive thinking (e.g., cognitive, behavioral, imagery). *Therapeutic modalities can help the client to replace or substitute irrational self-deprecating thoughts and images with more rational beliefs and images.* (See Appendix K.)

Help client prioritize problems:

- Assist the client to list problems from most to least urgent.
- Assist the client to find immediate solutions for the most troubling problems, postpone those that can wait, delegate some to significant others, and acknowledge those beyond the client's control. *Listing problems in priority helps to reduce their overwhelming effects and breaks them down into more manageable increments.*

Respond to the client's persistent self-deprecation with realistic, nonchallenging evidence:

"Your children phone you every day."

"I enjoyed reading your poems."

"I like the color of your shirt."

This encourages the client to focus on positive aspects of self.

Respond to delusional statements by stating your reality of the situation without arguing with client's reality.

Praise the client for adaptive coping (making rational decisions based on accurate judgment, solving own problems, demonstrating independence). *Genuine praise defines the client's adaptive behaviors and encourages continuance through positive reinforcement.*

Teach the client basic assertiveness skills *to assist the client in getting needs met and to cope with demands of the environment.* (See Appendix K.)

Encourage the client to describe his or her role performance (family member, student, employee) and satisfaction it brings self and significant others. *This promotes more functional role adaptation.*

Encourage the client to discuss feelings generated by ineffective coping (e.g., frustration, anger, inadequacy):
"It's OK to talk about your feelings. It helps you work through your problems."
Acceptance of feelings without judgment or retaliation helps the client to externalize emotions that may be a source of depression.

Inform family and friends that the client may direct anger toward them but that he or she is learning more constructive methods to deal with feelings. *Family members who are well informed are better able to use their energies to support the client rather than focus on their own reactions.*

Help family members cope with the client's troubling behaviors by including them in those areas of the treatment plan that are relevant to them. *Families who are aware of effective coping methods are more empowered and better able to manage family-client interactions.*

Assist the client to increase socialization and involvement in activities according to level of tolerance.
This provides opportunities to practice coping skills while reducing isolation.

Conduct a suicide assessment to prevent harm, injury, or death. (See Appendix J.)

Continue to support and monitor prescribed medical and psychosocial treatment plans.

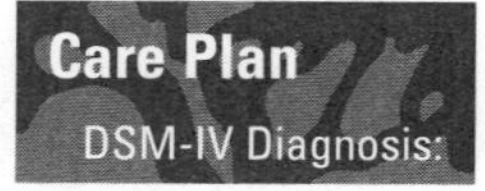
Care Plan
DSM-IV Diagnosis:

Depression (All Types)

NANDA Diagnosis: Hopelessness

A subjective state in which an individual sees limited or no alternatives or personal choices available and is unable to mobilize energy on own behalf

Focus:
For the client who experiences a sense of futility about his or her situation and the environment and thus perceives that life holds no meaning

NANDA Taxonomy
Pattern 7—Perceiving: A human response pattern involving the reception of information

ETIOLOGIC/RELATED FACTORS (RELATED TO)

Illness progression despite compliance with therapy
Long-term stressors
Illness-related regimen
Abandonment/isolation
Ineffective individual coping
Chronic low self-esteem
Fear/anxiety regarding illness/outcome of illness

DEFINING CHARACTERISTICS (AS EVIDENCED BY)

Verbalizes that life, situation, or status seems hopeless or futile:
"There's no sense in even trying."
"I can't do anything about it."
Frequent sighing, despondent content
Decreased or absent verbalizations
Decreased, saddened, flat, or blunted affect
Withdrawal from the environment
Behavioral demonstrations (e.g., turning away from speaker, closed eyes, lack of eye contact, shrugging shoulders)
Persistent despondent or "blue" mood or sense of impending doom
Physiologic symptoms of anxiety (tachycardia, tachypnea)
Decreased or absent appetite
Increased sleep
Lack of involvement in care
Passively receptive to care
Lack of involvement or interest in significant others

OUTCOME IDENTIFICATION AND EVALUATION

Expresses hopeful thoughts and feelings:
"My future looks brighter now."
"I feel more positive about my life."
Demonstrates hopeful, enthusiastic attitude and behaviors (erect posture, good eye contact, cheerful voice tone)
Participates willingly in daily activities and self-care
Exhibits brightened affect with broad range of expressions (smiles and laughs appropriately)
Engages in positive relationships with significant others or identified support persons
Sets attainable goals that indicate hope for the immediate future
Uses effective coping methods to counteract feelings of hopelessness (e.g., talks out feelings with staff, exercises daily, shares concerns with other clients in group meetings)

PLANNING AND IMPLEMENTATION

Nursing Interventions and Rationale

Conduct a suicide assessment. (See Appendix J.)

Encourage the client to verbalize feelings of hopelessness, despondency, and aloneness. *This gives the client the opportunity to vent and explore feelings realistically.*

Identify positive aspects in the client's world:
"Your family phones the hospital every day to ask about you."
"I see you washed your hair today and you're wearing a new shirt."
"The clients in group responded favorably to your comments."
Reflecting appreciation of the client's progress and participative efforts by staff, family, and supportive peers conveys hope and reduces alienation.

Assist the client to identify behaviors that promote hopelessness (morbid conversations, dwelling on negative ideas, avoiding interactions with staff, decreased participation in activities, procrastination) *to help the client develop an awareness of experiences that perpetuate negative themes.*

Teach the client to construct pleasant thoughts or images to combat hopelessness (being with a supportive person, recalling a previous successful experience, setting a future attainable goal). *Pleasant and positive thoughts, ideas, or images tend to inhibit or reduce the intensity of unpleasant, negative experiences and offer hope.* (See Appendix K.)

Encourage the client to engage in experiences that promote positive thoughts and feelings (communicate with staff, participate in activities, share experiences in supportive groups, phone concerned family members) *to discourage and interrupt hopelessness and alienation.*

Provide activities of interest to the client in which he or she can succeed. *Success encourages the client to repeat positive behaviors.*

Instruct the client in simple relaxation strategies (slow, deep breathing; relax muscles progressively from toes to head; listen to soothing music or relaxation tapes) *to assuage manifestations of anxiety such as rapid heart rate, rapid breathing patterns, and a sense of impending doom that may accompany feelings of hopelessness and alienation.* (See Appendix K.)

Encourage the client to participate in self-care and other milieu activities. *Clients who take an active role in their care and treatment are apt to feel more in control and hopeful about their outcome.*

Offer genuine praise for the client's efforts toward setting goals, initiating self-care, and participating in activities. *Praise promotes continuance of positive behaviors and decreases hopelessness and alienation.*

Inform the family that the client needs unconditional love, support, and encouragement. *Families have the power to give clients hope and strength through their unconditional love and acceptance.*

Continue to support and monitor prescribed medical and psychosocial treatment plans.

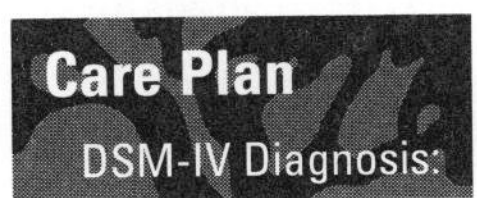

Depression (All Types)

NANDA Diagnosis: Powerlessness

A state in which an individual perceives that one's own actions will not significantly affect an outcome or perceives a lack of control over a current situation or immediate happening

Focus:
For the client who perceives that there is nothing he or she can do to change negative thoughts, feelings, behaviors, and circumstances

NANDA Taxonomy
Pattern 7—Perceiving: A human response pattern involving the reception of information

ETIOLOGIC/RELATED FACTORS (RELATED TO)

Lifestyle of learned helplessness
Reaction to chronic, recurrent illness
Illness progression despite compliance with treatment
Health care environment despite therapeutic value
Hopelessness
Ineffective individual coping
Impaired internal locus of control
Unmet role expectations (perceived or actual)

DEFINING CHARACTERISTICS (AS EVIDENCED BY)

Verbal expressions of having no control or influence over a situation or outcome:
"Nothing I do will improve my situation."
"I can't do one thing that will make my life better."

Demonstrates behaviors that reflect a loss of control over self and environment (apathetic toward staff, other clients, and environment; fails to assert self in order to get needs met; allows other clients to dominate or intimidate self; allows staff to make basic decisions, such as when to dress, what to wear, what to eat)

Expresses despair over illness and inability to see a way out of it or to help self get well in spite of compliance with treatment

Fails to participate in activities or meetings despite staff support and coaxing

Verbalizes dissatisfaction and disgust over inability to perform previous tasks, skills, or activities:
"I used to be so good at sports. Now I don't have the energy to play Ping Pong."

Expresses serious doubts regarding role and role performance:
"I'm not sure what my function is or what purpose I serve."
"My kids always turned to me for help. Now I'm useless to them."
"I've been a big disappointment to my friends."

Demonstrates dependence on others that may result in irritability, resentment, anger, or guilt

Accepts without resistance decisions made for him or her by staff and significant others

Fails to defend self, ideas, or opinions, in favor of others, when challenged

Demonstrates apathy or indifference about decreased energy level

OUTCOME IDENTIFICATION AND EVALUATION

Verbalizes feeling in control of self and situations:
"I was a help to my team in the volleyball game."
"It was tense in group when John got upset, but I handled it OK."

Questions or challenges decisions being made on his or her behalf.
"I'm sure I want to go back to live in that place."
"I want to know more about this medication."

Makes choices regarding management of care:
"I can do my own laundry."
"I prefer to attend the assertiveness training class today."

Verbalizes more realistic role expectations and goals for meeting them:

"I think I'll see my kids once a week instead of every day, and try not to do so much."
"I'm ready for a part-time job, but I can't manage full-time work right now."

Demonstrates internal locus of control by taking responsibility for care, situation, and outcome:
"I know I can help myself by taking my medications regularly."
"I think I can keep a part-time job if I get help as soon as I begin to feel bad."

PLANNING AND IMPLEMENTATION

Nursing Interventions and Rationale

Continue to monitor assessment parameters listed in the Defining Characteristics section.

Continue to consider etiologies listed in the Etiologic/Related Factors section.

Utilize principles of the nurse-client relationship. (See Appendix G.)

Observe for behaviors that indicate the client's sense of futility (e.g., shrugging shoulders, slouched posture, head lowered, lack of eye contact) *to intervene in the process before the client's sense of powerlessness becomes overwhelming.*

Determine situations/events that contribute to the client's sense of powerlessness, *to avoid or minimize situations that are out of the client's control.*

Accept the client's expressions of powerlessness without indicating that the perceptions are correct:
"I understand that you think you have nothing to say in group; your attendance is wanted, however."
"You're saying you can't play volleyball, but I noticed you got the ball over the net several times."
Acceptance of client's feelings and thoughts while focusing on behavior and capabilities builds trust and helps the client develop awareness of his or her strengths.

Assess the client's response to the treatment plan:
- Is the client passively compliant?
- Is the client willingly compliant and cognizant of the purpose of treatment?
  Passive compliance indicates powerlessness. Clients who are involved in their care and attempt to understand the reasons behind it are seeking more control over their illness and outcome.

Identify factors that may contribute to the client's loss of control (e.g., new environment, rules and regulations, sharing space, uncertainty about outcomes) *to reduce or minimize contributing factors.*

Help the client identify those things he or she can control and those he or she cannot, *to help the client gain an understanding of how to achieve successful outcomes.*

Explore with the client areas in the client's life that he or she has mastered. *Recalling past successes encourages future attempts to gain control.*

Provide opportunities for the client to exercise control in situations that he or she can manipulate (e.g., allow the client to decide where to place items in room; give the client choices of food, let the client decide where to sit during meetings). *Positive reinforcement promotes feelings of power and control.*

Do not offer choices where none exist (e.g., whether to take medications; engage in activities). *Choices should not include opportunities that interfere with the treatment plan.*

Slacken unnecessary restrictions whenever possible and safe, *to promote a sense of control.*

Identify the client's use of manipulative behavior and note its effect on other clients. *Clients may resort to manipulative methods to manage powerlessness because of distrust of others or fear of interpersonal closeness.*

Encourage the client to express needs openly and discuss ways needs can be met without use of manipulation. *This teaches the client positive strategies that promote control.* (See Appendix K, Assertive Training.)

Discuss with staff the importance of giving the client control *to ensure consistent approach to care.*

Assist the family with ideas and methods that empower the client in the home environment. *This promotes consistency in the treatment plan and assures the client that he or she has control over specific aspects of life.*

Recognize when the client begins to take responsibility for self and outcome ("I could prevent this by taking my medication regularly") rather than seeing self as a victim of circumstances ("Everything happens to me"). *This indicates that the client is developing an internal locus of control rather than attributing his or her experiences to external sources.*

Add responsibilities as the client progresses in self-care (assign one or two tasks per week) *to further develop the client's internal locus of control.*

Provide the client with a daily written schedule of activities which he or she is expected to attend and participate in. *The client's contribution in the milieu increases feelings of power over his or her situation and outcome.*

Assist the client to set attainable short-term goals (e.g., attend a meeting once a day for 1 week; be on time for each meal for 1 week) *to ensure achievement and promote sense of control.*

Continue to support and monitor prescribed medical and psychosocial treatment plans.

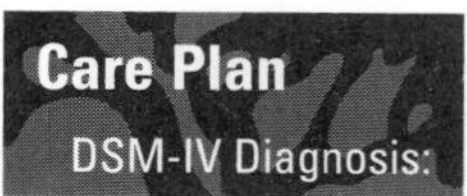

Depression (All Types)

NANDA Diagnosis: Self-care deficit

A state in which an individual experiences an impaired ability to perform or complete feeding, bathing, toileting, dressing, and grooming activities for oneself.

Focus:
For the client whose emotional or mental health is compromised to the extent that he or she cannot provide for basic self-care needs

NANDA Taxonomy

Pattern 6—Moving: A human response pattern involving activity

ETIOLOGIC/RELATED FACTORS (RELATED TO)

Depressed mood
Hyperactivity/distractibility (e.g., as in mania)
Decreased activity/energy
Apathy/withdrawal
Extreme or continuous anxiety
Perceptual or cognitive impairment
Developmental lag

DEFINING CHARACTERISTICS (AS EVIDENCED BY)

Inability to maintain appearance at satisfactory, age-appropriate level, e.g., unkempt hair, clothing, and appearance
Inadequate personal hygiene (foul body and mouth odor)
Infrequent, ineffective bathing or showering
Inadequate toileting (urine and stool stains found on undergarments)
Failure to launder clothing
Repeatedly wears soiled clothing
Unshaven facial hair (male)
Absence of makeup in female client who previously used it

OUTCOME IDENTIFICATION AND EVALUATION

Consistently performs self-care activities in accordance with ability, health status, and developmental stage (bathes, dresses, grooms, brushes teeth, toilets, launders clothes)

PLANNING AND IMPLEMENTATION

Nursing Interventions and Rationale

Continue to assess the extent to which self-care deficits interfere with the client's functions *to evaluate his or her strengths as well as areas that require assistance.*

Assist with personal hygiene, appropriate dress, grooming, and laundering until the client can function independently, *to preserve his or her dignity and self-esteem.*

Reduce environmental stimulation such as noise, lights, bright colors, and people during self-care activity times, especially for clients with hyperactivity, mania, anxiety, and perceptual or cognitive impairments. *A quieter environment is more soothing to the senses and tends to decrease the client's anxiety to allow better concentration on tasks.*

Make available only the clothing that the client is going to wear; and more clothing as the client's judgment and attention span improve. *Reducing the number of choices will minimize the client's confusion and simplify the selection process.*

Provide clean clothing and grooming and toileting supplies as needed; obtain the client's own clothing and supplies as quickly as possible. *The client will feel more comfortable and less confused if personal supplies are available.*

Establish routine goals for self-care, adding more complex tasks and increasing frequency as the client's condition improves (e.g., bathe or shower each day, brush teeth twice daily, comb hair every morning, wash clothes twice a week). *Routine and structure tend to organize the client's chaotic world and promote success.*

Initiate grooming and hygiene tasks when clients are best able to comply. *Depressed clients may have more energy and brighter affect later in the day, and clients with anxiety and hyperactive behaviors may be more attentive to self-care after taking medication.*

Encourage the client to initiate the activity of grooming even when he or she does not feel like doing so. *The very act of grooming and its results influence attitude.*

Provide privacy during self-care in accordance with safety factors, *to preserve the client's dignity.*

Protect the client from the ridicule and manipulation of other clients, *to prevent embarrassment and emotional or physical trauma.*

Praise the client for attempts at self-care and each successfully completed task, *to increase feelings of self-worth and promote continuity of positive behaviors.*

Teach the family the importance of promoting the client's self-care abilities. *This provides consistency between the hospital and home environment and assures the client's progress while decreasing the client's dependency.*

Continue to support and monitor prescribed medical and psychosocial treatment plans.

Nursing Process for

Mania

Universal Principles for Interactions and Interventions with Clients Who Are Experiencing Manic Episodes

- Continue to monitor assessment parameters listed under *Defining Characteristics.*
- Continue to consider the etiologic factors listed under *Etiologic/Related Factors.*
- Utilize principles of the *Therapeutic Nurse-Client Relationship* (Appendix G).
- Address clients' spiritual and cultural needs.

General Principles

- Protect the client from destructive behaviors toward self and/or others.
- Maintain adequate nutrition (which requires normal salt intake for clients on lithium), rest, and hygiene.
- Modify an environment that is overstimulating.
- Control hyperactive behavior.
- Provide goal-directed activities.
- Modify manipulative behavior.
- Promote appropriate socialization and support systems.
- Maintain physiologic and psychologic integrity.
- Teach the client how to identify psychosocial stressors and how to recognize, manage, and prevent symptoms.
- Educate clients about medication effects

Care Plans for Mania

DSM-IV Diagnoses

Bipolar I Disorder
Bipolar II Disorder
Cyclothymic Disorder

NANDA Diagnoses

Violence, risk for: self-directed
Violence, risk for: directed at others
Injury, risk for
Social interaction, impaired
Thought processes, altered
Coping, defensive
Nutrition, altered: less than body requirements
Self-care deficit

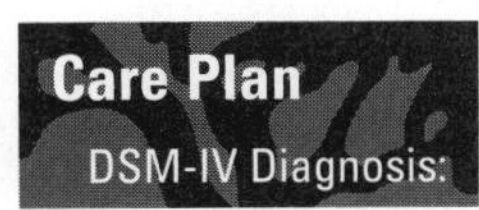

Mania (All Types)

NANDA Diagnosis: Violence, risk for: self-directed; Violence, risk for: directed at others

The state in which an individual experiences behaviors that can be physically harmful either to the self or others

Focus:
For the client with mania whose negative, uncontrolled thoughts, feelings, and behaviors pose a threat or danger to self or others

NANDA Taxonomy
Pattern 9—Feeling: A human response pattern involving the subjective awareness of information

RISK FACTORS

History of attempts to harm self or others during manic phase
History of another's death as a result of client's abuse
History of substance use/abuse
Makes overt attempts to harm self or others
Verbalizes intent to harm self or others
Demonstrates aggressive behaviors and mannerisms—hits/kicks objects; clenched fists, rigid posture, taut facial muscles
Exhibits increasing motor activity with agitation—paces back and forth, bumps into furniture/objects/people
Scans environment with angry, startled, or frightened facial expression
States that others in the environment are threatening or planning to harm or kill client
Verbalizes that he or she is omnipotent or destructive
Demonstrates inability to exercise self-control
States feeling threatened, closed in, or crowded

OUTCOME IDENTIFICATION AND EVALUATION

Verbalizes ability to recognize and describe early symptoms of escalating anxiety/agitation that may lead to violence, and takes necessary steps to interrupt them
Demonstrates absence of verbal intentions to harm self or others
Demonstrates absence of violent or aggressive behaviors

PLANNING AND IMPLEMENTATION

Nursing Interventions and Rationale

Instruct the client to seek out staff when experiencing feelings of agitation, hostility, or suspiciousness, *to help the client prevent violent episodes by redirecting negative feelings in a socially acceptable way, such as talking and exercising.*
Engage the client in gross motor activities such as walking or running, *to expend and refocus energy, decrease anxiety, and regain control and organization over behavior.*
Engage in brief, frequent contacts with the client throughout the day rather than getting involved in lengthy discussions, *as client can better tolerate short interactions. It also lets the client know that he or she is worthy of time and attention, even though his or her behavior is not always acceptable.*
Encourage journal writing or maintaining a log or diary to record feelings/symptoms on a daily basis, when capable, *to attempt to connect negative feelings with events that may invoke them and learn to manage or avoid such situations when possible.*
Conduct a suicide assessment, e.g., listen for verbal threats; observe threatening gestures, *to intervene early and prevent harm, injury or death.* (See Appendix J.)
Teach the client and family to recognize early signs/symptoms of escalating behavior and to seek appropriate help (medication, other resources, learned strategies, professional intervention), *to interrupt escalating behaviors before client reaches a full-blown manic state and/or violence.*
Praise client for efforts made to control anger or aggression directed at self or others. *Positive feedback reinforces repetition of functional behaviors.*
Administer prn medication when warranted, *to help calm client and reduce the risk of violent, destructive behavior.*
Seclude and restrain the client if necessary, according to hospital policy, *to protect client and others from harm.* (See Appendix L.)

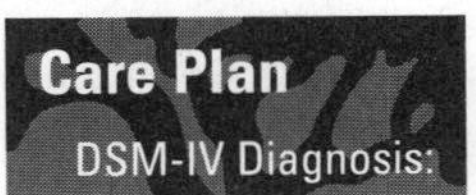

Mania (All Types)

NANDA Diagnosis: Injury, risk for

A state in which an individual is at risk for injury as a result of environmental conditions interacting with the individual's adaptive and defensive resources

Focus:
For the client who is susceptible to injury as a result of excessive interaction or collision with environmental obstacles due to impulsive, hyperactive, and/or intrusive behaviors

NANDA Taxonomy
Pattern 1—Exchanging: A human response pattern involving mutual giving and receiving

RISK FACTORS

Increased internal stimulation secondary to biologic alterations (e.g., neurophysiologic, genetic, structural)
Environmental stressors that exceed coping abilities
History of injury during manic phase
Hyperactivity/distractibility
Impulsivity/intrusiveness
Inattentive to environmental obstacles
Grandiosity (attempts feats beyond capabilities, e.g., jogging, jumping, tumbling, lifting heavy objects, punching hard objects with bare fists)

OUTCOME IDENTIFICATION AND EVALUATION

Maintains physical integrity
Demonstrates awareness of physical environment in proximity to body boundaries
Exhibits decreased hyperactivity (able to walk around environment more slowly)
Manifests reduced impulsivity (reacts more slowly appropriately to internal and external stimuli)
Avoids obstacles when moving around environment
Attempts activities within physical capabilities

PLANNING AND IMPLEMENTATION

Nursing Interventions and Rationale

Reduce or minimize environmental stimulation *to promote a quiet, soothing environment, which may assuage the client's internal stimulation, reduce the client's hyperactivity, and prevent accident or injury.*

Remove furniture with sharp edges or place as close to the wall as possible *to prevent accident or injury.*

Provide frequent, quiet time-outs, especially following a stimulating experience, *to calm the client by providing opportunities for rest and relaxation and reduce the risk for injury.*

Accompany the client on walks and provide other gross motor activities in an open, secure area *to expend and refocus energy.*

Praise client for efforts made to utilize energy productively and avoid injury. *Positive feedback reinforces adaptive behaviors.*

Engage the family in efforts to minimize the client's risk for injury and maximize safety. *Families who are included in relevant areas of the client's treatment plan are more empowered to help the client maintain a safe, secure environment.*

Continue to support and monitor prescribed medical and psychosocial treatment plans *to prevent escalating behaviors and subsequent injury.*

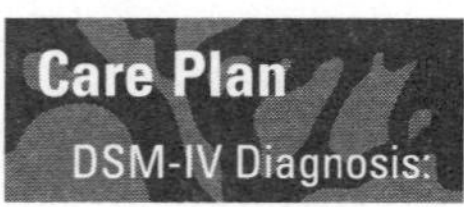

Mania (All Types)

NANDA Diagnosis: Social interactions, impaired

The state in which an individual participates in an insufficient or excessive quantity or ineffective quality of social exchange

---

Focus:
For the client who demonstrates hyperactive behavior that is incompatible with effective interpersonal interactions

NANDA Taxonomy
Pattern 3—Relating: A human response pattern involving established bonds

---

ETIOLOGIC/RELATED FACTORS (RELATED TO)

Expansive, irritable mood
Hyperactivity (motor/verbal)
Impaired judgment
Impulsivity
Altered thought processes (paranoia/grandiosity)
Biologic alterations (e.g., genetic, neurophysiologic, structural)

DEFINING CHARACTERISTIC (AS EVIDENCED BY)

Invades others' personal space and property
Interrupts others' conversations and activities
Uses critical, sarcastic, insulting, or sexually provocative dialogue
Engages in sexually provocative behavior in the presence of staff and clients, e.g., wears seductive, inappropriate clothing; tells lewd stories or jokes, makes obscene remarks about other's attributes
Damages or steals other people's possessions
Is unable to sit through or participate in group activities
Blames others without substantiation
Uses incomprehensible, rapid, forced speech pattern
Claims to be omnipotent or famous, e.g., "I'm God . . . Superman . . . the devil . . . the president."
Demonstrates flamboyant, excessively gregarious behavior
Changes clothing several times a day (often dresses in bizarre, garish attire with loud, bright colors that are mismatched or uncoordinated)
States that he or she has "racing" thoughts

OUTCOME IDENTIFICATION AND EVALUATION

Identifies self accurately to others
Listens to others converse without interrupting
Communicates with others by using appropriate language, tone, and speech pattern
Maintains adequate distance from others when interacting
Refrains from violating or damaging others' property
Dresses and grooms appropriately for age and status
Participates in individual, milieu, and group activities without outbursts or disruptions
Identifies escalating behaviors and takes steps to circumvent them
Acknowledges reasons for and necessity of compliance with medication regimen

PLANNING AND IMPLEMENTATION

Nursing Interventions and Rationale

Actively listen, observe, and respond to the client's verbal and nonverbal expressions. *Active listening signifies unconditional respect and regard for the client. It builds trust and rapport, guides the nurse toward problem areas, and encourages the client to express concerns and continue in the interactive process.*

Redirect negative behaviors in a calm, firm, nondefensive manner (suggest a walk, physical activity, or time-out). *This provides a healthier avenue to direct energy and prevents further escalation of behavior.*

Provide activities that are suitable to client's level of tolerance and capability and are noncompetitive, e.g., a brisk walk, physical exercise, stationary bicycle, *to avoid frustration and resultant outbursts or sense of failure.*

Initiate a verbal or written contract that clearly describes appropriate social behaviors, if warranted, *to assist client to comply with unit and milieu rules and to avoid disruptions that affect other clients and their attitude toward the client who has mania.*

Protect other clients from impact of negative behaviors *to prevent emotional and physical trauma.* (Increase staff-per-client ratio.)

Set limits on the client's intrusive, interruptive behavior:

"When you keep interrupting, it is difficult to stay on the topic, so please wait for your turn." "It's Sam's turn to speak now; when your turn comes, no one will interrupt you."

This helps the client develop awareness and attain/maintain control, and helps others to tolerate his or her presence.

Demonstrate appropriate role-modeling during one-to-one and group activities, *to promote change by example.*

Offer feedback concerning the effect of negative behaviors on others, when the client is able to be receptive. "Others leave the area when you interrupt them and behave in a disruptive manner." *Awareness of how others view him or her provides impetus for change.*

Assist the client to develop more productive ways to meet needs and achieve goals, e.g., activities, games, physical exercises, *so patient need not rely on dysfunctional nonproductive methods of meeting needs.*

Assist the client with tasks of eating, grooming, and hygiene. *This prevents ridicule from other clients and preserves dignity.*

Praise the client for attempting and using socially appropriate behaviors. "You spoke up in group very appropriately today." *This provides feedback, promotes subsequent appropriateness, and increases self-esteem.*

Help the client achieve effective, independent problem solving *to foster independence and decrease regression.*

Encourage the client to verbalize feelings rather than acting out. *This prevents negative consequences, defuses hostile feelings, and promotes impulse control.*

Initiate frequent, brief contacts with the client. *Brief contact allows continual monitoring of communication capabilities; the client cannot tolerate long interactions.*

Gradually engage the client in interactions with other clients, beginning with one-to-one contacts and progressing toward more formalized groups. *Level of tolerance must be considered for the client to succeed in socialization skills.*

Include the family in those aspects of the client's treatment plan that relate to socialization and interactive skills. *Families that are aware of the client's problems with social skills are better equipped to respond in a more effective way, and more willing to learn the social skills necessary for more successful family-client interactions.*

Assist the client in identification of escalating behaviors. "What do you feel just before you begin to act in a disruptive manner?" "What are some clues that let you know you're angry enough to act aggressively?" *This gives the client the opportunity to seek help from staff or engage in acceptable activity before losing control.*

Set constructive limits on manipulative behavior in accordance with the client's ability to comply. *Guidelines are necessary to maintain control.*

Administer routine prn medications judiciously *to reduce and minimize manic symptoms.*

Seclude the client and/or administer medication when the client is unable to maintain control. *Seclusion helps the client to regain control and composure and prevents harm to the client and others.* (See Appendix L.)

Continue to support and monitor prescribed medical and psychosocial treatment plans.

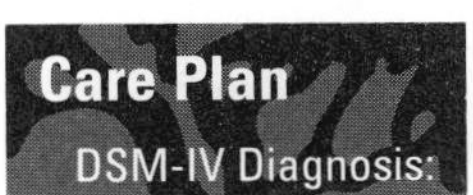

Mania (All Types)

NANDA Diagnosis: Thought processes, altered

A state in which an individual experiences a disruption in cognitive operations and activities

---

Focus:
For the client who has impaired judgment, insight, comprehension, perception, and problem-solving abilities and who may experience flight of ideas and delusions or ideas of reference

NANDA Taxonomy
Pattern 8—Knowing: A human response pattern involving the meaning associated with information

---

ETIOLOGIC/RELATED FACTORS (RELATED TO)

Ineffective processing and synthesis of internal and environmental stimuli

Anxiety secondary to the manic state

Low self-esteem

Psychosocial stressors

Biologic alterations (e.g., neurophysiologic, genetic, structural)

DEFINING CHARACTERISTICS (AS EVIDENCED BY)

Inaccurate interpretation of environmental events and incoming information (e.g., mistakes a friendly gesture as a potentially harmful or violent act)

Inaccurate belief about self or others (e.g., believes he or she was sent by God to save mankind—a delusion of grandeur, to compensate for feelings of low self-esteem)

Believes others in the milieu are planning to kill or harm him (delusion of persecution, represents fear or threat to the self-system)

Exaggerated, inappropriate, or disruptive behaviors and reactions directed toward the environment and others (e.g., laughs or talks too loudly, uses foul or sexually explicit language)

Inability to follow or comprehend the directions of others, unrelated to language or cultural differences
Confused about the circumstances surrounding admission to the mental health facility
Unable to see self as ill and in need of treatment:
"I'm only here to have my ankle checked. It's swollen." (Client is unaware the ankle was injured during manic episode.)
Impaired judgment or decision-making or problem-solving abilities (e.g., attempts activities or feats beyond capabilities; wears loud, garish, bizarre clothing combinations; has careless hygiene, bathing, and grooming habits)
Suspiciousness, anger, or fear projected toward the environment and others
Describes thoughts as "racing" (flight of ideas)
Rapidly shifts from topic to topic (flight of ideas)
Uses pressured speech (can not express thoughts quickly enough)
Is preoccupied with sexual, religious, political, or financial ideas (may be delusional)
Refuses to eat, drink, or take medication (may reflect persecutory thoughts that someone wants to poison him/her)

OUTCOME IDENTIFICATION AND EVALUATION

Expresses logical, goal-directed thoughts and ideas with absence of delusions
Solves problems and makes decisions appropriate for age and status
Demonstrates socially appropriate behaviors

PLANNING AND IMPLEMENTATION

Nursing Interventions and Rationale

Listen actively for key themes, meanings, feelings, and reality-oriented words or phrases, *to build trust, compare content and intent, meet the client's needs, and encourage the client to relate to others. Many clients resist becoming involved in a therapeutic alliance, so acceptance and perseverance are necessary.*

Assist the client to correct misinterpretations about the environment, self, and experiences, through recall of events and problem solving, *to encourage reality orientation:*

"Let's go back and discuss what happened one step at a time."

Convey acceptance of the client's need to hold onto the false belief while not agreeing with the delusion itself.

Therapeutic response

"I find that hard to believe, but it sounds as if it's troubling for you."

"I'm not sure what you mean, but I'm trying to understand how you feel."

Nontherapeutic response:

"If you really believe that, I won't disagree."

"Whatever you say is right."

Acceptance of the client and his or her needs and condition builds trust and preserves the client's dignity and self-esteem, whereas agreement with the belief system would imply that it is real and further confuse the client.

Focus on the meaning, feeling, or intent engendered by the client's delusions—not the content—*to help meet the client's needs, reinforce reality, and discourage false beliefs.*

Therapeutic response:

"It sounds as if you're feeling threatened. How can staff help you?"

"Do you mean that you're feeling sad or lonely?"

Nontherapeutic response:

"Describe those people you say are out to get you."

Avoid challenging the clients delusional system or arguing with the client, because *it may diminish trust, incite a volatile response, or force the client to cling to the false belief in order to preserve his or her dignity and self-esteem.*

Nontherapeutic response:

"I don't believe that and no one else does either."

"If you're really God, how come you got sick?"

Distract the client from the delusion at the first sign of anxiety or escalating behaviors by introducing a less volatile topic or suggesting an activity:

"Let's talk about today's activities for a while."

"I think a walk around the unit would be helpful now."

"It might be a good time to finish our Ping Pong game; we can talk again this afternoon."

Distracting the client from troubling delusions that threaten loss of control interrupts the client's volatile, agitated state and allows him or her to focus energies toward productive, less provocative activities. Discussion can resume when client is less agitated.

Gradually encourage the client to discuss his or her experiences prior to onset of the delusion, *to help the client identify threatening thoughts and feelings and connect them to real situations rather than to delusional content:*

"What happened just before you started thinking that your roommate was stealing your clothes?"

"When your wife phoned to say she wouldn't visit you today, how did it make you feel?"

Focus on real topics and events that anyone can relate to, such as the weather, movies, or music, and avoid volatile subjects such as sex, politics, or religion. *This distracts the client from focusing on delusional content and brings the client closer to a commonly shared reality.*

Offer praise as soon as the client begins to differentiate between reality-based and nonreality-based thinking. "What you're saying now is clear and makes sense." "The group's response to your statements showed that they understand your meaning." *Positive reinforcement increases self-esteem and encourages continued reality-based thoughts and behaviors.*

Teach the client to interrupt irrational thoughts or replace them with rational ones and to notify staff when irrational thoughts begin *in order to break the pattern of illogical thinking and prevent further impairment of thought processes.* (See Appendix K, Thought-Substitution/Thought-Stopping Strategies.)

Refrain from the use of touch with delusional clients, especially if thoughts reflect ideas of persecution, *because clients who are suspicious or paranoid may perceive touch as threatening, may misinterpret intentions, and/or may respond with aggression.*

Give simple, concrete explanations and avoid abstractions or metaphors.

Therapeutic response:

"It's time to get out of bed."

Nontherapeutic response:

"Time to rise and shine."

Clients with altered thought processes interpret abstractions concretely and will misunderstand the message.

Assist the client with hygiene, bathing, and grooming until judgment regarding basic needs returns, *to preserve dignity and self-esteem and prevent the client from becoming an object of ridicule.*

Allow the client to select his or her own food and drink, read the labels, and open his or her own unit-dose medication packets *to offer the client more control during those times when the client cannot be dissuaded from the belief that his or her food or medicine may be "contaminated" or "poisoned." (This is not an unspoken agreement that the delusion is factual but rather an attempt to provide the client with the nutrition needed to sustain life and the medication needed to encourage reality-based thoughts.)*

Therapeutic response:

"I don't believe your food is poisoned, but you may get yourself another tray of food today."

"This is the medication you've been taking all along. Read the name and open the packet yourself."

Nontherapeutic response:

"Of course the food isn't contaminated. Would we serve bad food to clients?"

"If you refuse your medication, I'll have to call your doctor and you'll probably get a shot."

Correct with simple, factual information the client's misinterpretation of others in the environment who the client may feel are threatening or dangerous:

"Those two clients are Tom and Joe, and they're talking about baseball."

"That's Dr. Smith who is here to see your roommate."

Such clarifying statements serve to allay the client's fears and suspicions about others in the environment and bring relief and security.

Clarify the client's identity and status and that of the caregiver *to counteract the belief that client and staff have other identities and purposes:*

"You're William Brown, and you're a client here at Hillview Hospital."

"I'm Sara Smith, the nurse assigned to this unit today."

Inform the client when his or her behavior is not acceptable and direct him or her toward activities or solutions that encourage more appropriate behaviors, in a firm but nonthreatening manner. *Note:* Irrational thoughts can invoke inappropriate behavior. If behavior escalates, the client may require seclusion or seclusion and restraint. (See Appendix L.)

Therapeutic response:

"Harassing other clients in the group activity is not acceptable here. I'll go with you for a walk around the patio, which will release some of that energy."

"Other clients are disturbed when you curse and talk about sex so much. This might be a good time to play that game of Ping-Pong on the patio."

These statements inform the client that although the behavior is not acceptable, the client is still worthy of help. Firm, nonthreatening directives guide the client whose thoughts and actions are out of control toward more appropriate methods by which to gain control. The client relies on the nurse and other caregivers to intervene in such circumstances and provide safety and security.

Nontherapeutic response:

"You're behaving badly and need to control yourself or someone is going to get hurt."

"If you continue to talk like that, no one here will want to be around you."

These statements indicate that the client has the power to control his or her behavior and, if not, he or she is threatened with painful, frightening consequences.

Teach the family about the dynamics underlying the client's altered thoughts and how to best respond to the client. *Families who are empowered with knowledge (within their capabilities) are better able to manage family-client interactions and are less fearful toward the client.*

Continue to support and monitor prescribed medical and psychosocial treatment plans, *to help manage anxiety and delusions and increase reality-based thoughts.*

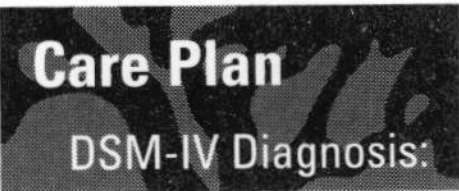

Mania (All Types)

NANDA Diagnoses: Coping, defensive

The state in which an individual repeatedly projects falsely positive self-evaluation based on a self-protective pattern that defends against underlying perceived threats to positive self-regard

Focus:

For the client with mania who defends against feelings of inadequacy, insecurity, anger, fear, and anxiety by using coping mechanisms in a maladaptive way, in an effort to increase self-esteem and raise self-concept/image

NANDA Taxonomy

Pattern 5—Choosing: A human response pattern involving the selection of alternatives

ETIOLOGIC/RELATED FACTORS (RELATED TO)

Irrational beliefs and assumptions, unrealistic perceptions of self and/or situation (long-standing)

Disturbed relationships (neglectful, domineering, overprotective, abusive)
Identity problems (self, sexual)
Goal obstacles (Goals may be unrealistic or unattainable.)
Social learning patterns
Impaired self-concept, self-esteem, self-image
Low impulse control
Knowledge deficit regarding coping methods
Stressors that exceed coping abilities

DEFINING CHARACTERISTICS (AS EVIDENCED BY)

Excessive use of makeup, jewelry, toiletries, color of clothing
Changes clothes several times a day
Restless, hyperalert
Hyperverbal
Confrontational, "testy" with staff and other clients
Blames others for unsubstantiated acts
Rationalizes when explaining behaviors, situations, or ideas
Swears, shouts
Becomes angry when intentions or activities are thwarted
Nonparticipative in activities with others (short attention span)
Difficulty interacting and communicating (boisterous, intrusive, boastful)
Delusional, grandiose, and boastful regarding identity/importance/knowledge, *or* may be delusionally paranoid:
"I'm God . . . Superman . . . the devil . . . the president."
"I know the secrets of the universe."
"Everyone wants to rob me of my powers."

OUTCOME IDENTIFICATION AND EVALUATION

Dresses appropriately in relation to status and situation, with minimal changes of clothing
Uses moderate makeup, jewelry, and other accessories
Waits turn to speak
Refrains from interrupting groups, conversations, activities
Uses nonoffensive, moderate speech (tone, amount, frequency)
Refrains from hyperactivity (able to sit still and engage in group and one-to-one conversation)
Uses defense mechanisms more adaptively
Explores beliefs, problems, and values with staff
Discusses perceived threats to self-system with staff
Ceases to "split" staff when feeling threatened or vulnerable; relies on staff for appropriate support
Recognizes when he or she has gained control and discusses this with staff
Expresses recognition of attempts by staff and other clients to help support him or her
Decreases manipulation of staff and clients
Adheres to prescribed facility regimen
Absence of delusional or boastful behaviors

PLANNING AND IMPLEMENTATION

Nursing Interventions With Rationale

Protect the client from embarrassment and ridicule that may occur during uninhibited behavior. *Behaviors such as undressing in public, sexually explicit acting out, and threats to others may be a source of embarrassment for the client following a manic phase. Staff awareness can intercept or prevent this, preserve dignity, and promote self-esteem through intervening on the client's behalf.*

State and restate, when necessary, in a calm matter-of-fact way all unit rules, dress codes, and makeup codes. *Repetition of rules may be necessary during a manic phase when the client has difficulty concentrating and is impulsive. When done in a nonthreatening, consistent way, this can serve as a stable external source of structure for the client. Authoritarian statements may antagonize the client, as clients with mania have low tolerance for authority.*

Therapeutic response:
"The television hours are from 6 to 10 PM, Tom. It's 11 PM and the TV will be off so that others can sleep."
"Here are two outfits, Sally. Select one and I'll put the other one away."

Nontherapeutic response:
"I've told you a dozen times why you can't watch TV, so turn if off now and get to bed."

Present a unified approach when interacting with the client, enforcing unit rules, and meeting client's needs. *A unified staff promotes structure and consistency for the client and diminishes confusion. It also reduces imposed isolation that individual staff may experience when not working as a team.*

Provide a mature role model for the client. *Acting-out behaviors by the client will decrease as he or she learns adaptive coping skills by identifying with positive staff behaviors.*

Inform the client that staff believes he or she is capable of meeting his or her own needs and that staff will help the client accomplish this:
"I know you want me to make your bed, but I think you can do it. I'll stay with you until you're through."
Staff expressions of support and belief in the client's ability increase the client's confidence, self-esteem, and sense of security.

Praise the client for attempts to achieve realistic goals. *Praise serves as a guide for expected behavior, and rewarded behavior tends to be repeated.*
"You were able to sit for 15 minutes in group today; that's a real improvement."
"You were able to get dressed and make your own bed before breakfast. That's a big accomplishment."

Encourage the client to express feelings and explore false self-assumptions and beliefs:
"You said you felt more important when you were telling others you were a hospital administrator. Let's discuss important aspects of going to college as you had been doing."

Through discussions with therapeutic staff members, the client gains insight, becomes more realistic, and is able to modify maladaptive responses.

Praise client for statements of realistic self-appraisal and insights:

"I'm glad you're aware that the symptoms recurred when you stopped taking the medication and that you see that relief of symptoms helps you manage your life."

Positive reinforcement strengthens and perpetuates insight and judgment.

Provide activities and opportunities for the client to interact with others in appropriate ways. *This allows the client to gain support, learn vicariously, and expend energy adaptively and encourages reality-based thinking.*

Support the family in their effort to effectively interact with the client in light of the client's defensive coping style. *Families need continued encouragement in maintaining appropriate family-client interactions.*

Set limits in a nonpunitive way on behavior that is unacceptable or threatening to staff and client (blaming swearing, confronting), *to help client regain control, prevent client from alienating others, and preserve his or her self-esteem.*

Continue to support and monitor prescribed medical and psychosocial treatment plans.

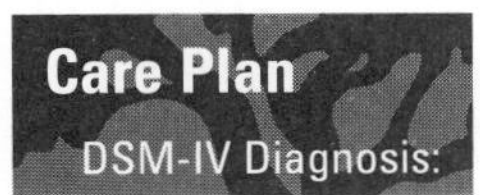

Mania (All Types)

NANDA DIAGNOSIS: Nutrition, altered: less than body requirements

The state in which an individual experiences an intake of nutrients insufficient to meet metabolic needs

---

Focus:

For the client whose nutritional state may be compromised because of hyperactive behaviors that distract the client from the social and physical functions of eating. There is also a danger of decreased salt intake, which could lead to lithium retention and subsequent toxicity (body will use lithium if blood sodium is insufficient).

NANDA Taxonomy

Pattern 1—Exchanging: A human response pattern involving mutual giving and receiving

---

ETIOLOGIC/RELATED FACTORS (RELATED TO)

Inadequate intake and hypermetabolic need secondary to the manic state

Loss of appetite secondary to constipation and/or urinary retention

Diarrhea and/or excessive perspiration

Paranoid delusion (belief that food is poisoned or contaminated)

Grandiose delusion (belief that food is unnecessary owing to the client's omnipotent state)

DEFINING CHARACTERISTICS (AS EVIDENCED BY)

At least 20% less than ideal body weight

Distracted from task of eating and drinking

Unable to sit through routine meals

Reported food and fluid intake less than recommended daily allowance

Appears wary or frightened when offered food

Frequently refuses to eat or drink

Dry mouth

Sore, inflamed buccal cavity

Pale mucous membranes and conjunctivae

Capillary fragility

Loose, dry skin turgor/decreased subcutaneous fat

Poor muscle tone

Fluid and electrolytes below normal levels

Hyperactive bowel sounds

Shakiness/tremulousness secondary to increased lithium level

Nausea/gastrointestinal upset secondary to increased lithium level

OUTCOME IDENTIFICATION AND EVALUATION

Consumes adequate daily calories per kilogram of body weight

Eats adequate amounts of different food groups

Fluid intake equal to output

Demonstrates and maintains ideal body weight

Has fluid and electrolyte levels within normal range

Exhibits no signs of lithium toxicity

Skin turgor and muscle tone reveal nutritional state commensurate with physiologic and metabolic needs

PLANNING AND IMPLEMENTATION

Nursing Interventions and Rationale

Offer frequent carbohydrate and protein snacks. *Protein is necessary for building and repairing body cells and tissues. Carbohydrates are needed for energy.*

Offer nutritious finger foods and sandwiches, *to provide convenient methods for eating and maintaining nutritional integrity.*

Offer easy-to-carry drinks that are high in vitamins, minerals, and electrolytes, *to provide convenient methods for hydration and nutrition and to maintain fluid and electrolyte levels.*

Regularly assess fluid and electrolyte status, especially sodium and lithium levels, *to prevent lithium toxicity.* (See Appendix M.)

Continually assess urinary output. *Polyuria is a common side effect of lithium because of polydipsia, and clients need to be kept well-hydrated.* (See Appendix M.)

Check time, frequency, and consistency of bowel movements *to determine client's bowel function and regularity. Liquid, diarrheal, or tarry stools may indicate possible impaction, dehydration, or ulcerative condition.*

Assess for abdominal pain or discomfort because *client may be constipated or obstructed.*

If warranted, examine abdomen for firmness *to assess for possible constipation.*

If warranted, auscultate abdomen in all four quadrants *to assess for presence and frequency of bowel sounds because hypoactive or absent bowel sounds may indicate serious pathology.*

Administer high-fiber foods unless contraindicated, increased amounts of liquids, and prescribed stool softeners *to prevent or relieve constipation and increase appetite and hydration.*

Examine the urinary bladder for firmness *to assess for urinary retention and need for increased fluid and/or catheterization.*

Assess delusional system in a simple, nonchallenging manner *as a possible reason for food and fluid avoidance, because the client may believe the food is poisoned or contaminated.*

Therapeutic response:

"You're not eating and seem troubled."

This statement lets the client know feelings of fear or threat to the self-system are acknowledged and accepted, and he or she is more likely to reveal the delusion.

Therapeutic response:

"I don't believe the food is poisoned but I know you do right now. I'll come with you to select your food and stay with you when you eat."

This statement reflects the nurse's understanding of the client's fear by offering to help the client select food that may be more acceptable and by remaining with the client throughout the meal. At the same time, by not agreeing with the client's false belief, the statement presents reality in a nonchallenging manner and allows the client to maintain control and dignity.

Nontherapeutic response:

"You can trust the food here. You know you have to eat."

This statement, although well-meaning, does not acknowledge the feelings generated by the delusion that the food may be poisoned. It challenges the client's false belief and intimates that the client has no alternative. The client is thus likely to cling to the delusion in an effort to preserve control and self-esteem.

Offer alternative selections of foods and fluids in a direct, calm manner versus an authoritarian, threatening approach *to provide variety and promote interest in eating without resistance.*

Reduce stimulation (noise, lights) when the client is ready to resume meals in the dining room *to promote a more relaxing atmosphere conducive to eating.*

Praise the client for any attempts to eat or drink *to promote continuity of positive behaviors.*

Educate the client, family, and significant others about the need for adequate nutritional intake *to maintain physiologic integrity and bowel and bladder function.*

Teach the client and significant others about the need for adequate sodium intake *to prevent lithium toxicity. Inform them that lithium is a salt and that reduced sodium intake can result in lithium retention with subsequent toxicity; thus salt should not be eliminated from the client's regular diet.*

Describe the signs of lithium toxicity to the client, family, and significant others and elicit their feedback *to ascertain that they are able to differentiate between the expected effects and toxic effects of lithium.* *(See Appendix M.)*

Continue to support and monitor prescribed medical, psychosocial, and dietary treatment plans *to maintain physiologic and psychosocial integrity.*

The Schizophrenias and Other Psychotic Disorders

Schizophrenia is not a single disorder but a group of related disorders characterized by disordered thinking and perceptions. It may manifest as withdrawal from reality, acute psychotic episodes, disorganized or regressive behavior, altered affect, impaired communication, and impaired interpersonal relationships. Schizophrenia is a disorder with psychotic symptoms; however, not all psychoses are schizophrenia.

Some individuals experience one or several schizophrenic episodes and recover completely; however, most people who suffer from schizophrenia have a chronic course of multiple exacerbations with only occasional incomplete remissions. Because the schizophrenias are so little understood by the public, people with chronic schizophrenia are frequently forced to live outside the mainstream of society in unhappy, unfulfilled lives, often joining the ranks of the homeless. Their families often suffer consequences of the disorder as well. The affected member may be seen as a burden to the family and society because of the pervasive, chronic nature of the disorder, which affects the individual's personality even during times of remission.

ETIOLOGY

Specific etiologic factors related to schizophrenia are listed in Box 4-1.

EPIDEMIOLOGY

It is estimated that about 200,000 new cases of schizophrenia are diagnosed each year in the United States, and 2 million worldwide. Approximately 1% of the U.S. population have schizophrenia.

The onset of schizophrenia usually occurs in late adolescence or early adulthood, and onset sometimes occurs after age 50, though less frequently. It is equally prevalent in males and females and is described in all cultures and socioeconomic classes. The incidence is higher in the lower socioeconomic classes, a finding that may be due in part to the multiple psychosocial stressors that prevail in this group. Marriage and fertility rates have substantially increased among persons with schizophrenia, and the number of children born to parents with schizophrenia is on the rise. The risk of becoming schizophrenic increases significantly when one or both parents have the disorder.

The mortality rate related to both natural causes and suicide is higher for individuals with the disorder than for others. It is estimated that 50% of people with schizophrenia attempt suicide, and a high percentage succeed. Schizophrenia is the costliest mental disorder in terms of loss of productivity; half the U.S. hospital beds designated for mental illness are occupied by persons with schizophrenia, with a cost equal to 2% of the gross national product.

ASSESSMENT OF SCHIZOPHRENIA AND OTHER PSYCHOTIC DISORDERS

The symptom pattern for schizophrenia is multifaceted. Symptoms seen in schizophrenia may also be seen in other mental disorders, so a careful history, complete with family factors and premorbid function, is necessary

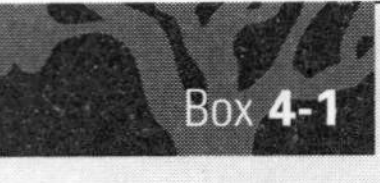

Box 4-1 Specific Etiologic Factors Related to Schizophrenia and Other Psychotic Disorders*

Biologic

Neuropathology

Dysregulation of neurotransmitters in the brain (dopaminergic hypothesis)
Neurodegeneration; cell loss or abnormal histology
Enlargement of ventricles of the brain
Cortical atrophy

Psychoneuroimmunology/Endocrinology

Slow viruses or other infectious agents cause immune dysfunction
Autoimmune dysfunction
Hormonal dysregulation

Genetic

Specific genetic markers probable in some studies
Incidence is considerably higher for children when one or both parents have schizophrenia or if one identical twin has the disorder

Psychosocial

Psychodynamic therapy

Distortion in infant-nurturer relationship affects ego organization and self-object differentiation

Learning theory

Disordered thinking, irrational reactions, and inadequate social skills are learned by imitating parental figures, resulting in symptoms and deficient interpersonal relationships

Family theory

Patterns of relating and communication among family members cause symptoms and resultant inability to form or maintain relationships

*Although a specific etiology for the schizophrenias has not been established, a combination of biologic, psychosocial, and environmental factors is implicated. Current research is directed toward biologic research studies.

to make the diagnosis. Distinguishing features include the following:

Psychotic symptoms during acute episodes (at least 1 month, active phase)
Functional disturbances (social, occupational, personal)
Symptom disturbances of at least 6 months' duration

Psychotic Symptoms

Definition of the term *psychotic* has historically been controversial and to date has not received universal acceptance. All definitions include presence of delusions or hallucinations. Symptoms of schizophrenia are often described as positive or negative, as follows:

Positive symptoms
Delusions
Hallucinations
Thought insertion; thought withdrawal
Disorganized thoughts
Incoherence
Pressured speech
Behavior (aggressive, agitated, bizarre)
Suicide ideation

Negative symptoms
Anhedonia
Flat affect
Alogia, poverty of speech
Poor eye contact
Poor grooming, hygiene
Decreased spontaneity and gestures
Apathy, lack of volition
Disturbed family relationships

Functional Disturbance

Functional disturbance refers to failure to perform or function at a level equal to previous performance levels or, in the case of a child, failure to achieve an expected level of performance related to age and stage of development. For example, the individual may fail to attain or maintain expected age-appropriate personal care and hygiene, may change communication patterns or decrease or cease communicating with others, or may stop going to school or work.

Period of Disturbance

Symptoms must be present for a 6-month period to make a diagnosis of schizophrenia, and psychotic symptoms must be noted for at least 1 week during an acute phase. Other disorders are ruled out before the diagnosis of schizophrenia is made.

Prodromal and Residual Phases

Symptoms occurring before an acute episode (prodromal phase) or after an acute episode (residual phase) are similar. The prodromal period may begin with the individual's withdrawal, isolative behavior, and lack of energy and initiative. He or she may complain of multiple physical symptoms (back pain, headache, gastrointestinal problems) or become excessively interested in subjects of a religious, occult, or philosophic nature. Peculiar behaviors may be noted by family and peers, who describe that the individual has noticeably changed.

The individual may seem confused or perplexed or have unusual perceptual experiences (e.g., sensing others in the room when no one is present, being controlled by a "force"). Ideas and beliefs become odd or eccentric, and self-care and personal hygiene deteriorate. Affect is blunted or inappropriate, and anxious or angry behaviors may be manifested. When interacting, the individual may be vague, digressive, and lack words to express his or her point or may be overelaborative and circumstantial. These symptoms may occur in the prodromal and residual phases.

Prepsychotic Phase

In the prepsychotic phase the individual may be passive, quiet, and obedient and prefer solitary activities over gregarious ones. He or she may be introverted, withdrawn, suspicious, or eccentric and usually has few, if any, close friends.

Acute Phase

Symptoms of the acute phase of schizophrenia vary widely. Disturbances occur in multiple psychologic and psychosocial areas, including the categories of thought, affect, perception, and behavior.

Thought disturbance. Thought disturbance may be manifested in three major areas: content, form, and process.

Content refers to dysfunctional beliefs, ideas, and interpretations of actual internal and external stimuli. Delusions are examples of disturbed thought content; some common types in schizophrenia are persecutory, grandiose, religious, and somatic. Some examples of delusions are as follows:

The client believes that stereo speakers, TV, or computers are controlling his or her thoughts.

Intergalactic electrical waves are beaming on the world, ready to destroy the client.

The client has the power to change the seasons.

The client has a demon in the stomach that causes sounds.

Other symptoms include thought broadcasting (thoughts or ideas are being transmitted to others), thought insertion (others can put thoughts into the client's mind), and thought withdrawal (thoughts can be taken from the client's mind).

Content disturbance is also noted by ideas of reference, which are beliefs that other people or messages from the media (TV, radio, or newspaper) are directly referring to the client. For example, two strangers may be across the room holding a conversation about the weather, and the client believes they are talking about him or her; the president of the United States gives a speech on TV about the space program, and the individual believes it is a message to become an astronaut.

The client's preoccupation with particular thoughts or ideas that are persistent and cannot be eliminated (obssesional thinking) also represents content disturbance; frequently, such thoughts are accompanied by ritualistic behavior. Schizophrenic clients often make symbolic references to actual persons, objects, or events. For example, the color red may symbolize anger, death, or blood to the client.

Form refers to incoherence, loose associations, tangentiality, circumstantiality, neologisms, word salad, echolalia, perseveration, verbigeration, and autistic and dereistic thinking, all of which are observable by staff as the client speaks or writes.

Process includes thought blocking, poor memory, symbolic or idiosyncratic association, illogical flow of ideas, vagueness, poverty of speech, and impaired ability to abstract (concrete thinking), reason, calculate, and use judgment.

Affective disturbance. Affective disturbance may be characteristically evidenced by flat (blunted) or inappropriate affect. The person with *flat affect* demonstrates little or no emotional responsivity. Facial expression is immobile, voice is monotonous, and the client describes not being able to feel as intensely as he or she once did or not being able to feel at all. *Inappropriate affect* is manifested by emotional expression that is incongruent with verbalizations, situation, or event; client's ideation and description do not match the affective display. For example, the individual may describe the death of a parent and laugh. Other affective manifestations may appear as sudden, unprovoked demonstrations of angry or overly anxious behavior, silliness, or giddiness. The person may be responding to internal stimuli at such times (hallucinations).

Persons with schizophrenia may demonstrate or express a wide range of emotions and say they feel terrified, perplexed, ambivalent, ecstatic, omnipotent, or overwhelmingly alone or that they do not feel anything at all. These clients are frequently not in touch with their feelings or have difficulty expressing them.

Note: Staff's knowledge of the action and adverse effects of antipsychotic medications is essential because affective displays may represent the manifestations of schizophrenia or may be a reaction to the medications. Interventions depend on the nurse's correct assessment. (See Appendix M.)

Perceptual disturbance. Perceptual disturbances may include hallucinations, illusions, and boundary and identity problems.

Hallucinations. A common perceptual dysfunction in schizophrenia is the hallucination, a sensory perception by an individual that is not associated with actual external stimuli. Although hallucinations may occur in any of the senses (hearing, sight, taste, touch, smell), the most common are auditory hallucinations. The voices that clients hear carry messages of various types but are usually derogatory, accusatory, obscene, or threatening. It is important for staff to thoroughly assess auditory command hallucinations in which voices tell the client to harm self or others, so that staff can initiate protective interventions. (See Appendix J.) In some instances clients describe the auditory hallucinations as thoughts or sounds rather than voices.

Visual, gustatory, tactile, and olfactory hallucinations are less common but do occur. Delusions may or may not accompany hallucinations; if they do, the delusional content usually parallels the hallucination, as if the client is attempting to "make sense" of the hallucination. (See glossary.)

Illusions. Occasionally the client may experience illusions, which are misinterpretations of actual external environmental or sensory stimuli. For example, as the sun is setting, the patient looks out a window and tells staff that the bush he sees is instead his grandfather. Differentiation by staff of illusions and hallucinations is often difficult and requires keen assessment. Illusions may also occur in any of the senses.

Boundary and identity problems. The schizophrenic client may seem confused and lack a clear sense of self-awareness in which the client is not sure of his or her own boundaries and sometimes cannot differentiate self from others or from inanimate objects in the environment. This is often frightening for the client. The client may also describe *depersonalization* or *derealization* phenomena. In depersonalization, individuals have the sense that their own bodies are unreal, as if they are estranged and unattached to the world or the situation at hand; derealization is the experience that external environmental objects are strange or unreal.

A client with schizophrenia may perceive a loss of sexual identity and doubt his or her own gender or sexual orientation. This may be frightening for the client and should not be interpreted as homosexuality by the staff.

Behavioral disturbance. Behavioral disturbances may be demonstrated by impaired interpersonal relationships. Because of the difficulties these clients have with communication and interaction, the individual is frequently emotionally detached, socially inept, and withdrawn and has difficulty relating to others. Forming a therapeutic relationship with schizophrenic clients is a challenge because of the detached affective responses, illogical thinking, and egocentrism, along with the many problems described previously. A concerted effort must be made to engage the schizophrenic client because the usual encouraging cues to continue interaction are often absent. The nurse is aware that during acute episodes the client may be more restricted in thought and speech production (alogia), so initiation of contacts by the nurse is imperative.

Psychomotor disturbances such as grimacing, bizarre posturing, unpredictable and unprovoked wild activity, odd mannerisms, and compulsive stereotypical or ritualistic behavior may be present, or the patient may stare into space, seem totally out of touch with the external surroundings or persons in it, and show little or no emotional response, spontaneous speech, or movement. Clients may appear stiff or clumsy, be socially unaware of their appearance and habits, and fail to bathe or wash their clothes. They may spit on the floor and in extreme cases may regressively play with or smear feces. Clients frequently demonstrate anxious, agitated, fearful, or aggressive behavior. Once again, staff's knowledge of the effects of antipsychotic medications is essential to distinguish between symptoms of the disorder and behavioral response to the drugs. (See Appendix M).

After an acute episode, clients almost always lack energy and initiative to engage in goal-directed activity. Interest and drive seem absent (impaired volition).

Another characteristic manifested in schizophrenia is *ambivalence* (opposing thoughts, ideas, feelings, drives or impulses occurring in the same person at the same time). For example, when asked to come to the group meeting, the client may step out of and reenter his or her room dozens of times, unable to make a decision. *Negativistic* behavior is usually demonstrated as frequent oppositions and resistance to suggestions.

There are several types of schizophrenia, and not all signs and symptoms previously mentioned occur in each type. Schizophrenia has a generally poor prognosis, with a chronic deteriorating course of multiple acute episodes interspersed with relative remissions. Prognosis is more favorable for paranoid and catatonic types.

DIAGNOSIS OF TYPES OF SCHIZOPHRENIA

Paranoid Type

Distinguishing features of Paranoid Type are (1) persistent delusions with a single or closely associated, tightly organized theme of persecution or grandeur and (2) auditory hallucinations about single or closely associated themes. Clients are guarded, suspicious, hostile, angry, and possibly violent. Anxiety is pervasive in this disorder. Social interactions are intense, reserved, and controlled.

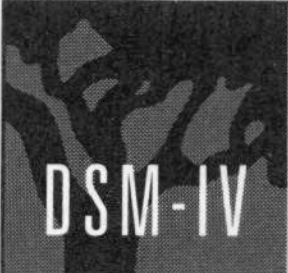

Schizophrenia

The essential features of this disorder are disordered thinking and perceptions.

DSM-IV Categories

Paranoid Type
Disorganized Type
Catatonic Type
Undifferentiated Type
Residual Type
Schizophreniform Disorder
Schizoaffective Disorder

Onset is later in life than other types, with less regressive behavior and a more favorable prognosis as a rule.

Disorganized Type

Disorganized Type was once called *hebephrenic,* and that label still exists in other classifications. The distinguishing features are grossly inappropriate or flat affect, incoherence, and grossly disorganized primitive and uninhibited behavior. These clients appear very odd or silly. They have unusual mannerisms, may giggle or cry out, distort facial expressions, complain of multiple physical problems (hypochondriasis), and are extremely withdrawn and socially inept. Invariably the onset is early, and the prepsychotic period is marked by impaired adjustment, which continues after the acute episode. Clients may hallucinate and have delusions, but the themes are fragmented and loosely organized.

Catatonic Type

The distinguishing feature of the Catatonic Type is marked disturbance of psychomotor activity. Once common, this type is rarely seen in the United States. The behavior of the catatonic client is either stuporous (psychomotor retardation) or excited (psychomotor excitation), or the client can alternate between the two states.

The client may be immobile or exhibit excited, purposeless activity. He or she may be out of touch with the environment and display catatonic negativism, mutism, and posturing. These individuals can be placed in bizarre positions (waxy flexibility), which they may rigidly maintain until moved by a staff member. It is as if they do not even feel their bodies. Careful supervision is required to prevent injury, promote nutrition, and support physiologic and psychologic functions.

Undifferentiated Type

Clients with a diagnosis of Undifferentiated Type display florid psychotic symptoms (delusions, hallucinations, incoherence, disorganized behavior) that do not clearly fit under any other category.

Residual Type

The Residual Type category is used when a client has had at least one acute episode of schizophrenia and is free of psychotic symptoms at present but continues to exhibit persistent signs of social withdrawal, emotional blunting, illogical thinking, or eccentric behavior.

Schizophreniform Disorder

Diagnostic criteria for Schizophreniform Disorder meet criteria for the positive symptoms of schizophrenia except for two factors: (1) duration of the illness is at least 1 month but less than 6 months, and (2) social/occupational function may be impaired.

Schizoaffective Disorder

Defining characteristics of Schizoaffective Disorder are demonstration of symptoms of both schizophrenia (delusions and/or hallucinations) and a mood disorder (major depressive, manic, or mixed).

OTHER PSYCHOTIC DISORDERS

Delusional Disorder

The presence of one or more nonbizarre delusions that persist for 1 month or more defines Delusional Disorder. Bizarre delusions are comprised of strange and markedly unusual or incredible content. *Example:* A person believes his brain was removed by alien beings and replaced by a computer that controls his life. Nonbizarre delusions, however, are plausible and could possibly exist in the individual's life. *Example:* A student believes there is a conspiracy to keep him from graduating from college. The following types of delusions are identified by their themes:

Erotomanic—The theme centers around belief that another person is in love with him or her, which in fact is untrue. The individual may go to great lengths to communicate with the loved object (stalking, phoning, spying).

Jealous—The belief is that the individual's lover or spouse is unfaithful without evidence to support the belief.

Prognosis for Schizophrenia

Favorable Course and Prognosis	Unfavorable Course and Prognosis
1. Good premorbid social, sexual, and work/school history	1. Poor premorbid history of socialization
2. Preceded by definable major psychosocial stressors	2. Early and insidious onset
3. Late and/or acute onset	3. No clear precipitating factors
4. Adequate support systems	4. Withdrawn and isolative behaviors
5. Paranoid or catatonic features	5. Undifferentiated and disorganized features
6. Family history of mood disorders	6. Few if any supports
	7. Chronic course with many relapses and few remissions

Grandiose—The theme focuses on the individual having an extraordinary or important undiscovered talent or special knowledge, that she or he knows an important or famous person, or, less frequently, that the person *is* a famous person.

Persecutory—The theme centers on the belief that the individual is a victim of conspiracy, poisoning, harassment, or cheating. The person frequently is angry or resentful or may be violent.

Somatic—The belief focuses on bodily sensations or functions. Most frequent somatic delusions include belief that the person has a foul odor emanating from a body part (mouth, vagina, skin), that insects or parasites are on or in the body, or that a body part is nonfunctional.

Brief Psychotic Disorder

The defining characteristic of Brief Psychotic Disorder is at least one of the following symptoms: hallucinations, delusions, incoherence and disorganized speech, or behavior disturbance (disorganized or catatonic). Symptoms last at least 1 day but less than 1 month.

Shared Psychotic Disorder

Shared Psychotic Disorder, a delusional disorder also known as *folie à deux,* develops in a person who has formed a relationship with another individual who has prominent Delusional Disorder.

INTERVENTIONS FOR SCHIZOPHRENIA AND OTHER PSYCHOTIC DISORDERS

Hospitalization

Hospitalization is necessary during acute episodes when the individual is a danger to self or others, has grossly disorganized and inappropriate behavior, or is unable to meet own basic needs for food, clothing, or shelter. At this time a diagnosis is made, and the client is stabilized on medication for the management of both positive and negative symptoms. The client also receives relief from psychosocial stressors, support, guidance, education, and help from staff in determining aftercare and rehabilitation possibilities.

Pharmacotherapy

During acute psychotic episodes medications are usually prescribed. The antipsychotics (also called *major tranquilizers* or *neuroleptics*) are used to change positive and negative symptoms, thus allowing the patient to become amenable to other interventions. These medications only treat the symptoms; they are not a cure. Many times people with chronic schizophrenia take antipsychotic medications on a long-term basis. The adverse effects of these drugs are many; most notable are extrapyramidal symptoms (EPS), some of which are irreversible. The most serious of these is called *tardive dyskinesia* (named because it is generally a later development in the course of drug therapy, although it may more rarely occur early in the treatment as well). The nursing staff needs to understand these symptoms and not mistake them for manifestations of the disorder, in which case the client would inadvertently be given a larger rather than a lesser dose! A potentially fatal, but rare, consequence of neuroleptic drug therapy is called *neuroleptic malignant syndrome* (NMS). Two newer, atypical antipsychotic medications currently used are Clozaril (clozapine) and Risperdal (resperidone). Both have minimal EPS and improved response to negative symptoms. Clozaril, however, requires frequent white blood cell counts because of the possibility of agranulocytosis and a critical reduction in leukocytes in some clients.

Antidepressants, lithium, valproates (Depakote), and carbamazepine (Tegretol) are sometimes given to clients with schizophrenia who exhibit disturbances of mood or whose family history is positive for mood disorders. (See Appendix M for complete information on medications.)

Psychosocial Therapy

Because a major characteristic of schizophrenia is the impaired ability to form and maintain interpersonal relationships, a major focus of interventions centers on helping the client enter into and maintain meaningful socialization within the client's ability.

Therapeutic nurse-client relationship. The nurse-client relationship is a therapeutic vehicle for the person with schizophrenia to attain a sense of acceptance and self-worth. Within the trusting relationship the client can learn and practice new skills, receive nonjudgmental feedback about progress, and gain support and encouragement in the process. Focus in on interpersonal communication, socialization skills, independence issues, and survival skills for posthospitalization. (See Appendix G.)

Group therapy. Some groups prove therapeutic for persons with schizophrenia. In general these individuals benefit from groups that provide support, education, and motivation rather than groups that emphasize gaining insight, problem solving on higher levels, or personality reconstruction.

Low-functioning individuals who may be psychotic are more successful in a low-stress group whose members receive positive reinforcement for even minimal functioning. The goals of these focus groups are realistic, meet the needs of the members, and address such issues as identification and support of strengths, hygiene/grooming, activities of daily living, socialization skills, motivation, self-esteem problems, and stress and anxiety reduction. (See Appendix K for anxiety-reducing strategies, e.g., deep-breathing and relaxation exercises.)

Family therapy. Support by family members can reduce relapses in clients with schizophrenia. Because the family often feels responsible for the disorder, nurses provide the family with education about the client's condition and concern for their difficult situation. Family support groups for parents of children with schizophrenia are often helpful. (See Appendix K, Family Therapy.)

Behavior Modification

Behavior modification techniques can be therapeutic for the client with schizophrenia. After a thorough assessment to identify strengths, abilities, and deficits, both client and staff target specific behaviors to be strengthened, modified, or eliminated. The program is successful when the client has full knowledge of the plan and is cooperative. Adaptive behaviors are rewarded or reinforced through praise, privileges, or actual tokens that may be exchanged for goods such as cigarettes or food. Maladaptive behaviors are negatively reinforced in the attempt to eliminate them by ignoring the behavior, removing something of value when a behavior is repeated, or having the client take "time out" from a situation. Behavior modification is generally more effective than insight-oriented therapy for this disorder.

DISCHARGE CRITERIA FOR SCHIZOPHRENIA AND OTHER PSYCHOTIC DISORDERS

Verbalizes absence or reduction of hallucinations and other sensory alterations (*Note:* Clients with chronic schizophrenia may never be entirely free of hallucinations but can learn to control them. Individuals who chronically experience hallucinations require closer supervision.)

Identifies psychosocial stressors, situations, and events that trigger hallucinations

Recognizes and discusses connections between increased anxiety and occurrence of hallucinations

Describes several techniques for decreasing anxiety and managing stress

Identifies family and/or significant others as support network

States methods for contacting physician, therapist, and agencies to meet needs

Describes importance of continuing use of medication, including dose, frequency, and expected and adverse effects

Discusses vulnerability in social situations and realistic ways to avoid problems

Verbalizes knowledge of responsibility for own actions and wellness

Describes plans to attend ongoing social support groups and rehabilitation or vocational training within limits

States alignment with aftercare facilities (home, board and care, halfway house)

Nursing Process for

Schizophrenia and Other Psychotic Disorders

Universal Principles for Interactions and Interventions with Clients Who Have Schizophrenia and Other Psychotic Disorders

- Continue to monitor assessment parameters listed under *Defining Characteristics.*
- Continue to consider the etiologic factors listed under *Etiologic/Related Factors.*
- Utilize principles of the *Therapeutic Nurse-Client Relationship* (Appendix G).
- Address clients' spiritual and cultural needs.

General Principles

- Maintain health and safety.
- Establish a trusting interpersonal relationship.
- Confirm the client's identity.
- Orient the client to reality.
- Assist the client to communicate to help him or her understand self and others and to be understood.
- Decrease demanding situations and psychosocial stressors.
- Help the client manage anxiety.
- Promote compliance with prescribed therapeutic regimen.
- Assist with activities of daily living.
- Promote social interaction.
- Regulate activity levels (hypoactivity/hyperactivity).
- Encourage/praise socially acceptable behaviors.
- Promote family involvement and understanding.
- Encourage responsibility for self.
- Teach the client how to identify psychosocial stressors and how to recognize, manage, and prevent symptoms.
- Educate client and family about potential side effects and toxic effects of antipsychotic medications.

Care Plans for Schizophrenia and Other Psychotic Disorders Based on Nursing Diagnosis

DSM-IV Diagnoses

Schizophrenia (all types)
Paranoid
Disorganized
Catatonic
Undifferentiated
Residual

NANDA Diagnoses

Sensory/perceptual alterations
Thought processes, altered
Social isolation
Communication, impaired verbal
Coping, defensive
Coping, ineffective family: disabling
Self-care deficit

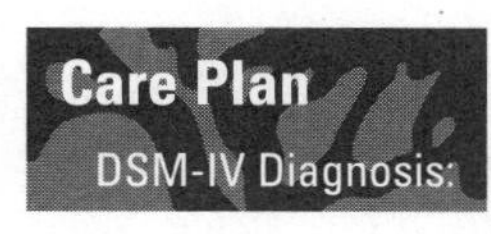

Care Plan
DSM-IV Diagnosis:

Schizophrenia (All Types)

NANDA Diagnosis: Sensory/Perceptual Alterations

The state in which an individual experiences a change in the amount or patterning of incoming stimuli accompanied by a diminished, exaggerated, distorted, or impaired response to such stimuli

Focus:
For the client who experiences sensory perceptions that are incongruent with actual stimuli. This may be demonstrated by hallucinations, illusions, or impaired awareness of self or environment.

NANDA Taxonomy
Pattern 7—Perceiving: A human response pattern involving the reception of information

ETIOLOGIC/RELATED FACTORS (RELATED TO)

Psychosocial stressors that are intolerable for the client and that threaten the client's integrity and self-esteem
Disintegration of boundaries between self and others and self and the environment
Severe and panic anxiety states
Loneliness and isolation (perceived or actual)
Powerlessness
Withdrawal from environment
Lack of adequate support persons
Inability to relate to others
Critical or derogatory, nonaccepting environment
Low self-esteem
Negative self-image, self-concept
Chronic illness and institutionalization
Altered thought processes
Disorientation
Derealization, depersonalization
Ambivalence
Biologic factors (neurophysiologic, genetic, structural)

DEFINING CHARACTERISTICS (AS EVIDENCED BY)

Inattentive to surroundings (preoccupied with hallucination)
Startles when approached and spoken to by others
Talks to self (lips move as if conversing with unseen presence)
Appears to be listening to voices or sounds when neither is present (cocks head to side as if concentrating on sounds that are inaudible to others)
May act upon "voices," commands (e.g., attempt mutilating gesture to self or others that could be injurious)
Describes hallucinatory experience:
"It's my father's voice and he's telling me I'm no good." (auditory)
"My mother just walked by the patio and I saw her go behind that tree." (visual)
"There's an awful taste in my mouth . . . like rotten eggs." (gustatory)
"I can feel my brain moving around inside my head." (somatic) "It's turning into a transmitter." (coupled with a delusion)
"There are things crawling under my skin." (tactile)
False perceptions occurring when client is falling asleep (hypnogogic hallucination) or waking from sleep (hypnopompic hallucination)
Misinterpretation of environment (illusion) (e.g., perceives roommate's teddy bear as his or her own dog, interprets a statue in the yard as his or her brother)
Describes feelings of unreality:
"I feel like I'm outside looking in, watching myself." (depersonalization)
"Everything around me became really strange just now." (derealization)
May voice concern over normalcy of genitals, breasts, or other body parts. "My breasts are distorted." "My penis is abnormal."
Misinterprets actions of others: "Sarah is coming at me with her tray; she wants to kill me."
Leaves area suddenly without explanation (may perceive environment as hostile or threatening)
Has difficulty maintaining conversations (cannot attend to staff member's responses and own hallucinatory stimuli at same time; confused and preoccupied)
Interrupts group meetings with own experience, which is irrelevant to the situation or event and has symbolic, idiosyncratic meaning only for the client
Demonstrates inability to make simple decisions, e.g., cannot decide which socks to wear or what foods to eat, whether to sit or stand during a group session (may indicate ambivalence or suspicion)

OUTCOME IDENTIFICATION AND EVALUATION

Note: The following criteria depend on severity of symptoms, client diagnosis, and prognosis. In some cases, staff expectations may be for modification of symptoms rather than for complete change of behavior.

Able to relevantly focus on conversations with others on the unit
Ceases to startle when approached
Ceases to talk to self
Seeks staff when feeling anxious or when hallucinations begin
Seeks staff or other clients for conversation as an alternative to autistic preoccupation
Refrains from harming self and others
Relates decrease or absence of obsessions
No longer expresses feelings of self or environment as being unreal or strange
Describes body parts as being normal and functional
Able to hold conversation without hallucinating
Remains in group activities
Attends to the task at hand (e.g., group process, recreational or occupational therapy activity)

States that hallucinations are under control. ("The voices don't bother me any more" or "I don't hear the voices anymore.")

Utilizes learned techniques for managing stress and anxiety (e.g., deep breathing and relaxation exercises). (See Appendix K.)

States realistic expectations for self and future ("I plan to live in a good board-and-care home and take one college class this semester.")

PLANNING AND IMPLEMENTATION

Nursing Interventions and Rationale

Establish rapport and build trust with client. *(The client must first trust the nurse before being able to talk about hallucinations and other sensory/perceptual alterations.)*

Continuously orient the patient to actual environmental events or activities, *to present reality.*

Call the client and staff members by their names *to reinforce reality.* "I'm Kathy, your staff person for today"; "These people are other hospital staff members and other clients."

Utilize clear, concrete (vs. abstract or global) statements. *Because of the client's misperceptions, altered thinking, and idiosyncratic symbolization, he or she may not understand the message.*

Use clear, direct verbal communication rather than unclear or nonverbal gestures (e.g., don't shake head yes or no, or point to indicate directions). *Unclear directions or instructions may be confusing to patient and promote distorted perceptions or misinterpretation of reality.*

Refrain from judgmental or flippant comments about hallucinations, *to avoid decreasing self-esteem.* (e.g., "Don't worry about the voices, as long as they don't belong to anyone real.")

Focus on real events or activities to *reinforce reality and divert client from the hallucinatory experience.*

Reassure the client (frequently if necessary) that he or she is safe and won't be harmed:

"You're in (name of facility) and you're safe. The staff is here to help you."

Alleviation of fear is necessary for the client to begin to trust the environment.

Observe for verbal and nonverbal behaviors associated with hallucinations (e.g., statement content, talking to self, scanning, eyes averted, staring, bolting and running from the room). *The nurse must recognize sensory-perceptual disturbance before he or she can intervene.*

Describe the hallucinatory behaviors to the client:

"Sue, you seem to be distracted while we're talking. Are you hearing voices?"

"You're staring at the ceiling, Sam. What do you see?"

The client may be unable to disclose perceptions, and the nurse can openly facilitate disclosure by reflecting observations of the client's behaviors.

Attempt to determine precipitants of the sensory alteration (stressors that may trigger the hallucination):

"What happened just before you heard the voices?" *The hallucination may occur after an anxiety-provoking situation. When such situations are identified, the client understands the connection and can begin learning to manage, avoid, reduce, or eliminate them.*

Identify, whenever possible, the need fulfilled by the hallucinations (e.g., loneliness, dependency, rejection, lack of interpersonal intimacy). *Hallucinations may fill the void that is created by the lack of satisfying human contact. Once the client's need is elicited, the nurse can begin to replace the hallucinations with a therapeutic interpersonal relationship and activities that meet some of the unfulfilled needs. Also, the client who feels understood is likely to experience decreased anxiety, which, in itself, reduces incidence of hallucinations.*

Modify the environment to decrease situations that provoke anxiety (e.g., excessively competitive, noisy, challenging activities):

"That was a noisy basketball game, Don. I know you're upset because you say you're hearing voices again. I'll go with you while you work on your model."

"You left the group, Bob. It was pretty demanding today. Let's go for a walk outside."

Decreased anxiety can reduce the occurrences of hallucinations.

Explore the content of auditory hallucinations to determine the possibility of harm to self, others, or the environment (auditory command hallucinations) *to prevent destructive behavior:*

"You seem frightened, Bob, and you say you're hearing voices. What do the voices that you hear say?"

When danger or violence is imminent, protect the client and others by following facility procedures and policies for seclusion or chemical or mechanical restraint to prevent harm or injury to client or others. (*Note:* These procedures are used only when less restrictive verbal and behavioral methods are unsuccessful. (See Appendix L.)

When it is determined that the client is *not* harmful to self or others, proceed as follows:

Recognize and acknowledge the feelings underlying the hallucination or other sensory experience rather than focusing on the content:

"You look sad, Nancy. You say the voices you hear keep telling you bad things about yourself. The staff is here to help you get relief from the voices."

"You seem frightened, Tom. Are you hearing voices now?"

When the client feels understood, anxiety and the sense of being alone are diminished, thus decreasing the hallucinatory experience.

State your reality about the client's hallucinatory experience:

Therapeutic response:

"I don't hear the voices you describe, Tom. I know you hear voices, but with time they may go away."

(Do not deny the existence of the client's experience.)

"I hear your voice and my voice, Tom, as we talk with one another."

This helps the client to distinguish the actual voices in order to promote reality.

Nontherapeutic response:

"There aren't any voices. Your father isn't here. You're making them up yourself."

Continuous reality orientation by staff helps to convince the client that the hallucinations (and accompanying delusion, if present) are not real. The client may then begin to let go of the importance attached to the experience.

Refrain from arguing or having lengthy discussions about the content of the client's hallucination:

Therapeutic response:

"We talked about the voices earlier, Tom. I'll walk to the activity room with you so you can continue with the project you started."

Nontherapeutic response:

"Tom, this is Miss Jenkins, a new nurse on our unit. Tell her what the voices say to you and what they tell you to do."

This encourages the client to focus on and defend the experience, which reinforces it and makes it more important to the client.

Teach the client techniques that will help stop the hallucinations.

Have the client sing, whistle, or play a musical instrument over the voices.

Tell the voices to "go away."

Describe disbelief in derogatory or negative messages that the voices carry. "I don't believe you're the devil, Tom."

Have the client seek another person in the environment for conversation.

Have the client tell a staff member when the voices are bothersome.

Have the client engage in an activity, exercise, or project when the voices began.

Such techniques distract the client from the hallucination, provide alternative competition for the hallucination, and give the client control.

Accept and support the client's feelings (sadness, fear, anger) underlying the hallucination: "I know the voices that you hear make you feel frightened, Sue. Staff is here for you. *"This conveys empathy and understanding and reduces fear and anxiety.*

Accept, within limits, hostile, quarrelsome outbursts without becoming personally offended. *The client's actions represent the client's own misery and are not a reflection of feelings toward staff.*

Set limits on behavior when necessary:

"Your cursing is interrupting the activity, Barbara. Take a 10-minute time-out in your room."

This helps to keep the environment safe and comfortable for all clients.

Praise the client's efforts to use learned techniques to distract from or manage hallucinations (e.g., by joining activities or using the techniques described previously). *Positive feedback increases self-esteem and promotes repetition of successful behavioral strategies.*

Encourage the patient to take medications. *Medication compliance controls psychotic symptoms.* (See Appendix M.)

Teach the client and family about the therapeutic effects of medications and the important role medications play in reducing psychotic symptoms. *Understanding may increase compliance.*

Discuss with client and family the adverse effects of medications and how to manage them in accordance with the client's treatment plan *to ensure the client's and family's understanding of the effects of medication, and provide comfort* (see Appendix M).

Provide environmental opportunities to expand the client's social network (start with one-to-one, add group activities when appropriate and the client is able to tolerate them). *Satisfying experiences with others tend to decrease/replace hallucinations.*

Provide a consistent, structured milieu. *Constancy and a dependable environment promote trust, safety, and a sense of well-being for disorganized clients.*

Discuss with the client and family realistic plans and goals for prevention and management of sensory/perceptual alterations. *This encourages the client to begin to practice and utilize any available personal skills and resources while in a safe environment.*

Provide group situations in which the client can learn and practice activities of daily living, communication skills, and social skills and begin to improve interpersonal relatedness and independence. *This increases feelings of adequacy, satisfaction, and self-esteem, which tends to decrease negative sensory/perceptual experiences.*

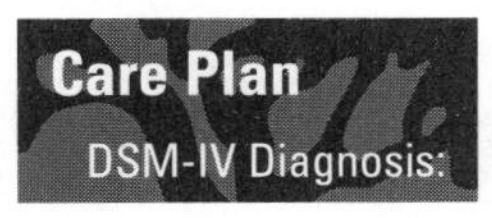

Schizophrenia (All Types)

NANDA Diagnosis: Thought processes, altered

The state in which an individual experiences a disruption in cognitive operations and activities

Focus:

For the client with thought disorders and inability to test reality, who experiences delusions, magical thinking, loose associations, ideas of reference, thought broadcasting, thought insertion, thought withdrawal, and impaired judgment, comprehension, perception, and problem-solving abilities

NANDA Taxonomy

Pattern 8—Knowing: A human response pattern involving the meaning associated with information

ETIOLOGIC/RELATED FACTORS (RELATED TO)

Impaired ability to process and synthesize internal and external stimuli

Disintegration of boundaries between self and others and self and the environment

Biologic factors (neurophysiologic, genetic, structural)

Sensory-perceptual alterations

Psychosocial/environmental stressors

DEFINING CHARACTERISTICS (AS EVIDENCED BY)

Inaccurate interpretation of incoming information (e.g., thinks others in the environment are spies or demons; believes the psychiatric intensive care unit is a prison; perceives others' benign statements or gestures as hostile or sexual overtures)

Inability to distinguish internally stimulated (autistic) thoughts from facts or actual events. (Client's statements reflect combined segments of reality and fantasy, such as "The president is our leader—he is the ruler of the universal life and death.")

Perceives that others in the environment can hear his or her thoughts (thought broadcasting)

Demonstrates neologisms, word salad, thought blocking, thought insertion, thought withdrawal, poverty of speech, or mutism. (See Glossary.)

Believes that his or her thoughts are responsible for world events or disasters (magical thinking, delusion):

"My thoughts are causing all those fires; they're burning up the world."

Thinks that he or she is omnipotent and capable of superhuman powers (delusion of grandeur):

"I'm a messenger for the devil and can destroy the universe."

Believes that others in the environment are plotting evil deeds against him or her (delusion of persecution):

"I know they're planning to capture me and use my brain for science."

Inappropriate reactions to others' communication and behavior and environmental events (e.g., laughs in response to sad or despondent content)

Incites fear or confusion in other clients

Inability to follow or comprehend others' communication or simple instructions, unrelated to language or cultural differences

Impaired ability to abstract, conceptualize, reason, or calculate. For example, the client may interpret the proverb "A stitch in time saves nine" as "It takes nine stitches to save time" (paralogical, concrete thinking).

Suspiciousness, anger, or fear directed toward environment or others in the environment manifested by hypervigilance or scanning with angry, frightened, or confused facial expression; withdrawal from activities and others in the milieu; outbursts of rage or fear; statements that reveal mistrust or hostility without apparent external basis

Distractibility, decreased attention span, or difficulty in concentrating on simple activities or events

Disorganized, incoherent, fragmented, illogical speech patterns (looseness of associations, tangential, circumstantial references) (See glossary.):

"The sea is the water hole of life, the sea of life; I want to marry in the sea."

Attachment of symbolic or idiosyncratic meanings to environmental events, objects, persons, or colors (e.g., the color purple symbolizes death); blondes represent goodness; a particular film star is revered as a savior)

Preoccupation with religious or sexual ideas manifested by chanting, preaching, praying, condemning, or making erotic references and gestures

Makes generalizations from specific or isolated events or persons:

"My mother has blue eyes and she's an alcoholic, so all blue-eyed women are alcoholics."

Demonstrates ambivalence through statements and behaviors:

"I want to kill my brother so he could live."

"I love everyone here so much, I want to leave right now."

Makes a violent gesture while verbalizing pleasant statements

States that the major influences in his life are God and the devil

Believes that information coming from the media or immediate environment refer to the client (ideas of reference):

"The president was referring to me when he spoke about the space program."

"The food trays are late because I wasn't ready to eat."

Interrupted sleep patterns or inability to fall asleep related to delusions or frightening thoughts

OUTCOME IDENTIFICATION AND EVALUATION

Demonstrates reality-based thinking in verbal and nonverbal behavior

Demonstrates absence of psychosis (delusions; incoherent, illogical speech; magical thinking; ideas of references; thought blocking; thought insertions; thought broadcasting)

Demonstrates the ability to abstract, conceptualize, reason, and calculate in accordance with developmental stage

Exhibits judgment, insight, coping skills and problem-solving abilities in accordance with developmental stage

Distinguishes boundaries between self and others and self and the environment

PLANNING AND IMPLEMENTATION

Nursing Interventions and Rationale

Assess own level of anxiety and employ anxiety-reducing strategies to reduce it to tolerable level. *Anxiety is transferable, and clients experiencing psychosis are extremely sensitive to external stimuli. The nurse's anxiety can increase the client's anxiety and foster altered thought patterns.* (See Appendix K.)

Approach the client in slow, calm, matter-of-fact manner, *to avoid distorting the client's sensory-perceptual field, which could foster altered thoughts and perceptions.*

Maintain facial expressions and behaviors that are consistent with verbal statements. *The client with altered thought processes may have a difficult time interpreting correct meanings if nurse misrepresents intent with a conflicting or "double" message.*

Examples of nontherapeutic or "double" messages:

The nurse smiles while discussing a serious matter with the client.

The nurse frowns and appears impatient while telling the client she/he accepts and understands his/her behavior.

Continue to assess the client's ability to think logically and to utilize realistic judgment and problem-solving abilities, *to determine the extent of cognitive impairment and progress made in use of logical thinking.*

Listen attentively for key themes and reality-oriented phrases or thoughts, *to elicit problem areas, to promote the client's willingness to relate to another person, and to help meet the client's needs.*

Interpret the client's misconceptions and misperceived environmental events in a calm, matter-of-fact manner, *to assist the client in correcting misconceptions or ideas of reference without challenging the client's belief system.*

"That's John, your new roommate; you met him this morning."

"Those clients are discussing the lunch menu; we're having chicken today."

"The president is talking about the astronauts; you're an interested citizen as I am."

Instruct the client to approach staff when frightening thoughts occur, *to provide safety and security, decrease anxiety, and prevent further cognitive impairment.*

When client is amenable, teach cognitive replacement strategies *to interrupt or displace irrational thoughts with realistic thoughts (may not be appropriate for all clients).* (See Appendix K.)

Refrain from touching a client who is experiencing a delusion, especially if it is persecutory type. *Clients who are suspicious, hostile, or paranoid may perceive touch as a threatening gesture and react aggressively.*

Utilize simple, concrete, or literal explanations and avoid use of abstractions or metaphors *because clients with altered thought processes interpret abstractions concretely and may misunderstand or misinterpret the meaning of the message:*

Therapeutic response:

"It's 10 o'clock and time for you to go to bed."

Nontherapeutic response:

"It's 10 o'clock and time to 'hit the hay."

Avoid challenging the client's delusional system or arguing with the client *because delusions cannot be changed through logic, and challenging the belief, no matter how irrational, may force the client to adhere to it and defend it.*

Distract the client from the delusion by engaging the client in a less threatening or more comforting topic or activity at the first sign of anxiety or discomfort *because dwelling on delusional content may increase the client's anxiety, aggression, or other dysfunctional behaviors:*

"This subject seems troubling for you; let's work on your jigsaw puzzle."

"You seem uncomfortable with this topic; let's walk out to the patio."

Focus on the meaning, feeling, or intent provoked by the delusion rather than on the delusional content, *to help meet the client's needs, reinforce reality, and discourage the false belief without challenging the client:*

Therapeutic response:

"I know that's troubling for you; I'm not frightened because I don't believe the end of the world is here."

Nontherapeutic response:

"Describe those people who are out to get you; what do they look like?"

Gradually encourage the client to discuss experiences that occurred before the onset of the delusion, *to help the client identify threatening thoughts, feelings, or events and associate them with reality rather than with the delusional content:*

"What happened just before you felt this way?"

"I noticed when you received that phone call, you became anxious and began to think those troubling thoughts."

Avoid pursuing the details of the client's delusion *so as not to reinforce the false belief and further distance the client from reality.*

Offer praise as soon as the client begins to differentiate reality-based and nonreality-based thinking. *Positive reinforcement increases self-esteem and encourages the client to identify and continue reality-based thoughts and behaviors.*

Respond to the client's delusions of persecution with calm, realistic statements:

Therapeutic response:

"At this time, you may believe your food is poisoned; I don't think your food is poisoned, but it sounds like you have some concerns, and the staff is here to help."

Delusions of persecution represent the client's fears or threats to the self-system in an environment he or she perceives as hostile. Focusing on the client's concerns, fears, and insecurity rather than on the content of the delusion promotes the client's trust and willingness to be helped.

Nontherapeutic response:

"Do you really believe a hospital would serve the clients poisoned food? There's no reason to be afraid to eat the food."

This statement challenges the client's belief by focusing on the delusional content (whether or not the food is poisoned) and forces the client to cling to the delusion in an attempt to justify it and protects his or her self-esteem. Also, the client's feelings and concerns are negated, which disrupts trust, blocks communication, and increases the client's fear, insecurity, and sense of isolation.

Respond to the client's delusions of grandeur or omnipotence in a calm, nonchallenging manner, focusing on the client's need to retain or regain control over his or her status or situation:

Therapeutic responses:

"When you say you are God and can change the world, it sounds like you're unhappy about being a client in the hospital and would like to change your situation."

"You're John Smith, a client in this hospital; it must be scary to think you're a messenger for the devil; in time, you may not believe this."

These types of responses present reality without challenging the client's belief system, focus on the client's intent and meaning behind the delusions (helplessness, powerlessness), and express the staff's desire to understand and help the client maintain safety, control, dignity, and hope at a time of vulnerability.

Nontherapeutic responses:

"You know you're not God and can't change the world."

"There's no such thing as the devil, so you can't possibly be his messenger."

These responses, while truthful, tactlessly challenge the client's belief system, threaten the client's self-esteem, overlook the meaning and intent behind the delusions (powerlessness, helplessness, fear, frustration), and negate his or her feelings, all of which may inhibit the client's trust and block communication.

Use simple declarative statements when talking to the client who demonstrates fragmented, disconnected, incoherent, or tangential speech patterns, which reflect loose associations:

Therapeutic responses:

"I want to understand you better; tell me again."

"I'm having trouble understanding you now; let's get a snack and we'll talk some more."

"It sounds as if you may be upset because your mom isn't here yet; it's 7 o'clock now; visiting hours aren't over until 8 o'clock."

These responses let the client know that you want to understand the message and meet the client's needs. This reduces anxiety and helps the client to collect his or her thoughts and engage in more goal-directed communication. Your responses do not place blame on the client, but rather they focus on your desire to pursue the meaning and intent of the client's communication and to help the client communicate more clearly. (Occasionally, the client may be able to write the message or make gestures to convey his or her needs.)

Nontherapeutic responses:

"You're just not making any sense at all; try to concentrate harder on what you want to say."

"I can't understand one word you're saying; go lie down and clear up your thoughts."

These responses reflect your frustration in trying to understand the client's message, place the blame for the behavior on the client, and challenge the client to remedy the behavior. Your desire to comprehend the client's message or meet the client's needs is absent, which may increase the client's anxiety and perpetuate dysfunction.

Offer the client clear, simple explanations of environmental events, activities, and the behaviors of other clients when necessary, *to assuage the client's suspiciousness and fear or mistrust of the surroundings and others and to prevent aggressive behavior:*

"That remark was not meant for you; it was directed to all of us in the community meeting."

"That noise is coming from the patio; the clients are playing volleyball."

"John got a little upset in the group meeting, so he raised his voice, but everything is OK now."

"You will not be harmed here."

"Those people are clients, not spies. They are deciding on an activity."

Remain silently and patiently with the client who demonstrates mutism or poverty of speech, without demanding a response. *The client will feel worthy even though he or she is unable to perform at the time.*

Therapeutic responses:

"I know your thoughts are troubling you now; let's wait a while and then continue our talk; I'll sit here with you."

"We don't need to talk now; I'd like to stay here with you."

These responses illustrate your understanding and acceptance of the client's inability to engage in a meaningful, goal-directed interaction at this time and your willingness to help meet the client's needs while offering comfort, safety, and companionship.

Nontherapeutic responses:

"I can't understand a word you say; I'll come back later after you've had a chance to rest."

"I know your thoughts are affecting your speech; try to concentrate on what you really want to say."

These responses focus on the client's inability to express his or her thoughts. Leaving the client at this time may increase anxiety and decrease self-worth, which could perpetuate symptoms. Asking the client to rest or concentrate harder places on the client the responsibility to "fix the problem" through unrealistic means.

Assess the client's nonverbal behavior *to meet the client's needs that cannot be conveyed through speech.*

Continue to support and monitor prescribed medical and psychosocial treatment plans.

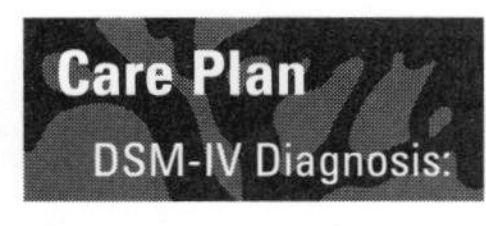

Schizophrenia (All Types)

NANDA Diagnosis: Social Isolation

The state in which an individual experiences aloneness that is perceived as imposed by others and as negative or threatening

Focus:
For the client who is isolated because of mental or emotional impairment. This does not refer to the voluntary solitude that one seeks for personal rejuvenation, the aloneness needed for creativity, or the loneliness experienced following a major loss.

NANDA Taxonomy
Pattern 3—Relating: A human response pattern involving established bonds

ETIOLOGIC/RELATED FACTORS (RELATED TO)

Altered sensory perception (hallucinations or illusions, which may result in mistrust of or rejection by other clients in the environment)
Altered thought processes (delusions, magical thinking, ideas of reference, thought blocking, thought insertion) (See Glossary.)
Impaired verbal communication (neologisms, word salad, loose associations, tangentiality, incoherence, poverty of speech, mutism) (See Glossary.)
Long-term illness, hospitalization, or environmental deprivation
Ineffective support systems (family, friends, work, school)
Unsatisfying or ineffective role/relationships
Unaccepted social values (may result in client behaving in manner incongruent with accepted social norms)
Impaired developmental stage (client may be socially inept and unable to perform age-appropriate tasks)
Decreased energy level
Fear or anxiety
Impaired volition
Impaired social interactions

DEFINING CHARACTERISTICS (AS EVIDENCED BY)

Withdrawal from the environment and from others in the environment
Isolates self in room or bed for most of the day and night
Difficulty in establishing bonds or relationships with others in the environment (fails to seek out or respond to others)
Verbalizations that indicate feelings of rejection from others in the environment:
"I guess I'm not wanted by the other clients in the group."
"The staff never seem to be available for me."
"No one ever seems to notice me."
"My family never visits me. They don't know I exist."
"I just wish people liked me more."
Inability to engage in social interactions or milieu activities
Inability to share or express feelings with others in groups or one to one
Verbalizes difficulty in engaging in social conversations:
"I have trouble talking to others on any subject."
"I'm really uncomfortable socializing with strangers."
"I don't have anything of interest to add to a discussion."
Relates history of inadequate or unsatisfactory relationships:
"I was never involved in a happy relationship."
"I could never seem to find anyone who really cared about me."
"My parents never approved of me."
Expresses a lack of purpose in life:
"Life holds no meaning for me."
"The days seem to drag by endlessly without meaning."
"I have no real plans or desires for my life."
Inappropriate or immature interests or activities for developmental level
Noncommunicative, with flat or dull affect and minimal or absent eye contact
Preoccupied with dysfunctional thoughts, activities, or rituals (may be responding to obsessions, hallucinations, or delusions). Remains in room, rearranging clothes:
"I'm not really a client; I'm here to meditate for all mankind."
Inability to concentrate or make decisions
Expresses feeling "useless" or "worthless":
"I'm no good to anyone."
"I just don't seem to matter."
"I'm not worth talking to."
Demonstrates physical inactivity
Verbalizes decreased or lack of energy:
"I don't feel like getting involved in groups or discussions."
"I don't have the strength to get out of bed just to talk to people."
Changes in appetite or eating habits (overeats or undereats)

OUTCOME IDENTIFICATION AND EVALUATION

Verbalizes willingness to engage in social interactions and activities with others in the environment:
"I plan to come to community meeting this afternoon."
"I'm going to contact my staff person for a one-to-one discussion after lunch."
Engages in social activities with others in the environment (meals, exercises, crafts, games, outings)
Expresses pleasure derived from social conversations and activities with other clients, staff, and significant others:
"I liked talking to my roommate today."
"I got a lot out of my meeting with my staff person."
"Bowling yesterday was fun."
"It was good to see my family."
Spends most of time out of room, involved with others in the environment

Expresses belief that he or she can make meaningful contributions to social discussions and activities:
"The group seemed to like my input."
"I helped my bowling team win last night."

PLANNING AND IMPLEMENTATION

Nursing Interventions and Rationale

Assess the extent of the client's self-imposed isolation *to plan strategies to break the pattern of withdrawal with interactions and activities.*

Assist the client to meet basic needs during times of social withdrawal (sleep, nutrition, personal hygiene) *to promote the client's physical health and well-being.*

Structures each day to include planned times for brief interactions and activities with the client *to help the client organize times to engage with others and to let the client know participation is expected and that he or she is a worthwhile member of the community.*

Spend brief intervals with the client each day, engaging in meaningful, nonchallenging interactions, *to ease the client out into the community by first developing trust, rapport, and respect.*

Discuss with the client anything of interest to him or her, such as items in the client's room, favorite activities, or hobbies, *to encourage the client's social skills and decrease social isolation.*

Identify the client's significant support persons (other clients, family), and encourage them to seek out the client for interactions, phone conversations, activities, and visits. *A strong network of supportive individuals will increase the client's social contacts, enhance social skills, promote self-esteem, and facilitate positive relationships.*

Help the client differentiate social isolation and a desire for solitude or privacy. *The client may occasionally choose to be alone at appropriate times.*

Assess the client's self-concept (sense of worth, self-esteem) and coping abilities and how they relate to social isolation. *Low self-esteem and maladaptive coping strategies may result from and/or perpetuate social isolation.*

Act as a role model for social behaviors in one-to-one and group interactions (maintain good eye contact, appropriate distance, calm demeanor, and moderate voice tone) *to help the client identify appropriate social skills for age and status.*

Engage other clients and significant others in social interactions and activities with the client (card games, meals, sing-along) *to promote social skills in a safe setting.*

Help the client to seek out other clients with similar interests with whom the client can socialize. *Shared or common interests promote more enjoyable socialization, which is likely to be repeated.*

Praise the patient for attempts to seek out others for interactions and activities and to respond to others' attempts to engage the client in interactions and activities *to promote continued positive social behaviors:*
"It was beneficial for you to seek out John for a game of cards."
"Your participation in group today was helpful."
"Your consent to go with Sally and Bob to lunch was a positive step."

Provide the client with stimulation from recreational and other milieu activities *to expose the client to social activities and increase opportunities for socialization.*

Provide the client with graded activities according to level of tolerance and cognitive and affective functioning: (1) meal planning, (2) simple games with one staff member, (3) simple group activities, (4) process group interactions, *to gradually expose the client to more complex interactive exercises and activities.*

Provide the client with outings (e.g., to shopping malls, grocery stores, day care centers, pet shops, museums, the zoo) *to encourage a variety of interactive experiences outside the hospital community and reduce social isolation.*

Intervene with the client demonstrating compulsive acts, hallucinations, delusions, or impaired verbal communications by remaining with the client during acute dysfunctional phases and engaging in brief, calm social contacts with the client throughout the day *to demonstrate your understanding of the client's limitations and fill the client's social void.*

Keep all appointments for interactions with the client *to promote the client's trust and self-esteem, which enhance socialization.*

Encourage the client to engage in social activities that are within his or her physical capabilities and tolerance *to provide the client with successful social experiences that are likely to be repeated.*

Continue to support and monitor prescribed medical and psychosocial treatment plans.

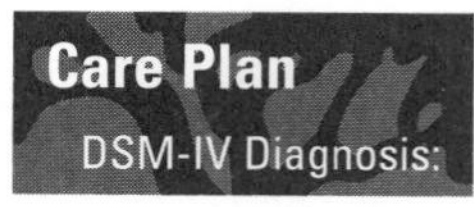

Schizophrenia (All Types)

NANDA Diagnosis: Communication, impaired verbal

The state in which an individual experiences a decreased or absent ability to use or understand language in human interaction

Focus:
For the client whose altered thought content and withdrawal from reality often result in misinterpretations that affect the ability to communicate verbally or to use language in a meaningful way. The client's comprehension of others' communication is also compromised.

NANDA Taxonomy
Pattern 2—Communicating: A human response pattern involving sending messages

ETIOLOGIC/RELATED FACTORS (RELATED TO)

Disturbances in form of thinking (autistic)

Altered thought processes (e.g., delusions, magical thinking) (See Glossary.)

Poverty of speech/mutism
Sensory/perceptual alterations (e.g., hallucinations)
Disturbances in structure of associations (e.g., neologisms, word salad, perseveration) (See Glossary.)
Obsessive thoughts (e.g., sexual, religious)
Inability to reason, abstract, calculate, or problem solve
Impaired insight or judgment
Inability to distinguish self from environment or from others in the environment
Panic anxiety state
Inability to distinguish internally stimulated thoughts from actual environmental events or commonly shared knowledge
Withdrawal from environment into self/lack of external stimulation
Regression to earlier developmental level

DEFINING CHARACTERISTICS (AS EVIDENCED BY)

Loose (or tangential) associations:
"It's 5 o'clock in the morning and I am dawn of the new age."
Neologisms:
"There are no *cornerfrocks* here, only *doppel skirts.*"
Word salad:
"Sit to seagreen underwear." "Jump out winter sludge."
Clang associations (use of words that may rhyme or are similar in sound but not meaning: "ping-a-long," "the man can," "ding-dong")
Vague, obscure speech that gives little information and may be repetitious
Echolalia (the client repeats words that are heard—may reflect the client's inability to distinguish boundaries)
Use of symbolic references or idiosyncratic meanings (attributed to names, objects, events, people, or shapes). *Examples:*

- Client may state that the color red means *dead* or *blood;* all blue-eyed people are relatives; cross-shaped objects have magical powers. "My name is Dawn Eve—dawn of the universe, Eve of the garden where Adam is waiting."

Verbalizes concrete or literal interpretations in relation to abstract terms. *Example:*

- Client interprets the proverb "People who live in glass houses shouldn't throw stones" as "houses made of glass will break if they're struck with stones."

Use of circumstantiality (digression of inappropriate thoughts into ideas); perseveration (repetition of same word or idea in response to different questions); stereotypy (continuous repetition of speech or activities); verbigeration (meaningless repetitions of speech); circumlocution (a roundabout way of speaking to reach desired goal) (See Glossary.)
Repetitious ritualistic verbalization of religious or sexual topics that are socially inappropriate (may chant or preach endlessly from the Bible or other holy book)
Addresses others in the environment with odd or idiosyncratic phrases, titles, or identifications that hold meaning only for the client:
"Lily Pureface," "Green Goddess," "Funny Man," "Mary from the Sanctuary"
Accuses staff and other clients of plotting or planning to harm or kill him or her:
"I know Liz has poisoned my food."
Accuses others in the environment of reading his or her thoughts:
"I'm sure Tim knows what I'm thinking right now."
Claims to be able to read the thoughts of others:
"I have telepathic powers and can read minds."
Introduces self to others as an omnipotent figure with superhuman powers:
"I'm king of the universe and have been sent here to heal the world."
Speaks minimally or not at all for long periods of time (poverty of speech, mutism)
Uses speech that is vague and obscure and gives little or no information (poverty of content)
Responds inappropriately or irrationally to rational statements or questions posed by others. *Example:*

- Staff may ask client what he or she would like for lunch and client may respond:
"Bricks and sticks on white copper sand."
"Delicious turmoil of life's bread and guts."
(Examples of loose associations)

Claims that his or her thoughts are responsible for events, cause events to occur, or can prevent an occurrence via magical means:
"I willed those wars to happen and they did."
"The menu was changed to chicken because of my thoughts."
Converses with voices emanating from radio or television
Talks, perseverates, or mumbles incoherently to self with no apparent external stimuli
Frequently interrupts group sessions with verbal outbursts that may or may not be reality-based

OUTCOME IDENTIFICATION AND EVALUATION

Communicates thoughts and feelings in a coherent, goal-directed manner
Demonstrates reality-based thought processes in verbal communication
Displays meaningful and understandable verbal communication
Demonstrates verbal communication that is congruent with affect and other nonverbal expressions
Recognizes that increased anxiety states exacerbate impaired verbal communication
Identifies psychosocial stressors that increase anxiety and perpetuate impaired verbal communication
Initiates strategies to decrease anxiety and promote coherent, meaningful verbal communication
Responds coherently in group sessions without frequent inappropriate verbal interruptions

PLANNING AND IMPLEMENTATION

Nursing Interventions and Rationale

Assess the extent to which the client's impaired verbal communication interferes with his or her ability to get others to understand the meaning behind the message. (Note reaction of other clients to client's communication attempts. Do they appear confused, frightened, offended?) *This observation will serve as a basic guideline for helping the client and peers to learn alternate methods of communication, develop trust and patience, and better meet each other's needs.*

Demonstrate a calm, patient demeanor rather than attempting to force the client to speak coherently *to decrease the client's fears and anxieties about the inability to communicate needs and to demonstrate acceptance of client.*

Actively listen to and observe verbal and nonverbal cues and behaviors during the communication process *to piece together each method of communication to understand better the intent of the client's message and demonstrate a willingness to meet the client's needs.*

Use communication strategies such as restatement, clarification, and consensual validation *to help reveal the intent of the client's message:*

"When you say. . . , do you mean. . . ?"
"I'm not sure what you mean by. . . . Tell me again."
"Are you saying. . . ?"
"Please explain that again."

Acknowledge the client's inability to use the spoken word while encouraging alternative methods to convey messages (gestures, writing, drawing) *to demonstrate empathy, develop trust, and encourage the total communication process:*

"I know you find it difficult to speak now; perhaps you can tell me with a gesture or sign."
"Although you're not able to speak now, you may be able to write your thoughts."
"If you're having trouble expressing yourself now, you can try again in a few minutes. I'll still be here."

Instruct the client to seek assistance from staff when experiencing communication problems. *Staff can help facilitate the communication process.*

Anticipate the client's needs until he or she can communicate coherently and meaningfully *to provide safety, comfort, and support.*

Act as a liaison between client and peers while the client is unable to speak coherently *to facilitate the communication process and decrease alienation from other clients.*

Assign staff persons who are familiar with the client's methods of verbal and nonverbal communication and encourage clear intershift reports *to facilitate consistency and increase opportunities to understand the meaning behind the client's actions and expressions.* (For example, a delusional system with the persistent theme of achieving world peace may reflect the client's fear of war and death. The nurse can communicate this to other caregivers so that staff can consistently provide a calm, low-stimulation environment for the client in a collaborative effort to meet his or her needs.)

Encourage the client to approach other clients for conversations *to practice communication skills in a safe setting.*

Assist the client to listen and engage in actual conversations (one-to-one interactions with staff and peers, group meetings, and activities) *to encourage the client to respond to reality rather than to own inner (autistic) thoughts.*

Assess the effects of the client's cultural and spiritual background on dysfunctional speech patterns to individualize client care *because talk of a religious or spiritual nature may not all be aberrant.* (For example, a client may pray or speak to deceased relatives more frequently as anxiety escalates, but during periods of higher functioning some of those behaviors may be culturally appropriate and provide comfort.)

Teach the client strategies to use whenever he or she initially experiences impaired verbal communication *to decrease anxiety, which may exacerbate symptoms, and to promote more functional speech patterns.* (For example, practicing slow, deep breathing and progressive relaxation; replacing or interrupting irrational, negative thoughts with realistic ones; taking periods of time-out; seeking out a supportive person; engaging in a simple exercise or activity.) (See Appendix K.)

Praise the client's attempts to speak more coherently and to engage in more meaningful conversations with others *to increase self-esteem and promote continued functional speech patterns.*

Continue to support and monitor prescribed medical and psychosocial treatment plans.

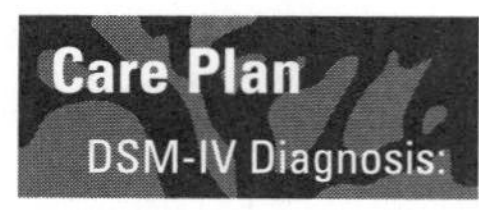

Schizophrenia (All Types)

NANDA Diagnosis: Coping, defensive

The state in which an individual repeatedly projects falsely positive self-evaluation based on a self-protective pattern that defends against underlying perceived threats to positive self-regard

Focus:
For the client who copes by defending against perceived threats to the self-system, e.g., persistently blaming, accusing, or threatening others, generally in a hostile manner. Underlying this behavior is often a negative self-concept.

NANDA Taxonomy
Pattern 5—Choosing: A human response pattern involving the selection of alternatives

ETIOLOGIC/RELATED FACTORS (RELATED TO)

Depletion of adaptive coping strategies
Moderate to severe anxiety states
Altered thought processes
Perceived threats to self-system (integrity, self-esteem)
Low self-esteem

Sensory/perceptual alterations
Developmental impairment secondary to personality disorder (Axis II diagnosis)
Suspicion and mistrust of persons and situations in the environment secondary to schizophrenic process (Axis I diagnosis)
Misinterpretations of actual environmental events and activities
Inability to interpret or express emotions
Inability to displace angry or hostile feelings constructively
Inability to get needs met through direct communication channels
Impaired reality testing
Ambivalent/mistrustful family dynamics

DEFINING CHARACTERISTICS (AS EVIDENCED BY)

Projection of blame, hostility, or responsibility on others:
"You made me late for group today."
"It was all your fault that I got caught smoking."
Hypersensitivity to slightest criticism (leaves group in middle of discussion, angers easily when confronted)
Grandiosity (may be delusional):
"I'm the smartest person in this room."
"I'm the nephew of the president of the United States."
Superior attitude toward others:
"I shouldn't be here; I'm not sick."
"I know more about psychiatry than my doctor does."
Difficulty establishing and maintaining relationships (makes no friends on the unit; other clients leave when client enters room)
Hostile laughter and ridicule of others
Takes other clients' cigarettes or other belongings, then denies it and/or projects behavior to others
Sabotages own treatment and therapy with overt defensive behaviors (fails to attend groups or acts out during group activities to elicit negative attention)
Feelings of being persecuted (may be delusional):
"I feel as if everyone here is against me."
"I just know my roommate wishes I was dead."
Paranoid ideation/ideas of reference:
"Those clients are always whispering. I'm sure it's about me."
"Everyone I see on TV is talking about me."
Abuses drugs and/or alcohol during unit passes and brags about behavior to other patients

OUTCOME IDENTIFICATION AND EVALUATION

Utilizes coping strategies in a functional, adaptive manner in appropriate situations
Demonstrates trust in staff and other clients in the environment (seeks out staff for one-to-one interactions), participates with clients in groups and activities)
Expresses feelings appropriately through verbal interactions with staff and other clients
Displaces the energy of anxiety toward physical exercise and group activities
Accurately interprets environmental events and behavior of others in the environment
Meets own needs through clear, direct methods of communication
Demonstrates absence of hypersensitivity, suspiciousness, or paranoia during interactions with others
Demonstrates absence of verbal abuse, threats, or ridicule or physically aggressive behavior directed at others

PLANNING AND IMPLEMENTATION

Nursing Interventions and Rationale

Accept hypersensitivity, ideas of reference, and paranoia as part of the client's impaired self-system and altered reality-testing *to establish trust and begin a therapeutic working relationship.*
Demonstrate calm, nonjudgmental, nonthreatening demeanor in all interactions *to diminish the client's perceived threats to self-system and encourage more adaptive coping.*
Assure the client who exhibits mistrust, suspicion, or paranoia that the environment is safe *to decrease the client's anxiety, build trust, and present reality:*
"You're in the hospital and you're safe here."
"Those people are clients; they're planning an activity."
Refrain from attacking or challenging the client's delusional system. *It may alienate the client, diminish trust, and force the client to defend the delusion in an effort to justify the belief and thereby preserve self-esteem.*
Engage the client in frequent, brief contacts; avoid whispering or laughing; refrain from arguing; inform the client of schedule changes; gently question irrational beliefs of grandiosity or paranoia; and speak in a calm, clear concise manner *to establish a therapeutic, trusting relationship and reduce ambivalence, suspicion, and other defensive behaviors.*
Inform the client gently, but firmly, when you do not share his or her interpretation of an event, even though you acknowledge the client's feelings, *to help the client focus on actual vs. perceived situations:*
"The group is not against you, although you think so now; your cursing upsets them."
"Sam didn't take your cigarettes; you gave the last one to Jeff last night."
"It's OK to feel bad about not getting your pass. The staff is not to blame."
Refocus conversations to realistic topics when the client begins to misinterpret events and the behaviors of others *to encourage reality-based thinking and minimize defensive behaviors.*
Offer feedback whenever the client resorts to defensive coping behaviors (blaming or threatening others, using angry voice tones, cursing or shouting, acting aggressively) *to help the client identify maladaptive behaviors and their effects on others in the environment:*
"We were having a nice conversation, but now you seem angry; I'm wondering what happened."
"The group is upset with your shouting. They find it hard to concentrate on the discussion."

"Sam is tired of you blaming him for taking your cigarettes. What are your feelings about this?"

Encourage the patient to participate in milieu activities, e.g., leisure activities, occupational and recreational activities, one-to-one and group sessions, *to assuage anxiety, gain insight into stressors that incite defensive coping behaviors, and acquire more adaptive coping skills.*

Help the client select activities that are most rewarding and generally result in success *to increase self-esteem and reduce incidents of defensive coping to meet needs.*

Teach the client behavioral strategies, e.g., slow deep-breathing exercises, progressive muscle relaxation, simple physical exercises, *to divert anxiety-producing energy toward constructive activities and reduce incidents of defensive coping.* (See Appendix K.)

Praise the client for using more adaptive methods to meet needs *to increase self-esteem and ensure continuity of functional behaviors:*

"Your cooperation in group today was appreciated."

"You expressed yourself clearly and quietly. It was nice that you didn't shout or curse."

Continue to demonstrate concern and caring for the client during times of anxiety, suspiciousness, and mistrust. *Suspicious clients respond well to staff who display concerned, interested attitudes, and it may provide the impetus for the client to change or modify dysfunctional behaviors.*

Refrain from touching the client during times of increased anxiety, paranoia, and impaired reality testing *to prevent client from misinterpreting motives and possibly reacting with aggression.*

Help the client associate maladaptive behaviors with thoughts and feelings that precipitate them *to give the client the opportunity to interrupt the sequence and replace negative behaviors with learned relaxation strategies.* (See Appendix K.)

Never challenge, threaten, or use unnecessary force with a client who is verbally insulting. *The client may react with violence to protect the self-system.*

Suggest trying writing or drawing as a means of communication *to offer constructive alternative methods to express feelings and meet needs that would decrease anxiety and minimize defensive coping.*

Construct a written behavioral contract with the client, listing acceptable behaviors, expected outcomes, methods by which to achieve them, and consequences of unacceptable behaviors in clear, concrete terms. *Written contracts serve as permanent, visual reminders for clients who find it difficult to respond to verbal directives.*

Set limits in a calm, direct, matter-of-fact manner when the client begins to demonstrate behaviors that are out of control (accuses, blames, curses, threatens, exhibits hostile or aggressive acts) *to prevent injury to the client and others and give the client the opportunity to choose more functional methods to get needs met.*

"You may remain in the volleyball game if you do not shove other clients."

"Threatening others is not acceptable even if you say you're joking. Let's discuss other ways to deal with your feelings."

"It's OK to leave the group when you feel anxious, but slamming the door shut is disruptive; let's talk instead."

Be aware that verbal abuse and persistent anger are signals of the client's potential for violence, and inform the client of the consequences of his or her behavior *to prevent injury to the client and others and to offer the client another opportunity to choose alternative means to get needs met.* (See Appendix L.)

Continue to support and monitor prescribed medical and psychosocial treatment plan.

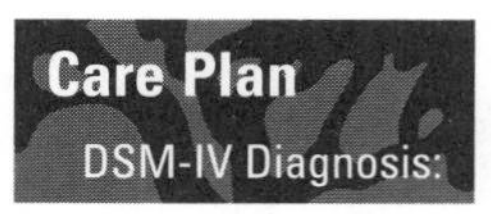

Schizophrenia (All Types)

NANDA Diagnosis: Coping, ineffective family disabling

The state in which the behavior of a significant person (family member or other primary person) disables his or her own capacities and the client's capacities to effectively address tasks essential to either person's adaptation to the health challenge

Focus:
For the family and significant persons of a chronically ill client who demonstrates dysfunctional behaviors owing to lack of cognitive, physical, or psychologic resources needed to cope with the effects of mental illness

NANDA Taxonomy
Pattern 5—Choosing: A human response pattern involving the selection of alternatives

ETIOLOGIC/RELATED FACTORS (RELATED TO)

Extremely ambivalent family relationships (members vacillate between withdrawal from and solicitude toward the ill person)

Significant persons unable to express feelings of guilt, anger, frustration, or despair

Ineffective or maladaptive coping strategies used by significant persons

Denial by significant persons of psychosocial and financial impact of illness on client, family, and community

Disintegrated client and family role/relationships

Resistance or refusal of significant persons to participate in client's treatment and care

Physically, developmentally, or emotionally impaired significant persons

Defensive or uncooperative significant persons

Knowledge deficit of significant persons regarding illness and management

Family enmeshment, overinvolvement, solicitude, extreme worry regarding client, illness, and management of care

DEFINING CHARACTERISTICS (AS EVIDENCED BY)

Inattention to the client's basic needs by significant persons:
- Client exhibits unkempt, unclean appearance on various admissions.
- Client demonstrates progressive weight loss, poor skin turgor, broken skin, and dental cavities.
- Client's clothes are dirty, shabby, or sparse.

Failure of significant persons to attend to client's needs for love and companionship:
- Absence of visitors during hospitalization
- Client statements such as "No one cares about me," "Everyone I know eventually leaves me," and "I'm not wanted at home anymore."

Failure of significant persons to assist client in management of illness:
- Refusal to accompany client on follow-up treatments
- Neglects to help client comply with medication regimen after discharge
- Uncooperative with staff regarding client's placement after discharge

Inappropriate or mixed reactions by significant persons toward client's illness and effects of illness on client, family, and community:
- Family members display little or no emotion when discussing client's illness and treatment and the effects of the illness on all their lives.
- Family members express conflicting, emotionally charged content, e.g., criticism, disappointment, solicitude, worry, overprotectiveness, or overinvolvement.

Preoccupation of significant persons with negative thoughts and feelings regarding client's illness and management of care:
- Family members describe feeling overwhelmed with anger, anxiety, fear, guilt, or despair.
- Family members state they are unable to dismiss thoughts of personal inadequacy and hostility toward client.

Withdrawal of significant persons from client during time of need (intolerance, rejection, abandonment, desertion)

Demonstrations of overprotective behavior or overinvolvement by significant others toward client, which fosters client's dependency (enmeshment):
- Family constantly reminds staff of their devotion to the client; phones the unit several times a day; visits day and night and hovers around the client; acts as the client's protector in the milieu; makes demands on staff on the client's behalf.

Alternate displays of rejection and overprotection by significant persons toward client (ambivalence).

Distortion of reality by significant persons regarding the client's illness, e.g., extreme denial about its existence or severity:
- Family members carry on usual routines, disregarding the client's needs.
- Family members act indifferent or apathetic toward serious information given to them about client and illness.

Decisions and actions by family that are detrimental to client's and family's social or economic well-being. (Family accumulates debts that do not include cost of client's care, treatment, or placement.)

Signs of agitation, depression, aggression, or hostility demonstrated by significant others

Ineffective or neglectful relationships among family members, which disintegrate the family support system

Client's development of helplessness, inactivity, and dependence on significant persons and society

Impaired ability of family members to restructure meaningful lives or to individualize owing to prolonged involvement with client.

OUTCOME IDENTIFICATION AND EVALUATION

Significant persons will:

Verbalize realistic perception of roles and responsibilities regarding client and client's illness, care, and treatment.

Express thoughts and feelings about responsibility to client, openly and frequently, in a therapeutic environment.

Demonstrate improved communication, problem-solving, and decision-making skills in relating to other family members and health-care personnel regarding client's illness and treatment.

Exhibit effective coping strategies in dealing with client's illness and management of care.

PLANNING AND IMPLEMENTATION

Nursing Interventions and Rationale

Assess the family's current level of functioning and contrast with their level of functioning prior to the onset of the client's illness *to determine the degree of the family's dysfunction over time and assist them to develop a realistic plan to support the client according to their tolerance and capabilities.*

Assess and promote the readiness and willingness of individual family members to participate in client's management of care. *Aftercare of clients must include family if the client is to succeed in meaningful interpersonal functioning.*

Examine the extent of expressed family emotions, enmeshment, or disintegration regarding the client, the illness, and management of care. *Clients from families who are overinvolved, enmeshed, of overprotective or who consistently express criticism, disappointment, hostility, solicitude, extreme worry, or anxiety are at high risk for relapse.*

Encourage family members to join therapeutic family groups. *Anger, despair, frustration, guilt, or powerlessness can be expressed with others who share similar emotions. Realistic expectations and goals regarding the family's role in the client's illness and treatment can be discussed.* (See Appendix K, Family Therapy.)

Teach family members the facts about the illness (and that it could strike any family), including its course and chronicity, and the expected effects of the illness on the family and its role in the community. *Dispel myths, decrease stigma, enlist cooperation of capable family members, promote adaptive coping skills, and encourage the family to rejoin society armed with accurate information and decreased embarrassment about the client and the client's illness.*

Promote family involvement in the hospital environment, e.g., attend groups, family therapy meetings, conferences with client; confer with caregivers as often as necessary; attend in-service seminars; review current literature on the client's illness, treatment, and research. *This encourages healthy family involvement and participation in the client's hospital domain, which could be continued after discharge, informs the family of all facets of the client's illness and management, illustrates that care of the client is a team effort so the family will not feel isolated and overwhelmed, and offers hope through the client's success in a therapeutic environment.*

Encourage family involvement in behavioral management programs that specifically address the client's problems *to help the family acquire strategies that can positively influence the client's life and strengthen the family system.*

Inform the family of the community services and personnel available to assist them when the client's symptoms and behavior are difficult to comprehend or manage, e.g., hospital treatment team (nurse, physician, social worker, occupational therapist), aftercare services (local mental health meetings, day treatment groups, night hospitals, sheltered workshops, rehabilitation services, private therapists). *This assures the client and family of the availability of qualified help and support, reduces feelings of isolation and powerlessness, encourages use of services to enable clients to remain in the community, relieves the family of its burdens, and strengthens the family system.*

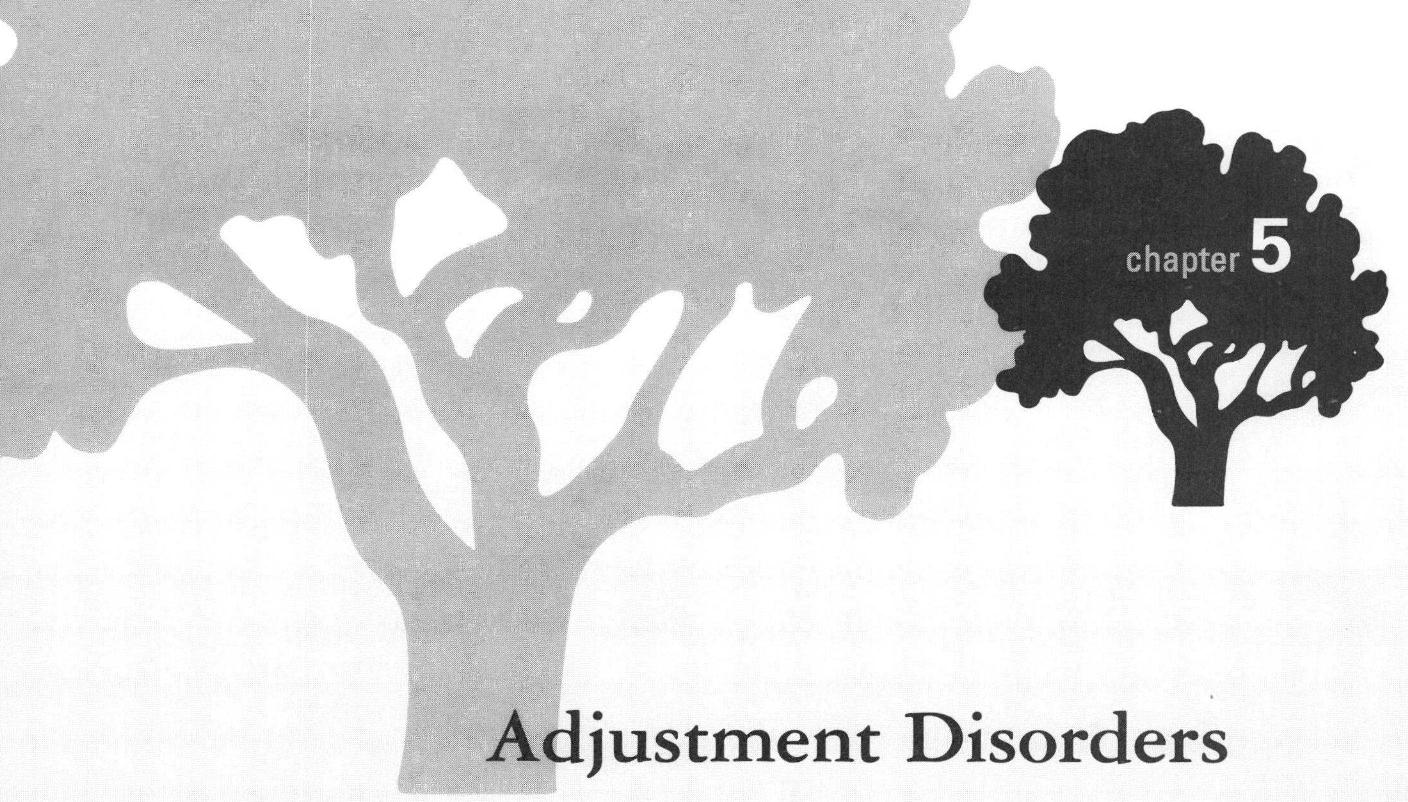

Adjustment Disorders

Adjustment disorders represent a group of diagnostic categories that describe a maladaptive reaction to a clearly identifiable stressor event or events. Stressors may be a single event such as the ending of a personal relationship, several events such as serious business or marital problems, recurrent events such as those associated with seasonal jobs or business crises, or ongoing circumstances such as living in a high-crime neighborhood or working with difficult people. Stressors may affect a single individual, a whole family, a larger group, or an entire community, as in a natural disaster. Some stressors may accompany specific developmental events such as beginning school, leaving one's home of origin, getting married, becoming a parent, or retiring (Box 5-1).

An adjustment disorder is not an exacerbation of a preexisting mental disorder that has its own set of criteria, such as an anxiety disorder or a mood disorder. However, an adjustment disorder can coexist with another Axis I or Axis II diagnosis if the latter does not account for the pattern of symptoms that have occurred in response to the stressor event. An adjustment disorder, by definition, occurs within 3 months after the onset of the stressor and resolves within 6 months of the cessation of the stressor or its effects, but it may be prolonged if the problem and its consequences are persistent and enduring, such as a chronic, disabling illness, long-term marital strife, or a divorce (Box 5-2).

Not only are adjustment disorders associated with an increased risk of suicide attempts and suicide completion but also an adjustment disorder may complicate the course of illness (e.g., decreased compliance with the medical regimen or increased length of hospital stay) in people diagnosed with a medical condition.

In a multiaxial assessment, the nature of the stressor is indicated by listing it on Axis IV (e.g., marital, divorce, work, or academic problem). Table 5-1 compares the stressors and symptoms of adjustment disorder, posttraumatic stress disorder, and acute stress disorder; adjustment disorder responses and bereavement responses are compared in Box 5-3.

ETIOLOGY

Specific etiologic factors related to adjustment disorders are listed in Box 5-4.

EPIDEMIOLOGY

Adjustment disorders are common and may occur in any age group; men and women are equally affected. Epidemiologic features vary widely because of the types of population studied and the assessment methods used, but here seems to be a higher incidence of adjustment disorders in individuals from disadvantaged life circumstances than in the general population in that they experience a high rate of stressors (e.g., the results of poverty, unemployment, crime, unwanted pregnancies, malnutrition, single parenthood, drug abuse, and other physical and psychologic abuses).

The percentage of people in outpatient mental health treatment with a diagnosis of adjustment disorder ranges from approximately 5% to 30%.

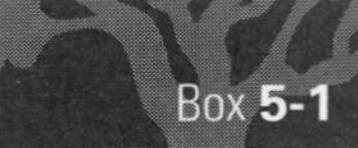

Box 5-1

Stressors and Their Relationship to Developmental Stages

Childhood: Separation from significant others; preschool
Adolescence: Graduation from high school; life choices
Adulthood: Intimacy; marriage; parenthood; career building
Adult Midlife: Financial/emotional care of young and old
Adult Old Age: Loss of job/spouse; possible major illness

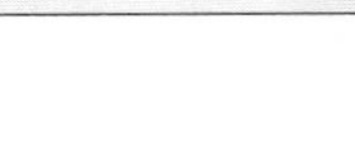

Box 5-2

Course of Illness

Onset of Disturbance: Within 3 months of identified stressor
Duration of Disturbance: No longer than 6 months after the cessation of stressor and effects*
Onset in Acute Event: Usually immediate or within a few days
Duration of Disturbance: Relatively brief (a few months).*

*Adjustment disorder may persist if stressor or its effects are prolonged.

Table 5-1

Comparison of Adjustment Disorder, Posttraumatic Stress Disorder, and Acute Stress Disorder

Disorders That Are Preceded by Stressors	Intensity of Stressor	Types of Symptoms
Adjustment disorder	Various levels of severity	Wide range of possible symptoms
Posttraumatic stress disorder	Severe	Specific constellation of symptoms
Acute stress disorder	Severe	Specific constellation of symptoms

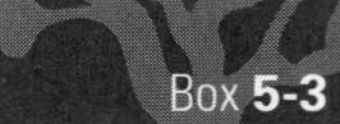

Box 5-3

Responses of Adjustment Disorder and Bereavement

Adjustment Disorder: Responses to stress are generally unexpected
Bereavement (Grief): Responses to stress are generally expected (e.g., death of a loved one)*

*A diagnosis of adjustment disorder may be made if the response in bereavement is in excess of or more prolonged than what is typically expected.

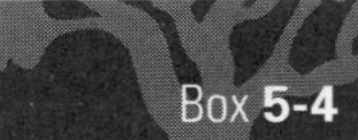

Box 5-4

Etiologic Factors Related to Adjustment Disorders*

Biologic/Genetic

Physiologic response to crisis and stress such as acute or chronic illness or injury that requires a biologic adjustment

Biochemical

Activation of adrenaline and other neurotransmitters as noted in stress adaptation and crisis models

Psychodynamic

Maladaptive ego defenses or lack of ego strength at critical life stages; inability of the ego to adapt/adjust to crises

Psychosocial

Psychologic/emotional responses to crisis and stressor events; inability to use existing coping methods or create new ones. These may be influenced by timing, intensity, or repetition of the stressor event

A chronic, debilitating illness may require both physical and psychologic adjustments to the ongoing stressors.

Developmental

Stressors experienced at critical developmental stages of adolescence, adulthood, adult midlife, and adult old age.

Cultural

Sociocultural adjustment, response to illness, and meaning of illness vary among individuals from different cultures.

An individual's culture may determine whether the reaction to the stressor is expected or exceeds the usual response.

*Although a specific etiology for adjustment disorders has not been established, a combination of factors is implicated. The current research emphasis is biologic.

DIAGNOSIS OF ADJUSTMENT DISORDERS*

Adjustment Disorder with Depressed Mood

The defining characteristics of adjustment disorder with depressed mood are depressed mood, tearfulness, sadness, and feelings of hopelessness or helplessness. More serious responses are melancholia, regression, psychophysiologic decompensation, and depersonalization.

Adjustment Disorder with Anxiety

The defining characteristics of adjustment disorder with anxiety are worry, nervousness, jitteriness, and, in children, fears of separation from major attachment figures, resulting in myriad symptoms.

Adjustment Disorder with Mixed Anxiety and Depressed Mood

The defining characteristics of adjustment disorder with mixed anxiety and depressed mood are symptoms of both anxiety and depression, as described in the previous two categories.

Adjustment Disorder with Disturbance of Conduct

The defining characteristics of adjustment disorder with disturbance of conduct is a disturbance in conduct in which there is violation of others' rights or of major age-appropriate societal norms and rules such as truancy; vandalism; reckless driving; substance abuse; fighting and other inappropriate forms of anger, aggression, and impulsivity; and defaulting on legal responsibilities.

Adjustment Disorder with Mixed Disturbance of Emotions and Conduct

The defining characteristics of adjustment disorder with mixed disturbance of emotions and conduct combine emotional symptoms such as depression and anxiety with a disturbance in conduct, as described previously.

Adjustment Disorder, Unspecified

The defining characteristics of adjustment disorder, unspecified, are not classifiable in any of the other subtypes, such as physical complaints, social withdrawal, school or work problems, or other psychosocial stressors.

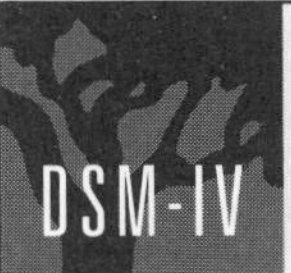

Adjustment Disorders

The essential characteristic of adjustment disorders is the development of clinically significant behavioral or emotional symptoms in response to an identifiable psychosocial stressor

DSM-IV Categories

Adjustment Disorder with Depressed Mood
Adjustment Disorder with Anxiety
Adjustment Disorder with Mixed Anxiety and Depressed Mood
Adjustment Disorder with Disturbance of Conduct
Adjustment Disorder with Mixed Disturbance of Emotions and Conduct
Adjustment Disorder, Unspecified

*Adjustment disorders are coded according to the subtype that best characterizes the predominant symptoms.

INTERVENTIONS FOR ADJUSTMENT DISORDERS

Hospitalization

Adjustment disorders are typically treated on an outpatient basis unless the stressor or its consequences are greater than the individual's ability to cope and short-term acute care is necessary. A variety of therapeutic techniques may be employed by an interdisciplinary team, depending on the professional preference, assessment of problem, and desired outcome.

Somatic Therapy

Medications are used sparingly for these clients because adjustment disorders are expected to resolve after the immediate cause is identified and processed. Also, practitioners prefer to observe the client without the effects of medications because in some cases symptoms of adjustment disorder may progress to include symptoms of a major mental disorder. Benzodiazepines may be used to treat clients with adjustment disorder who manifest symptoms of anxiety. Antidepressants may be used to treat clients with adjustment disorder who experience symptoms of depression. The literature shows that research studies are needed to evaluate the use and effectiveness of medications in treating clients with adjustment disorder, especially those with underlying mood disorders.

Psychosocial Therapies

Nurse-client relationship therapy.
Refer to Appendix G.

Adjunctive therapies. Recreational therapies may be useful for clients diagnosed with adjustment disorder, whether they are in an outpatient or inpatient setting. Leisure activities promote socialization and help clients become more comfortable with others who may have similar problems, even if they do not all share the same diagnosis. Recreational therapies also inspire clients to engage

*In an adjustment disorder, the response is considered maladaptive because of noted impairment in social, academic, or occupational functioning or because the resultant symptoms or behaviors exceed normal, usual, or expected responses.

in more self-directed pursuits that may build confidence and increase self-esteem. Exercise can be a constructive anxiety-reducing outlet for some clients; others may prefer relaxation strategies. Occupational therapy may help clients whose crises are related to role changes or who may have some residual dysfunction as a result of a concomitant physical disability. In any case, the client's developmental stage, capabilities, presented problems, and preferences should all be considered before any of the adjunctive therapeutic activities are initiated.

Supportive therapies. Clinical nurse specialists, social workers, physicians, and psychologists are prepared and trained to manage the care of clients with adjustment disorders via a therapeutic interdisciplinary team approach. A variety of treatment options is available for outpatients, depending on professional preference, assessment of problems, and desired outcomes. Cognitive therapy, brief strategic therapy, and other types of behavioral interventions may be used effectively in combination with psychodynamic, psychotherapeutic, or interpersonal approaches. Family therapy may be selected when the identified stressor is a crisis within the family system. Group therapy may also be used.

Other therapies. Biofeedback, psychodrama, hypnosis, meditation, visual imagery, and journal writing are other therapeutic modalities that may be helpful for clients with adjustment disorders, depending on individual problems and client and practitioner preference. (See Appendix K.)

DISCHARGE CRITERIA FOR CLIENTS WITH ADJUSTMENT DISORDERS

Verbalizes absence of thoughts of self-harm
Verbalizes realistic perceptions of self and capabilities
Sets realistic goals and expectations for self and others
Identifies psychosocial stressors and potential crises
Describes plans and methods to minimize stressors
States realistic/positive methods to cope with stressors
Identifies signs and symptoms of adjustment disorder
Contacts appropriate sources for validation/intervention
Utilizes learned techniques to prevent/minimize symptoms
Verbalizes knowledge of therapeutic/nontherapeutic effects and potential problems of prescribed medications
Makes and keeps follow-up appointments with appropriate staff
Expresses feelings openly, directly, and appropriately
Engages family/significant others as sources of support
Structures life to include appropriate outlets/activities
Verbalizes plans for future with absence of suicidal thoughts

Nursing Process for

Adjustment Disorders

Universal Principles for Interactions and Interventions with Clients with Adjustment Disorders

- Continue to monitor assessment parameters listed in *Defining Characteristics.*
- Continue to consider the etiologic factors listed in *Etiologic/Related Factors.*
- Utilize principles of the *Therapeutic Nurse-Client Relationship* (Appendix G).
- Address clients' spiritual and cultural needs.

General Principles

- Maintain health and safety
- Protect client from self-destructive behavior
- Assist client to anticipate situations that produce stress and to recognize effects of stressful situations
- Teach client effective coping methods to manage stressors and to minimize stressor effects whenever possible
- Help client identify emerging signs of adjustment disorder
- Instruct client to contact appropriate sources for help as soon as symptoms occur
- Promote compliance with prescribed therapeutic regimen
- Engage client/significant others in therapeutic effects and problem areas of prescribed medications
- Teach client about therapeutic/nontherapeutic effects and problem areas of prescribed medications
- Encourage client to express thoughts and feelings openly and appropriately
- Reinforce symptom prevention measures with client and support system
- Assess client continually for self-destructive thoughts and behaviors and for future goals and plans

Care Plans for Adjustment Disorders Based on Nursing Diagnosis

DSM-IV Diagnoses

Adjustment Disorder with Depressed Mood
Adjustment Disorder with Anxiety
Adjustment Disorder with Mixed Anxiety and Depressed Mood
Adjustment Disorder with Disturbance of Conduct
Adjustment Disorder with Mixed Disturbance of Emotions and Conduct
Adjustment Disorder, Unspecified

NANDA Diagnoses

Coping, ineffective individual
Grieving, dysfunctional

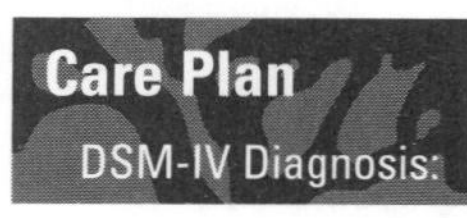

Adjustment Disorders (All Types)

NANDA Diagnosis: Coping, ineffective individual

The state in which an individual demonstrates impairment of adaptive behaviors and problem-solving abilities in meeting life's demands and roles

Focus:
For the client experiencing maladaptive responses to an identifiable stressor event, as demonstrated by impairment in social, academic, or occupational functioning, and behaviors that exceed the normal expected response to the stressor. Symptoms of anxiety, depression, or conduct disturbances may also be present. Stressors can be acute or chronic; psychosocial, physical, or developmental; singular or multiple.

NANDA Taxonomy
Pattern 5—Choosing: A human response pattern involving the selection of alternatives

ETIOLOGIC/RELATED FACTORS (RELATED TO)

Impaired reactions to developmental conflicts. *Examples:* Graduation from high school, leaving home for college, marriage, parenthood, retirement.
Maladaptive responses to psychosocial stressors. *Examples:* Marital problems, divorce, job dissatisfaction, business failure, moving to a new environment.
Residual effects of physical or psychiatric illness/disability
Depletion of previously existing coping methods and inability to attain new ones
Premorbid life-style of negative coping methods
Developmental lag
Ineffective or absent resources
Dysfunctional family system
Ineffective problem-solving skills
Knowledge deficit regarding crisis management
Lack of insight regarding own abilities and limitations
Unrealistic expectations of self and others
Low self-esteem
Negative role modeling
Unresolved grief in response to crisis or stressor event

DEFINING CHARACTERISTICS (AS EVIDENCED BY)

Verbalizes inability to cope with stressors/conflicts:
"I can't make it without my significant other."
"I'll never find another job that satisfies me."
"My marital problems are ruining my life."
"I can't adjust to this new place; it's depressing."
Demonstrates nonacceptance of health-status change
- Withdrawal from social functions
- Loss of appetite/weight unrelated to disability/illness
- Saddened affect with intermittent crying spells
- Self-destructive behavior (smokes, stays up all night)
- Anger or blame directed toward family or friends
- Unable to work or perform activities of daily living

Demonstrates ineffective capacity to problem solve or establish goals (i.e., cannot make simple choices or decisions)
Exhibits increased dependency on others to complete work and fulfill needs. *Examples:*
Child depends on parents to complete school assignments and household chores.
Adolescent overspends allowance and borrows money from family and friends, rather than work for it.
Adult uses fiancé, spouse, or family members to support him or her financially and emotionally.
Older adult relies on grown children to provide basic needs even though capable of performing own daily tasks.
Demonstrates inability to adjust to maturational changes:
- *Child:* regression during toilet-training process
- *Adolescent:* depression due to body changes (e.g., acne, unfulfilled body image)
- *Adult:* depression about weight gain due to pregnancy
- *Older adult:* depression following "normal" changes of aging

Demonstrates inability to meet role expectations
- *Child:* regression at birth of new sibling
- *Adolescent:* anxiety when attempting intimacy
- *Adult:* depression with own performance as parent
- *Older adult:* depression following retirement from cherished job/profession

Manifests alterations in societal participation (i.e., isolates/withdraws from social scene, refuses to engage in community activities)
Fails to follow societal/unit rules of conduct. *Examples:*
Child demonstrates temper tantrums and other acting-out behaviors upon perceiving needs to be unmet.
Adolescent steals others' belongings and engages in physical fights with individuals perceived to be "enemies" or opponents.
Adult commits violent or illegal crimes and misdemeanors with apparent unconcern about consequences of actions.
Expresses self-destructive thoughts, plans, gestures
Demonstrates noncompliance with therapeutic regimen, including refusal to take prescribed medications
Verbalizes knowledge deficit regarding stress prevention skills and ability to minimize stressors when they occur
Describes symptoms of grief responses to stressor events and crisis situations
- Frequent sighing
- Sad, despondent feelings
- Negative, hopeless thoughts
- A sense of powerlessness
- Ambivalence, anger
- Low self-esteem
- Yearning and protest
- Inability to plan future goals

OUTCOME IDENTIFICATION AND EVALUATION

Verbalizes ability to cope with stressors/conflicts:

"I can make it now; my friends have given me the support and strength to go on without (significant other)."

"I know I have the talent to be successful in another job; I've done it before."

"Maybe divorce isn't the worst thing in the world; it's better than struggling in an unhappy marriage."

"I miss my family and friends, but moving to a new place is an exciting opportunity to meet new people."

Demonstrates acceptance of health change status. *Examples:*

- Decrease in depressive symptoms (laughs and engages with others more often)
- Increase in appetite
- Normal weight maintained
- Return to normal sleep patterns
- Healthy expressions of anger
- Others not blamed for health change
- Normal activities/interests resumed
- Absence of self-destructive behavior

Demonstrates decreased dependency on others to meet needs. *Examples:*

Child completes schoolwork and household tasks with minimal supervision.

Adolescent works for allowance and spends within means.

Adult supports self and family or significant other adequately.

Older adult is supportive adjunct to grown children and grandchildren *or* significant others, as age and circumstances allow.

Demonstrates effective adjustment to maturational changes. *Examples:*

Child achieves mastery of stages (e.g., trust, autonomy, initiative) without significant regression.

Adolescent achieves puberty and identifies with appropriate role models, with minimal conflicts and stress.

Adult accepts generative processes (e.g., pregnancy, weight gain) with absence of midlife crisis.

Older adult accepts normal changes of aging with integrity versus despair.

Meets role expectations with minimal stress. *Examples:*

Child accepts changes (e.g., preschool, school, new sibling) with minimal regression.

Adolescent achieves healthy peer relationships with minimal anxiety and conflict.

Adult exhibits strong, flexible parenting and other mentor skills and successful job/career performance.

Older adult accepts retirement as part of life and transfers productivity to alternate worthwhile activities.

Actively participates socially with family, friends, and community groups

Follows societal or unit rules of conduct. *Examples:*

Child is directable and adaptive with minimal acting-out or oppositional behaviors.

Adolescent gets along well with peers and accepts adult supervision and directives, with minimal opposition.

Adult refrains from hostile, illegal acts toward society or other clients.

Demonstrates absence of self-destructive behaviors

Complies with therapeutic regimen, including medication

Verbalizes knowledge and plan to prevent stress and minimize inevitable stressors when they occur

Demonstrates stress prevention/reduction skills:

- Physical exercise/activities
- Writing in a log or journal
- Cognitive therapeutic strategies
- Reframing techniques
- Assertive response behaviors

(Refer to Appendix K, Psychiatric Therapies.)

Cites knowledge of appropriate community resources for ongoing follow-up care, as necessary

- Self-help groups
- Day treatment program
- Individual or group therapy

PLANNING AND IMPLEMENTATION

Nursing Interventions and Rationale

Encourage discussion of feelings and emotions (such as anger, fear, sadness, guilt, hostility) according to developmental level, with the client, *to help client identify actual object of stress/crisis and develop the trust to begin to work through unresolved issues.*

Provide physical outlets for healthy release of pent-up anger/anxiety and hostile feelings (e.g., punching pillows, running, jogging, simple stretching and breathing exercises, as appropriate). *Physical exercise is a safe and effective method to reduce stress/tension.*

Promote independent behaviors, role, and life-style experienced by the client prior to adjustment disorder symptoms.

- *Child:* Assign simple age-appropriate tasks related to school and home with appropriate rewards/tokens for each completed task.
- *Adolescent:* Construct, with the adolescent, a written daily log/diary of completed school/household work, and the amount of money or privilege earned for each task.
- *Adult:* Encourage adult support groups (e.g., cognitive, behavioral, brief strategic, assertive, relational, retirement planning, psychodrama, or process groups, as appropriate). Suggest family therapy for all age groups as it applies to individual situations.

Increased responsibility for age-appropriate life tasks and roles promotes coping skills, self-esteem, and independent functioning. Also, the individual's success or failure depends on his or her choices. (Refer to Appendix K, Psychiatric Therapies.)

Assist client (if inpatient) to adhere to unit rules and discuss consequences of noncompliance. Carry out consequences in a matter-of-fact manner if unit rules are broken.

- *Child:* Facilitate chair time (time-out) or reduction in rewards, privileges. Engage in role playing and role modeling as appropriate.
- *Adolescent:* Deny a special recreational activity such as a group outing or field trip. Engage in role playing and role modeling. Facilitate behavioral contracts as necessary.
- *Adult:* Deny movement to higher level of privilege in the unit. Engage in individual, group, family, or didactic therapies, appropriate to coping/adjustment problem. Adults who continue to be noncompliant with unit rules or do not engage in milieu programs may be recommended for alternative treatment (e.g., partial hospitalization, crisis centers, rehabilitation facilities, or discharged to own support system).

Adjustment problems related to conduct disorders require clear guidelines and directives by the staff to increase client compliance and coping. Also, other clients are entitled to a safe, nondisruptive, therapeutic milieu, without fear of manipulation.

Help clients recognize those aspects of their lives in which they have maintained control and order. *Awareness of personal control during critical developmental stages decreases powerlessness and enhances self-esteem. It also provides hope that the individual can transfer those abilities to resolve present conflicts/stressors.*

Identify, with the client, the stressor or stressor event that precipitated the maladaptive coping and other symptoms of adjustment disorder, and assist the client through the problem-solving process.

- Prioritize possible alternative coping methods appropriate to client's age and life circumstances.
- Discuss positives and negatives of each alternative (e.g., suggest that the client construct a double column on a sheet of paper and write positives on one side and negatives on the other, for each alternative coping method).
- Choose the best alternative method and apply it to the identified problem, first in a role-play situation, then in actual life.
- Evaluate the effectiveness of the alternative method (e.g., did the method minimize the stressor and its effects?).
- Develop awareness of areas of limitations and learn effective responses that create more distance between the self and the stressor or stressor event. (Refer to Appendix K, Assertiveness Training Skills.)
- Continue to consult with therapists/staff for assistance and modification of plan, as necessary.

Identifying stressors or stressor events that result in maladaptive coping and continued negative consequences is the first step in formulating effective alternative solutions and coping methods.

Provide realistic praise for client's attempts at adaptive coping and finding solutions for adjustment problems, even when they are not always successful. *Positive reinforcement for continued attempts at adaptive coping skills promotes hope and repetition of effective, desirable behaviors.*

Encourage client to discuss life-style prior to health status change, including coping methods used during those times. *Identification of client's strengths, support system, and healthy coping style is useful in facilitating adaptation to current change or loss.*

Give client permission to express normal grieving emotions (such as fear, anger, sadness) related to health status change and actual or perceived loss. *Some people may not be aware that anger, fear, and sadness are normal, healthy responses to critical life crises that need to be expressed, although their persistence may indicate a more serious depressive disorder that requires further treatment.*

Teach the client and family/significant others about the emotional, psychologic, and physiologic responses to stressors and stressor events, as appropriate, and provide understandable current reading material regarding adjustment disorders and related symptomatology. *Appropriate knowledge empowers clients and their families and increases hope, cooperation, and compliance. Information can also result in preventive measures that can minimize or eliminate future stress-related problems.*

Locate (with client and family) community resources that are geared to each individual's adjustment crisis (e.g., health status change, marital discord, maturational or developmental crisis, occupational or academic problem). *Community resources provide a wide variety of professionals (e.g., community health nurses, social workers, psychologists, marriage and family counselors, school and occupational counselors, and clergy who are available for ongoing help with adjustment problems.*

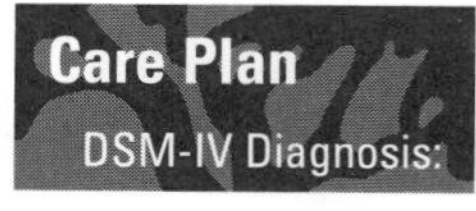

Adjustment Disorders (All Types)

NANDA Diagnosis: Grieving, dysfunctional

The state in which an individual or group experiences prolonged unresolved grief and engages in detrimental activities

Focus:

For the individual who demonstrates a sustained or prolonged detrimental response approximately several months to a year following a loss of a loved one or valued occupation, object, or life-style. Individuals in clinical settings are often at high risk for dysfunctional grieving because they frequently experience unsuccessful emotional and/or societal reintegration after a loss.

NANDA Taxonomy

Pattern 9—Feeling: A human response pattern involving the subjective awareness of information

ETIOLOGIC/RELATED FACTORS (RELATED TO)

Physical/Psychologic

Loss of body or psychologic functioning as a result of a physical or mental/emotional disorder or trauma

Situational

Changes in life-style or status, such as unanticipated death of a loved one; unwanted or unplanned pregnancy; complications of childbirth; a physically or mentally ill family member; divorce; loss of career, finances, or occupation; victim role (rape, robbery, abuse)

Maturational

Losses associated with aging (e.g., eyesight, hearing, mobility). Also includes forced retirement, death of spouse or old friends, and leaving own home to live with grown children or moving to a retirement home or skilled nursing facility.

Other Losses

Multiple or cumulative losses

Feelings of guilt and loss of self-esteem engendered by ambivalent or difficult relationships with the deceased

Lack of support systems

History of vulnerability as noted by response patterns associated with crisis or stressor events such as loss.

DEFINING CHARACTERISTICS (AS EVIDENCED BY)

Verbal expressions of distress (grief symptoms) regarding loss, change, or stressor event (e.g., anger, guilt, sadness, crying, labile mood, yearning and protest, sighing) inappropriate to normal stages of grieving

Alterations in functioning (e.g., loss of appetite, libido, sleep, concentration, and pursuit of tasks). Also, notable fatigability and anxiety (agitation, irritability).

Statements about unresolved issues and inability to move forward in life, with negative dream patterns, reliving of past experience, and idealization of previous lifestyle or of the deceased.

Excessive, inappropriate anger projected toward self and other family members and friends, rather than focusing anger appropriately toward the loss.

Continued ambivalence and loss of self-esteem are indicative of high risk for self-destructive behavior, as noted by the following statements.

"I should have died instead of him/her."

"He/she was so wonderful; I was the bad one."

"It was my fault that he/she died; I don't deserve to live."

Unsuccessful adjustment/adaptation to the loss (e.g., prolonged denial, delayed emotional response, precoccupation with loss experienced by others)

Social isolation or withdrawal (e.g., failure to resocialize with current friends, develop new relationships/interests, restructure life following the loss)

Idealization of the deceased or lost valued object, situation, role, status, or occupation, with concomitant nonacceptance of current life circumstances

OUTCOME IDENTIFICATION AND EVALUATION

Acknowledges the loss and expresses feelings/emotions associated with the loss experience (e.g., anger, sadness, guilt) appropriate to the grief process

Demonstrates a decreasing response in the intense pain associated with the grief process, appropriate to the stages of grieving

Demonstrates increased functional abilities (e.g., sleep, appetite, sexual activity, concentration, and pursuit of tasks)

Attempts to resolve issues associated with the loss in a healthy, meaningful way; discusses both positive and negative qualities (realistically) about the deceased or lost object, status, or occupation

Moves forward and beyond the grief experience in a timely manner (e.g., makes future plans, seeks others for socialization, experiences healthy dreams, focuses on more positive aspects of life)

Resolves ambivalence and self-blame about loss or lost valued object or concept, with concomitant increased self-esteem.

Seeks support persons and community resources (e.g., self-help groups, counseling, clergy) as needed

PLANNING AND IMPLEMENTATION

Nursing Interventions and Rationale

Identify the tasks of mourning that must be accomplished (acknowledging the loss, experiencing the pain, adjusting to the loss, reinvesting, and goal setting) for the individual, *to establish client's place on the grief continuum and begin to help with grief work and reintegration of life.*

If denial persists and the individual continues to disavow feelings associated with the loss, assure client that feelings/emotions are normal, healthy responses to loss and should be expressed in a safe, nurturing environment. *Unexpressed feelings result in pent-up emotions that may be directed inward and eventually lead to depression or other disorders.*

If anger is excessive and inappropriately expressed, help client and family understand that anger is a normal response to loss and powerlessness that needs to be vented, but that it is best to channel it toward the loss and its actual consequences, rather than project it toward self or others. *Such assurance provides structure and control for the client's emotional expressions while still giving permission to vent.*

Note: A diagnosis of adjustment disorder may be made if the response in bereavement (grief) is in excess of or more prolonged than what is typically expected (e.g., if the individual remains fixed in one stage of the grief process for an extended period of time or if the normal symptoms of grief become exaggerated).

Encourage the client and family to talk about both positive and negative qualities of the deceased or lost object, status, or role. *Realistic appraisal of the loss gives the client a clearer perspective of the situation, minimizes idealization, and promotes acceptance of current life circumstances.*

Engage the client in motor activities (e.g., brisk walks, jogging, physical exercise, volleyball, exercise bike). *Physical exercise provides a safe, effective method for expending anxious energy, anger, and tension.*

Assess the client's level of functioning:

- sleep
- appetite
- dream patterns
- sexual activity (if appropriate)
- socialization

Increase in functioning indicates successful movement toward health and reintegration and decrease in grief pain and despair.

Evaluate whether the individual is goal directed and making future plans or regressing and withdrawing from life. *Goals and plans for the future are indicators of health and reintegration, whereas regression and withdrawal signify that the client is at risk for depression and needs further evaluation and follow-up care.*

Continue to engage the individual in social activities and meaningful interpersonal interactions. *People experiencing grief and loss need to be involved with others to minimize isolation and withdrawal and to regain trust that others will help bear the pain of grief and that "life goes on."*

Identify effective supports in the family and community (e.g., self-help groups, individual and group counseling, clergy) for the grieving individual. *Appropriate support can help clients more readily do the grief work that will move them toward health and integrity.*

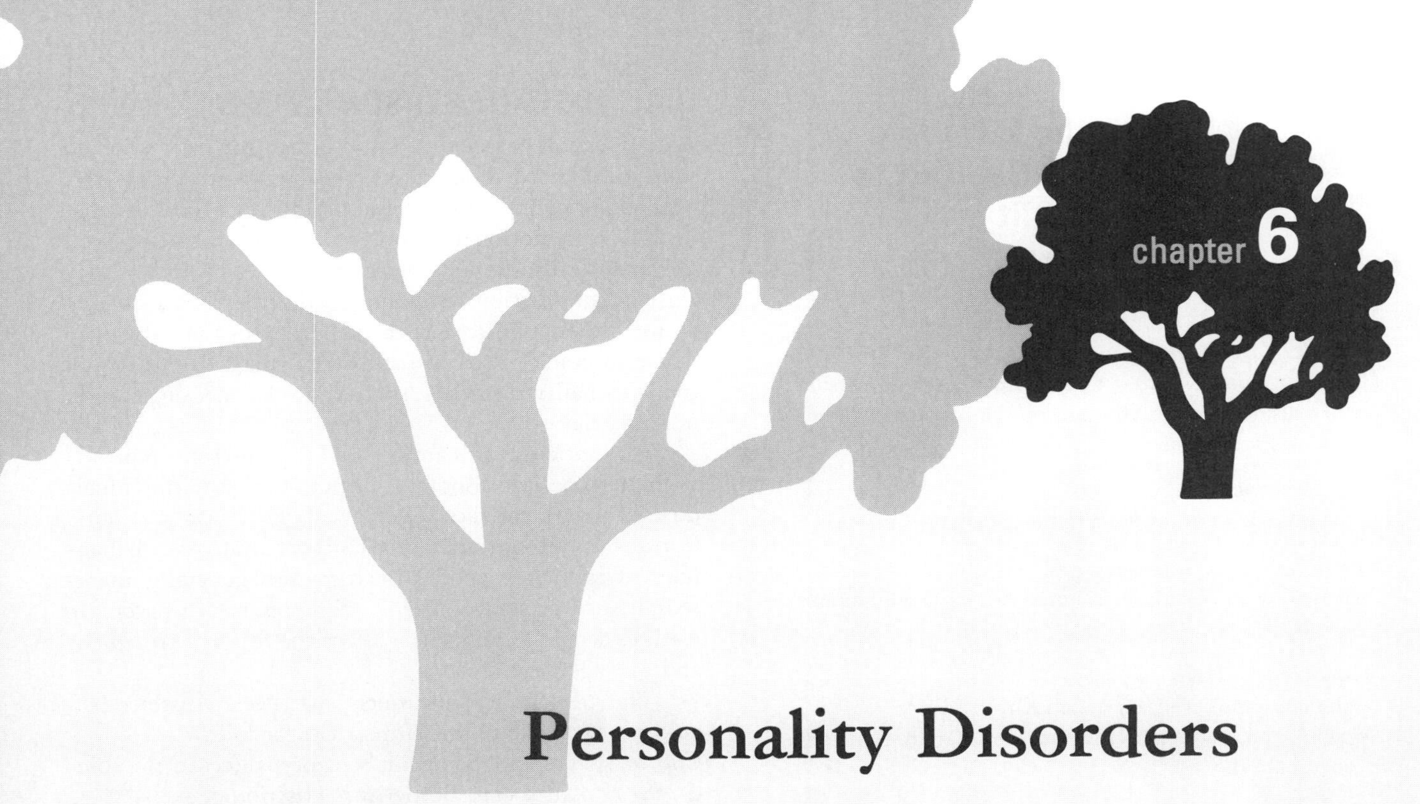

Personality Disorders

Personality is that unique and distinctive human quality that defines and determines the essence of a person's character—what he or she is really like. An individual's personality serves to distinguish him or her from everyone else in the world yet at the same time reflects qualities that are commonly noted in all individuals.

Personality traits are specific features or behavioral patterns that make up an individual's overall personality. Personality traits are defined in the DSM as "enduring patterns of perceiving, relating to and thinking about the environment and oneself." Traits represent an individual's lifelong style of viewing and interacting with the world. They begin to emerge early in life, develop over time, and are manifested within a broad range of experiences and social situations.

Personality disorders develop when those enduring, deeply ingrained traits or patterns become maladaptive and inflexible and cause difficulty for the person in relating to, working with, or loving others. The disorders are stable over time and eventually lead to distress and impairment. Frequently a personality disorder may be annoying to others or troubling to society or the law yet not viewed as a problem by the person with the disorder. Because the behavior has been so long-standing, it often feels "comfortable" (ego-syntonic) to the individual. Therefore, the person believes that he or she is right and the world is wrong and attempts to manipulate the environment to fit his or her needs.

Another factor that promotes resistance to change or treatment is that these individuals rarely experience the pain and discomfort of anxiety as a cue to their maladaptive behavior or its consequences. This lack of anxiety reinforces their perceptions that change is unnecessary, and they may seek treatment only when they become depressed because others can no longer tolerate the dysfunctional behaviors and proceed to make it difficult for them to continue to function in the same manner. In other words, societal demands exceed their ability to cope.

Personality disorders manifest during adolescence or early adulthood and persist throughout life, but generally a person is 18 years old before a formal diagnosis of personality disorder is assigned.

ETIOLOGY

Specific etiologic factors related to personality disorders are listed in Box 6-1.

EPIDEMIOLOGY

In general, definitive epidemiologic statistics are not clearly specified because individuals with personality disorders are not usually formally diagnosed. Incidence is higher among those whose first-degree relatives have personality disorders or related disorders. Antisocial, schizoid, and obsessive-compulsive personality disorders occur more often in men, whereas borderline, dependent, and histrionic personality disorders are more common in women.

Diagnosis of personality disorders has increased since the 1980 edition of the *Diagnostic and Statistical Manual* was published, in which criteria were revised to be more specific and to produce standardized classification.

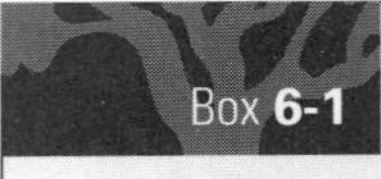

Box 6-1 Specific Etiologic Factors Related to Personality Disorders*

Biologic

Genetic/Hereditary

Higher incidence when first-degree relatives have personality disorder or related disorder. Concordance higher in monozygotic twins.

CNS Dysfunction

Higher incidence in minimally brain-damaged people.

Hormonal

Increased levels of androgens noted in people with aggressive tendencies.

Neurotransmitters

High endorphin levels associated with passivity.

Dopamine and serotonin arousal systems (aggression and impulsivity).

Psychodynamic

Early impulse/object choice relation and/or fixation at psychosexual development stage.

Psychosocial/Environmental

Poor parental/child bonding; environment encourages disorder (e.g., poverty, stressors); deviant behaviors learned from others in the environment.

*Although a specific etiology for personality disorders has not been established, a combination of biologic, psychosocial, and environmental factors is implicated. (Current direction is toward biologic research).

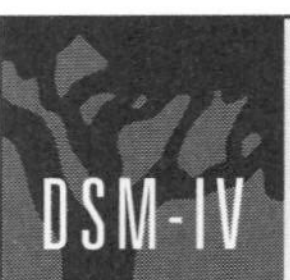

DSM-IV Personality Disorders

Regardless of the type of personality disorders diagnosed, most clients tend to manifest self-focused and self-serving behaviors.

DSM-IV Categories

Paranoid Personality Disorder
Schizoid Personality Disorder
Schizotypal Personality Disorder
Antisocial Personality Disorder
Borderline Personality Disorder
Histrionic Personality Disorder
Narcissistic Personality Disorder
Avoidant Personality Disorder
Dependent Personality Disorder
Obsessive-Compulsive Personality Disorder
Personality Disorder Not Otherwise Specified

DIAGNOSIS OF PERSONALITY DISORDER

A diagnosis of personality disorder is made only when an individual has demonstrated maladaptive characteristics over a long period and when signs and symptoms of other mental or emotional disorders are not demonstrated. Personality disorder is a separate entity, although it may exist in conjunction with another disorder. For example, an individual admitted with major depression as an Axis I diagnosis may also have an Axis II diagnosis of one of the personality disorders, such as borderline, dependent, or antisocial.

Psychotic features are generally not present in people with personality disorders, although these individuals do not always tolerate reality well. However, psychotic features may be present in clients with an Axis I diagnosis in which psychotic features are generally manifested, such as schizophrenia. The presence of psychotic features would significantly affect the focus of treatment and management of care.

The personality disorders have been clustered according to characteristic similarities, as follows:

Cluster A Paranoid, Schizoid, Schizotypal (eccentric, cold)
Cluster B Antisocial, Borderline, Histrionic, Narcissistic (emotional, erratic, dramatic)
Cluster C Avoidant, Dependent, Obsessive-Compulsive, Passive-Aggressive (anxious, fearful)

Paranoid Personality Disorder

The distinguishing features of Paranoid Personality Disorder are pervasive, long-standing suspicion and distrust of others and expectations of being threatened, harmed, exploited, or degraded. These individuals are secretive, guarded, and devious; they search for hidden meanings in harmless or benign remarks or situations. They are invariably argumentative, hostile, defensive, and stubborn. They are acutely aware of rank and power and frequently jealous of superiors and authority figures. Rigid and uncompromising behaviors make it difficult to work with these individuals in groups. A persistent search for injustice that is directed toward them permeates their lives. They hold grudges and refuse to forgive others.

Schizoid Personality Disorder

The distinguishing features of Schizoid Personality Disorder are a lifelong, pervasive, voluntary withdrawal from familial and social relationships and restricted emotional expression. These individuals have no close friends or confidants and have little or no desire for intimacy or sexual contact with another person. They prefer solitary activities and seem lonely, isolated, and eccentric. They appear aloof and cold and seldom, if ever, express strong emotions or respond to others with gestures or smiles.

Schizotypal Personality Disorder

The distinguishing features of Schizotypal Personality Disorder are odd or strange appearance, ideations, and behaviors and an inability to attain or maintain relatedness. These individuals have peculiar beliefs; experience magical thinking, bizarre fantasies, and unusual perceptions; and are extremely uncomfortable in the company of strangers. They tend to be suspicious, commonly experience ideas of reference, and may believe that they have special powers or insight. Affect is generally bland or silly, and interpersonal interactions are impaired.

Antisocial Personality Disorder

The distinguishing features of Antisocial Personality Disorder are an enduring pattern of violation of social norms and an inability to conform to them that results in impaired life functioning. Antisocial Personality Disorder is common in first-degree relatives of those with the disorder. The pattern may include a generally irresponsible attitude toward duties, obligations, and the rights of others; lying; cheating; stealing; running away from home; drug abuse; and unusual sexual behavior. Criminal activity and disregard for the rights of others are prevalent. In fact, up to 75% of people in prisons have been diagnosed with this disorder.

These individuals may be witty, charming, seductive, and manipulative to get their needs met, yet they invariably lack a social conscience or feel remorse about mistreating others. Reckless, demanding, cunning, conning, abusive, and aggressive behaviors are common. Interpersonal skills are generally ineffective, with resultant difficulties in sustaining close, warm, or lasting relationships. These individuals are often incapable of leading self-supporting, independent, rewarding lives and seldom have success in meeting the needs of others. Manipulation and impulsivity are hallmarks.

Many people with antisocial characteristics have manipulated the environment to achieve political or economic power. Most likely, they were exposed to a lifestyle in which such traits were considered necessary adjuncts to success.

Borderline Personality Disorder

The distinguishing features of Borderline Personality Disorder are a pervasive disturbance in self-image, mood, and affect; impulsivity; and an excessive need state, with resultant unstable, ineffective interpersonal relationships. Individuals with borderline personality disorder appear to be in a perpetual state of crisis. During periods of extreme stress, they may experience transient psychotic symptoms that are generally not severe enough to warrant a formal diagnosis of psychosis.

These individuals may demonstrate disturbances in identity, sexual orientation, and value-belief system and may make poor choices in career goals, friends, or romantic partners. They invariably experience chronic feelings of boredom and excessive fears of abandonment, whether real or imagined. They tend to manipulate the environment to satisfy their needs and assuage their fears.

Persons with this disorder often display sudden, unpredictable outbursts of anger as a result of their labile and unstable mood and affect. Their anger is often intense and uncontrolled and may be demonstrated as general irritability, temper tantrums, verbal abuse, physical assaultiveness, anxiety, or depression.

Because of intense feelings of ambivalence (two opposing feelings occurring at the same time), these individuals tend to view others as either "all good" or "all bad" at any given time and are unable to perceive others as being able to integrate these characteristics. Because affected individuals see the world only in terms of "black and white," they can act on only one extreme feeling at a time. This defense process, known as *splitting,* is considered a hallmark of the borderline personality.

Often, these individuals tend to overidealize people or groups in a momentary effort to get close, but, because of their fear and distrust of attachments, they just as quickly devalue them as an expression of rejection. They also tend to project their own feelings of discomfort onto others to protect themselves from any anxiety that may be provoked by such feelings. These manipulative, dysfunctional behaviors distance the individuals from others and perpetuate unstable, unsatisfying relationships.

Impulsive behaviors may lead the individual to activities that are self-damaging, such as excessive shopping sprees, shoplifting, casual sex, binge eating, or substance abuse. In more severe cases, self-mutilation and other suicidal gestures are common, generally because attempts to manipulate others have failed or because of intense anger or feelings of depersonalization, described by the individual as "numbness" or "detachment." Often, during these times, pain is not felt.

Histrionic Personality Disorder

The distinguishing feature of Histrionic Personality Disorder is an excessively dramatic, extroverted or flamboyant, attention-seeking display of emotions. These individuals need to be the center of attention, want immediate gratification, and exhibit poor tolerance for frustration. They constantly seek approval, praise, and reassurance from others and often resort to crying spells, temper tantrums, or accusations when their needs are not met.

Although the individuals may readily form relationships, their ingenuine, superficial, and egocentric charm generally dissipates quickly when others tire of their immature, histrionic behaviors. Once they form a relationship, they either attempt to control their partner or become dependent. Seductive, coy, and flirtatious behaviors are common in this personality disorder. These individuals are impressionable, demonstrate poor judgment, and are easily influenced by others.

Narcissistic Personality Disorder

The distinguishing features of Narcissistic Personality Disorder are a grandiose sense of self-importance and feelings of entitlement. These individuals believe that they are unique and thus deserving of special treatment and consideration. They actively seek praise or approval from others, are hypersensitive to evaluation, and become humiliated or enraged by others' criticism. They may hide their feelings of shame or anger by outwardly appearing indifferent.

These individuals often lack empathy for others and may exploit people to get their own needs met or for self-aggrandizement. Interpersonal relationships are generally disturbed and ineffective because "friendships" and romantic or sexual encounters are formed primarily to serve the individual's own needs.

Avoidant Personality Disorder

The distinguishing features of Avoidant Personality Disorder are excessive shyness and timidity and hypersensitivity to negative evaluation or rejection by others, which usually results in social withdrawal. Close, interpersonal relationships are rare with these individuals because they require, prior to making any commitments, a guarantee of constant, unconditional acceptance without the threat of criticism.

The extreme shyness and timidity these individuals experience often leads to avoidance of social situations, which greatly interferes with attaining and maintaining lasting friendships, as well as their choice of occupation. Individuals with this disorder generally avoid any new situation that may involve potential risk, danger, or difficulty, even though the possibilities are remote.

Unlike persons with Schizoid Personality Disorder, who socially isolate themselves with no desire to engage with others, these individuals may have strong desires for social contact, acceptance, and affection but are unable to reach out and relate to people. As a result, their interpersonal relationships are severely restricted.

Dependent Personality Disorder

The distinguishing features of Dependent Personality Disorder are extreme submissiveness toward others and a pattern of dependence on others to assume responsibility for their lives. These individuals generally lack self-confidence, cannot make decisions for themselves, and require constant reassurance and advice. They avoid leadership roles and find it extremely difficult to initiate or complete a project or task. These people intensely dislike being alone and consistently seek others on whom to depend. In fact, it is not uncommon for them to tolerate unhappy or even abusive relationships to satisfy their strong dependency needs.

Obsessive-Compulsive Personality Disorder

The distinguishing features of Obsessive-Compulsive Personality Disorder are exaggerated orderliness, perseverance, stubbornness, indecisiveness, and restricted emotionality. These individuals tend to be rigid, inflexible, and perfectionistic and often fail to complete projects because of their inability to achieve their own high performance and outcome standards. They are invariably preoccupied with correct form, rules, details, and efficiency and usually appear overconscientious when involved in a task. They generally insist that a project be done their way; if not, they prefer to do it themselves.

These individuals are not generous with material goods, praise, or affection and find it almost impossible to part with even worn-out or worthless possessions. Because of their rigidity, inflexibility, stubbornness, and selfishness, close, warm friendships are difficult for them to maintain.

Personality Disorder Not Otherwise Specified

This category is reserved for personality functions that do not meet criteria for any specific personality disorder; for example, a personality disorder that consists of features of more than one disorder (mixed personality). These combined personality functions can cause significant clinical impairment in one or more important areas of functioning; for example, social or occupational. Examples include depressive personality disorder and passive-aggressive personality disorder.

INTERVENTIONS FOR PERSONALITY DISORDERS

Long-term psychotherapy may be effective in bringing about behavioral changes, but the long-standing, enduring traits or patterns that are inherent in all personality disorders may be obstacles to treatment. Characteristic features and behavioral styles that have become ingrained in the very core and fabric of the individual will naturally be resistant to change.

Behavioral, cognitive, group, and family therapy, and assertiveness training have proven helpful in symptom management and modification. Medications are administered when necessary for such symptoms as anxiety, depression, and uncontrolled rage or aggression.

A person who has a personality disorder (Axis II) is generally not in need of hospitalization unless suicide threats, gestures, or attempts are present, or the personality disorder occurs in conjunction with a major Axis I disorder.

DISCHARGE CRITERIA FOR PERSONALITY DISORDERS

Controls impulses to manipulate others to meet own needs
Demonstrates ability to postpone immediate gratification
Verbalizes anger without acting out
Utilizes learned strategies to reduce anger
Refrains from harming self or others
Identifies dependent, interdependent, and independent behaviors
Demonstrates independent thinking, such as decision making
Verbalizes realistic goals toward independence

Expresses needs and opinions assertively
Demonstrates ability to overcome procrastination, negativism, and resistance
Identifies events or situations that trigger anxiety and obsessions/compulsions
Manages anxiety with multiple stress-reducing techniques
Employs cognitive and behavioral techniques to control obsessions/compulsions
Initiates and completes projects effectively
Recognizes own mistrust and projection
Validates perceptions with others
Seeks interaction and socialization with others
Refrains from idealizing, blaming, and devaluing others
Demonstrates respect for the needs and rights of self and others
Voices realistic appraisal of own talents and achievements

Nursing Process for

Personality Disorders

Universal Principles for Interactions and Interventions with Clients with Personality Disorder

- Continue to monitor assessment parameters listed in *Defining Characteristics.*
- Continue to consider the etiologic factors listed in *Etiologic/Related Factors.*
- Utilize principles of the *Therapeutic Nurse-Client Relationship* (Appendix G).
- Address client's spiritual and cultural needs.

General Principles

- Maintain health and safety.
- Establish a trusting relationship.
- Protect client from injury to self or others.
- Assess client's functional and dysfunctional behaviors.
- Focus on client's strengths, assets, and accomplishments.
- Assist client to control impulsive and aggressive behaviors.
- Teach strategies to reduce impulsivity and aggression.
- Encourage client to verbalize anger rather than act in aggressive or passive-aggressive manner.
- Provide mature, assertive role modeling.
- Teach client strategies to manage anxiety and obsessive-compulsive behaviors.
- Assist client to recognize manipulative behaviors.
- Set limits on manipulative behaviors when necessary.
- Encourage client to seek others for interactions and socialization.
- Provide opportunities to learn and practice interactive and socialization skills.
- Engage client in cognitive-behavioral activities that promote realistic self-appraisal and increase self-esteem.
- Reinforce expressions of positive feelings and behaviors.
- Reinforce realistic thoughts, perceptions, and appraisals.
- Teach assertive behaviors.
- Provide opportunities to practice assertiveness.
- Assist client to reduce procrastination and resistance.
- Help client to identify dependent, interdependent, and independent behaviors.
- Reinforce independent, responsible behaviors.
- Facilitate independent thinking, such as decision making.
- Provide opportunities to practice decision making.
- Praise client for respecting needs and rights of self and others.
- Assist client to formulate realistic, attainable goals.
- Teach the client how to identify psychosocial stressors and how to recognize, manage, and prevent symptoms.

Care Plans for Personality Disorders Based on Nursing Diagnosis

DSM-IV Diagnoses

Paranoid Personality Disorder
Schizoid Personality Disorder
Schizotypal Personality Disorder
Antisocial Personality Disorder
Borderline Personality Disorder
Histrionic Personality Disorder
Narcissistic Personality Disorder
Avoidant Personality Disorder
Dependent Personality Disorder
Obsessive-Compulsive Personality Disorder
Personality Disorder Not Otherwise Specified

NANDA Diagnoses

Coping, defensive (Behaviors)
- Mistrust/suspicion
- Anger/aggression
- Assaultive/destructive
- Blaming/projecting
- Passive/aggressive
- Impulsivity
- Lying
- Narcissistic/antisocial
- Irresponsibility
- Maladaptive denial

Self-esteem disturbance (Behaviors)
- Dependency
- Isolative/withdrawn/avoidant
- Abandonment fears/attention seeking
- Hysteria
- Seductive
- Jealousy
- Hypersexual
- Rigid and perfectionistic

Coping, ineffective individual (Behaviors)
- Splitting
- Idealizes
- Devalues
- Manipulation
- Intense, unstable relationships
- Boredom
- Restricted affect and humor

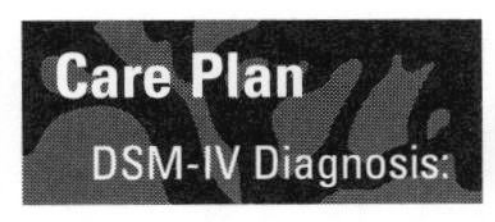

Personality Disorders (All Types)

NANDA Diagnosis: Coping, defensive

The state in which an individual repeatedly projects falsely positive self-evaluation based on a self-protective pattern that defends against underlying perceived threats to positive self-regard.

Focus:
For the client whose behavior patterns or personality traits result in lifelong ineffective interpersonal relationships owing to denial of problems, weaknesses, failures; projection, blame and responsibility; hypersensitivity, anger, aggression, lying; and perceived grandiosity or superiority over others

NANDA Taxonomy
Pattern 5—Choosing: A human response pattern involving the selection of alternatives

ETIOLOGIC/RELATED FACTORS (RELATED TO)

Personal identity disturbance
Self-esteem disturbance
Depletion of effective coping methods
Low impulse control
Role-relationship disturbance
Ineffective problem-solving skills
Lack of insight and judgment
Self-centeredness
Perceived threat to self-system
Life-style of defensive behaviors
Developmental conflicts
Psychosocial stressors
Environmental stressors
Knowledge deficit regarding adaptive coping methods

DEFINING CHARACTERISTICS (AS EVIDENCED BY)

Mistrust/Suspicion

Interprets others' words or actions as demeaning or threatening:
"What did you mean by that remark—were you making fun of me?"
"Why were you and the other clients laughing when I came into the room?"
"I didn't get chosen as group leader because they're all out to get me."

Views benign remarks or events as if they contained hidden meanings or messages:
"My check bounced because the bank deliberately held back money from my account."
"The board and care manager warned me to pay my rent on time; he's just looking for a reason to throw me out."
"The phone company sent me another notice; they take advantage of my emotional problems."

Avoids confiding in others for fear they may use the information to harm or belittle him or her:
"I'm afraid to tell anyone how I feel; they may turn against me."
"I don't trust anyone enough to tell them my personal thoughts."
"How can I ever be sure what I say will not be used against me?"

Demonstrates hypervigilant or extremely cautious behaviors toward persons perceived as threatening or hostile:
- Scans the environment during group meetings and activities
- Observes other clients from a distance

Verbalizes suspicion that others are saying rude, vulgar things about him or her:
"I just know they're spreading horrible rumors about me around here."
"They're probably making up all kinds of ugly, dirty stories about me."

Anger/Aggression

Reacts impulsively with anger toward people, groups, or situations perceived as threatening or belittling:
"How dare you spend all that time talking to Bob; you're supposed to be my staff person."
"I'm very angry at you for ignoring my comments in group today; you gave Sue lots of time to talk."
"I hate you for not choosing me to be community leader."

Bears long-term grudges toward others for slights, insults, or injuries:
"I wasn't invited personally to join the card game, so I want nothing to do with them."
"I'll never forgive my sister for treating me badly when we were kids."
"I'll never speak to my mother again; she always criticizes me."

Assaultive/Destructive

Engages in physical fights with other clients for no apparent reason:
"I hit Jack because his bragging really irritated me."
"Sue's attitude really made me mad so I tore up her diary."
"If you come anywhere near me, I'll punch your face in."
"You think you're so smart, but I bet I can beat you up."
"I messed up Jane's room because she made me mad."

Relates history of child or spouse abuse:
"Sure, I beat my kids; it'll make them tougher."
"Every once in a while my husband and I get into a real fistfight."

Blaming/Projecting

Avoids accepting blame for actions or inaction, even when blame is warranted:

"Don't blame me for not cleaning the dining room; there were still clients in it at 9 PM."

"It wasn't my fault that I missed the 7 o'clock activity; staff should have reminded me."

"I don't understand why the group is so mad at me all the time; what did I do?"

Blames others for own thoughts, feelings, or behaviors:

"It was Jack's idea to go AWOL; he wanted us to smoke some pot."

"You never cared about me; I'm not one of your favorite clients."

"Everything was perfect today until *you* came in and started to tell everyone what to do."

"The other clients are just jealous of me. That's why they don't talk to me."

"You didn't help me get my laundry together; how can I wear clean clothes?"

Passive/Aggressive

Expresses indirect resistance toward fulfilling responsibilities, based on covert aggression:

"It's too hard for me to be the client leader. I can't wake up everyone in time for community meeting every day."

Reacts resentfully, resistively, and oppositionally to others' demands and requests:

"Your idea seems OK, Sue, but I don't think we can fit it in at this time."

Procrastinates when asked to complete a task, project, or activity:

"I'll get going on that project eventually; just give me some time."

"I know I keep promising to take my turn at cleaning the craft room; I'll try to get to it today."

"Next time, I'll be sure to bring the tools we need to complete that project."

Uses subtle sarcastic remarks in lieu of overt anger:

"Jim, I thought you might like this sandwich; you're such a good eater." (Jim is overweight.)

"You're such a good nurse; you're always so busy; I hardly ever see you." (client to nurse)

Obstructs and thwarts the efforts of others by failing to do own share:

"I know I signed up to bring the dessert; I just didn't feel good."

"I just didn't find the time to do that favor you asked me to do."

Avoids obligations by conveniently "forgetting" (e.g., forgets important appointments, birthdays, special events, names):

"I can't understand how I forgot to prepare my half of the speech for today's meeting."

"Sue, I can't believe I forgot to get your magazine when I was out on pass; I did remember Jack's cigarettes."

Demonstrates intentional inefficiency:

"No, I just didn't have enough time to call the board and care home."

"I tried to bake the cake, but I'm not good at it, so I brought some doughnuts."

Withholds information (conveniently "forgets"):

"I'm sorry Kate, I guess I forgot to tell you about the meeting."

"I forgot Jim was going home today; I would have told you if I remembered."

Impulsivity

Engages in impulsive acts without regard for consequences:

"I don't know why I started doing drugs again; I suddenly got the urge."

"Bill collectors are always after me; I'm a compulsive spender."

"I have several unpaid speeding tickets; I can't resist driving fast."

"I have no regular home address; I like to get up and go."

Lying

Verbalizes untruths to staff and other clients:

"I would never 'cheek' my medications; I always take them when I should."

"I swear that I attended the assertiveness group yesterday; you just didn't see me."

"Sue said I lied about smoking her cigarettes; I never take anyone else's things."

"John insisted that he saw me eating his snack, but it wasn't me."

Narcissistic/Antisocial

Demonstrates self-important, grandiose behaviors:

- Takes command of community meetings and activities
- Interrupts groups or individuals in an authoritarian manner
- Exaggerates achievements and talents:

"I'm the best client leader in the world."

"If it wasn't for my organizational skills, nothing would get done around here."

"I almost became a psychiatrist so I understand most of the client's problems."

Verbalizes belief that he or she is entitled to special treatment or privileges:

"I simply have to play my radio at night or I can't fall asleep."

"I deserve a pass; I'm a model client."

"I don't care if there isn't enough space in the meeting room; I'm going in anyway."

Ignores hospital rules and policies as if they do not apply to him or her:

- Leaves the unit without telling staff or signing out
- Smokes in nonsmoking areas
- Makes phone calls when he or she should be attending group activities

Exploits others to meet own needs:

- Asks other clients to give up contact time with staff in order to have staff's time for self
- Feigns friendship with roommate to gain something (e.g., more closet space, the bed near the window)

Cannot express feelings or emotions

Lacks empathy and understanding for others:

"I don't feel sorry for Sam just because his wife left him; other people have gone through the same thing."

"I can't worry about these other clients; I have better things to do."

Irresponsibility

Exhibits irresponsible, insensitive behaviors toward others and the environment:

- Fails to clean room, pick up clothes, remove dirty dishes or ashtrays after use
- Leaves shower or bathroom messy or dirty after use
- Eats food or snacks that belong to other clients

Neglects to fulfill obligations or duties:

"Why should I have to help clean the craft room? That's what they pay housekeepers for."

"Oh, well, I missed the relationship meeting; I hope someone else took the minutes."

Fails to recognize consequences of irresponsible actions:

"I don't see why Joe is so mad at me for 'borrowing' two lousy dollars; I intend to pay him back."

"So what's the worst thing that could happen if I smoke a little marijuana at the board and care home?"

Maladaptive Denial

Fails to recognize own weaknesses or limitations:

"I don't have any problems with the other clients; they all love me."

"No one can say I don't do my share of work around here, even if I'm not a regular client."

Denies client role and reason for hospitalization:

"I'm only here for a rest; I had to get away from my crazy family."

"I can't imagine what the other clients here are going through; I try to help them whenever I can."

Denies consequences of actions:

"I don't know why everyone is so 'crazy' because I was AWOL."

OUTCOME IDENTIFICATION AND EVALUATION

Mistrust/Suspicion

Establishes trusting relationships with staff, peers, and significant others:

- Expresses meaningful thoughts and feelings to trusted clients and staff
- Participates in group meetings and activities
- Shares personal confidences with a special person
- Verbalizes trust in clients, family, and staff

Demonstrates decreased or absent suspicious behaviors toward others and the environment:

- Accurately interprets meanings of others' words or behaviors
- Refrains from searching for "hidden" messages or agenda in others' statements or actions
- Ceases to believe that others' statements or behaviors refer to client
- Ceases to believe that others are making up "lewd," "vulgar" stories about client
- Ceases to interpret others' words or actions as demeaning or threatening to client

Demonstrates absence of scanning, guarding, or hypervigilant behaviors

Anger/Aggression

Exhibits decreased or absent verbal expressions of anger

Exhibits decreased or absent aggressive outbursts or demonstrations

Refrains from bearing grudges against significant others, clients, or staff:

"I think it's time I gave my parents another chance."

"I'm not mad at Kate any longer; she didn't mean to hurt me."

"I realize the staff was only trying to help me when they put me in seclusion."

Demonstrates assertive rather than aggressive behaviors

Assaultive/Destructive

Ceases to engage in physical fights or altercations with others

Demonstrates absence of violent or destructive behaviors

Verbalizes desire to seek help for abusive behaviors

Blaming/Projecting

Accepts blame or share of blame when warranted:

"It wasn't only Jack's idea to leave the unit; I also wanted to go."

"I know now that it was my angry behavior that drove people away; it wasn't that they didn't care."

"The meeting was postponed because of my lateness."

"I'm sorry for accusing staff of being 'bossy' and 'protective'; I've been acting like a child."

"I admit I did my share to mess up the clients' lounge and I apologize."

Ceases to blame others for own behaviors:

"I realize that no one made me smoke the marijuana; I wanted to smoke."

"It was my problem with alcohol that broke up my marriage, not my wife's nagging."

"I started the fight with my bad temper; Paul was just defending himself."

Passive/Aggressive

Directly expresses anger, irritation, and frustration without resorting to indirect or covert responses:

- Ceases to use humor, sarcasm, or messages with "hidden" meanings when expressing anger, irritation, or frustration:

"I'm angry that staff is too busy to give me much time today."
- Verbalizes angry feelings overtly (e.g., "I'm feeling angry about . . ."; "It made me angry when . . ."; "I was angry because. . . ."

Ceases to use indirect behaviors as covert expressions of aggression to resist fulfilling responsibilities:
- No longer resists others' reasonable ideas, wishes, or responsibilities
- Ceases to withhold critical or relevant information from staff

Refrains from procrastinating when asked to complete a task, project, or activity (e.g., begins and ends work on time)

Completes full share of work in client community so that others' efforts are not obstructed

Fulfills client duties and obligations willingly:
- Cleans up after self without being urged
- Takes turns with other clients at group tasks

Demonstrates efficiency and reliability:
- Attends groups and activities
- Arrives on time to groups and activities
- Participates satisfactorily in groups and activities

Demonstrates assertive rather than passive-aggressive behaviors:
- Uses "I" messages, eye contact, and congruent verbal and facial expressions in communicating with others

(See Appendix K, Assertive Behaviors.)

Impulsivity

Verbalizes decreased need to act impulsively

Utilizes learned techniques to control impulsive behaviors (e.g., slow, deep breathing; counting to 5 before responding to stimulus; see Appendix K, Deep Breathing Techniques)

Demonstrates significant decrease or absence of impulsive acts or behaviors (e.g., refrains from speeding, shopping, spending, moving from place to place, taking drugs)

Lying

Makes truthful statements to staff and clients

Refrains from using lies or fabrications to meet needs

Shares information relative to health and safety of self and others (does not withhold information)

Narcissistic/Antisocial

Demonstrates absence or significant reduction in self-important, grandiose behaviors:
- Refrains from interrupting or "taking over" group activities
- Resists exaggerating or flaunting own talents and achievements
- Praises others' talents and accomplishments

Exhibits consideration for others rather than demonstrating self-entitlement:

"I'll turn off my radio at 9 PM so others won't be disturbed."

"Since I've already been on a field trip, I'll give up my window seat to another client."

Obeys hospital rules and policies:
- Informs staff when leaving the unit
- Smokes only in designated smoking areas
- Makes phone calls at times other than during scheduled activities

Meets own needs without exploiting others

Facilitates genuine interpersonal relationships

Expresses feelings and emotions more readily (e.g., "I'm feeling sad . . . angry . . . anxious . . . happy.")

Expresses empathy and understanding for others:

"I feel sorry for Sam since his wife left him."

"It was difficult for Jane to be client leader; she was nervous."

"Jack had a tough day; I know what it's like when visitors don't show up."

"It's sad that Ken has no place to go when he's discharged."

Irresponsibility

Demonstrates mature, responsible behaviors toward self and others:
- Maintains neat, clean personal environments (e.g., room, clothing, and self)
- Completes fair share of client responsibilities (e.g., helps set up for meals and activities, relays messages regarding meeting times and places)

Fulfills client role and obligations:
- Engages in therapeutic treatment regimen
- Participates in milieu groups and activities

Verbalizes awareness of consequences of actions:

"I'm going to pay back the money I borrowed from Jack as soon as possible; I don't want to ruin our relationship."

"I'll wait for my break to smoke; if I smoke in my bathroom, my roommate and I could get into trouble."

Accepts accountability for own behavior:

"It was my job to help the group prepare for the party; I just didn't go to enough meetings."

"I should have been dressed and ready for my appointment with the social worker. Now I'll have to wait to select a board and care facility."

Maladaptive Denial

Recognizes own limitations and weaknesses:

"I realize I haven't done my share as a client."

"I admit that I have problems being accepted by other clients."

Accepts consequences of actions:

"I don't blame that staff for being angry that I left the unit without telling anyone. I deserve to be placed on restrictions."

"I understand now that the other clients resented me because I didn't act like a client."

Accepts client role and need for treatment:

"I realize now that I'm here because I need help with my emotional problems."

"I can understand what the other clients are going through; I'm going through similar experiences."

PLANNING AND IMPLEMENTATION

Nursing Interventions and Rationale

Mistrust/Suspicion

Identify your own level of anxiety and use strategies to reduce it. *Anxiety is transferable; an anxious nurse could foster the client's mistrust and suspicion.*

Approach the client face-to-face, *not* from behind. *The client is likely to become startled if he or she cannot immediately see the approaching person. Face-to-face contact decreases incidences of suspicion and mistrust.*

Utilize a calm, matter-of-fact manner when interacting with the client *to create a secure, nonthreatening environment:*

- Low, steady voice tones, *not* high-pitched or urgent ones
- Slow, smooth body movements, *not* sudden or erratic ones

Initially, assign the same staff person(s) to work with the client *to establish consistency and trust.*

Engage the client in brief one-to-one interactions initially, progressing to longer interactions, informal groups, and finally more structured groups and activities. *This sequence gives the client more opportunities to establish trust and develop interpersonal relationships.*

Employ assertive, *not* aggressive (authoritarian) responses *to provide clear directives, increase the client's trust in staff and the environment, reduce suspicion and hostility, and help the client to interpret the meaning of his or her behavior:*

Therapeutic responses:

- "I noticed that you sat alone during lunch and seemed upset when you looked at Jane and me." ("I," *not* "you," statements.)
- "Eye contact" (meeting the client's eyes with a calm, unemotional facial expression, without constantly staring) so as not to seem demanding or threatening
- Facial expression congruent with verbal responses (e.g., maintaining an unemotional facial expression and affect while relating facts and meaning regarding a benign incident or situation)

Nontherapeutic responses:

- "*You* shouldn't feel threatened just because Jane and I sat together at lunch today." (Implies something is wrong with the client.)
- Smiling inappropriately with little or no eye contact while giving the client serious directives
- Acting impatiently or angrily while asking the client to clarify the meaning of his or her behavior

(Refer to Assertive Therapy, Appendix K.)

Offer the client clear, simple explanations of environmental events, activities, and the behaviors of other clients when necessary *to assuage the client's doubts, fear, and suspiciousness and to promote trust:*

"That remark was not meant for you, Tom; it was directed to everyone in the group."

"I noticed you looked uneasy at the community meeting, Sue; the other clients were pleased that you came."

"Joe, the clients were laughing at a funny story that Sam told them; they weren't laughing at you."

Inform the client in a direct, matter-of-fact manner that you do not share his or her interpretation of a statement or event, while acknowledging feelings, *to foster realistic rather than irrational thoughts and conclusions:*

"I know you think we planned to change your staff person, Pam, but actually she was assigned to another unit."

"Mark, I know you believe that Jim and Jack don't want to sit with you, but they need to sit in the front of the bus because sitting in the back makes them nauseous."

Assist the client to interpret statements or events more concretely *to discourage concerns that they contain "hidden" meanings or ulterior motives directed toward the client:*

"John, it's very likely that your landlord sends a notice to anyone who is late with the rent."

"Sue, the phone company has no way of knowing about your mental disorder; they just want a payment."

"Jack, the clients don't leave dirty ashtrays around just to upset you, although it can be annoying."

Clarify the meanings and intent of remarks or situations that are misinterpreted by the client *to provide factual information that will promote the client's trust.*

"John, the board and care manager told the social worker that you will not be thrown out of the facility as long as your rent is paid."

"Joe, your check bounced because there wasn't enough money in your account, not because the bank stole your money."

"When Jane said she was 'sick and tired,' she did not mean that *you* made her 'sick and tired,' Tom."

Assure the client that, although other clients and staff discuss him or her, they are *not* spreading vicious, ugly rumors, *to decrease anxiety that may perpetuate suspicious behaviors while increasing self-esteem by assuring the client that he or she is thought about in a positive way:*

"Jack and Joan do talk about you, Sue; but they have not spoken about you in an unkind way."

"Sarah did say she had lunch with you, Ann, and she also said she enjoys spending time with you."

Direct conversation toward reality-based topics when the client gets bogged down in irrational beliefs or paranoid ideations *to reestablish logic and decrease suspicious thoughts and perceptions:*

"Sam, a few minutes ago you were talking about movie stars; let's talk about your favorite movies."

"Jane, just before the meeting we were discussing music. I'd like to hear about your record collection."

Identify the client's expressions and behaviors during interactions:

"Joe, I notice that you hesitate when you begin to talk about your problems with me."

"Sarah, you have a puzzled look on your face; I wonder if you believe what I'm saying."

"John, I wonder if you are uneasy about sharing your experiences with the group."

Clarification of the client's suspicions helps to expose areas of mistrust and gives the client and opportunity to challenge them.

Set limits on the duration and frequency of the client's suspicious concerns during one-to-one and group interactions *to discourage perpetuation of negative behaviors:*

"Jane, I know you have concerns about some things, and staff will listen for about 10 minutes each shift. The rest of the time needs to be spent in scheduled activities."

Share a benign, nonthreatening personal fact or feeling with the client *to establish rapport and trust and encourage the client to confide in the staff.*

Therapeutic responses:

"I'm a student nurse; I like to help others."

"I sometimes feel sad when others have problems."

"I also get upset once in a while."

Nontherapeutic responses:

"I know *just* how you feel; I'd feel the same way in your situation."

"I worry too when I think people are talking about me."

"It's normal not to trust banks or any big businesses."

The nurse could not *possibly know how the client feels, and agreeing with the client in this case justifies his/her suspicions. The client relies on the nurse to present and interpret reality.*

Assure the client that anything discussed with staff is confidential information and will be shared *only* with staff persons who are responsible for the client's treatment and care. *Assurance of confidentiality promotes trust and encourages the client to share thoughts, feelings, and beliefs that are relevant to his or her treatment and care.*

Note: Clients who reveal suicidal thoughts or plans must be advised that such intents will be shared with other appropriate staff and physician in order to protect the client. (See Appendix J.)

Explore situations in which the client often feels suspicious, and discuss alternative problem-solving methods *to provide the client with more realistic and appropriate methods to deal with situations that provoke suspiciousness:*

"John, at other times when people were laughing, what did you do to determine whether they were laughing at you? Sometimes asking people directly to explain that behavior can prevent misinterpretation."

"Joe, rather than assume others are saying bad things about you, what about talking to a trusted staff person or client about your concerns first?"

"Sue, have you thought about approaching the board and care manager with your concerns about being evicted? You may find out if there actually is a problem."

Discuss with the client the consequences of not validating actual meanings behind situations or events that provoke suspiciousness *to prevent the client from misinterpreting situations or events and to promote trust in others and the environment:*

"By not finding out what actually *is* happening, you will continue to feel left out."

"Your feeling of isolation may not go away if you don't ask about situations that seem troubling to you."

Assist the client to examine and clarify his or her own thoughts and beliefs *to help the client evaluate thoughts and beliefs more accurately and realistically and thus avoid misinterpretation:*

"What do you think about the incident that happened in group today?"

"Think more about what happened in the community meeting."

"What do you actually believe about the clients' responses to you during the activity?"

Encourage the client to raise healthy doubts about his or her suspiciousness and erroneous beliefs *to help the client challenge and analyze his or her beliefs more closely and realistically and to reduce suspiciousness:*

'"Do you really believe the telephone company disconnected your phone because of your mental illness?"

"Is it actually possible that everyone here is saying bad things about you?"

"I find it hard to believe that the staff can't be trusted with information that will help you."

Offer the client feedback when, as a result of the client's doubts and suspicions, he or she erroneously accuses others of behaviors *to increase the client's awareness that his or her behaviors can affect others in a negative way and result in rejection by others:*

"When you say Jack has spread vicious rumors about you, he gets upset."

"Tom said he felt hurt when you accused him of taking your share of the staff's time."

Praise the client for efforts made toward correct interpretation of the meanings and intent of others' responses and situations *to build self-esteem and trust, encourage continued efforts through positive reinforcement, and decrease paranoid thinking:*

"I was impressed with your clear understanding of the group's response today."

"The clients appreciated your accurate interpretation of their remarks during the community meeting. I could tell by the way they all listened to you."

Engage the client in activities, crafts, or exercises during unstructured or "free" time *to distract the client from preoccupation with suspicious thoughts and beliefs and fill the time with activities that bring quick rewards and increase self-esteem.*

Anger/Aggression, Assaultive/Destructive

Approach the client in a calm, nonthreatening manner to prevent an increase in angry feelings and possible violent behavior.

Set limits on the client's behavior if it appears that anger may escalate to physical aggression or violence *to establish control and guidelines for the client and to promote safety:*

- Suggest to the client that he or she take "time out." "Jane, that is not acceptable behavior; some time in your room may help you gain control."
- If "time-out" does not relieve the client's feelings, offer prn medication.
- Seclusion and/or restraint may be the least restrictive intervention.

(Refer to Guidelines for Seclusion and Restraint, Appendix L.)

Assure the client that he or she is entitled to angry feelings but may not impose angry outbursts on other clients *to help the client manage behaviors that interfere with other clients' rights or disrupt milieu activities, while acknowledging anger:*

"John, I realize you're angry, but cursing in group is not acceptable behavior."

"Pam, I know you're upset that the chocolate pudding is gone, but slamming your tray down in the cafeteria is disruptive and won't be tolerated."

"Sue, I know you're upset that your visitors didn't come, but yelling at the other clients is not appropriate."

Give the client feedback regarding impulsive, angry outbursts *to illustrate the negative effects of volatile behavior on the client and others:*

"Sam, your screaming and yelling during the community meeting upsets you and the other clients."

"Kate, your roommate asked the staff to change her room because your episodes of rage frighten her."

"Ted, staff are concerned because your anger is interfering with your progress and is disruptive to others."

"Tom, the group stops listening to you when you scream and wave your arms like that. Instead, they get anxious."

"Mark, I will not continue our conversation when you curse like that."

Teach the client quick, effective strategies *to reduce the physical manifestations of anger:*

- Walk away from the immediate area to a less stimulating environment
- Slow, deep-breathing techniques
- Progressive relaxation exercises
- Visual imagery

(See Appendix K.)

Assist the client to put angry feelings into words during one-to-one interactions *so that the client can express feelings in a nonthreatening setting and avoid directing anger toward other clients:*

"Ted, when you feel angry, talk about your feelings with staff."

"Jane, you seemed upset at lunch today; you slammed your tray down hard; let's discuss your feelings."

"Sarah, you say you're not angry, but you shouted at several people this morning; let's talk about your feelings during our session today."

Encourage the client to identify situations or events that generate angry feelings *to help the client connect behaviors to specific anger-producing stimuli and begin to take steps to manage or prevent impulsive, angry outbursts:*

"Tom, I noticed you were calm until the topic of intimacy came up in group; then you immediately began to shout."

"Jim, you seemed relaxed until your roommate spoke to someone else; then you cursed and stomped out of the room."

Discuss with the client possible fears or frustrations that may provoke impulsive, angry outbursts *to help the client recognize that anger can be a response to a real or imagined threat:*

"Jim, when your roommate talks to other people, you lose your temper. Do you feel ignored or left out?"

"Jane, it seems that whenever other clients talk about their boyfriends, you get angry. Are you feeling lonely or sad?"

Assist the client to clarify the intent of situations he or she perceives as threatening *to promote reality and avoid angry outbursts.*

"Jim, when your roommate talks to other clients, it doesn't mean he's forgotten you; he speaks to you often."

"Jane, it's OK to feel sad or lonely when others discuss their boyfriends, but they don't do it to make you mad."

Help the client to reevaluate the perceived threat involved in the anger-producing situation before reacting explosively *to extend the time between the anger-producing stimulus and the client's response and to give the client more opportunity to control anger:*

"When a situation begins to anger you, count to five before reacting and think of what is upsetting about the situation."

"If discussing intimacy upsets you because you don't have a relationship now, think of ways to work on your relationships with others instead of getting angry."

"Use your learned strategies when you begin to feel anger; then rethink the situation."

(See Appendix K.)

Use assertive responses with clients who resort to angry outbursts to get their needs met. *Assertive responses set limits for the client and tend to reduce anger, whereas aggressive or authoritarian responses challenge the client and may provoke anger.*

Therapeutic responses:

"John, I asked Bob to be the group leader because it was his turn; you were the leader last week."

"Jane, Sue talked more than you in community meeting today because she had many concerns, as you did yesterday."

"Sam, I spoke with Tom a lot today because he needed my help; I also help you."

Nontherapeutic responses:

"John, don't be so selfish; you know it's not your turn to be group leader."

"Jane, you're being unreasonable; Sue talked more because she has more problems than you."

"Sam, you're acting childishly; Tom needed me more than you did today."

(Refer to Assertive Response Behaviors, Appendix K.)

Engage the client in a physical exercise program to be used throughout the day, especially before and after stress-producing experiences. *Physical activities help redirect anger-producing energy toward productive, psychomotor activities.*

Examples:

- Stationary bicycle
- Brisk walks
- Exercises
- Sing-alongs
- Ping-Pong
- Volleyball

Assure client that he or she need not resort to angry outbursts to get needs met *to decrease the fear and frustration that accompany unmet needs and to promote more socially acceptable behavior:*

"Jack, it's not necessary to scream at staff; we'll help you when you need us."

"Sue, you don't need to bang on the door of the nurses' station; we'll open the door when we see you."

"Ted, the group will listen to you better if you speak without cursing."

Discuss with the client how angry outbursts can discourage social relationships and foster threats of loneliness and abandonment *to increase the client's awareness of the consequences of negative behaviors:*

"When you direct your frustrations toward others in an angry way, they won't want to be around you and the very thing you fear (abandonment) may occur."

Initiate a written contract that sets limits on the client's angry outbursts with strategies to help reduce their frequency *so the client can have access to a tangible reminder of acceptable milieu behaviors and ways to maintain them.*

Engage the client in cognitive or behavioral strategies and therapies *to manage anger effectively, increase self-esteem, and express angry feelings in more socially acceptable ways.*

Examples:

- Role play
- Behavioral therapy
- Thought substitution or stopping
- Cognitive therapy
- Assertive responses
- Process or focus groups

(See Appendix K.)

Praise the client for efforts made to manage angry feelings and express self in a socially adaptive manner *to promote continued efforts and increase self-esteem:*

"It was a positive decision to approach me to discuss your feelings before attending community meeting."

"The staff has noticed a significant improvement in your behavior since you began cognitive therapy."

"You are really making an effort to use exercise and physical activity to manage your anger."

Blaming/Projecting

Make short, frequent contacts with the client throughout the day *to establish a trusting interpersonal relationship.*

Assess the client for potential for violence to self or others *to protect client and others from harm or injury.*

Refrain from reacting with anger or hostility to the client's accusations *to decrease the client's feelings of alienation and discourage blaming and projection.*

Collaborate with staff to ensure consistent responses when the client refuses to accept blame or blames and accuses others, *to clarify unacceptable or maladaptive behaviors with the client.*

Use assertive responses to gently challenge the client's false accusations ("I" vs. "you" messages, eye-contact, congruent facial and verbal expressions) *to discourage validation of the client's beliefs and accusations without inciting anger or aggression.*

Therapeutic responses:

"I don't think it was Jack's idea to go AWOL, Jim; he never mentioned wanting to leave."

"I find it hard to believe that the other clients are jealous of you, Sue; I've seen nothing to indicate that."

"I don't believe it's up to me to do your laundry, Jack; all clients do their own laundry."

"I care about you and all the clients equally, Jane; I can't always give everyone all the time they want."

Nontherapeutic responses:

"You know you deliberately missed the 7 o'clock activity, Sam; *you've* done it before."

"*You* could have cleaned the dining room even if there were clients in it, Tom; *you* just didn't want to do it."

"*You* know better than to believe I have favorite patients, Kate; what makes *you* think that?"

"*You* and every single client here must do his or her own laundry, Jack; that's the rule."

The wrong responses convey an accusatory, harsh tone that may incite defensiveness and anger in the client and diminish the client's trust and self-esteem.

Refrain from responding prematurely in the assessment process to the client's accusatory or "disgruntled" remarks that reflect his or her dissatisfaction (e.g., "I don't know why I have to go to every meeting; this place expects too much"; "This food is terrible; you'd think they would hire a decent cook"). *Allowing the client to vent negative feelings in the initial stages of an admission helps the staff to assess the degree of anger and plan interventions accordingly.*

Engage the client in groups that encourage social interactions (e.g., community meetings, relationship groups, outings) *to increase social skills, build trust among peers, and discourage blaming and projection.*

Assist the client to identify when blaming or projection is hurtful or threatening to others *to help the client recognize the negative impact of his or her accusations and blame on others:*

"Tom, the clients are upset because you've been saying they take your belongings."

"Sue, when you say that everything was fine until I came into the room, I feel annoyed."

"Kate, allowing Pam to take the blame for not reminding you about your responsibility in the group project will hurt your friendship."

Assist the client to analyze his or her belief system and situations that result in blaming others *to promote a more realistic belief system and decrease the incidence of blaming or accusing others:*

"John, you say you missed the meeting because Sarah didn't remind you. Actually I told you several times about the meeting."

"Pam, you say it was Sue's idea to leave the unit without permission, yet you left as well."

"Tom, you're telling me everything was fine until I came into the room. What do you think happened when I came into the room?"

Engage the client in milieu activities that are productive and rewarding (e.g., physical exercise, sports, or arts and crafts) *to build self-esteem and self-worth and reduce opportunities for blaming.*

Assign the client milieu responsibilities (e.g., have him or her notify clients for meetings and groups, ask him or her to plan activities with staff) *to occupy the client's time with activities that increase sense of responsibility and self-worth and to promote awareness of positive versus negative behaviors.*

Praise the client whenever he or she accepts responsibility for actions and refrains from blaming or accusing others *to increase self-concept and self-esteem and reinforce positive behaviors:*

"Joe, taking responsibility for the meeting starting late was the right thing to do."

"Kate, it was good to hear you say you left the dining room a little messy without blaming anyone else."

"Jack, the group said they appreciated your apology for playing the radio so loud."

Passive/Aggressive

Observe nonverbal behavioral clues that may indicate anger (e.g., avoids group activities and one-to-one interactions; procrastinates when asked to complete a project or task; resists or rejects suggestions or ideas; conveys a sense of impatience, frustration, or boredom; uses sarcasm often disguised as humor). *Assessment of passive-aggressive behaviors is the first step toward helping the client connect behaviors with angry feelings.*

Assist the client to identify and label angry feelings underlying passive-aggressive behaviors *to promote awareness of physical and emotional sensations of anger and begin to develop management strategies:*

"Sue, what were you actually feeling when you left in the middle of our interaction?"

"Joe, when you told the group you were 'bored' with the discussion, what kinds of emotions were you experiencing?"

"Jane, describe what you were feeling when you ignored me today."

Assist the client to recognize the negative effects of passive-aggressive behavior on self and others *to reduce the frequency of insensitive or hostile remarks:*

"Ted, when you use sarcasm with humor, the other clients tend to avoid you."

"Kate, did you notice the group's irritation when you said you found the group boring?"

Help the client identify the source of angry emotions *in order to deal directly with the cause and avoid displacing hostile feelings toward others:*

"Joe, you were very sarcastic in group today; perhaps you're angry because your folks didn't visit you?"

"Kate, you've been avoiding people all day; are you still upset because you haven't been discharged yet?"

Teach the client strategies to express repressed anger in accordance with the treatment plan *to help the client demonstrate anger through acceptable channels.*

Examples:

- Physical exercise or activity (stationary bike, Ping-Pong)
- Use punching bag, batakas with supervision
- Art or music therapy
- Express angry feelings in a nonthreatening setting (e.g., talk, cry, or shout in presence of trusted staff member)

Encourage the client to express anger directly rather than using sarcasm, avoidance, procrastination, or ignoring others or responsibilities *to get needs met from appropriate sources, reduce anxiety, and prevent aggression that may occur from built-up anger:*

"John, tell staff when you feel angry or irritable so we can help you deal with the cause of your anger."

"Sarah, it's better to express your anger when you begin to feel it rather than let it build up."

Assure the client that expressions of anger will not bring retaliation or chastisement from staff *so the client will not fear the consequences of baring feelings:*

"John, it's OK to express angry feelings; staff are here to help you cope with them."

"Kate, expressing anger with staff is therapeutic and not wrong."

Assist the client to identify areas of procrastination and ineffective performance *to help the client develop an awareness of dysfunctional behaviors and their effects on others:*

"Donna, you haven't begun your share of the art project; the other clients can't continue without your help."

"Sally, you didn't collect the names we need to elect a client leader; the group can't vote without a list of names."

Point out to the client the positive results of initiating projects and performing tasks effectively *to illustrate that the rewards of initiating and completing tasks are greater than covert acts of aggression:*

"Donna, your work on the quilt contributed to your group's prize; could that be part of the reason that you're feeling so good today?"

"Steve, you said at the community meeting that you're feeling happier than you have for a long time. Did the compliments you receive for leading the group contribute to that feeling?"

Acknowledge those experiences regarding hospitalization that commonly cause anger, irritation, or resentment (e.g., being away from a familiar living situation, sharing space with others, talking to strangers about problems) *to assure the client that anger related to loss of control and feelings of powerlessness is a normal, human emotion and can be expressed openly.*

Share with the client some similar experiences that provoked anger, resentment, or irritation in you *to assure the client that certain events or experiences promote similar responses in most people.*

Explore with the client situations, topics, or experiences that result in feelings of anger, resentment, or irritation *to determine causes and begin to plan strategies that will best help the client in each situation.*

Engage the client in groups and activities *to help disclose angry feelings and learn to cope with them and communicate them more effectively.*

Examples:

- Behavioral therapy
- Cognitive therapy
- Assertive therapy
- Process or focus groups
- Role play (sociodrama)

(Refer to Appendix K.)

Praise the client for efforts made toward direct expression of anger versus use of passive-aggressive behaviors *to increase self-esteem and reinforce direct expression of anger:*

"Sue, you expressed your angry feelings clearly in group today."

"Jack, it was good that you told me how angry you were when I forgot our meeting."

"Kate, your verbalizing your anger in assertive therapy today was helpful."

Impulsivity

Assess the degree and destructiveness of the client's impulsivity *to determine its effects on the client and others and to protect the patient and others from harm.*

Protect the client and others from injury when the client loses control as a result of impulsive behaviors *to prevent injury to the patient and others.*

(Refer to Guidelines for Seclusion and Restraint, Appendix L.)

Ask the following questions:

- What type of problems result from the client's impulsive behaviors (e.g., alcohol or drug abuse, spending or credit card abuse, driving too fast with unpaid speeding tickets, drunk driving citations, moving from place to place with no permanent home base, changing jobs for a variety of reasons, trouble with the law or legal system)?
- What type of resources and support systems are available for the client (e.g., family and friends, employers, conservator, Veterans Administration system, insurance, religious affiliates, parole officer)?
- How can the hospital setting and health care personnel collaborate with other resources and systems to help the client meet his or her needs (e.g., social service referral, short-term inpatient milieu therapy, outpatient therapy, county mental health services, legal system)?

Assist the client to recognize feelings that precede impulsive acts (e.g., anxiety, anger) *to prevent subsequent impulsive acts.*

(See Passive-Aggressive Interventions in this chapter.)

Teach the client strategies to increase the time between the stimuli that trigger feelings and the impulsive actions *to control and reduce impulsive behaviors by interrupting the stimulus-response cycle.*

Examples:

- Slow, deep-breathing exercises
- Relaxation techniques
- Count slowly to 5 as soon as feelings that precede impulsive behaviors emerge
- Remove self from stimuli (take time out) when there is a sense that feelings are escalating out of control
- Occupy free time with meetings, activities, and groups

(See Appendix K for Deep-Breathing and Relaxation Strategies.)

Collaborate with the client and interdisciplinary team members to identify the best therapeutic approach to the client's impulsive life-style *to best meet the client's needs through the multidisciplinary approach.*

Engage the client in an appropriate therapeutic regimen in the hospital or in the community that will help the client modify impulsive behaviors *to best meet the client's needs.*

Examples:

- Chemical dependency rehabilitation program
- Classes for drunk driving
- Legal counseling
- Family counseling
- Groups that deal with addictive behaviors (gambling, drinking, prostitution, spending, shoplifting, speeding)

Lying

Assess the degree, frequency, and consequences of the client's use of lies to meet needs, *to plan interventions to eliminate lying.*

Challenge the client's lies by pointing out the discrepancies in the client stories *to make the client aware of lies and discourage their use:*

"Paul, you say you never cheek your medications, yet you were refused a pass last week because of that."

"Sarah, you told your doctor that you attend every group; you didn't attend the assertiveness training group today."

"Jane, staff saw you taking Sue's cigarettes out of her jacket pocket, although you say you don't take other people's things."

"Mark, the snack you were eating had John's name on the label, so John was correct about you eating his snack earlier."

Teach the client to approach staff directly to get needs met rather than resorting to lies or fabrications, *to assure the client that needs will be met without the use of lies and that lies are not acceptable:*

"Paul, if you have problems with taking your medication, talk to staff or your doctor about it; not taking it will not solve your problem."

"Sarah, it's better to discuss the reasons you don't attend assertiveness training group rather than tell your doctor you never miss it."

"Jane, when you run out of cigarettes, let staff know; taking them from another patient is not acceptable."

"Mark, if you want a snack, tell staff or check it on your menu. Don't take another client's food."

Inform the client of the effect of his or her lies on others *to illustrate negative consequences of lies and reduce lying behaviors:*

"Mark, lying about eating John's snack makes it difficult for him to trust you."

"Jane, taking Sue's cigarettes made her angry and could hurt your relationship."

"Paul, cheeking your medication is serious; staff will have to put you on a behavioral contract."

"Sarah, lying about attending the assertiveness training group will not gain trust; it will hurt your treatment and progress."

Initiate activities that build the client's self-esteem *to discourage use of lies and fabrications to gain attention and meet needs.*

Examples:

- Physical activities (e.g., Ping-Pong, volleyball)
- Arts, crafts, music
- Games (e.g., Scrabble, chess)

Construct a behavioral contract that clearly describes acceptable behaviors and consequences of lying *to establish guidelines and help set limits on the client's use of lies.*

Assure the client that direct, truthful behaviors are more rewarding than lying, *to reinforce continuity of open, honest interactions:*

"Mark, requesting a snack from staff instead of taking another client's food is appreciated by everyone."

"Jane, admitting that you took Sue's cigarettes is a big step toward regaining her trust."

"Paul, sharing your concerns about medication effects rather than cheeking them was beneficial in changing the dosage."

"Sarah, apologizing for not being truthful about attending the assertiveness training group has helped your relationship with staff and other clients."

Engage the client in activities *to help develop his or her awareness of the benefits of truthfulness versus the negative results of lying.*

Examples:

- Role play, sociodrama
- Behavior modification
- Cognitive therapy
- Assertiveness training
- Process and focus groups

(See Appendix K.)

Praise the client for efforts made toward use of open, honest interactions and reduction or absence of lying *to build self-esteem and reinforce repetition of truthful behaviors:*

"Jane, the staff say they have noticed your efforts to be direct and honest."

"Sarah, the staff and clients say they appreciate your truthfulness."

(See Ineffective Individual Coping Care Plan in this chapter for additional intervention.)

Narcissistic/Antisocial

Assess the client's level of narcissism and grandiosity *to determine how behaviors interfere with the client's role and his or her interactions with other clients and to plan interventions.*

Assure the client that he or she does not have to resort to narcissistic or antisocial behaviors to get needs met, *to decrease the client's concerns about meeting needs and to discourage narcissistic behaviors:*

"Pam, it's not necessary to interrupt groups to make your needs known; it's more effective for you to ask staff for assistance."

"Tom, breaking hospital rules will not get you the kind of attention you need."

Assist the client to recognize the negative effects of self-centered behaviors on others *to help the client develop an awareness of the results of his or her behavior and begin to modify it:*

"Sam, the rest of the group gets upset when you occupy their time with long, exaggerated stories."

"John, staff doesn't appreciate it when you walk into their private areas without asking permission."

"Joe, playing music after 9 PM disturbs the other clients."

Encourage the client to challenge his or her narcissistic beliefs *to present reality and help the client decrease feelings of entitlement and exaggerated self-importance:*

"Jack, the other clients find it hard to believe the stories you tell about your accomplishments."

"Jane, what makes you believe you should have more privileges than the other clients?"

"Kate, you have done a commendable job as client leader; other clients have also done well."

Confront the client with his or her attempts to exploit other clients to meet own needs, *to make the client aware of negative behaviors and reduce their frequency:*

"Jeff, it seems as if you're only nice to John when you want a favor from him."

"Sarah, you offered to make your roommate's bed and clean the room just before you asked for $10. She says you ignored her before that."

Initiate a written contract that sets limits on the client's antisocial behaviors *to give the client a tangible reminder of acceptable milieu behaviors and methods to achieve them.*

(Contracts may not always be effective with these clients because contracts provide opportunities for further manipulation. Also, it is difficult for staff to monitor behaviors.)

Encourage the client to participate in milieu activities *to help modify narcissistic, self-important behaviors through the cooperative group process.*

Examples:

- Physical games (e.g., Ping-Pong, volleyball, shuffleboard)
- Intellectual games (e.g., Trivial Pursuit, Scrabble)
- Other group activities (e.g., bingo, arts and crafts, sing-alongs)

Engage the client in therapies that will help him or her recognize and manage narcissistic, grandiose, and exploitive behaviors, *to reduce negative behaviors through education and practice.*

Examples:

- Role play (sociodrama)
- Behavioral therapy
- Assertiveness training
- Cognitive therapy
- Group therapy

(Refer to Appendix K.)

Demonstrate appropriate, mature behaviors through role modeling *to expose the client to acceptable, effective interpersonal interactions.*

Use role modeling to express feelings and emotions such as joy, sadness, or laughter in a variety of appropriate situations. *It is difficult for persons with narcissistic and antisocial personality traits to get in touch with feelings and express emotions. The nurse can facilitate this through role modeling.*

Give positive feedback whenever the client expresses self in relation to others and situations outside the self (e.g., laughs with others in response to a humorous situation, feels sad or cries in response to others' misfortune) *to let client know that expressing feelings toward others is acceptable and beneficial to one's emotional health:*

"Joan, it's good to see you laughing with the other clients; the community meeting was fun today."

"Barbara, it's OK to cry when you feel sad for other people; it can be healthy to release emotions."

Inform client directly when actions are inappropriate or interfere with the rights of others *to help client control unacceptable behaviors by setting limits:*

"Paul, it's not acceptable to put your arm around other clients or to touch them, unless it's part of a game or activity."

"Sarah, taking cigarettes, snacks, or anything else that belongs to other clients is not tolerated."

Praise the client for relating to others without use of narcissistic, grandiose, or exploitative behaviors *to reinforce appropriate behaviors and increase self-esteem:*

"Sally, you really were an equal team member in the volleyball game."

"Jim, staff appreciate that you knock on the door and wait for us to respond before walking into staff areas."

"Sam, the other clients were happy with your cooperation in group today; you didn't interrupt anyone."

"Jane, it was a nice gesture to give someone else the opportunity to lead the community meeting."

Irresponsibility

Evaluate the effects of the client's irresponsible behaviors on the client's progress and interactions with others in the milieu *to plan appropriate interventions.*

Inform the client in a calm, direct manner each time he or she demonstrates irresponsible, insensitive behaviors *to increase the client's awareness of negative behaviors:*

"John, you didn't clean the shower after you used it; that's the responsibility of every client here."

"Mark, the group waited 20 minutes for you to lead the meeting; you didn't tell us you were out on pass."

Point out the consequences of the client's irresponsible actions on other clients *to illustrate the overall negative impact of irresponsible behaviors on the milieu:*

"Pam, Joe loaned you money that you promised to pay back the next day. When you didn't, he was unable to pay his way into the movie."

"Bob, hiding marijuana in your room caused serious problems for your roommate."

Construct a verbal or written behavioral contract with the client, listing specific responsibilities and obligations that he or she is expected to achieve and behaviors that are restricted, *to promote responsible behaviors and set limits on irresponsible actions.*

Examples of client expectations:

- Maintain neat, clean room and client areas
- Wash shower and bathtub after use
- Attend all meetings and activities
- Be on time for all meetings and activities
- Inform other clients and staff when unable to keep appointments and commitments

Client restrictions:

- Borrowing money, clothing, cigarettes, or other valued items from other clients

- Smoking or keeping illegal drugs in or around hospital area
- Having alcoholic beverages in or around hospital area

Maladaptive Denial

Assess situations in which the client uses maladaptive denial *to determine areas of conflict that are too anxiety-provoking for the client to confront and that prevent progress. Examples of possible causes of denial:*

- Fear of mental illness and its outcome
- Client role and responsibilities
- Low self-esteem
- Limitations, weaknesses
- Resistance to treatment regimen or compliance
- Guilt or shame

Assist the client to identify threats that precipitate denial *to help the client confront conflicts that inhibit compliance with treatment and movement toward health:*

"Paul, staff realizes the other clients often ask your advice; you are also a client and need help, too."

"Steve, it's difficult for you to admit that you have a mental health problem, yet it's the first step toward getting better."

"Mark, you say you're not a 'regular' client, yet you're experiencing what many clients experience."

"Sam, it may be true that your family has problems and you're here because it was difficult for you to cope as well."

Explore with the client the consequences of resistance or refusal to admitting the need for treatment, *to help the client recognize the negative results of noncompliance:*

"Paul, attending groups and meetings is part of your treatment plan; to ignore that will delay your progress."

"Mark, saying you're not a 'regular' client doesn't mean you don't need therapy. Your chances for recovery are better with treatment."

"Kate, leaving the hospital without telling staff tells us that you're not taking your client role seriously. That will make it harder for you to recover."

Teach the client anxiety-reducing strategies to manage threats to the self-system *to diminish use of denial and increase compliance with treatment plan.* (See Appendix K.)

Provide opportunities for the client to express feelings of fear, low self-esteem, guilt, shame and so on, *to help the client bring fears and conflicts out into the open and reduce the incidence of denial:*

"John, staff is here to listen to your feelings about your illness and hospitalization."

"Kate, it will help staff with our treatment approach if you talk about your concerns with us."

Help the client recognize that the unrealistic "optimism" of denial does not reduce his or her illness or symptoms, *to promote the client's awareness that denial is ultimately not useful or conducive to the client's health and well-being:*

"Jack, your inability to allow yourself to be treated as a client may reduce anxiety for a short while, but your illness needs to be treated in order to reduce painful symptoms and behaviors."

"Tom, ignoring or negating your problems will not make you feel better; that's what the treatment plan is for."

Allow the client to use defenses such as denial when he or she is unable to cope in a more functional way, *to decrease overwhelming anxiety.*

Identify expressions of fear, guilt, shame, etc., as possible signs of progress, *to encourage the client to continue to express feelings that provoke denial and offer hope for movement toward recovery.*

Challenge the client's belief that weaknesses are synonymous with illness, *to present the client with more theoretically sound explanations for illness:*

"There are several theories of mental illness, Pam, but a mental disorder is not a weakness of character."

"John, a mental disorder is as real as a physical illness; both can be treated and neither are considered weaknesses."

Encourage the client to participate in groups and activities within the milieu, *to distract the client from the use of denial by reducing anxiety through pleasurable activities.*

Engage the client in cognitive and behavioral therapy groups, *to share feelings with other clients, elicit helpful feedback through the group process, and reduce maladaptive denial. Examples:*

- Behavioral therapy
- Cognitive therapy
- Assertiveness training
- Role-play/sociodrama
- Process/focus groups

(Refer to Appendix J.)

Praise the patient for a reduction in or absence of maladaptive denial and for compliance with treatment regimen:

"John, talking about your illness and problems shows real progress."

"Pam, bringing your concerns out in the open is a big step in coping with them more effectively."

"Kate, admitting that you need help as other clients do is a sign of growth."

"Mark, sharing your guilt about your illness in group today is a sign of strength."

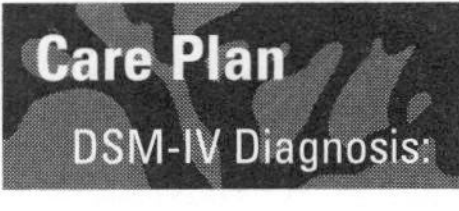

Personality Disorders (All Types)

NANDA Diagnosis: Self-esteem disturbance

The state in which an individual has negative self-evaluation/feelings about self or self capabilities, which may be directly or indirectly expressed

Focus:

For the client who demonstrates a life-style of overt or covert behavior patterns that reflect a negative self-concept. Behaviors may manifest as dependency or jealousy, among others, and may greatly interfere with the patient's ability to function at an optimal developmental stage.

NANDA: Taxonomy

Pattern 7—Perceiving: A human response pattern involving the reception of information

ETIOLOGIC/RELATED FACTORS (RELATED TO)

Personal identity disturbance
Disturbance in self-perception/self-concept
Powerlessness
Lack of insight/judgment
Ineffective problem solving
Perceived abandonment/rejection
Developmental conflicts
Psychosocial stressors
Environmental stressors
Role/relationship disturbance
Life-style of dependence/avoidance
Perceived victimization
Knowledge deficit regarding effective social skills

DEFINING CHARACTERISTICS (AS EVIDENCED BY)

Dependency

Demonstrates dependency on others to get needs met.

Appears frequently at nurses' station with nonurgent requests. Asks for help with tasks that can easily be done by client:

"I need help with my laundry; I can't do it alone."

"Could you get my cigarettes for me? They're in my room."

Demonstrates inability to make decisions without an excessive amount of advice from others, procrastinates:

"I just can't make up my mind; please help me decide what I should do."

"What should I do now—make my bed, get dressed, take a shower?"

Needs constant reassurance from others:

"Am I doing this right?"

"Is this OK?"

"Should I take my medication now?"

Allows others to make important life decisions:

"You decide what board and care home I need."

"I wish you would call my husband and tell him I can't see his mother anymore."

Lacks self-confidence or belittles own abilities and assets:

"I just can't seem to do anything right; you do it so much better."

"I'm a flop and a failure as a wife and mother."

"I don't blame my husband for leaving me; I'm not even attractive."

Manifests difficulty in initiating projects:

"How should I get started on my assignment?"

"It's too hard to begin this project on my own."

Fears abandonment, is uncomfortable when alone:

"I'll die without my husband to take care of me."

"I can't imagine leaving my mother's home."

"Why does everyone always leave me alone?"

Isolative/Withdrawn/Avoidant

Demonstrates inability to form close, personal relationships with others:

- Avoids social contact in the milieu
- Remains isolated in room for long periods
- Responds minimally when approached
- Exhibits cool, detached behavior toward others
- Rejects intimacy with one significant partner
- Referred to as a "loner" by significant others
- Easily hurt by criticism
- Fears being embarrassed or humiliated (e.g., blushes or cries when others offer praise or criticism)
- Exaggerates risks or danger in ordinary situations or events:

"I'm not going on the field trip. The bus could skid and go over a cliff in the rain."

- Arrives late for milieu activities and/or leaves early

Abandonment Fears/Attention-Seeking

Demonstrates frantic efforts to avoid actual or perceived abandonment:

- Makes frequent appearances at the nurses' station, often with nonurgent requests
- Makes unreasonable demands for staff's time and attention:

"I hate to bother you during your lunch hour, but I won't take up much of your time."

"Why do you only talk to me for a few minutes and then leave?"

- Seeks contact person or other staff members with a sense of urgency that is incongruent with the actual need:

"I really *need* to see you now—I'm out of clothes."

- Demands that staff call attending psychiatrist several times throughout the day:

"I *have* to see my doctor; I know he or she is in the hospital now."

"Can you call my doctor at home? There's something I forgot to ask."

"I saw my doctor leave the unit without talking to me; could you *please* catch the doctor before he or she leaves the hospital?"

- Questions loyalty of friends and family members:

"I doubt that my best friend will be waiting for me when I get out of here."

"I'm scared that my father will give up on me and *never* let me back in the house again."

- Telephones significant others for reassurance many times throughout hospitalization

Hysteria

Responds in dramatic, urgent, or exaggerated manner toward persons or situations that do not warrant such reactions:

"I absolutely *must* see my doctor right now."

"If I don't get my weekend pass, I'll just *die*."

"You simply *have* to speak to my roommate; I *can't* tolerate her abuse for one more day."

(These responses are accompanied by an increase in voice tone, gestures, and intense emotional expressiveness.)

Seductive

Exhibits seductive, flirtatious, or teasing behaviors with sexual overtones (may be directed toward favored person or toward the milieu in general)

Examples:

- Gazes suggestively and poses seductively
- Wears tight, scanty, or revealing clothing
- Engages in romantic fantasies regarding favored person(s)
- Discusses personal or sexual topics
- Makes excuses to see the favored person(s) as often as possible
- Writes love notes to objects of affection

Jealousy

Expresses extreme feelings and thoughts of jealousy regarding suspected infidelity of spouse, sexual partner, staff, or other clients:

"I can't even trust my wife with my own brother or father."

"I'm sure my husband is attracted to most of the female clients when he visits me."

"I realize my boyfriend flirts with all the nurse here; I'll bet he's going out with the whole neighborhood while I'm in here sick."

"My roommate thinks she's so great and that everyone loves her; I can't stand her."

"Everyone thinks Tim is so wonderful; he's really a big phony."

Accuses staff members of giving more attention to other clients or spending more time with them

Makes frequent phone calls home to check up on spouse or partner

Hypersexual Behavior

Makes frequent sexually suggestive statements, generally in an attempt to increase self-esteem:

"Why should anyone care if I put my arms around Mary; after all, I am a man."

"It's no big deal that the staff caught us in bed together; it's normal."

"I don't know why I can't even kiss someone I like just because we're in a hospital."

"Gosh, Jane, that blouse really shows off your figure; it makes me get ideas."

Behaves in a sexually provocative manner:

- Winks, thrusts hips or chest in suggestive manner
- Tells sexually oriented stories and jokes
- Sits next to individuals in ways that result in physical contact

Rigid and Perfectionistic Behaviors

Is unable to complete tasks owing to fear of substandard performance and product:

"I just can't finish my assignment; I don't have enough time to do it right."

"It will take me forever to do justice to this project; I'd rather not try it at all."

Is preoccupied with details to such a degree that activities and projects go uncompleted:

"I don't know if I can finish this project; there are so many details that need my attention."

"I want to complete my activities, but I have other things on my mind."

Demonstrates excessive rigidity regarding values, ethics, and morals, so that task performance and completion are inhibited.

Examples:

- Preoccupied with verbal or written accounts of ethical or moral issues to the exclusion of assigned tasks or projects
- Discusses spiritual beliefs during activity times without regard for task assignment

OUTCOME IDENTIFICATION AND EVALUATION

Dependency

Verbalizes independent statements:

"I can take care of my own basic needs."

"I'm going to take shower an do my laundry today."

Demonstrates independent behaviors:

- Approaches nurses' station only when necessary
- Performs self-care and other tasks without help

Makes decisions related to illness and treatment:

- Discusses possible change in medication dose with nurses and physician
- Plans and organizes daily tasks and activities

Makes decisions unrelated to illness and treatment:

- Enlists family or friends to take care of personal business (e.g., pay rent and bills, feed pets, and water plants) during hospital stay
- Chooses own place to live after discharge

Verbalizes self-confidence in abilities and assets:

"I know I'm a darn good parent."

"When it comes to my work, I'm very capable."

"I've always been a good artist."

Demonstrates confidence in abilities and tasks:

- Initiates and completes projects successfully

Expresses comfort in spending time alone:

"I actually enjoy having some time to myself."

"I love my family, but it's good to be alone once in a while."

Makes independent choices regarding life-style:
"I need to leave my parents' home and be on my own."
"I'm no longer afraid to live without a man/woman."

Isolative/Withdrawn/Avoidant

Seeks social contact with clients and staff
Spends majority of time in client areas rather than alone in room
Responds with brightened affect when approached
Initiates interactions with others
Participates with others in milieu activities
Arrives at milieu activities on time and stays for entire session
Engages in conversations and dialogue with others
Forms close personal relationship with a significant other
Accepts constructive criticism without crying or retreating
Accepts praise without blushing or retreating
Seeks praise for accomplishments
Attends outdoor activities and field trips without expressing exaggerated risks or dangers

Abandonment Fears/Attention-Seeking

Approaches nurses' station only when necessary
Approaches staff at convenient times rather than during their breaks or lunch hour
Seeks staff's time and attention for relevant reasons rather than benign requests
Acknowledges loyalty of family and friends:
"I know my family and friends care about me."
"I'm sure that my family and friends will always be there for me."
Refrains from frequent telephone calls to family or friends
Ceases to make frequent requests of staff to contact attending physician
Makes requests of staff without an exaggerated sense of urgency
Expresses comfort in spending time alone rather than feeling fearful or anxious:
"I actually enjoy being alone once in a while."
"The times I spend by myself are peaceful."

For the Client with Borderline Personality Disorder with Intense Abandonment Fears:
No longer requires a "transient object" (e.g., picture, note, or stuffed animal) when left alone

Hysteria

Demonstrates absent or decreased dramatic or exaggerated affect when interacting with others:
- Low to moderate voice tone
- Appropriate emotional response that is congruent with the situation

Seductive Behavior

Responds appropriately toward others, with absence of seductive, flirtatious, or teasing behaviors:
- Refrains from using sexually provocative dialogue
- Assumes appropriate positions rather than seductive or suggestive body language
- Ceases to demonstrate provocative or suggestive gestures or expressions
- Stops seeking out favored staff person or physician for personal, "romantic" reasons

Resists wearing tight-fitting, revealing clothing that is inappropriate to the setting
Reports absence of romantic notions, daydreams, or fantasies directed toward others in the environment

Jealousy

Demonstrates absence or reduction in jealous behaviors:
- Decreases number of phone calls to significant others during hospitalization
- Refrains from accusing partner of infidelity or flirting with others
- Ceases to accuse staff of giving more time and attention to "all the other clients"

Verbalizes trust toward significant partner:
"I really do trust my wife/husband/fiancé."
"I have faith in my partner; I know he or she will be loyal to me while I'm in the hospital."

Hypersexual Behavior

Refrains from making lewd, sexually provocative statements
Resists touching others in a sexually suggestive manner
Demonstrates appropriate behaviors with absence of sexually provocative gestures, poses, or expressions
Ceases to wear scanty, revealing clothing

Rigid and Perfectionistic Behaviors

Completes tasks without fear of substandard performance and product
Accomplishes assignments with absence of preoccupation with details
Completes activities and projects without being diverted by rigid moral and ethical preoccupations
Demonstrates flexible versus rigid, perfectionistic behaviors:
- Makes sufficient time for all scheduled activities and projects
- Reacts in calm, matter-of-fact manner to imperfect, substandard task or project

PLANNING AND IMPLEMENTATION

Nursing Interventions and Rationale

Dependency

Assess client's level of dependence *to collect data from which to plan interventions and measure client's level of progress against expected outcomes.*

Formulate a nursing care plan, outlining the client's basic needs and activities of daily living, *to determine and encourage appropriate independent behavior. List the following:*
- Activities the client can perform independently (independent)

- Activities with which client requires help (interdependent)
- Activities client needs nurse to perform (dependent)

Positively reinforce client's independent behavior *to encourage continuity of appropriate independent behavior:*

"Pam, I see you showered and put on some makeup this morning."

"Tom, you made out your own menus without help for three days."

"John, you were on time for all the group activities today."

"Jim, start to do your laundry and I'll be here if you need help."

Establish clear boundaries between nurse and client and client and others *to prevent the client from becoming enmeshed or dependent on others to get needs met:*

- Separate nurse's duties from client's responsibilities:

"Pam, I'll set the trays on the table and you and the other clients can arrange the napkins and utensils."

"Paul, I'll put your clothes in your room and you can fold them and put them away."

- Distinguish between the client's responsibilities and the responsibilities of other clients:

"Ken, it's your turn to clean the clients' dining room; Bob volunteered to empty ashtrays and wash out the coffeepot."

"Sarah hasn't been here long enough to be client leader, Beth, but you can handle it."

Encourage independent decision making in accordance with client's level of progress *to increase client's self-worth and self-esteem.*

Examples:

- When client asks, "What shall I do now?" you can reply with the statement, "What are some of the things you want to do now?"
- If the client cannot make up his or her mind about which activity to attend, you can ask, "What do you think would be most beneficial to you now?"

Clarify with the client both negative and positive feelings that accompany dependency *to illustrate that there are more negative aspects connected to dependency and to discourage dependent behavior:*

"Ken, how do you feel when you do something for yourself? Do you feel that way when others do things for you?"

Identify with the client the positive results of independent behaviors and accomplishments *to reinforce continuance of independent behaviors:*

"Sam, the clients really enjoyed the article you wrote in the clients' newsletter."

"Jane, the placemats you made for the clients' holiday meal brightened their day."

"Ken, your planning Sam's farewell party was a nice surprise for everyone."

"Sue, your starting the sing-along was appreciated. Will you do it again when the group is together?"

Offer the client choices whenever possible, *to increase independence and control over management of care.*

"Are you going to take your shower now or after the community meeting?"

"You choose which game to play during activity time."

"You can select the clients' prizes at the bingo game tonight."

Encourage the client to make decisions regarding his or her own care and treatment whenever feasible, rather than ask staff's permission, *to increase independence, judgment, and decision making.*

Examples:

- If the client asks, "Is it OK if I go to my room to rest?" ask the client, "Do you want to rest?" and if response is yes, encourage the client to restate: "I *am* going to my room to rest."
- If the client asks, "Can I take my shower now?" ask client, "Do you want to shower now?" and if response is yes, have the client restate: "I *prefer* to take my shower now."
- If the client asks, "Is it OK if I attend Dr. Jones's lecture instead of playing bingo?" ask client what she or he wants to do, then, based on client's reply, encourage the client to state: "I *want* to attend Dr. Jones's lecture this afternoon."

Increase decision-making opportunities as the client progresses *to foster problem-solving and critical thinking:*

"When you leave on your pass today, what are the things you'd like to do?"

"You'll need to decide between staying in your parents' home and going back to independent living."

"After you're discharged, it will be up to you to return for follow-up treatment."

Respond with approval to the client's efforts toward independent decision making *to reinforce continued independent behaviors:*

"Pam, it was good that you made a decision about where to live after you are discharged."

"Tom, it's good that you arrived at the decision to pay your bills while you were out on pass."

Demonstrate respect for the client's feelings, even when he or she is unable to perform independently, *to assure the client that he or she is worthwhile and accepted:*

"Donna, it's OK to feel bad that independent living didn't work out for you this time."

"Kate, you're saying you're feeling frustrated, but it's OK to ask for help with difficult tasks."

"Jane, you're feeling mad at yourself for not having decided where to live when you're discharged. You can begin working on that tomorrow. How can we help?"

Engage the client in physical activities that offer quick rewards *to increase energy level and promote self-esteem.*

Examples:

- Brisk walks
- Exercises
- Stationary bicycle

- Ping-Pong
- Volleyball

Help the client set realistic, attainable goals *to avoid failure to meet goals, provide hope for behavioral change, and increase feelings of independence and control over life.*

Therapeutic responses:

"Ted, it's good that you're making plans for your discharge; what did you think about the board and care homes you visited?"

"Sally, I know you want your own apartment; what are your thoughts about independent living for a while?"

"Pam, your desire to become a psychiatrist makes me think that you would like to do something to help people feel better."

These statements are based on the nurse's judgment of the client's capabilities, rather than based on the client's wishes and desires, and more closely reflect achievable goals.

Nontherapeutic responses:

"Ted, if you really want to live by yourself, give it a try."

"Pam, you way you want to become a psychiatrist; why not talk to a college counselor about the course work?"

"Sally, you can do almost anything if you put your mind to it."

Gradually help the client to decrease secondary gains (e.g., assistance from others, avoidance of responsibilities) that accompany dependent behaviors *to discourage continuance of dependent behaviors:*

"Paul, since you've been on time for the morning community meeting for three days, you don't need to be awakened by staff anymore."

"Ken, you've made progress; staff thinks you're ready for the responsibility of client leader."

Teach the client to challenge unrealistic beliefs (e.g., failure, unattractiveness, lack of initiative) by pointing out factual information *to replace unrealistic, self-defeating thoughts with facts, decrease negative self-concept, and promote self-worth.*

Therapeutic responses:

"Susan, you say you haven't succeeded at anything in your life, yet your children visit you and phone you every day."

"Jeff, you say you never had ambition; you've achieved a bachelor's degree in history, which is an accomplishment."

"Kate, you keep saying you're unattractive, yet I've heard clients and staff compliment your hairstyle and taste in clothes many times."

These statements challenge the client's unrealistic, negative beliefs by presenting actual facts versus opinions in an effort to replace negative beliefs with realistic, factual information.

Nontherapeutic responses:

"Susan, how can you say you're unsuccessful? You have a nice family."

"Jeff, anyone with a college degree has to be successful."

"Kate, you have the prettiest blue eyes; I find that very attractive."

These statements are based on opinion rather than fact and seem extreme and contrived, which may foster the client's fears of failure and negative self-concept.

Challenge the client's exaggerated fears of abandonment and perceived consequences with factual information *to illustrate the client's actual capabilities and strengths.*

Therapeutic responses:

"Sarah, you say you 'can't make it' without your husband, yet you left him to enter the hospital for help and you've done well for three weeks."

"Pam, no doubt your mother has helped you; she will continue to be supportive even if you live apart from each other."

"Tom, you stated that you're hesitant to leave your roommate because you don't want to be alone, even though you fight a lot. Is being alone more stressful than tolerating the fighting?"

These responses gently challenge the client's fears and suggest that they may be unwarranted. This allows the client to reexamine fears of abandonment and consequences.

Nontherapeutic responses:

"You know, Sarah, you really don't feel you need a man to make your life complete; you're doing fine without one."

"Pam, everyone has to leave his or her mother behind; it's part of growing up."

"Tom, you can always get another roommate; why put yourself through all that stress?"

These statements tend to chastise the client rather than challenge the belief system, which may perpetuate the fears rather than decrease them.

Assist the client to evaluate resources that will encourage and promote independence *so that client can use reliable sources of help when necessary:*

"Sam, the social worker is an appropriate person to help you inquire about places to live."

"Tom, the pharmacist teaches a class for clients every Tuesday; he may be another source of information about medication effects."

Identify with the client and family the strength and assets of the family unit and the client's contribution to the functioning of the family *to reinforce the importance and value of the client's role as a family member.*

Discuss with the client and family the family behaviors that are no longer necessary but continue to interfere with the client's need for independence, *to gain an understanding of ways the family may contribute to the client's dependency and offer rationale for change:*

"It may be that John can now make more decisions for himself, since he is taking the new medication that helps him to function more independently."

"It's understandable for the family to be concerned about Pam wanting to try independent living; her doctor and staff believe she's capable of doing it with your support."

Assist the family to work with the client, doctor, and staff in promoting and encouraging the client's independent behaviors *to foster more autonomous family functioning for all members:*

"It's to everyone's benefit that we all work together with John so he can reach goals that are achievable."

"Everyone will gain when Pam's goals for independent living are successful; she needs our support to do it."

Engage the client in appropriate group, cognitive, and behavioral therapies *to increase self-esteem and foster independent functioning and behaviors, resulting from support, acceptance, and the universality of group dynamics.*

Examples:

- Role play
- Cognitive therapy
- Assertiveness training
- Process groups

(See Appendix K.)

Problem solve with the client to mutually identify the following:

- Problems that realistically require some assistance
- Goals that the client can achieve independently
- Issues that need to be deferred to other sources
- Alternative solutions for each problem
- Solutions that consider both positive and negative points, *to maximize the client's independent functioning and minimize dependent behaviors.*

Praise the client for efforts made toward independent functioning *to increase self-esteem and reinforce independent behaviors:*

"Jeff, your leading the community meeting in Ken's absence showed real initiative."

"Pam, making the final decision to find a roommate rather than move back in your parents' home was a big step for you."

Isolative/Withdrawn/Avoidant

Assess the degree of the client's isolation and level of progress in the program. *The client may be newly admitted and need time to adjust to the facility and milieu.*

Make short, frequent visits to the client's room *to let the client know that staff is caring and empathetic and understands that long, drawn-out interactions may be overwhelming.*

Provide assistance with basic needs and activities of daily living, as needed, *to maintain self-respect and increase self-esteem:*

- Initially accompany the client to the shower, laundry room, and other new places
- Provide the client with toothbrush, toothpaste, comb, and hairbrush
- Offer literature, magazines, writing paper, and pencils
- Provide the client with a copy of the milieu structured activities

Provide the client with his or her own clothing and valued personal belongings, as feasible, *to reinforce the client's self-identity and promote comfort.*

Engage in short, simple verbal interactions with the client *to begin to draw the client into the therapeutic community:*

"Here's the new toothbrush I promised you."

"I see you have pictures in your room."

"Is there anything else you need?"

"Did you fill out your menu for the day?"

Sit with the client for brief periods, interrupting silence only if it appears uncomfortable for the client (fidgets, paces, has worried or strained facial expression) *to allow the client to feel safe in an interpersonal relationship.*

Gradually increase time of one-to-one interactions with the client *to promote socialization and decrease periods of isolation.*

Example:

Begin with 5-minute, one-to-one interactions; progress in increments of 5 minutes until the client can engage in a 20-minute interaction without demonstrating discomfort or verbalizing the need to withdraw.

Encourage the client to *gradually* join other clients *to decrease social isolation and increase healthy socialization skills.*

Begin in the dining room. Have the client first sit near the door, then graduate to a more populated, central area; progress to an informal or casual group setting; participate in one-to-one games with trusted staff, eventually including one or two trusted clients; progress to noncompetitive group activities (e.g., exercise, drawing, cooking, singing); attend a didactic class (e.g., cognitive or assertive therapy); participate in more structured formal or process groups.

Promote involvement in physical activities (e.g., exercise, walking, Ping-Pong) *to increase the client's energy level and social accomplishments.*

Provide the client with plants or pets, if appropriate, *to promote expressions of love and nurturing through contact with nonthreatening living things.*

Set limits on naps and the amount of time spent in room *to ensure that the person will sleep at night and be awake and rested for daytime milieu activities.*

Provide the client with a balanced nutritional regimen *to prevent dehydration, constipation, and deterioration of physical health.*

Gradually promote closeness, if appropriate, in accordance with team assessment of client's tolerance, *to demonstrate warmth and caring and decrease isolation.*

Example:

Allow the client more space when beginning the interaction, gradually narrow the space between yourself and the client to arm's length, and progress to comfortable social distance.

Facilitate nonverbal expression of painful feelings (e.g., writing, drawing, typing, playing piano, singing, painting, physical exercise) *to provide a release of painful feelings when the client cannot verbalize them.*

Engage the client in casual conversations at intervals throughout the day *to show interest and promote ease in social interactions.*

Example:
Call the client by name, ask how he or she is doing, discuss nonthreatening topics of interest, share a cup of tea.

Accept the client's refusal to join staff or group in every activity or interaction, without personalizing it, *to prevent personal feelings from interfering with the therapeutic relationship and to role model acceptance of the client's resistance.*

Role model social and interactive skills *to illustrate healthy, effective socialization skills for the client's benefit.*

Avoid placing the client in social situations or activities where he or she may fail or feel uncomfortable *to prevent decreasing self-esteem and further withdrawal from others.*

Provide the client with opportunities to discuss situations that may influence social withdrawal and isolation *to allow the client to accept painful experiences and move on with life:*

"Tom, what makes it difficult for you to join the community?"

"Bob, what situations cause you to want to leave groups and activities?"

"Pam, how can staff help you feel more comfortable here in this community setting?"

Point out situations that seem to result in the client's withdrawing from the milieu *to prepare the client to begin to manage environmental stressors that promote isolation:*

"Jack, I notice that when there's too much noise you tend to leave the client areas."

"Pam, whenever the clients get into a 'heated' discussion, you retreat to your room."

"Sue, it seems that you find it difficult to attend group activities after a meeting with your doctor."

Problem solve with the client methods to manipulate the environment or modify situations *to facilitate increased participation in milieu activities and decrease isolation.*

Examples:

- Reduce stimuli (e.g., lower volume settings on radio, stereo, television; reduce lighting)
- Accompany the client to a less stimulating area and assign less stressful activity with fewer people

Collaborate with doctor and staff to schedule intense one-to-one interactions during times that do not interfere with milieu groups and/or activities, *to decrease the client's withdrawal from the community and promote participation and socialization.*

Demonstrate respect and interest in the client's desire for aloneness and isolated activities (e.g., reading, painting, listening to music or favorite radio or television program, or praying), as long as the client participates in the therapeutic regimen, *to validate the client's life choices and increase self-worth and self-esteem:*

"Bob, I think it's good to enjoy such valuable interests and hobbies as long as you also participate in the treatment plan."

"Jane, it's important to be alone occasionally; you also need to attend community meetings."

"Kate, reading and painting in your room can be therapeutic; so are group activities and interactions."

"Sue, your faith is important to you, and staff can help you plan your day so you will have time to pray."

Explore with the client realistic and unrealistic components of the client's perceptions about situations and events that cause him or her to withdraw, *to distinguish between rational and irrational thoughts and begin to challenge irrational ones:*

"Joe, you say you left because Tom seemed to criticize you; I didn't see it that way; let's discuss it with Tom."

"Sue, your face turned red and you walked away when the group complimented you; it's OK to accept praise for a job well done."

"Kate, holding hands was part of the group activity; it doesn't mean anything more."

"Ann, you cried when Jane shared information that you felt was personal; staff agrees you need to talk to Jane, then join the group."

Involve family, friends and other support systems in the client's social activities *to strengthen the client's social network and decrease alienation and isolation:*

"Pam, your sister and brother-in-law are coming to visit you this evening; perhaps they can join the family group activity."

Praise the client for efforts made toward contacting others, attending groups, participating in activities, and decreasing withdrawal and isolation, *to reinforce continued socialization:*

"Kate, you attended all group activities this week; your participation contributed to their success."

"Sam, returning to the community meeting after talking to your doctor showed real progress."

Abandonment Fears/Attention-Seeking

Assess the frequency and intensity of the client's attempts to seek out staff for unreasonable nonurgent demands or requests, to plan interventions that minimize abandonment fears and interrupt attention-seeking behaviors.

For the Client with Borderline or Mixed Personality Disorders with Exaggerated Fears and Dread of Abandonment:

Leave the client with a symbolic or "transient" object (e.g., a note, card, or picture) *to help bridge the gap between actual contacts and relieve the intensity of abandonment fears.*

Assure the client that everything necessary is being done for his or her treatment and care, while acknowledging concerns, *to relieve the client's fears of being alone, ignored, or abandoned:*

"Paul, we realize you worry about your care; staff meet regularly to discuss your treatment plan and progress."

Address the client's major concerns, whenever possible, *to reduce attention-seeking behaviors.*

Assure the client that staff are available to meet needs when necessary, *to reduce the client's fears of abandonment and interrupt attention-seeking behaviors.*

Therapeutic responses:

"Kate, staff are here when you need our assistance; seeking us out for things you can do yourself is not necessary."

"Paul, it's not necessary to approach the nurses' station so often; staff will be available when you need us."

Nontherapeutic responses:

"Kate, you know better than to bother the staff with unnecessary requests; we're not going to leave you."

"Paul, standing in front of the nurses' station all day is very irritating to the staff. We're not going anywhere."

These statements reflect a parental disapproval that may result in exacerbation of the client's abandonment fears and attention-seeking behaviors.

Teach strategies that help the client cope with the feelings of urgency that accompany perceived abandonment, *to assuage irrational feelings and emotions that magnify or distort fears of abandonment.*

Examples:

- Slow, deep-breathing exercises
- Relaxation techniques
- Count slowly to 5 before seeking staff
- Take a brisk walk
- Use visual imagery

(See Appendix K.)

Assist the client to replace perceived fears of abandonment with actual situations, *to focus the client on reality and discourage attention-seeking behaviors:*

"Jane, you say you're afraid of being left alone; actually, you're seldom alone with the staff so near."

"Paul, it seems you have a real concern about being alone; in reality there's always someone close by."

"Kate, you say you hate to be alone; staff are here when you need us."

"Sue, you say you're afraid your friends will leave you, yet they visit you almost every night."

"Joe, you're worried that your dad won't let you live at home when you leave here, yet he phones every day asking when you'll be able to go home."

Help the client structure activities throughout the day, *to minimize periods of free time and discourage attention-seeking behaviors.*

Plan with the client solitary activities he or she is interested in pursuing *to maximize the client's periods of aloneness and reduce the need to seek others to fill each moment of free time.*

Examples:

- Writing letters
- Riding a stationary bicycle
- Keeping a diary

Develop a behavioral contract with the client that sets limits on attention-seeking behaviors *to help the client gain control over dysfunctional patterns and develop self-sufficiency.*

Examples:

- Set up a schedule with the client for times the client may approach the nurses' station.
- Have the client address problems to assigned staff person only.
- Limit personal telephone calls to three per day; have client decide on times.
- Construct a list with the client that defines urgent versus nonurgent concerns for requests.

Encourage the client to participate in therapeutic group activities *to maximize strengths and capabilities and to learn strategies for coping with abandonment fears through the dynamics of the group process.*

Examples:

- Role play, sociodrama
- Behavioral therapy
- Cognitive therapy
- Assertiveness training
- Process or focus groups

(See Appendix K.)

Gently challenge the client's fears of abandonment *to illustrate the client's actual capabilities and strengths:*

"Kate, you often say you can't bear to be alone, yet you accomplish a lot during those times."

"Paul, you may think you need to be around people all the time, but you are quite capable on your own."

"Mark, you have concerns about free time, yet you do good things for yourself when you're alone."

Engage family and friends in therapeutic sessions with the client and appropriate therapist *to address the client's concerns about loyalty of loved ones and reduce fears of abandonment.*

Consult with appropriate sources (e.g., social services, adjunctive therapists, and psychiatrist) for collaborative solutions to problems *to minimize the client's attention-seeking behaviors and fears of abandonment.*

Use assertive responses *to help set limits on the client's unreasonable demands for time and attention:*

"Kate, I can't talk now; we'll talk in 45 minutes."

"Sam, I'll help you when you need it; you don't need my help to wash your clothes."

"Mark, you spoke with your doctor just a few minutes ago; we'll call her office after the 2 o'clock activity."

"Sarah, we spent a good deal of time together this morning; I'll plan to spend time again with you in 2 hours. We can plan about 15 minutes talking at that time."

"John, your frequent use of the telephone is interrupting your treatment; we need to set up a phone schedule."

Praise the client for decreased attention-seeking behaviors and ability to cope with free time without making unreasonable demands on staff, *to reinforce repetition of positive behaviors and increase self-esteem:*

"Jane, staff have noticed your efforts to work out some problems on your own before you seek us out."
"Paul, it shows real progress that you don't need to approach the nurses' station so often."
"John, your decreased use of the telephone is a sign of growth."
"Mark, making less demands on staff's time shows you're able to be alone successfully."

Hysteria

Assess the frequency and intensity of the client's melodramatic or exaggerated responses *to plan interventions that will help the client subdue his or her reactions.*

Assure the client that it is not necessary to resort to dramatic or exaggerated behaviors to get needs met, *to reduce the incidence of hysterical responses:*
"Jane, it's not necessary to respond so dramatically; staff will listen to your concerns."
"Tom, responding in such an exaggerated way isn't necessary; the doctor already agreed to give you a pass."
"Sue, staff will speak to your roommate about your concerns; there's no need to be talking in this manner."

Point out to the client the incongruence between the actual situation and the client's response *to help the client adapt his or her responses to match the intensity of the situation and refrain from overreacting:*
"Sue, your roommate left her laundry on your bed for five minutes to answer the phone; your screaming that she 'abused' you is an overreaction."
"Tom, your weekend pass was granted three days ago; yelling that you'll 'die' if you don't get it is an exaggerated response."

Inform the client of the negative impact of his or her hysterical behavior on others *to encourage the client to reduce overly dramatic responses:*
"Jane, your responding in this manner is troubling to the other clients."
"Tom, it bothers the other clients when you respond so dramatically to simple events."
"Sue, screaming demands at the staff annoys us."

Teach the client therapeutic strategies *to interrupt hysteric responses and expend emotional energy constructively.*
Examples:
- Slow, deep-breathing techniques
- Relaxation exercises
- Count slowly to 5 before responding
- Physical exercises and activities
- Biofeedback

(See Appendix K for deep-breathing and relaxation strategies. See Glossary for *biofeedback* definition.)

Use role play in formal and informal situations *to teach the client to modulate overreactions and dramatic responses.*
Examples:
- Create a hypothetical situation between nurse and client (formal).
- Demonstrate appropriate responses to events that occur in client areas such as dining room or lounge (informal).
- Discuss the client's feelings and perceptions after the role-play exercises.

(See glossary for *role-playing* definition.)

Engage the family and client in therapeutic group sessions with an appropriate therapist *to discuss the family's interaction pattern and its influence on the client's hysterical behavior. (See Appendix K.)*

Encourage the client to approach assigned staff for one-to-one interaction whenever he or she feels overwhelmed by a sense of emotional urgency *to talk out feelings with a trusted staff person and avoid displaying hysteric behaviors in the client setting.*

Instruct the client in therapeutic groups *to learn strategies to reduce hysteric, dramatic responses through the dynamics of group process.*
Examples:
- Role play, sociodrama
- Behavioral therapy
- Cognitive therapy
- Assertiveness training
- Process or focus groups

(See Appendix K and Glossary.)

Praise the client for efforts made to reduce or eliminate hysteric, melodramatic responses *to increase self-esteem and reinforce repetition of positive behaviors:*
"Jane, your responses lately have been appropriate to the situation and show real maturity."
"Tom, staff have said that they appreciate your efforts to react to situations without being overly dramatic."
"Kate, the clients have commented favorably on your attempts to respond in moderation."

Seductive Behavior

Assess the degree and frequency of the client's seductive behaviors *to plan interventions that interrupt and minimize seductive patterns.*

Inform the client that staff will meet needs related to hospitalization but will not accept seductive behaviors, *to assure the client that needs will be addressed, while setting limits on inappropriate, disruptive behaviors:*
"Jack, staff are available to help you with your problems, although your suggestive behaviors will not be tolerated."
"Pam, staff cares about your well-being, but flirting with other clients or staff is not allowed."
"Jane, staff request that you ask your assigned staff person for help and stop seeking out male staff."

Explain to the client the negative reactions of others toward his or her seductive behaviors *to make the client aware of the impact of behaviors on others and take steps to eliminate them:*
"Jack, the other clients want you to stop your sexual advances; it makes them uncomfortable."

"Pam, your continuous flirting is annoying to the other clients, and they ask that you stop."

"Donna, staff and clients are uncomfortable when you wear such tight clothing; we request that you stop."

"Mark, sending seductive notes to other clients angers them and must stop."

Collaborate with staff to plan treatment strategies for the client's seductive behaviors *to assure consistency in the management of care.*

Assign a staff person who can be firm about the client's seductive behaviors yet flexible enough to accept the client's vulnerabilities. *Clients with seductive behaviors need a balance of structure and discipline and acceptance and understanding. Rigid disapproval decreases self-esteem and inhibits trust.*

Engage the client in therapeutic group sessions with an appropriate therapist *to discuss seductive behaviors and problem solve effective management strategies.*

Praise the client for positive qualities and behaviors *to increase self-worth and diminish the need for seductive behaviors:*

"Jack, you were a very effective client leader during the community meeting."

"Pam, it was thoughtful of you to lend your sweater to Kate when she said she was cold."

"Jane, your suggestions for the group activity today were very helpful."

"Mark, sharing your visitor's time with your roommate was very considerate."

Use role play with the patient in one-to-one situations *to illustrate the inappropriateness of seductive behaviors and teach the client mature, appropriate interpersonal skills.*

Discuss the role-play exercises with the client *to elicit his or her perspective of the different behaviors and their effects on client and nurse.*

Examples (nurse to client):

"When I responded to your request with suggestive behaviors, how did you feel? Did you feel valued or devalued as a person?"

"How did you think I reacted when you interacted with me without using a seductive approach? Was I more, or less, receptive to your actual needs?"

Engage the client in milieu activities *to help the client use free time productively and refrain from using seductive behaviors to promote self-worth and meet needs.*

Engage the client in therapeutic group activities *to build self-esteem and learn mature methods of interacting through the dynamics of the group process.*

Examples:

- Role play, sociodrama
- Behavioral therapy or cognitive therapy
- Assertiveness training or process groups

(See Appendix K and Glossary.)

Construct a behavioral contract, if necessary, *to help set limits on the client's seductive behaviors and direct the client toward mature, effective interactions.*

Examples (consequences vary according to hospital policy):

- Refrain from using seductive behaviors (e.g., flirting; teasing; suggestive statements, poses, or gestures).
- Cease wearing tight, revealing clothing; must wear undergarments.
- Stop sending sexually provocative notes or messages to staff or clients.

Give the client positive feedback whenever he or she refrains from seductive behaviors or ceases to wear revealing clothes, *to increase self-esteem and reinforce repetition of positive mature behaviors:*

"Donna, staff have noticed that your choice of clothing is appropriate and not suggestive."

"Mark, the clients are pleased that you've stopped sending seductive notes to them."

"Jane, approaching your staff person for assistance, instead of seeking out male staff, shows real progress."

"Jack, refraining from making sexual advances is a sign of growth and maturity."

Jealousy

Assess the degree and potential for injury to the client and others as a result of the client's jealousy *to plan interventions that will protect the client and others from harm.*

Protect the client and others from injury when the client loses control as a result of jealous rage *to prevent injury to the client and others.*

(See Appendix L.)

Evaluate situations that provoke the client's jealousy and loss of control *to plan interventions that will assist the client to manage jealous thoughts and behaviors* (whether jealousy is justified or out of proportion to the actual situation).

Encourage the client to put jealous thoughts into words *to prevent the client's behaviors from escalating to uncontrolled rage and aggression and to provide opportunities for client self-expression:*

"Pam, you seem to become agitated each time your husband visits you; let's discuss it."

"Ted, it may be helpful to talk about your jealous thoughts with staff, to clarify some points."

Assist the client to challenge unwarranted or exaggerated jealousy by helping the client separate facts from misperceptions, *to discourage jealousy:*

"Paul, you say your wife is out with other men every night while you're in the hospital, yet she visits you every night and works all day."

"Sarah, you tell us how your husband flirts with the nurses when he visits you; none of the nursing staff has observed that."

"Jack, you say staff spends more time with other clients; let's talk about the time we spend with you."

"Karen, the others probably like Joan and Tim because they are good-natured and helpful."

Provide activities (e.g., occupational therapy, therapeutic recreation) that increase the client's self-worth and control, *to decrease jealousy that may stem from a low self-concept and powerlessness.*

(See Glossary for definitions.)

Suggest physical outlets *to divert anger-producing energy toward productive, rewarding activities.*

Examples:

- Stationary bicycle
- Brisk walks
- Ping-Pong, volleyball, shuffleboard

Discuss with the client and family the situations and behaviors that provoke anger, jealousy, and rage, *to problem solve and modify those behaviors and situations and prevent or reduce jealous episodes among family members.*

Engage the client in the milieu and group therapies *to encourage ventilation of feelings and input from peers, nurses, and adjunctive therapists that will increase client's self-esteem and control and reduce jealousy.*

Examples:

- Community meetings
- Behavioral therapy
- Cognitive therapy
- Assertiveness training
- Role play
- Relationship groups

(Refer to Appendix K.)

Praise the client for successful management of jealous thoughts *to reinforce positive behaviors:*

"Paul, it shows real progress that you haven't made any jealous accusations about your wife for a week."

"Sarah, it was good to hear you tell the group that you no longer feel jealous of the nurses when your husband comes to visit you."

"John, you deserve credit for bringing your feelings of jealousy out into the open; that's the first step toward resolving them."

Hypersexual Behavior*

Assess the extent and frequency of the client's hypersexual behavior *to plan interventions that interrupt or eliminate hypersexual behaviors.*

Inform the client that staff will meet needs but that hypersexual behavior will not be tolerated, *to assure the client that problems will be addressed while setting limits on disruptive, hypersexual behavior:*

"Sam, staff wants to help you, but placing your arm around clients or touching them in a suggestive manner is not allowed here."

"Jack, we're here to assist you with your problems, but talking to others in a sexually provocative way will not be tolerated."

"Kate, staff wants to help you, but it's against hospital policy to lie in bed with another client or engage in sex; it may get you dismissed from the hospital."

"Pam, staff care about you, but kissing other clients, or anyone else here, is not acceptable."

Construct a behavioral contract to set limits on the client's hypersexual behavior *to help the client control disruptive behavior and to teach appropriate, effective methods of interacting.*

Examples (consequences vary according to hospital policy):

- Refrain from demonstrating inappropriate sexual behaviors (e.g., hugging, kissing, touching in sexually provocative manner, lying in bed with other clients).
- Cease using sexually suggestive body language, gestures, or poses.
- Stop sexual, lewd dialogue or innuendo.

Engage the client in therapeutic sessions with an appropriate therapist *to work on problems associated with hypersexual behaviors and learn to replace them with mature, effective interactions.*

Point out the negative impact of the client's hypersexual behavior on other clients and staff *to illustrate the disruptive effects the behavior has on the milieu and to encourage the client to reduce or eliminate the behavior:*

"Jack, when you use sexual language in front of others, they tend to leave the area."

"Pam, your frequent kissing and hugging attempts are annoying to the other clients and they ask that you stop."

"Kate, lying in bed with another client was upsetting to everyone and cannot be repeated or you may be dismissed from the hospital."

Collaborate with staff to ensure consistent management of the client's hypersexual behaviors. *Clients with long-standing inappropriate behaviors require consistent treatment strategies.*

Assign a staff person who can be firm about the client's hypersexual behavior, not intimidated by it, and flexible enough to address problem areas. *Clients with hypersexual behavior patterns require firm control and direction yet need acceptance to preserve their feelings of self-worth.*

Praise the client for positive qualities and behaviors *to increase self-esteem and diminish the need for hypersexual behaviors:*

"Kate, showing the new client around the unit was very considerate."

"Jack, offering your place at the card game to Joe was generous."

"Pam, it was nice of you to take notes at the community meeting."

Encourage the client to participate in physical activities *to direct sexual energy toward productive physical activities and reduce the incidence of hypersexual behavior.*

Examples:

- Aerobic exercises (unless contraindicated)
- Brisk walks
- Stationary bicycle
- Jump rope
- Volleyball, Ping-Pong

*Hypersexual behavior is generally more intensely manifested than seductive behaviors and may be noted in clients with mania and antisocial personality disorder. See Sexual and Gender Identity Disorders, Chapter 11, for additional information.

Engage the client in therapeutic group activities *to build the client's self-esteem, help the client learn mature, effective methods of interacting, and reduce or eliminate hypersexual behaviors.*

Examples:

- Behavioral therapy
- Cognitive therapy
- Assertiveness training
- Process and focus groups
- Role play

(See Appendix K and Glossary.)

Give the client positive feedback whenever he or she refrains from hypersexual behaviors *to build self-esteem and reinforce repetition of mature, positive behaviors:*

"Jack, staff have noticed that you no longer use sexual terms when you interact with others."

"Kate, you've made real progress; your behaviors are mature and appropriate."

"Pam, the other clients say they enjoy being around you since you've stopped trying to kiss them."

"Sam, refraining from touching and hugging other clients shows growth and maturity."

Rigid and Perfectionistic Behaviors

Assess the frequency of the client's inability to complete tasks or projects owing to concerns that the task performance or finished product will be imperfect or substandard, *to plan interventions that will enhance task completion.*

Assess the extent of the client's preoccupation with details *to determine the level of rigidity and perfectionism that inhibit task completion.*

Assess the degree of client's rigid preoccupation with values, ethics, and morals *to determine if it is a possible source of task incompletion or substandard performance.*

Assure the client that completion of a task, project, or activity is more valued than the quality of the product or performance *to reduce the client's fear of imperfection and encourage task completion:*

"Pam, it's more important to finish the volleyball game than to win it; your participation is needed for that."

"Sue, the art therapist is not concerned with artistic ability; your interpretation of the completed drawing is valued."

Assist the client to set limits on rigid preoccupations with values, ethics, and morals *to make time for task performance and completion:*

"Tom, staff agree that it's appropriate to spend 15 minutes each shift on your spiritual beliefs and the remainder of the time on completing assigned projects."

"Kate, it's acceptable to take 10 minutes each shift to discuss your ethical views with your staff person. The rest of the time needs to be spent on therapeutic activities."

Construct a written behavioral contract *to provide the client with a tangible reminder of the amount of time required for task performance and completion.*

Assign the client one task or project at a time, to be completed within a specific time frame:

"Pam, your job is to collect each person's contribution to the collage, including your own, by 2 PM next Monday."

"Jack, your assignment is to read the first section in the cognitive therapy book by Friday at 10 AM."

"Sue, you're expected to be up and dressed by 8 AM every morning. Tomorrow we'll discuss other responsibilities."

"Mark, this week you'll be responsible for cleaning and tidying up your room. Next week, you can begin to do your laundry."

Clients with rigid, perfectionistic qualities generally prefer to complete an assignment to the best of their abilities before moving on to the next project. Time constraints are necessary to minimize the client's preoccupation with details and promote task completion.

Engage the client in group activities in which each person's contribution is required for the task or project to reach completion, *to enhance the client's performance through the dynamics of the group process.*

Examples:

- Community jigsaw puzzle
- Preparing food for picnic or barbecue
- Development of collage or poster
- Sing-along session

Encourage the client to attend structured groups to develop an awareness of rigid, perfectionistic qualities and attempt *to overcome the constraints they place on task performance and completion.*

Examples:

- Role play, sociodrama
- Behavioral therapy
- Cognitive therapy
- Assertiveness training
- Process or focus groups

(See Appendix K and Glossary.)

Engage the client and family in therapeutic sessions with an appropriate family counselor *to discuss rigid and perfectionistic interactions within the family that inhibit the client's ability to complete tasks and to suggest alternate methods for enhancing performance and project completion.*

Encourage the client to select activities, tasks, and projects that he or she chooses to perform and complete *to help the client accept responsibility for finished products.*

Praise the client for successful completion of assigned tasks, projects, or activities *to reinforce repetition of positive behaviors and foster reduction in rigid, perfectionistic qualities:*

"Pam, you successfully completed your job of collecting the collage contributions from the clients on time."

"Jack, you were well prepared for group Friday morning after reading your cognitive therapy assignment."

"Sue, staff noticed you were dressed and ready for the day by 8 AM every day for 1 week."

(Refer to Impaired Social Interactions Care Plan in Chapter 2 for additional interventions for clients whose preoccupations with details or rituals are the result of an obsessive-compulsive disorder.)

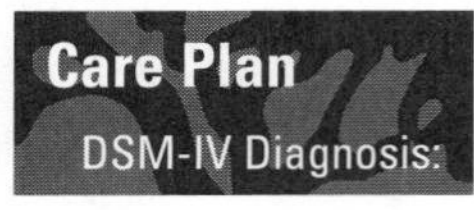

Personality Disorders (All Types)

NANDA Diagnosis: Coping, ineffective individual

The state in which an individual demonstrates impairment of adaptive behaviors and problem-solving abilities in meeting life's demands and roles

Focus:
For the client whose behavior patterns or personality traits result in significant impairment in coping with personal, social, or occupational demands or stressors. The characteristic features are generally typical of the person's long-term functioning and are not limited to isolated episodes of illness.

NANDA Taxonomy
Pattern 5—Choosing: A human response pattern involving the selection of alternatives

ETIOLOGIC/RELATED FACTORS (RELATED TO)

Depletion of coping methods/resources
Disturbance in self-concept/low self-esteem
Low impulse control
Ineffective or absent support systems
Ineffective problem-solving skills
Lack of insight/judgment
Knowledge deficit regarding societal rules, norms, interactions
Fear of abandonment/isolation
Perceived self-victimization
Self-involvement
Life-style of dependence
Developmental conflicts
Psychosocial stressors

DEFINING CHARACTERISTICS (AS EVIDENCED BY)

Splitting

Splitting is a hallmark defense mechanism of individuals diagnosed with borderline personality disorder.

Expresses conflicting alternate responses of acceptance and rejection at different times toward individuals or groups.

Examples:

During a morning session with her psychiatrist, Jane tells the doctor she "loves" his or her approach. Later that afternoon, Jane vents her rage at her doctor's "incompetence."

The following are typical splitting statements:

"I like you so much better than all the other nurses; you're so understanding and they don't seem to care at all."

"You're the only staff person here who really notices me; no one else will even talk to me."

"I hate the day staff; the nurses are so bossy and cold; the evening people are much nicer and friendlier."

"I thought you were my friend, but now I see the only one I can really count on is my roommate."

"I'm so mad at my roommate I could scream; she was so much nicer when we first met; I guess you're my best friend now."

"Don't you dare tell the staff about my wish to die; I don't trust anyone but you."

Idealizes—A Component of Splitting

Exaggerates others' attributes and capabilities:

"You're so wonderful; I just adore your personality; you're nicer than anyone I've ever known."

"I love the way you deal with clients; I want to be exactly like you someday."

"I just admire Kate so much; she's more like a nurse than a client; she's so helpful to me."

"My life was in complete ruins until I found Dr. Smith; he's a god to me."

Devalues—A Component of Splitting

Demeans, degrades others; typically follows idealization (see first example under Splitting for a typical statement that includes both idealizing and devaluing):

"I'm afraid to tell anyone here how I feel; they'll all turn against me."

"I don't trust anyone enough to tell them my personal thoughts."

"I'm sure that whatever I say here will be used against me."

"My doctor is a pompous fool; he thinks he knows everything."

"You're the worst nurse I ever saw; how did you ever get a job in a psychiatric hospital?"

"You don't know the first thing about helping people; I feel sorry for all your clients."

"You're the lowest form of life; you promised to be my roommate and now you're going to room with that [curses] moron."

"I hate you more than I've ever hated anyone in my life. I should have known you didn't care when you chose Sue for your partner."

"If you tell anyone about my suicidal thoughts, I'll always think of you as a dirty traitor who can't be trusted."

Manipulation

Manipulates others and the environment in order to meet own needs:

"You're the sweetest nurse in the whole world; I know you'll help me get a weekend pass."

"If you'll just watch out for the staff while I stay in my girlfriend's room, I'll do your laundry for a week."

"Couldn't you spare me one of your cigarettes? After all, I defended you when Sue complained about you to the other clients."
"Since you were out sick yesterday, do you think we could have more time to talk today?" (client to staff)
"If I can't be client leader I'll just have to leave this place and go where I'm wanted."

Intense/Unstable Relationships

Expresses intense, extremely emotional responses toward interpersonal relationships:
"The relationship between me and my boyfriend is so exciting; we're either hugging or kissing or yelling and screaming at each other."
"My girlfriend and I can be completely in love one minute; then before you know it we're tearing each other apart; it's maddening but never dull."
"My roommate and I fight constantly, but we really love each other to death."

Boredom

Verbalizes feelings of boredom frequently:
"I can't stand this place; there's nothing to do here."
"I wish something exciting would happen; I'm tired of the same old stuff."
"I hate following a routine every day; it's tiresome."
"There's nothing in this hospital that interests me; the staff, the clients, and the activities are all boring."
"If I don't find something exciting to do in this place very soon, I'm really going to go crazy."
"If I have to attend craft group one more time, I'll scream."
Demonstrates bored behaviors (rule out depression):
- Frequent sighing respirations or yawning during group activities
- Disinterested facial expressions throughout meetings
- Leaves room in middle of group function or activity for no apparent reason

Restricted Affect and Humor

Demonstrates lack of humor and restricted range of emotions, which the client may view as normal (ego-syntonic):
"I'm glad I can remain unemotional about my problems."
"It's just not in me to express my feelings."
"I see nothing funny about these jokes that all the other clients were laughing about."
Remains aloof and detached during situations that normally warrant strong emotional responses, such as joy and sadness
Displays indifference or disinterest toward the praise or criticism of others (e.g., blunted affect, no eye contact)

OUTCOME IDENTIFICATION AND EVALUATION

Splitting

Expresses consistent responses toward groups and individuals rather than the conflicting "splitting" responses of acceptance and rejection:
- Interacts with others as if they are multifaceted rather than either "all good" or "all bad"
- Demonstrates significant reduction in extreme, alternate responses toward groups or individuals

Idealizes

Refrains from idealizing or exaggerating others' attributes or capabilities, expresses more realistic view of the qualities of others:
"I don't always agree with my doctor, but she has always been there to help me."
"My roommate gives some good advice, but she's also a client with her own problems."
"You're a caring nurse and I appreciate that, even if I don't always agree with you."

Devalues

Ceases to devalue, degrade, or demean others; resists making rude, cruel, or derogatory statements directed toward others; responds in a mature manner:
"I'm very upset with my doctor for not issuing my pass as he promised, but I'll deal with it."
"I'm angry at you [nurse] right now for not keeping our appointment; let's talk about it."
"Now that I've had a chance to think about it, I don't believe my roommate is a 'dirty traitor' for telling the staff I was suicidal."
"After being here a while, I feel that the staff mean well and can be trusted."

Manipulation

Refrains from use of manipulation to get needs met:
- Makes requests clearly and openly without apparent hidden messages
- Ceases to use covert bribes or threats when interacting with others

Demonstrates significant reduction in manipulative behaviors as a way to meet needs:
- Engages in mature, open interpersonal interactions
- Expresses needs directly without apparent ulterior motives or agenda

Exhibits congruent verbal and behavioral expressions

Intense/Unstable Relationships

Expresses feelings toward relationships in realistic, moderate terms, with absence of intense, volatile emotions:
"My boyfriend and I no longer scream at each other one moment and kiss and make up the next."
"My girlfriend and I have a much more calm and stable relationship now."
"My husband and I have our ups and downs, but they are not as emotionally charged as they used to be."

Demonstrates calm, consistent emotions when interacting with others

Boredom

Verbalizes increased feelings of interest and excitement toward milieu groups and activities:

"I really get a lot out of the groups and activities."

"There's always something to do during our free time, like riding the stationary bicycle or listening to a relaxation tape."

Demonstrates increased interest in scheduled groups, activities, and individuals:

- Participates in milieu activities without signs of boredom (e.g., frequent sighing, yawning, or sleeping)
- Displays brightened or animated facial expression while engaged in groups and activities
- Initiates interactions with staff and clients frequently, rather than avoiding social contact

Restricted Affect and Humor

Demonstrates a wide range of emotional responses from joy to sadness

Expresses heightened interest and emotions toward the praise and criticism of others (e.g., animated affect, eye contact, increased feeling tone):

"I'm really interested in others' opinions about me, even though it is hard to hear some negative comments."

"Thank you for the compliment; it's important to me."

"I'm not happy about being criticized; in fact, it's upsetting."

Displays increased humor in appropriately humorous situations:

"The jokes that John told during lunch were funny."

"I laughed at Jane's stories along with everyone else."

PLANNING AND IMPLEMENTATION

Nursing Interventions and Rationale

Splitting

Assess the degree and frequency of the client's attempts to divide others through the defense mechanism of "splitting" *to determine the extent of dysfunctional behaviors and plan appropriate interventions to counteract the splitting.*

Feed back observations that gently challenge the client's perceptions that individuals or groups are either "all good" or "all bad" *to correct the client's distortions and reduce the incidence of splitting.*

Therapeutic responses:

"Donna, you say the evening staff treats you badly, but just last week you had good things to say about them."

"Ted, you're angry at me now, but this morning you said our discussion really helped you."

"Pam, you get really upset with your assigned staff nurse when she's with other clients; at other times you can't wait to talk to her."

"Kate, you say no one else here cares about you as I do; what are some things the staff has done to show they care?"

"Bob, you're telling me I haven't helped you at all, but yesterday you said you really appreciated my understanding."

"Jane, you seem angry with your doctor now; at other times you say she helps you a lot."

"Tom, you're asking me not to tell anyone else about your suicidal feelings because you don't trust them; each staff member is here to help you so we all need to be aware of your feelings."

Nontherapeutic responses:

"Donna, *how* can you say the evening staff treats you badly when they gave you a birthday party last week?"

"Ted, what did *I* do to make you so angry? You seemed OK during our discussion earlier."

"Jane, you know your doctor means well. She would be hurt if she knew how upset you are."

These responses defend against the client's accusations and place you in a vulnerable position. The responses fail to point out behaviors that would challenge the splitting attempts.

Develop a contract with the client stating that the client will approach only his or her assigned staff nurse on each shift for requests, questions, and so on *to prevent the patient from splitting staff to get needs met:*

"Donna, you say Kim told you it was OK to have a cigarette now; that's my role as your staff person and you'll have to wait 10 minutes when we go to the patio as a group."

"Mark, your request of me to phone your doctor at home to order a pass for you for tomorrow needs to be discussed with Sally, your staff person."

Assist the client to redirect angry or ambivalent feelings through constructive activities.

Examples:

- Physical exercise
- Art and music therapy
- Relaxation techniques

(See Appendix K for relaxation techniques.)

Assist the client to take responsibility for getting needs met *to place expectations for care on the client and discourage the client from splitting the staff:*

"Kate, you say the staff isn't meeting your needs. What do you feel we could do that would meet your needs?"

"Jim, how can you assist the staff to best meet your needs?"

For the Client Who Is Ready to Confront the Source of the Problem:

Assist the client to recognize the benefits of refraining from splitting to get needs met *to encourage mature, functional responses:*

"Donna, understanding that nobody can please everyone all of the time will greatly improve your relationships with others."

"Mark, the knowledge that most people are not either all good or all bad is helpful in your interactions and important to your recovery."

Engage the client in progressive, nonthreatening situations in which he or she can practice mature, effective response without splitting *to develop mastery of effective responses and gradually reduce splitting behaviors.* Begin with one-to-one nurse-client interactions; gradually include one or two trusted clients; proceed to informal group setting (e.g., dining room); progress to more structured group (e.g., community meeting); finally, engage client in formal group discussions.

Encourage the client to keep a record of times when he or she used mature, effective responses versus ineffective splitting responses *to compare and contrast difference in the effects of the two types of responses on others and to foster continued use of mature, effective responses.*

Praise the client for attempts to reduce splitting responses and to use mature, effective communication:

"Donna, your efforts to communicate in a mature, responsible way have been noticed by staff and clients."

"Mark, clients and staff have said they appreciate your hard work in changing your method of interaction."

Positive reinforcement promotes repetition of effective responses.

Idealizes—A Component of Splitting

Challenge the client's idealistic views with realistic responses *to correct the client's unrealistic exaggerated perceptions.*

Therapeutic responses:

"Donna, you say I'm better than all the other nurses; good nursing care is the goal for all of us."

"Jim, your doctor isn't a 'god,' but it's clear that you're satisfied with his care."

"Sue, I know you often go to your roommate for advice, but she's also a client and needs help from the staff as you do."

Nontherapeutic responses:

"Donna, thanks for the compliment, but the other nurses try hard, too."

"Jim, lots of clients think of their doctors as 'gods.'"

"Sue, it's good that you admire your roommate so much, as long as you realize she doesn't know everything."

These responses encourage the client's idealistic views and fail to correct the distortion.

Engage the client in therapeutic groups *to help the client explore splitting behaviors and their effects on self and others through the dynamics of the group process.*

Examples:

- Role play, sociodrama
- Behavioral therapy
- Cognitive therapy
- Assertiveness training
- Process and focus groups

(See Appendix K and Glossary.)

Devalues—A Component of Splitting

Use firm directives to set limits on the client's attempts to devalue persons or groups *to stop the client's verbal attacks.*

Therapeutic responses:

"Pam, your angry words directed toward others are not appropriate and won't be tolerated."

"Sue, you cannot remain in group if you curse and accuse people."

Nontherapeutic responses:

"Bob, what makes you think your doctor is a pompous fool?"

"Mark, how dare you say I'm a bad nurse after all I've done for you?"

These responses defend against the client's accusatory remarks and place you in a vulnerable position. The responses fail to clarify consequences for the client's unacceptable behavior.

Manipulation

Assess the extent and frequency of the client's manipulative behaviors *to recognize situations that provoke manipulation and plan interventions to reduce it.*

Direct attention to the client's manipulative behavior *to help the client develop an awareness of manipulation and take steps to reduce it:*

"Mark, whenever you give me all those compliments, you usually want something from me."

"Bob, what makes you think I can give you extra attention today because I was out sick yesterday?"

"Sam, asking John to 'watch out' for staff while you sneak your girlfriend into your room is taking advantage of John."

Explore consequences of manipulative behavior with the client *to inform him or her of its negative effects on others:*

"Mark, when you compliment people because you want something from them, they are not likely to trust what you say."

"Bob, when you say I *owe* you extra time because I was out sick yesterday, it annoys me."

"Sam, asking John to 'watch out' for staff while you sneak your girlfriend into your room would cause trouble for all of you."

Assist the client to mobilize feelings of anxiety, when appropriate:

"Sam, what feelings do you experience when you realize your behavior can seriously harm your friendship with John?"

"Mark, when people no longer believe your compliments, how does that make you feel?"

Individuals with long-standing use of manipulative behaviors generally fail to experience anxiety. Activating anxiety can help the client to anticipate the threat of consequences of manipulative behaviors and eventually learn to control them.

Refrain from responding to the client's manipulative behaviors such as self-pity, flattery, sexual innuendo, risqué jokes, or use of vulgar language. *Negative reinforcement of inappropriate behavior reduces the chances of its being repeated.*

Assist the client to clarify needs when he or she uses manipulation *to determine what needs the client is trying to meet through manipulative methods:*

"Pam, when you say Jane *owes* you a favor because you defended her in group, what do you really need from Jane?"

"Ted, you use a lot of flattering remarks with your staff persons; what do you actually expect from them?"

Assure the client that his or her needs will be met without resorting to manipulative behaviors *to reduce the incidence of manipulative behaviors:*

"Jane, staff will spend an appropriate amount of time with you when you need it; it's not necessary to threaten to leave the hospital."

"Paul, when you have a request, the best way to get results is to ask your assigned staff person directly rather than telling everyone you're being ignored."

Refrain from being judgmental while the client examines his or her manipulative behavior, *to demonstrate confidence in the client's attempts to recognize, reduce, and eventually eliminate manipulative behavior.*

Engage the client in therapeutic and didactic group activities *to teach more effective, socially appropriate methods of interacting with others.*

Examples:

- Milieu therapy
- Behavioral therapy
- Process and focus groups
- Cognitive therapy
- Assertiveness training

(See Appendix K and Glossary.)

Set limits on the client's manipulative behaviors when it interferes with the client's progress and the rights and safety of others *to help the client control dysfunctional behaviors and realize that there are consequences for breaking rules:*

"John, telling vulgar stories to get others to pay attention to you is not appropriate and will not be tolerated."

"Donna, your frequent complaints about staff to the other clients are not helping you or them; from now on, direct all your comments to staff."

Construct a behavioral contract *to help the client set limits on his or her manipulative behaviors when other methods fail.*

Document the client's methods of manipulation and effective nursing strategies *to ensure consistent interventions among staff members.*

Demonstrate consistency in limit setting and follow-through. *Inconsistency places you in a vulnerable position and encourages manipulative behavior.*

Express your willingness to admit your errors:

"Jane, I did forget that you signed up for the field trip; I'm glad you reminded me."

"Donna, I'm sorry I'm late for our meeting; I'll do my best to give you the time you need."

Clients who use manipulative methods are quick to recognize others' mistakes and will use them to gain control of a situation or interpersonal relationship.

Assist the client to identify when needs are actually met and situations in which he or she is treated with respect and dignity *to help the client recognize that needs can be met while he or she engages in appropriate interpersonal interactions:*

"Sarah, you got to go on the field trip after all without having to use unpleasant words or behaviors."

"Bob, your staff person spent some extra time with you today, and you requested it politely."

Relate staff's expectations of the client's behavior in a clear, direct manner *to avoid any chance of the client claiming misunderstanding as an excuse to manipulate and also to model direct communication.*

Teach the client strategies to delay need gratification *to provide time for the client to problem solve a method of interaction rather than automatically respond in a manipulative manner to meet needs.*

Examples:

- Relaxation techniques (See Appendix K.)
- Counting to 5
- Thinking about consequences of behavior
- Discussing alternative behaviors with staff

Engage the client in the treatment planning process *to increase motivation, participation, and self-esteem, which will diminish the need for manipulation:*

"Paul, how do you think we can help meet your needs?"

"Sarah, what do *you* feel is most helpful for you here?"

"Jane, what can *you* do to meet your needs?"

Provide mature role modeling in interactions with the client and others *to teach the client socially acceptable behaviors that yield positive results and to help the client use effective behaviors rather than manipulative methods.*

Examples:

- Demonstrate respect and consideration toward others. (See Therapeutic Nurse-Client Relationship, Appendix G.)
- Use assertive behaviors such as "I" messages, eye contact, congruent verbal and facial expressions.

(See Appendix K.)

Assist the client to perceive manipulative behavior and its results realistically *to help the client recognize that manipulative behavior is not satisfying and can be self-defeating:*

"Sue, when you say things to make people feel sorry for you, they see you as a victim. How do you *really* want to be treated by others?"

"John, when you tell vulgar jokes, ask yourself if you get the response and respect from others that you really want."

Explore with the client the problems in interpersonal relationships that develop as a result of manipulative behavior *to reinforce the client's awareness of behavior because he or she may have difficulty learning from experience:*

"John, the other clients are avoiding you because your vulgar jokes offend them; what can you do to improve your relationship with them?"

"Donna, the staff want to meet your needs; it's difficult to know if we do when you say we avoid you. How can we improve communication?"

Discuss with the client alternative ways of relating to others that do not include flattery, intimidation, invoking guilt, and so on, *to teach the client that clear, direct, assertive methods of interacting yield positive results and improve interpersonal relationships:*

"Bob, when you want a favor from me, ask me directly; for example, say, 'I need a favor,' rather than tell me the reasons why you think I owe you a favor. I'd be more likely to agree because the approach is honest and doesn't make me feel guilty."

"Sue, it's easier to tell the other clients the reasons why you would make a good client leader than to flatter them with compliments and gifts. People resent it when they feel forced to do something and are likely not to vote for you."

Spend time with the client when he or she is not using manipulative methods to be noticed *to illustrate to the client that needs can be met through socially acceptable behaviors.*

Engage the client in a group that helps individuals who manipulate to confront one another through role play or sociodrama (see glossary) *to foster the client's awareness of the negative effects of manipulation on self and others.*

Include family in therapeutic counseling sessions *to teach family members strategies that disrupt the client's manipulative behaviors and promote cooperation in treatment planning.*

(See Appendix K, Family Therapy.)

Praise the client for behaviors that are free from manipulative methods and that indicate consideration and respect for others:

"Donna, asking me to spend more time with you without telling me why I should shows real progress in communication."

"Sam, staff noticed that you no longer tell vulgar stories to gain attention. It is much more pleasant to spend time with you."

"Pam, it's a positive sign that you've stopped giving compliments when you want something. We have all noticed it."

Behaviors that are positively reinforced are likely to be repeated.

Promote continued mature behavior and feelings of self-worth *to increase self-esteem and personal growth:*

"John, you're dealing with your new role as client leader with more confidence."

"Sarah, your relationships with other clients show caring and consideration."

"Donna, your communication with staff is clear and honest and reflects growth."

Provide situations in which the client takes responsibility for choices and decisions to reduce dependency on others to satisfy needs and to learn to be self-reliant rather than manipulate others to gain support and acceptance:

"John, as client leader, *you* are responsible for getting the other clients together to choose the activity for tonight."

"Paul, there are several alternative places for you to live when you leave here; the final decision is *yours.*"

"Kate, whatever *you* choose to make for the cooking session will be OK with the group."

Intense Unstable Relationships

Assess the intensity and frequency of the client's emotional expressions *to plan interventions that will help the client modify his or her intense responses.*

Feed back observations of the client's intense responses in his or her interpersonal relationships *to help the client develop an awareness of his or her extreme emotional expression and how incongruent it appears to others.*

Therapeutic responses:

"Sarah, one minute you tell me how much you love your boyfriend, and the next minute you're ready to kill him."

"Donna, you say you adore your roommate, but you also say you fight with her all the time."

Nontherapeutic responses:

"Sarah, how can you say you love someone and then feel as though you want to kill him?"

"Donna, it's impossible for you to adore someone that you fight with all the time."

These responses negate the client's feelings and invoke doubts that he or she is capable of love.

Gently challenge the client's perception that extremes of feelings and emotions are necessary components in a relationship *to illustrate that relationships can survive without the drama of intense, extreme responses:*

"Bob, what makes it necessary for you and your wife to react so intensely to express your feelings to each other?"

"Mark, how come you and your girlfriend find it necessary to express such intense emotions in your relationship?"

"Sarah, what do you think your relationship with your boyfriend would be like without the extremes of emotions?"

Assist the client to recognize that extreme emotional responses can be more harmful than beneficial to a relationship *to help the client understand that dramatic, volatile emotions can foster instability in a relationship:*

"Sarah, when you and your boyfriend react to each other with such intense emotions, it's likely to put a strain on your relationship."

"Donna, the extreme emotions that you and your roommate express to each other may prove to be stressful to your relationship."

Teach the client strategies to increase the time span between the stimulus and the client's responses *to give the client an opportunity to choose an alternative, less volatile response and thus reduce the incidence of intense emotional expressions.*

Examples:

- Slow, deep breathing
- Relaxation techniques
- Count to 5 slowly
- Physical exercises and activities

(See Appendix K for deep-breathing and relaxation strategies.)

Engage the client and his or her partner in appropriate therapeutic counseling sessions *to discuss intense emotional responses, their effects on the relationship, and methods to modify or control them.*

Praise the client and his or her partner for attempts to control excessive emotional responses:

"Donna, you and your roommate have modified your extreme responses to each other very well. The improvement in your relationship is evident."

"Bob, it's obvious that you and your wife are really working on modifying your intense emotional responses."

Positive reinforcement increases self-esteem and promotes repetition of appropriate responses.

Act as a role model by responding to colleagues and clients within a socially appropriate emotional range *to teach the client socially appropriate emotional expressions and to discourage the use of extreme, intense responses.*

Relate to the client the benefits of responding within a socially appropriate emotional range *to reinforce the client's socially appropriate emotional responses:*

"Bob, you say you and your wife have never been happier. The change in your responses to each other has enhanced your relationship."

"Donna, it's good to see you and your roommate getting along so well. The work you've been doing to modify your emotional reactions has helped your relationship."

Engage the client in therapeutic and didactic groups *to teach the client how to modify extreme emotional responses through group dynamics and feedback.*

Examples:

- Role play, sociodrama
- Behavioral therapy
- Cognitive therapy
- Assertiveness training
- Process and focus groups

(See Appendix K and Glossary.)

Boredom

Assess the degree and frequency of the client's boredom *to plan interventions that will interrupt periods of boredom.*

Assure the client that occasional feelings of boredom are natural and acceptable *to acknowledge the client's right to genuine feelings of boredom:*

"Pam, it's OK to be bored once in a while."

"Jack, being in a hospital can occasionally be boring."

"Sam, it can seem boring at times when you're away from home."

"Sue, feelings of boredom do occur every once in a while in everyone."

Engage the client in therapeutic activities *to interrupt excessive moments of boredom with productive, rewarding activities and to release pent-up emotions underlying bored behaviors.*

Examples:

- Physical exercise
- Recreational activities (e.g., Ping-Pong, volleyball, shuffleboard)
- Arts, crafts, board games
- Field trips and outings

Provide the client with a variety of activities *to promote interest in the milieu and discourage boredom. The greater the selection of activities, the more likely the client is to participate.*

Feed back observations of the client's demonstrations of boredom *to help the client develop an awareness of his or her frequent use of bored behaviors:*

"John, you often make the comment that you're 'bored.' Are you aware of that?"

"Sue, you frequently fall asleep during the community meeting."

"Kate, from your expression, I wonder if you're really interested in the group discussion."

"Jane, you often leave before the activity is over."

"Pam, I notice you seldom participate in the group functions."

Assist the client to recognize the feeling state that accompanies expressions of boredom *to help the client identify the source of boredom:*

"John, when you say you're 'bored,' what feelings are you experiencing?"

"Sue, just before you fall asleep in group, how do you feel about what's happening?"

"Kate, when you seem uninterested during the meetings, what are you feeling?"

"Jane, how do you feel as you leave a group activity before it's over?"

"Pam, what do you feel when you sit quietly while the rest of the group participates?"

For the Client Who Has Difficulty Naming Feelings (Alexithymia):

Help the client name the feeling that accompanies expressions of boredom:

"Jane, when you leave in the middle of a meeting, are you feeling anxious or fearful?"

"Sue, do you feel frustrated or angry just before you fall asleep in group?"

"Pam, could it be that you're not participating in group because you're feeling fearful or anxious?"

"Kate, when you seem uninterested during the activities, are you feeling anxious or afraid?"

"John, when you say you're 'bored,' might you be feeling angry or frustrated?"

Labeling the feeling is the first step toward understanding the emotions underlying "bored" behaviors. Boredom is often a way to deny feelings.

For the Client Who Is Ready to Explore Threats to the Self-System:

Explore with the client possible threats that provoke feelings underlying "bored" behaviors *to help the client identify threats:*

"Jane, what is it about the group process that you find threatening or scary?"

"John, what causes you to feel frustrated?"

"Sue, you said you felt angry when you fell asleep during the group; let's discuss what makes you feel angry enough to fall asleep during the activities."

"Pam, it may help to talk about the anxiety that prevents you from joining the group."

Enlist the client in therapeutic groups *to explore further the threats that promote "bored" behaviors through the dynamics of group interaction.*

Examples:

- Role play, sociodrama
- Behavioral therapy
- Cognitive therapy
- Assertiveness training
- Process and focus groups

(See Appendix K and Glossary.)

Assist the client to confront threatening situations that result in the use of bored behaviors, *to help the client challenge his or her perception of the threat:*

"Sue, let's talk about the possible reasons for your anger during the group. The group can help you with this."

"Jane, you say you leave meetings because you're afraid to share your feelings; the group would accept that."

"Pam, the anxiety you feel about performing in group activities is understandable and can be dealt with."

"Kate, having fears about your role as a client is not uncommon; we can discuss it."

Assist the client to understand the therapeutic effects of milieu activities on his or her treatment and recovery, *to help the client recognize that excitement and entertainment are not the major foci for treatment and to encourage more realistic expectations:*

"John, not all activities may be interesting to you, but they are important in your treatment and progress."

"Kate, being bored with crafts is understandable, but it's the social process that's most helpful to your recovery because it helps you learn to cope with different kinds of experiences."

"Pam, playing bingo may not be as exciting as other activities; however, being part of the client community is therapeutic."

"Joe, there are more entertaining events than walking around the lake, but interacting with one another during the activity is important."

Praise the client for refraining from use of bored behaviors and for expressing actual feelings:

"John, you haven't mentioned being bored for several days. It's a real sign of progress that you're discussing your feelings."

"Sue, the staff and clients have noticed that you stay awake during the meetings and talk about your frustrations."

"Kate, talking about your fears rather than ignoring the group is a step forward in your recovery."

"Jane, we've noticed that you stay until the end of the meetings; discussing your anxiety with the group has helped."

Positive reinforcement promotes continuity of effective behaviors.

Restricted Affect and Humor

Assess the client's range of emotional expressions and ability to display humor (keeping in mind the effects of mental illness and medications on one's mood and affect) *to help the client express feelings and emotions when he or she is capable of doing so.*

Encourage the client to participate in pleasurable activities such as games, sports, and field trips *to expose the client to others who are responding with a wide range of emotions.*

Assure the client that it's OK to sometimes refrain from emotional displays but that at other times it's beneficial and acceptable to express emotions, *to demonstrate acceptance while giving the client reasons to express emotions and permission to do so.*

Assist the client to accurately perceive humorous situations and statements by pointing out their humorous aspects *to help the client experience the joyful feelings promoted by humor and continue to seek it on his or her own:*

"Sam, when Tom imitated that famous comedian during the activity today, it was really funny."

"Donna, did you notice how funny it was when all the clients told a different version of the same story at the recreational activity?"

"Mark, the group and staff really enjoyed the part in the movie where everyone thought the main character was a king instead of a butler."

"Jane, the joke that John told at dinner tonight was humorous."

Engage the client in frequent individual discussions that include interjections of humor *to continue to expose the client to humor and to draw the client out of his or her detached, withdrawn state.*

Use role playing to demonstrate to the client a wide range of expressions, such as joy, sadness, and laughter, *to expose the client to an appropriate range of emotions in a nonthreatening environment and encourage continued use of a broad emotional range.*

Assure the client that it's acceptable and beneficial to display emotions that are congruent with feelings, situations, and circumstances *to help the client release emotions and understand the benefits of their use:*

"Kate, it's OK to express sadness when your roommate is discharged; you're going to miss her and you need to talk about your feelings."

"Mark, laughter is a healthy expression of positive feelings and can help you feel better."

Engage the client in therapeutic groups *to participate with others in exercises and discussions that bring out a wide range of emotional expressions.*

Examples:

- Art and music therapy
- Cognitive therapy
- Assertiveness training
- Process and focus groups

(See Appendix K and Glossary.)

Praise the client for displaying humor and using a wider range of emotional expressions *to increase self-esteem and reinforce continuity of positive behaviors:*

"Jack, staff really notice your efforts to participate more in group and share amusing stories."

"Kate, it's nice to see you laughing with others more often."

"Donna, your ability to smile and joke with others shows real progress."

"Mark, showing that you felt sad when your roommate left is a big step toward your goal to express yourself more."

"Tom, it showed real improvement when you accepted John's compliment with a smile and a 'thank you.'"

"Sarah, it's good to see your growing interest in the group activities."

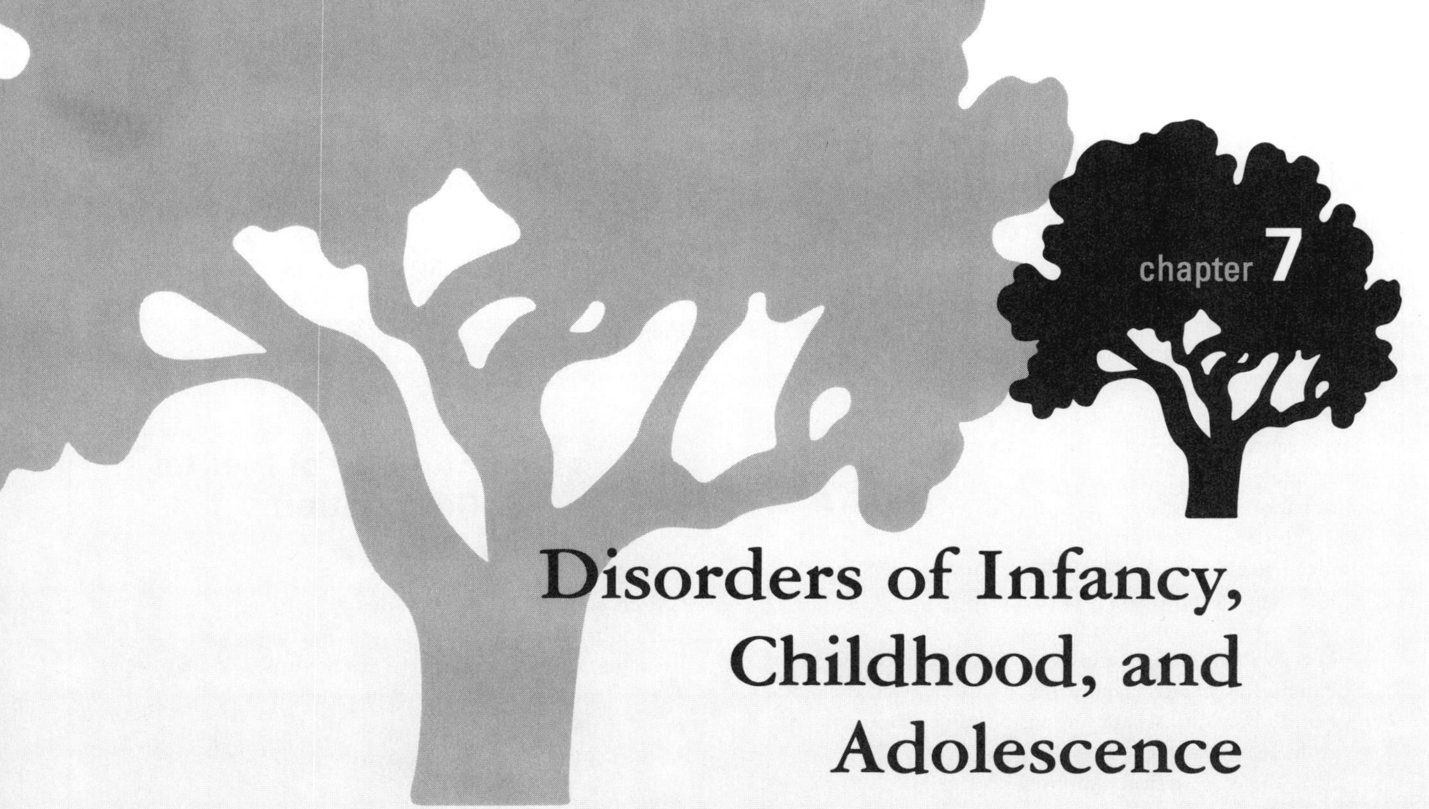

Disorders of Infancy, Childhood, and Adolescence

Mental and emotional disorders may occur at any age; some are identifiable even in infancy (e.g., reactive attachment disorder and developmental disorders). The defining characteristics for several disorders—schizophrenia, mood disorders, psychoactive substance use disorders, organic mental disorders, somatoform disorders, adjustment disorders, sexual disorders, and personality disorders—with a few intrinsic exceptions, are generally the same for children and adolescents as they are for adults. Diagnosis of personality disorder is usually reserved for people over age 18 but may be assigned earlier if maladaptive characteristics of the disorder have been stable, inflexible, and crystallized.

Children and adolescents have the inevitable task of progression through developmental stages that result in physical, mental, emotional, and sexual changes. Cultural, subcultural, social, and interpersonal influences play an important part in successful coping, adaptation, and integration of these factors by all individuals on the journey to adulthood.

Ideally the following developmental tasks are achieved during maturation:

- Evolution of identity (self, gender, in relation to family and society)
- Individuation and independence from parental control
- Clarification and prioritizing of values, beliefs, and interests
- Establishment of meaningful relationships with individuals of same and opposite sex
- Achievement of intimacy
- Understanding and appropriate expression of emotion
- Development of meaningful purpose in life
- Building of competence and honing of skills
- Determination of career goals, life-styles

EPIDEMIOLOGY AND ETIOLOGY

Because of the heterogeneity of disorders for children and adolescents, these categories are included under specific classifications when appropriate. Some general statistics appear in Box 7-1.

MENTAL RETARDATION

Mental retardation refers to a deficiency in intellectual function coupled with an impairment of adaptive function. Intellectual function is measured by means of standardized intelligence tests that yield an intelligence quotient (IQ); people scoring below 70 are considered to be mentally retarded (Box 7-2). IQ is believed to be a relatively stable factor that generally defies remediation.

Adaptive function is the individual's ability to perform effectively in accordance with expectations for age and culture in the following areas: communication, daily living skills, social skills, social responsibility, and independence.

Epidemiology

Approximately 1% of the U.S. population is mentally retarded, and the disorder is about 1.5 times more common in males than in females. The diagnosis is made before

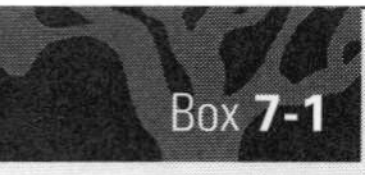

Box 7-1 Epidemiology for Disorders of Infancy, Childhood, and Adolescence

Ten to 12% of all children have mental or emotional disorders severe enough to be disabling as adults.
Only 5 to 7% receive adequate mental health intervention.
Disorders of boys outnumber those of girls 2:1 before adolescence; girls equal or outnumber boys during and after adolescence.
Emotional disturbances increase in children ages 9 to 12 years and 13 to 16 years.
Prolonged stressors increase incidence prevalence:
- Parental marital discord; divorce
- Overcrowded living conditions
- Low socioeconomic status
- Parental psychiatric condition or trouble with the law
- Family breakup, separation, foster home placement of child or adolescent
- Child abuse (physical, emotional, sexual)

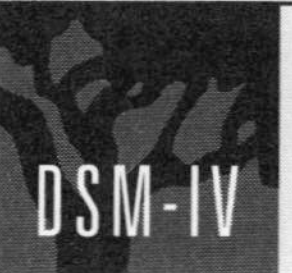

DSM-IV Mental Retardation

Note: *These are coded on Axis II.*

Mild Mental Retardation
Moderate Mental Retardation
Severe Mental Retardation
Profound Mental Retardation
Mental Retardation, Severity Unspecified

18 years of age; the highest incidence occurs during school years, with a peak between ages 10 and 15. The percentages of the retarded population can be categorized as follows: mild, 85%; moderate, 10%; severe 3% to 4%; profound, 1% to 2%.

Etiology

The specific etiology of mental retardation may be directly attributable to one or more of the factors listed in Box 7-3. A combination of factors (biologic, psychosocial, environmental) appears to be influential in many cases.

Mild Mental Retardation

Approximately 85% of the retarded population belong in the mild category and often are not noticed as "different" from the general population of school children until well into school years. They usually can learn vocational and social skills sufficient to support themselves and achieve academically to approximately the sixth-grade level.

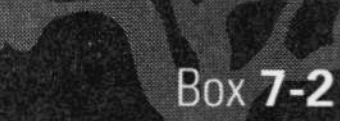

Box 7-2 Severity of Mental Retardation

Mild	IQ 50–55 to approximately 70
Moderate	IQ 35–40 to approximately 50–55
Severe	IQ 20–25 to approximately 35–40
Profound	IQ Below 20–25

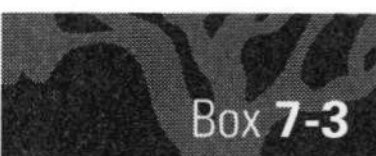

Box 7-3 Etiology of Mental Retardation

Biologic (25%)
Chromosomal (Down syndrome)
Metabolic (phenylketonuria)
Prenatal factors (rubella, cytomegalovirus, toxoplasmosis)
AIDS, syphilis, other viruses and infections
Enzyme deficiencies
Accidents (head trauma, near-drowning)

Psychosocial
Lower socioeconomic groups
Social deprivation
Inadequate medical care
Lack of intellectual and language stimulation
Living with a parent who has a psychiatric disorder

Cases with no known cause are usually mild

Moderate Mental Retardation

The moderate group comprises 10% of the retarded population; they can learn to take care of themselves with supervision and may be able to perform at jobs in sheltered environments or in the regular job market under strong guidance. They usually are educable to about the equivalent of grade 2 in school and live in group homes or with family.

Severe Mental Retardation

Individuals who are severely retarded are recognizable early in life (3% to 4% of retarded population) because they fail to develop adequate motor skills or speech for communication. They may eventually learn to talk, tend to basic hygiene, and perform simple tasks with close supervision.

Profound Mental Retardation

Approximately 1% to 2% of the retarded population are included in the profound category. They have very limited

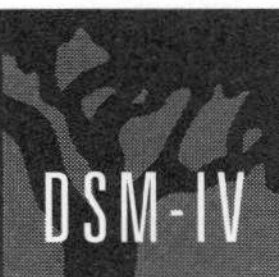

DSM-IV Learning Disorders

DSM-IV Categories
Reading Disorder
Mathematics Disorder
Disorder of Written Expression

sensorimotor function, may have other physical handicaps, and require constant care and supervision; with supervision they may learn to perform simple tasks.

LEARNING DISORDERS

A diagnosis of learning disorder is noted when individuals are unable to achieve designated scores on standardized tests of reading, math, or writing proficiency for specified ages, level of education, and IQ. In addition, the lack of these skills hinders progress in school and interferes with activities that require the skills. Disturbances in sensory, perceptual, or cognitive processing may underlie the disorder and are often found in conjunction with other medical conditions such as fetal alcohol syndrome, birthing traumas, or neurologic disorders. The individual with deficiency in skills frequently has low self-esteem and self-concept, negative self-worth, and concomitantly inept social skills.

Reading Disorder

The defining characteristic of Reading Disorder, commonly referred to as *dyslexia,* is inability to achieve specific scores on standardized tests that measure reading comprehension, speed, and accuracy. In addition, the skill deficiency interferes with school progression and daily living activities in which the skills are required. When reading aloud, the person may omit, substitute, or distort content, and the process is usually slow. Reading disorder is usually associated with math and writing disorders.

Mathematics Disorder

Mathematics Disorder is noted when an individual is unable to achieve specific scores on standardized tests that measure mathematics competence. The deficiency interferes with progress in school and daily activities in which the skills are important. Math competence includes several skills, including recognizing and naming math symbols and signs, changing written problems with math symbols, understanding math concepts and terms, learning tables, and following sequences. Math disorder is commonly associated with writing and reading disorders.

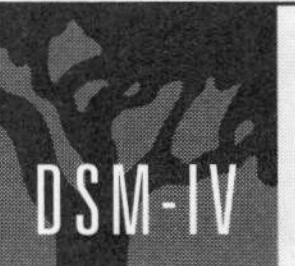

DSM-IV Motor Skills Disorder

DSM-IV Category
Developmental Coordination Disorder

Disorder of Written Expression

The defining characteristics of Disorder of Written Expression are inability to achieve standardized test scores and the resultant interference with school progress and daily activities that require writing skills. The disorder is manifested by difficulty organizing content into paragraphs; multiple errors in grammar, spelling, and punctuation; and poor handwriting. Written expression disorder is usually associated with reading and math disorders.

MOTOR SKILLS DISORDER

Developmental Coordination Disorder

The defining characteristic of Developmental Coordination Disorder is impaired motor coordination, but a diagnosis is made only in the absence of an underlying medical condition and only if the impairment significantly interferes with progress in school or with daily activities. Impairment is age-specific (e.g., babies—crawling, walking; toddlers—climbing, buttoning; school-age children—throwing or catching a ball, printing words).

COMMUNICATION DISORDERS

Expressive Language Disorder

Expressive Language Disorder is noted when expressive language development is impaired. Manifestations of the problem are poverty of speech, short sentences, leaving out parts of sentences, limited variety of speech, and use of unusual wording.

Phonological Disorder

Phonological Disorder is evidenced by nonuse or misuse of sounds of speech for an expected age, as evidenced by sound omissions, sound substitutions, or sound distortions. Examples include omitting the last consonant (*tru* instead of *truck*), use of the letter *b* instead of *p (bretty),* and use of *ax* for the word *ask.* The individual's cultural background (with its specific sound differences) must always be assessed in this regard to avoid misdiagnosis.

Stuttering

The defining characteristic of Stuttering is impaired flow and pattern of speech, resulting in discontinuous

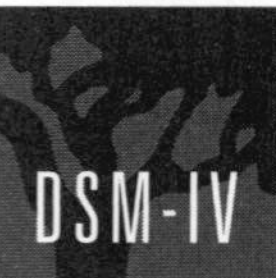

Communication Disorders

DSM-IV Categories
Expressive Language Disorder
Mixed Receptive-Expressive Language Disorder
Phonological Disorder
Stuttering
Communication Disorder

sentences. Manifestations are varied and may include repeated words or sounds ("can-can-can-can-I . . ."), prolonged sounds ("the sssssssun is warm"), pauses in speech, and other impairments.

PERVASIVE DEVELOPMENTAL DISORDERS

The term *pervasive* is used to describe this category of disorders in which several areas of development—social interaction, verbal and nonverbal communication, behavior, and activity—are severely affected. Pervasive developmental disorders are represented in the DSM-IV by Autistic Disorder, Rett's Disorder, Childhood Disintegrative Disorder, and Asperger's Disorder. Each disorder results in severely impaired social function.

Autistic Disorder

Autistic Disorder has been known by other names in the past, including infantile autism, Kanner's syndrome, childhood schizophrenia, and symbiotic psychosis.

Onset usually occurs before age 3, with a course that is generally lifelong, although changes can and do occur in some individuals (e.g., improvement of social and language skills at about 5 to 6 years, improvement or decline in cognitive and/or social skills at puberty, and escalation of negative behaviors such as aggression and opposition at puberty). Rarely are people with Autistic Disorder able to become totally independent because of their impaired IQ, language skills, and social skills, with the result that most affected individuals require a lifelong structured environment and close supervision. Four to five children per 10,000 births are affected by Autistic Disorder.

Etiology Biologic and prenatal, perinatal, and postnatal situations and conditions (e.g., anoxia at birth, encephalitis, chromosomal anomaly, phenylketonuria, maternal rubella) may cause brain dysfunction.

Autistic Disorder is a severe form of pervasive developmental disorder. Symptoms include the following:

1. *Impaired social interaction* (two of the following must be present for diagnosis):
   a. Unaware of feelings or needs of others; treats other people as objects
   b. At distressful moments, fails entirely to seek solace from others or seeks comfort in unusual ways (rather than wanting hugs, may walk in circles or stereotypically repeat a phrase)
   c. Does not imitate significant others' actions (waving good-bye) or imitates out of context of situation
   d. Impaired social play or total lack of it (plays alone or engages others only as objects)
   e. Severely impaired ability to form peer relationships (either shows no interest in others or lacks awareness or understanding necessary to interact socially)
2. *Impaired verbal and nonverbal communication* (one of the following must be present for diagnosis):
   a. Total lack of any mode of communication
   b. Presence of abnormal nonverbal communication (inappropriate and out-of-context posturing, facial expression, gazing, gesturing; e.g., fails to smile at or move toward parents or significant others when greeted; does not cuddle when held, may stiffen instead)
   c. Fails to engage in imaginative play
   d. Abnormal speech *process* (monotone; singsong quality; unusual pitch, rhythm, rate) or *content/form* (echolalia—repetition of speech of other persons, television, or radio; irrelevant or idiosyncratic use of words; e.g., "want to run the dasher" meaning "I want to take a bath")
   e. Inability to begin or successfully maintain conversations with others
3. *Unusual or bizarre activities and interests* (one of the following must be present for diagnosis):
   a. Ritualized, stereotyped behaviors (head-banging; rocking; body spinning; hand or arm flapping)
   b. Intense preoccupation with specific objects (flicking light switches on and off persistently; watching record spin for hours without playing music; rubbing or spinning one part of a toy instead of using as intended; carrying one object constantly; e.g., jar lid or particular piece of clothing)
   c. Need for sameness in environment (e.g., upset when furniture is moved from usual spot) and in routine (e.g., must take same route every time when traveling to grandparent's house)

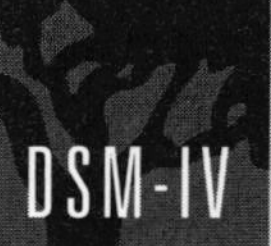

Pervasive Development Disorders

DSM-IV Categories
Autistic Disorder
Rett's Disorder
Childhood Disintegrative Disorder
Asperger's Disorder
Pervasive Developmental Disorder Not Otherwise Specified

d. Lacks variety of interests or is preoccupied with one interest (e.g., looks through one book only, repeatedly)

Up to half of autistic children are also mentally retarded at a moderate, severe, or profound level. Interestingly, some children with Autistic Disorder possess unusual or extraordinary abilities or "islands of genius." For example, a severely retarded person who is unable to make correct change in a store may be able to calculate an extraordinary range of numbers but unable to understand their significance, or an individual may be able to play a musical instrument without ever taking lessons or being able to read music.

Rett's Disorder

Defining characteristics of Rett's Disorder are a period of normal functioning prenatally, perinatally, and up to age 5 months, followed by development of multiple deficits: decelerated head growth, loss of acquired hand skills and substitution of stereotyped hand-wringing or hand-washing movements, changes in social interaction (loss of interest in interpersonal engagement at first, may engage later in course of disorder), and severe problems that develop in coordination and language development, both receptive and expressive.

Childhood Disintegrative Disorder

In Childhood Disintegrative Disorder there is a period of normal development for up to 2 years, followed by marked loss of skills before age 10. Loss of skills includes two of the following five areas: language (receptive and expressive), socialization, control of bowel or bladder, play, and motor skills. This disorder has been known in the past by other terms (disintegrative psychosis, dementia infantilis, Heller's syndrome).

Asperger's Disorder

Hallmarks of Asperger's Disorder are marked and prolonged impairment in socialization and the development of stereotypical, repetitive behaviors. The individual fails to use social regulators such as smiling directly at others or looking into a person's eyes when talking. There is a lack of sharing with others, and age-appropriate relationships do not develop. Behaviors and interests are frequently stereotypical, rigid, and repetitive (e.g., incessant hand tapping, preoccupation with daily air flights into the city) and of little or no interest to others. Social interaction is severely impaired.

ATTENTION-DEFICIT AND DISRUPTIVE BEHAVIOR DISORDERS

Attention-Deficit/Hyperactivity Disorder

Children who have Attention-Deficit/Hyperactivity Disorder are commonly referred to as being "hyperactive." They have developmentally inappropriate problems in maintaining attention and are impulsive and hyperactive. These difficulties may manifest as inability to stay with a task to completion, listen to the teacher, and finish chores at home. Affected children comment out of turn or cannot wait for a turn, do not follow directions, interrupt others continually, have difficulty staying in a seat, and are constantly on the go.

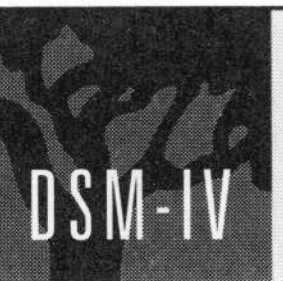

Attention-Deficit and Disruptive Behavior Disorders

DSM-IV Categories

Attention-Deficit/Hyperactivity Disorder
- Combined Type
- Predominantly Inattentive Type
- Predominantly Hyperactive-Impulsive Type

Conduct Disorder

Specify type: Childhood-Onset Type/Adolescent-Onset Type

Oppositional Defiant Disorder

Disruptive Behavior Disorder Not Otherwise Specified

Subtypes Some individuals demonstrate symptoms of both inattention and hyperactivity-impulsivity; others have one pattern more than another.

- Combined Type
- Predominantly Inattentive Type
- Predominantly Hyperactive-Impulsive Type

Conduct Disorder (Solitary Aggressive Type)

Conduct Disorder, characterized by persistent patterns of serious misconduct at home, at school, and in the community, is manifested by violation of the basic rights of others and basic rules, laws, or norms (verbal and physical aggression toward other people, animals, and property); stealing; rape; assault; lying; cheating; truancy from school; use of drugs and alcohol; callous disregard for others' feelings; blaming others for own transgressions; and lack of appropriate empathy, remorse, or guilt. If maladaptive behavior persists into adulthood, conduct disorder is changed to a diagnosis of antisocial personality disorder.

Oppositional Defiant Disorder

A pattern of defiance, hostility, and negativity characterizes Oppositional Defiant Disorder. Behaviors may include loss of temper; arguments with adults; defiance and refusal to adhere to adult rules; show of anger, resentment, or vindictiveness; swearing and use of obscenities; and deliberately annoying others.

FEEDING AND EATING DISORDERS OF INFANCY OR EARLY CHILDHOOD

Identifying characteristics of feeding and eating disorders are disturbances in feeding and/or eating during the early years of a child's life. Pica, Rumination Disorder, and

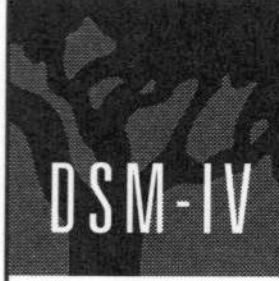
DSM-IV

Feeding and Eating Disorders of Infancy or Early Childhood

DSM-IV Categories
Pica
Rumination Disorder
Feeding Disorder of Infancy or Early Childhood

Box 7-4

Age-Significant Substances for Pica

Infants and young children	Paint, plaster, string, hair, cloth
Older children	Sand, insects, animal droppings, pebbles, leaves
Adults	Clay or soil

Feeding Disorder of Infancy or Early Childhood are disorders included in this section. Note that Anorexia Nervosa and Bulemia Nervosa are covered in the chapter on eating disorders.

Pica

The hallmark of Pica is the persistent eating of substances that have no nutritive value, and this behavior is inappropriate for the specific developmental level or cultural practice. Several factors affect this disorder. Poverty, developmental delay, neglect, and inadequate parental supervision increase the risk. Specific ingested substances vary with age (Box 7-4). This disorder tends to increase when associated with mental retardation.

Rumination Disorder

Defining characteristics of Rumination Disorder are repeated regurgitation and rechewing of food that has been swallowed by an infant or child who had normal functioning before the occurrence of this behavior. The child brings food back up into the mouth without retching and either rechews and reswallows or expels the food. Malnutrition may occur with weight loss or failure to gain weight, and there is a reported 25% death rate with this disorder.

Feeding Disorder of Infancy or Early Childhood

The defining characteristic of Feeding Disorder of Infancy or Early Childhood is a persistent failure to eat adequately, with resultant failure to gain weight, or loss of weight, before age 6 years.

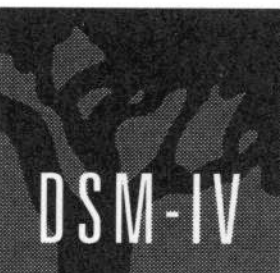
DSM-IV

Tic Disorders

DSM-IV Categories
Tourette's Disorder
Chronic Motor or Vocal Tic Disorder
Transient Tic Disorder
Specify if: Single Episode or Recurrent
Tic Disorder Not Otherwise Specified

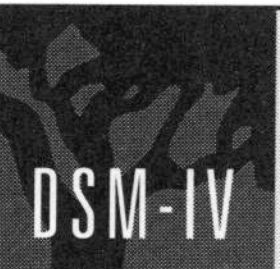
DSM-IV

Elimination Disorders

DSM-IV Categories
Encopresis
With Constipation and Overflow Incontinence
Without Constipation and Overflow Incontinence
Enuresis (Not Due to a General Medical Condition)
Specify type: Nocturnal Only/Diurnal Only/ Nocturnal and Diurnal

Table 7-1

Tic Manifestations

	Motor Tics	Vocal Tics
Simple	Coughing Neck jerking Eye blinking Shrugging of shoulders Facial grimaces	Throat clearing Grunting sniffing Snorting Barking
Complex	Grooming behaviors Jumping Stamping Facial gestures Smelling an object	Repeating words out of context Obscene words/ swearing (coprolalia) Repeating own words (palilalia) Repeating others' words (echolalia) Imitation of others' behaviors (echokinesia)

TIC DISORDERS

A *tic* is a stereotyped vocalization or motor movement that occurs rapidly and suddenly in a nonrhythmic manner. (See Table 7-1.)

Tourette's Disorder

Distinguishing characteristics of Tourette's Disorder are multiple motor and vocal tics that present several times a day at irregular intervals. Frequently individuals with Tourette's disorder experience obsessions and compulsions, hyperactivity, self-consciousness, and depression in addition to the tic disorder.

ELIMINATION DISORDERS

Enuresis

The defining characteristic of Enuresis is repeated urination voluntarily or involuntarily during the day or night into bed or clothing, past the age of expected continence (5 to 6 years). Physical causes must be ruled out before this diagnosis is made. *Primary enuresis* refers to the disturbance when it is not preceded by a year of urinary continence, and *secondary enuresis* refers to the disturbance when at least 1 year of continence precedes the disorder.

- *Nocturnal*—The most common type occurs during REM sleep, usually in the first third of total sleep, at night.
- *Diurnal*—Occurs during the day and is more common in females; may be due to reluctance to use public toilet.

Encopresis

The defining characteristic of Encopresis is repeated defecation voluntarily or involuntarily, into clothes or areas other than appropriate toilet facilities. Physical causes must be ruled out before the diagnosis is made.

- With constipation and overflow incontinence
- Without constipation and overflow incontinence

OTHER DISORDERS OF INFANCY, CHILDHOOD, AND ADOLESCENCE

Separation Anxiety Disorder

When separated from the major figure of attachment (primary caregiver), the child may experience severe to panic levels of anxiety. Symptoms that are unrealistic and persistent may include worry that the parent will not return or will have an accident while away, refusal to go to school, refusal to go to sleep when parent is not near, clinging behaviors, nightmares about separating from parent, physical symptoms (nausea, vomiting, headache, stomachache), or pleading not to be separated.

Selective Mutism

The defining characteristic is failure to speak when speaking is expected, even though the person speaks in other situations. For example, a child may not speak to playmates during school but talks at home. Before a diagnosis is made, the behavior must persist past the beginning of a new class (1 month) and must interfere with educational and social functioning.

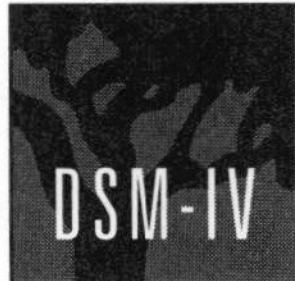

Other Disorders of Infancy, Childhood, or Adolescence

DSM-IV Categories

Separation Anxiety Disorder
Specify if: Early Onset
Selective Mutism
Reactive Attachment Disorder of Infancy or Early Childhood
Specify type: Inhibited Type/Disinhibited Type
Stereotypic Movement Disorder
Specify if: With Self-Injurious Behavior
Disorder of Infancy, Childhood, or Adolescence Not Otherwise Specified

Reactive Attachment Disorder of Infancy or Early Childhood

Reactive Attachment Disorder is characterized by age-appropriate, markedly disturbed social relationships, manifested either by (1) failure to respond to or initiate interactions with others (apathy; lack of spontaneity, visual tracking, curiosity, or playfulness) or (2) indiscriminate socializing (overfamiliarity with strangers, displays of affection toward them, or requests for attention from strangers).

In addition, evidence exists for one of the following regarding negligent or punitive care of the child: (1) disregard of child's needs for affection, comfort, and stimulation (emotional needs); (2) disregard of child's needs for food, clothing, and shelter (physical needs); (3) disregard of protection from abuse or danger; (4) frequent changes in primary caregivers, leading to unstable attachments.

Etiology Reactive Attachment Disorder is caused by pathogenic care of the infant by the primary caretaker. There may be a lack of bonding or a poor parent-infant fit because of problems that exist with one or both members of the dyad (e.g., poor parenting skills, low socioeconomic status, deprivation, presence of mental retardation or physical anomaly in the child).

Stereotypic Movement Disorder

Diagnosis of Stereotypic Movement Disorder is made when an individual persistently and repetitively performs a nonfunctional motor behavior in a driven way. Examples of behavior include biting self, playing with fingers, head-banging, waving hands, rocking, and picking at skin or body orifices. The disorder often occurs in conjunction with mental retardation or in individuals who are institutionalized and receive little stimulation.

INTERVENTIONS FOR DISORDERS OF INFANCY, CHILDHOOD, AND ADOLESCENCE

Hospitalization

Children with diagnoses of Mental Retardation, Autistic Disorder, and other serious pervasive developmental disorders are frequently able to live at home if the family is willing to commit to lifelong care of the individual. Severely disordered individuals may be institutionalized because of excessive daily challenges created by the dysfunction and the disruption it causes within the family system.

Specific developmental disorders are usually identified in the educational setting and are treated on an outpatient basis unless they are concomitantly associated with other mental or emotional disorders.

Parents and other caretakers must be particularly alert for signs of physical illnesses that may otherwise be overlooked because of the child's inability to communicate pain or discomfort.

Therapy

Behavior modification is often a therapy of choice for these age groups, but an important factor is the child's developmental stage. For instance, regressive behavior is common during disordered episodes of childhood and adolescence. The astute therapist is not only familiar with normal growth and development but also prepared to help the client manage the additional developmental setbacks coupled with psychotic disorder(s).

Therapeutic play is often used with younger children or those who are unable to effectively communicate by verbal responses. Group therapy can be an important vehicle for assisting behavioral changes, particularly with adolescents. Group play is usually incorporated into therapy to reinforce the development of interpersonal relationships and peer skills.

Family therapy is usually necessary when childhood disorders are severe. Intervention always includes education of the parents and other members of the family concerning the child's normal growth and development, behaviors to expect in association with the diagnosis, and identification of realistic expectations for the child's ability to function at home and in the community. Bonding issues are addressed, and parenting skills are assessed and taught when necessary. Emotional support must be provided for all family members, and emphasis is placed on expanding the family's social support network, which may include agencies, support groups, and religious or other affiliations.

Pharmacotherapy

Medications may be used when other therapies do not adequately manage behaviors. Acting-out behaviors often respond to methylphenidate (Ritalin), clonidine, and select antidepressants.

DISCHARGE CRITERIA FOR DISORDERS OF INFANCY, CHILDHOOD, AND ADOLESCENCE

Engages in self-care within level of capability
Demonstrates emotional control within capacity
Attends to tasks, schoolwork, and performance without undue anger or frustration
Exhibits healthy self-concept and self-esteem
Demonstrates functional eating habits and behaviors appropriate for age and stature
Utilizes cognitive, communication, and language skills to make self understood and get needs met
Demonstrates interactive skills appropriate for level of development
Verbalizes satisfaction with gender identity and sexual preference
Interacts meaningfully with staff, peers, and family within capability
Seeks attention and assistance appropriately from significant persons and refrains from undue to unnecessary interactions with strangers
Adheres to treatment regimen, including medication as needed
Plays appropriately with peers
Engages in educational and vocational programs within capacity
Utilizes adaptive coping techniques and stress-reducing strategies
Responds satisfactorily to others' attentions and requests
Utilizes community resources to enhance quality of life
Engages in ongoing individual and family therapy

Disorders of Infancy, Childhood, and Adolescence

Universal Principles for Interactions and Interventions for Disorders of Infancy, Childhood, and Adolescence

- Continue to monitor assessment parameters listed in *Defining Characteristics.*
- Continue to consider the etiologic factors listed in *Etiologic/Related Factors.*
- Utilize principles of the *Therapeutic Nurse-Client Relationship* (Appendix G).
- Address clients' spiritual and cultural needs.

General Principles

- Provide for safety and comfort, health and nutrition.
- Identify stages of growth and development.
- Assess cognitive, mental, emotional, and social communication and language function.
- Assist with activities of daily living as needed.
- Encourage independence in all activities within the individual's capacity.
- Promote self-esteem and maintain the individual's dignity.
- Support the therapeutic treatment plan including milieu, medical, adjunctive, individual, and group and family therapies.
- Provide intellectual stimulation and special education when necessary.
- Promote mental and emotional stability.
- Facilitate socialization through interactions with staff, peers, and parents.
- Encourage appropriate communication.
- Provide opportunities for formal and informal education.
- Promote satisfying and appropriate play with peers.
- Modify behavior and set limits with a firm, kind approach.
- Assist in education of entire family system to promote understanding and tolerance concerning disorders.
- Promote opportunities for vocational enhancement.
- Facilitate community involvement in meeting needs of client and family.

Care Plans for Disorders of Infancy, Childhood, and Adolescence Based on Nursing Diagnosis

DSM-IV Diagnoses

Attention Deficit and Disruptive Behavior Disorders
Mental Retardation (Axis II)
Pervasive Developmental Disorders

NANDA Diagnoses

Violence, risk for: directed at others
Violence, risk for: self-directed
Growth and development, altered

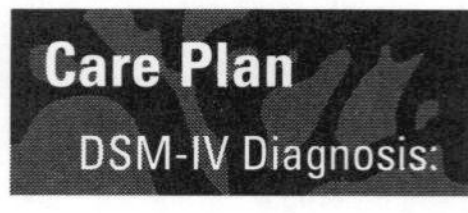

Care Plan

DSM-IV Diagnosis: **Attention Deficit and Disruptive Behavior Disorders**

NANDA Diagnoses: Violence, risk for: self-directed Violence, risk for: directed at others

The state in which an individual experiences behaviors that can be physically harmful either to self or others.

Focus:
For the child or adolescent who demonstrates a persistent pattern of behaviors, e.g., conduct and oppositional disorders that violate the rights of others, including potentially physically aggressive or violent acts directed toward self, persons, or property

NANDA Taxonomy
Pattern 9—Feeling: A human response pattern involving the subjective awareness of information.

RISK FACTORS

Overt, aggressive acts directed toward others and the environment.
Examples:
- Throws food tray and other objects in presence of others
- Shouts, curses loudly in classroom or group activity
- Threatens to harm staff members, peers, and family members

Self-destructive behavior (active)
- Suicidal thoughts, gestures, plans

History of destructive or violent behaviors self-directed or directed at others
Frequent use of curse words or obscene language without obvious provocation
A pattern of resistance, defiance, or opposition toward authority figures, rules, and regulations.
Examples:
- Frequent incidents of running away from home, foster home, or institution
- Frequent incidents of sexual promiscuity or acting-out behaviors

A pattern of cruel, hostile, or destructive behaviors.
Examples:
- Cruelty to animals
- Starting fires

Inability to attend to tasks or activities with concomitant hyperactivity (rule out mania).
Examples:
- Easily distracted during schoolwork and in group activities
- Wanders restlessly around classroom or unit, intrusive to others

Frequent loss of temper (low impulse control)
Low frustration tolerance
Examples:
- Angers easily during task performance
- Gives up in anger before task is completed

Impaired social or school functioning
Examples:
- Lies, steals, cheats
- Truant; disruptive in classroom

History of alcohol, drug, or tobacco use
History of alcohol-dependent father or absent father or father-figure
History of rejection or abuse by parents or parental figures
History of harsh or inconsistent discipline or management of care by parents or parental figures
Frequent shifting of parental figures (foster parents, stepparents, relatives)
Frequent shifting of residences (homes, institutions)
Low self-esteem
Powerlessness

OUTCOME IDENTIFICATION AND EVALUATION

Verbalizes awareness of factors and situations that precipitate violent behaviors
Relates understanding of negative effects of aggressive or violent behaviors
Avoids situations that precipitate aggressive or violent behaviors
Expresses anger in appropriate ways.
Examples:
- Physical activities and exercise
- Sports, hobbies
- Talking to staff members or peers

Utilizes defense mechanisms adaptively to rechannel or reduce angry feelings.
Examples:
- Displacement
- Compensation
- Sublimation
- Identification

(See Appendix I for defense mechanisms defined.)
Uses assertive rather than aggressive communication with adults and peers (i.e., "I" statements, *not* "you" statements)
Participates in stress-reducing strategies to redirect and reduce angry feelings.
Examples:
- Deep-breathing exercises
- Relaxation techniques
- Thought stopping or substitution exercises
- Visual imagery
- Positive affirmations via cognitive therapy

(Refer to Appendix K for Assertiveness Training and Therapeutic Strategies.)
Demonstrates absence of hostile, aggressive threats and gestures directed toward environment
Demonstrates absence of suicidal ideation, gestures, plans

Identifies and utilizes resources and support systems effectively.

Examples:
- Trusted, significant adults
- Staff members
- Social worker
- Teacher(s)
- Counselor/therapist

Initiates own behavioral contract to manage anger and avoid aggressive, violent behavior (in the hospital and at home)

PLANNING AND IMPLEMENTATION

Nursing Interventions and Rationale

Assess cues and warning signals such as behavioral changes, escalating anger or anxiety, hyperactivity, recently disrupted family, or chronic dysfunctional family life. *The child or adolescent's impulsive or violent reactions to stressful situations may be preceded by behavioral cues or changes. The nurse's keen assessment skills can prevent harm or injury to the client or others.*

Demonstrate acceptance of painful feelings that generally underlie the child's or adolescent's behaviors, while not condoning the specific behavior. *Anger and aggression often signify a cry for help or a defense against a reality that the child or adolescent finds intolerable. Acceptance of feelings validates self-worth, even though disruptive or inappropriate behavior is not acceptable.*

Therapeutic response:

"Billy, yelling and swearing in the cafeteria is not acceptable behavior. Finish your lunch without using this behavior and we'll talk about your feelings then."

If child or adolescent cannot stop using inappropriate behaviors:

"Billy, since you are still yelling and cursing, you'll have to leave the cafeteria and finish your meal later. We'll talk about your feelings then."

Nontherapeutic response:

"Billy, you know better than to yell and curse like that. We cannot tolerate it and you'll have to stop if you want to be accepted in this unit."

The incorrect response intimates that the client, his feelings, and his behaviors are all equally undesirable and unacceptable. This could diminish his self-esteem because it does not separate the behavior from the client and his feelings. It may ultimately create a barrier to further communication between the nurse and the client.

Investigate the client's past suicide attempts and violent acts directed toward others to determine the potential seriousness of present behaviors (threats, gestures, plans); note severity of threatening behaviors (on a scale of 1 to 10, with 1 being least severe and 10 being most severe) and availability of means. *Knowledge of previous patterns of violence may help you assess the client's tolerance for stress so that action can be taken to prevent subsequent destructive acts.*

Initiate a "show of force" with the child or adolescent who cannot control anger and when risk of violence is imminent, *to help the young client manage volatile feelings and behaviors and prevent harm or injury to self and others.*

(Refer to Appendix L for information on "Show of Force.")

Initiate suicide precautions and/or seclusion and restraint protocol if client's aggressive behavior escalates to 8 to 10 on the severity scale, and cannot be managed safely through other methods *to protect client and others from harm or injury.*

(See Appendixes J and L.)

Maintain a therapeutic environment with external controls such as suicide precautions or behavioral contract with clear, specific rules and consequences *to assist the client until he or she is able to use internal controls to modify or reduce inappropriate, aggressive, or destructive behaviors.*

Approach the adolescent with respect; avoid a judgmental and/or authoritarian attitude. *Adolescents are attempting to meet the developmental task of identification and avoid feelings of role confusion; thus they need approval and acceptance from adults as much as they need direction and limit setting.*

Avoid use of teenage jargon when interacting with adolescents. *Adults who try to be hip and use teen terminology generally create distance and distrust between themselves and the adolescents, who need adult role models they can count on when they are out of control.*

Clarify teenage expressions or jargon that are unclear, rather than acting as if you understand everything that is said. *Adolescents respect honesty, as they often come from troubled or dysfunctional families in which honesty is rare or nonexistent. Honesty builds trust when used tactfully and appropriately.*

Avoid "why" questions with children and adolescents. *"Why" questions tend to intimate that the client is wrong to think, feel, or behave a certain way, which invalidates the individual. With the adolescent, "why" questions tend to evoke defensiveness or intellectualization rather than awareness and exploration. With the young child, "why" questions tend to evoke the response "because" with a concomitant "bad feeling."*

Therapeutic response:

"Sarah, what happened just before you threw your tray on the floor?"

"Jimmy, how come you reacted so strongly in group today?"

Nontherapeutic response:

"Sarah, *why* did you throw your tray?"

"Jimmy, *why* were you so angry in group today?"

Use open-ended questions instead of closed-ended questions *to allow the child or adolescent to explain feelings, thoughts, or actions, rather than be confined to yes or no. Open-ended questions are nonjudgmental and allow the child or adolescent to be the expert about himself or herself.*

Therapeutic response:

"Mark, what are your thoughts about your contract?"

"Susan, how do you feel when the group focuses on you?"

Nontherapeutic response:

"Mark, do you think your contract is fair?"

"Susan, does it upset you to be the focus of attention?"

Observe and listen for nonverbal cues that may be symptoms of increasing anxiety, anger, or agitation, for example, looking down or away from the interviewer; long, frequent pauses; stuttering; flushed face; wringing hands; or looking bored, frustrated, or troubled. *Keen observations and listening skills can alert the nurse-interviewer to impending aggressive or violent behavior so preventive interventions can be taken.*

Teach the child or adolescent simple stress-management strategies *to redirect the energy generated by anger and anxiety toward healthy, functional anxiety-reducing activities and exercises.*

Examples:

- Deep-breathing exercises
- Relaxation techniques
- Thought-stopping exercises
- Visual imagery
- Positive affirmations and other cognitive strategies

(Refer to Appendix K.)

Engage the client in physical activities *to utilize physical energy in healthy, productive activities that increase self-fulfillment and reduce uncontrollable anger and anxiety.*

Examples:

- Ping-Pong
- Volleyball
- Stationary bicycle
- Brisk walking or running

Engage the client (with his or her input) in more satisfying, alternative outlets to redirect angry feelings (e.g., physical activities such as pillows or batakas to pound; soft balls to throw at inanimate objects; use of time-out or "quiet/alone time"; remain with staff member to talk it out). *Satisfying alternative outlets to cope with anger or stress reduce the need to direct angry feelings toward the environment in the form of aggressive or violent behaviors. Physical outlets help relieve pent-up tension, frustration, and anxiety. Staff members can help the client express feelings and begin to recognize the value of appropriately handling anger. The child or adolescent may initially view time-out as punitive but will eventually consider it a helpful way to gain control over angry, volatile feelings, as he or she takes more and more responsibility for initiating own "quiet/alone times."*

Provide individual or group counseling that includes the presence of significant others approved by the child or adolescent (e.g., parent(s), best friend, sibling(s), group of same sex or with same problem, or mixed group of teens). *Individual sessions provide opportunities for the client to vent personal problems and conflicts with a trusted nurse. Group work offers opportunities for increased insight and understanding of self and others and for group support. Discussion and practice sessions can be continued at the group's own pace. Angry feelings can be expressed and explored in a controlled setting with professional group facilitators.*

(See Appendix K, Group Therapy.)

Contract for confidentiality with the adolescent (i.e., state that information shared with staff will not be discussed with parents, foster parents, or anyone else unless teen gives permission to do so), explaining that the only exception would be if the adolescent threatens or plans to harm self or others, in which case protective actions would be taken, including talking with significant others after making the same contract with them. *Assurance of confidentiality between client and staff builds trust and self-worth in adolescents who have found few role models to trust. It also opens up channels of communication that can be used to further explore and manage angry feelings.*

Engage the client in role-playing situations in individual and group sessions *to provide opportunities for the child or teenager to reverse roles with trusted staff and group members, who portray significant others with whom the client can ventilate pent-up emotions. (Facilitators must be trained in role play and sociodrama theory and strategies.) (Examples of role playing appear in a later intervention.)*

Help children and adolescents clarify values through exploration of self-awareness (values clarification exercises). *Values clarification exercises help children and teens develop a value system by questioning, learning, and trying out alternative value systems. When values and beliefs are incongruent with behaviors, the individual experiences conflict, confusion, and ambivalence. Thus building a strong, positive value-belief system can influence behaviors and reduce the incidence of aggressive or violent episodes.*

Help adolescents compare and contrast their own values and beliefs with others, noting similarities and differences, by devising exercises in which the youngster can state "I strongly agree" or "I strongly disagree" to increase awareness of feelings, thoughts, and ideas regarding adolescent issues (e.g., relationships with peers, parents, foster families; body image; sexuality). *These exercises help the adolescent develop a greater awareness of own values, express own values, problem solve alternative values, and select from alternative values with consideration of the consequences.*

Inform the adolescent that occasional emotional outbursts are normal reactions to accumulated feelings of anxiety, confusion, and ambivalence *to assure clients that all adolescents experience unpredictable emotional highs and lows related to hormonal activity, adjustment to puberty, and pending adulthood. Such explanations offer the adolescent hope that he or she is like any other adolescent and thus need not experience overwhelming guilt, embarrassment, or shame each time he or she cannot control angry outbursts.*

Therapeutic response:

"This is upsetting for you; it would be for most people your age."

"It's OK to feel angry; what else about that makes you mad?"

Nontherapeutic response:

"Try not to get so angry about these things."

"Don't feel so upset about this; it's not necessary."

These incorrect responses infer that the adolescent's feelings or reactions are wrong or exaggerated, which could result in shame, embarrassment, or guilt and inhibit further communication.

Role model assertive communication skills *to teach the adolescent to express his or her needs and negotiate workable compromises instead of responding with aggressive communication to get needs met.*

Examples of assertive responses:

- "I" statements (e.g., "I feel," "I want," "I don't want," "I like," "I don't like," "I am willing to").
- "I'm angry at your behavior"; "I'm upset with the way your room is messed up."

Examples of nonassertive responses:

- "You" statements (e.g., "You make me so mad." "You're sloppy." "Your room is a mess.")

These unassertive responses tend to diminish self-esteem and evoke aggressive or defensive responses in the individuals to whom they are addressed.

(Refer to Appendix K for assertive communication skills.)

Teach the adolescent to use coping mechanisms appropriately *to adapt more effectively with stress, anger, anxiety, and frustration and to manage uncontrolled outbursts and aggression:*

- *Displacement* of anger/aggression through physical exercises, activities (punching bag, batakas, clay therapy)
- *Compensation* for perceived deficiencies by excelling in schoolwork, arts, crafts, sports, music
- *Sublimation* of aggressive feelings through hobbies, sports, recreation (video games, boxing, baseball)
- *Identification* with trusted adults and peers who role model mature, assertive behaviors

Child/Adolescent Counseling

Engage the client in ongoing counseling with a supportive child/adolescent therapist to help the young client adapt to changes and disruptions in his or her life, such as transition from family home to foster family home, from one foster family to another, or from a home to an institution. *Children and adolescents with ongoing conduct disorders and behavioral problems are often shifted form one place of residence to another and need help to learn how to respond and adapt to different environments, some of which may be dysfunctional.*

Help the child and adolescent respond and cope with unstable or shifting environments through role-playing situations. *Role playing helps the client practice responses and behaviors in simulated real-life family situations. Role playing can be used to help young clients explore different responses and behaviors, choose those behaviors that yield more positive results, and begin to problem solve as they incorporate learned concepts of values clarification and assertive responses in the role-playing exercises.*

Role-play exercise without use of learned concepts:

Nurse (role playing parent figure):

"Jimmy, your room is still a mess [loud, angry voice]; you promised to clean it before you went to school today."

Jimmy [client playing himself]: "You're always yelling at me [loud, angry voice]; why can't you let me do what I want with my own room?"

Role-play exercise with use of learned concepts:

Nurse [role-playing parent figure]: "Jimmy, your room is still a mess [loud, angry voice]; you promised to clean it before you went to school today."

Jimmy [client playing himself]: "Mom, I realize I didn't clean my room when I said I would [calm, low to moderate voice]; I'll get to it right away."

The first role-playing situation illustrates the client's lack of assertive communication in response to his "mother's" angry statement. Instead Jimmy matches his "mother's" emotion with an equally angry response, which only perpetuates the volatile situation. The second role-playing situation illustrates the client's use of assertive communication in response to his "mother's" angry remark, which reflects the young person's growing awareness that words have the power to change a negative situation into a positive one. As the child or adolescent gains more satisfying results through assertive communication, he or she will incorporate those skills into his or her own value system and continue to use them in subsequent relationships with peers and other adults.

Note: Role playing can be used in a variety of situations with young clients, some of which include providing opportunities for risk taking and problem solving as the child makes the transition into adolescence and the adolescent moves into adulthood. Separation from family, gaining independence, forming peer groups, developing intimate relationships, and expressing unique values and interests while adhering to social norms when necessary are all critical skills for a successful, satisfying life. For the young client with a conduct disorder whose significant adult role models and home life are not always stable, role playing can be a helpful, yet challenging adjunct to the client's overall therapy.

Practice assertive behaviors with adolescents in individual and group settings, using situations that occur in everyday life, progressing from simple, nonthreatening situations to more difficult, threatening situations. *This type of simulated role playing helps prepare the adolescent for similar real-life events with the individuals in his or her life and avoids explosive emotional encounters with significant others.*

Give the adolescent honest feedback regarding the effectiveness or ineffectiveness of learned assertive responses used during role-play practice sessions *to support and strengthen the client's successful responses and discourage unsuccessful communication.*

Behavior Modification Systems

Construct a behavior modification system, such as a token system in which the child or adolescent earns tokens that can be exchanged for personal items or benefits contingent on the client's behaviors. *Behavior modification systems reinforce positive behaviors by offering personal rewards as incentives. (Some systems include loss of tokens for negative behaviors such as lying, stealing, aggression, violence.)*

Design a level system in which young clients gain access to more privileges, consistent with improved behaviors. *The level system is a behavior modification system that offers higher client status along with more privileges, contingent on the client's behavior. (Some level systems include demotion to lower levels for negative behaviors or regression to earlier level behaviors.)*

Construct a written behavioral contract (when appropriate) that clearly states which behaviors are acceptable and which behaviors are unacceptable. Describe specific consequences expected for each unacceptable behavior while adhering to reward systems for acceptable behaviors. Include a time frame in which consequences begin and end. *Children and teens need to test limits as part of learning about themselves and acceptable behaviors in different situations. Firm, fair limit setting tends to promote trust and to prevent acting-out, disorganized, or violent behaviors. Although certain behaviors may be negotiable, stipulating those that are and are not acceptable teaches young people to learn how to set their own limits, a necessary adult skill.*

Family Education and Therapy

Engage families and foster families in ongoing family therapy sessions with and without the identified client. *Family members need to be aware of the effect each of their roles has on the client's dysfunctional behavior and on the dysfunctional behavior of the family as a unit. The child's or adolescent's behavior is a reflection of the entire family's dysfunction, and it is generally the entire family system that needs therapy.*

(See Appendix K, Family Therapy.)

Praise the child or adolescent and their families or foster families for engaging in more functional, socially appropriate interactions that produce positive relationships and reduced or absent aggressive or violent episodes. *Positive feedback reinforces repetition of functional, appropriate behaviors.*

ETIOLOGIC/RELATED FACTORS (RELATED TO)

Cognitive, mental, emotional deficits
Biologic/psychologic/sociologic factors

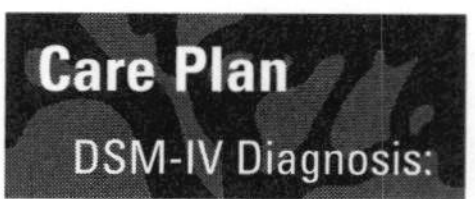

Mental Retardation or Pervasive Developmental Disorders

NANDA Diagnosis: Growth and development, altered

The state in which an individual demonstrates deviations in norms from his or her age group

Focus:
For the child or adolescent with a developmental disorder who demonstrates a predominant disturbance in the acquisition of cognitive language, motor, or social skills, such as a general delay (mental retardation) or a failure to progress in a specific area (speech, motor skills) or in multiple areas in which there are qualitative distortions (pervasive disorder, e.g., autism)

NANDA Taxonomy
Pattern (6)—Moving: a human response pattern involving activity

DEFINING CHARACTERISTICS (AS EVIDENCED BY)

Mental Retardation

Demonstrates significantly below-average intellectual functioning (IQ of 70 or below or clinical judgement in infants)

Mild Mental Retardation—Preschool Childhood

Demonstrates social and communication skills that may be indistinguishable from children of the same age (ages 0 to 5 years)
Participates appropriately in children's games, activities
Interacts socially with children of average intelligence

Mild Mental Retardation—Adolescence

Demonstrates social and communication skills slightly below abilities of peer group
Exhibits deficits in academic abilities in contrast to peers that are noticeable in classroom situations that require problem solving beyond the individual's capacity

Mild Mental Retardation—Young Adulthood

Demonstrates social and vocational skills adequate for minimum self-support:

- Able to care for self (grooms, cooks, cleans own home)
- Establishes intimate relationship consistent with social abilities
- Performs at skilled job commensurate with educational/social skills

Demonstrates ability to live independently with minimal support, but requires guidance and assistance during times of unusual social, emotional, or economic stress

(May live in an independent living complex supervised by managers who are trained to assist developmentally challenged tenants in crisis or emergency situations)

Moderate Mental Retardation—Childhood

Demonstrates ability to talk or learn to communicate during preschool years with greater effort than children of same age

Moderate Mental Retardation—Adolescence

Demonstrates ability to care for self with moderate supervision and guidance

Displays difficulty adhering to social conventions, which disrupts peer relationships

Exhibits pronounced intellectual impairment (unlikely to progress beyond second-grade level)

Moderate Mental Retardation—Young Adulthood

Demonstrates ability to improve skills with individualized social, occupational, or vocational training

Performs unskilled or semiskilled work under close supervision (in sheltered workshop or competitive job market)

Requires extra supervision and guidance during times of stress or crisis

Needs the structure and supervision of a group home

Severe Mental Retardation—Childhood

Displays poor motor development during preschool period (e.g., uncoordinated, slow, or hesitant)

Acquires little or no communicative speech during preschool period

Exhibits ability to learn to speak and perform simple hygiene skills during schoolage years

Severe Mental Retardation—Adolescence

Demonstrates only limited ability to learn the alphabet and master simple counting

Displays ability to learn sight-reading of some "survival" words (e.g., *men, women,* and *stop*)

Severe Mental Retardation—Adulthood

Demonstrates ability to perform simple tasks under close supervision.

Examples:

- Housework
- Short, simple errands
- Unskilled job
- Simple games and activities

Demonstrates ability to live in group homes or with family under close supervision

Profound Mental Retardation—Childhood

Displays minimal capacity for sensorimotor functioning

Requires highly structured environment with constant aid and supervision to perform self-care (some may not achieve this goal)

Performs simple task under close, individualized supervision by a caregiver

Profound Mental Retardation—Adolescence

Demonstrates some improvement in motor development, self-care, and communication skills with continued training

Profound Mental Retardation—Adulthood

Resides in group home, intermediate care facility, or with family

Performs simple tasks under close supervision in day programs or sheltered workshops (some may not achieve this goal)

Pervasive Developmental Disorders (Autistic Disorder)

Impaired Social Interactions

Demonstrates marked lack of awareness of the existence or feelings of others.

Examples:

- Treats others as if they were pieces of furniture or other inanimate objects
- Fails to notice the distress of other individuals
- Lacks awareness of the need for others' privacy

Displays absent or abnormal comfort-seeking behaviors when ill, hurt, tired, or distressed.

Example:

- Seeks comfort in a bizarre, stereotypical manner (e.g., says, "Go, go, go" or other type of term whenever hurt)

Exhibits impaired or absent modeling of others' social behaviors.

Examples:

- Fails to wave good-bye
- Does not imitate parents' domestic activities (e.g., dusting, sweeping)
- Copies others' actions in robotic, out-of-context manner

Demonstrates absent or abnormal social play.

Examples:

- Does not actively engage in simple games
- Manifests solitary play activities
- Responds to other children in play only as "mechanical aids"

Displays impaired ability to engage in peer friendships.

Example:

- Lacks awareness of conventions of social interactions (e.g., reads or recites phonebook to uninterested peers)

Impaired Verbal and Nonverbal Communication and Imagination Activity

Demonstrates absent mode of communication.

Example:

- Lack of verbal babbling, facial expression, gestures, mime, or spoken language

Displays abnormal, nonverbal communication, as in use of eye contact, facial expression, body posture, or gestures, to initiate or modulate social interactions.

Examples:
- Fails to anticipate being held
- Stiffens when held
- Does not look at the person or smile when making a social approach
- Fails to greet parents or visitors
- Has a fixed stare in social situations

Manifests absence of imaginative activity.

Examples:
- Lack of playacting of adult roles, fantasy characters, animals
- Absence of interest in imaginative stories or events

Demonstrates marked abnormalities of speech, including pitch, volume, rate, rhythm, stress, and tone (e.g., monotonous tone, questionlike melody, or high pitch)

Displays marked abnormalities in the form or content of speech, including stereotypical and repetitive use of speech.

Examples:
- Immediate echolalia (repeats the words of others)
- Repetition of television commercials in mechanical manner
- Use of "you" when "I" is meant (e.g., states "you" want a drink while actually meaning "I" want a drink)
- Uses idiosyncratic words or phrases (e.g., states "go fast riding" to mean "I want to ride in the car")
- Makes frequent irrelevant statements (e.g., starts talking about baseball during a conversation about music)

Demonstrates marked impairment in the ability to initiate or sustain a conversation with others despite adequate speech.

Example:
- Indulges in lengthy monologues on one topic regardless of others' interjections

Markedly Restricted Repertoire of Activities and Interests

Displays stereotyped body movements (e.g., hand-flickering, hand-twisting, hand-flapping, head-banging, spinning, or complicated, bizarre, whole-body movements)

Manifests persistent preoccupation with objects or parts of objects.

Examples:
- Sniffing or smelling objects
- Repetitive feeling of texture of materials
- Spinning wheels of toy cars and trucks
- Attachment to unusual objects (e.g., insists on carrying around article of clothing or piece of string)

Displays marked distress over trivial environmental changes (e.g., when a vase or lamp is moved from its usual place or position to another).

Examples:
- Cries, screams, or stamps feet
- Repeats words that generally indicate trouble or distress

Demonstrates unreasonable insistence on following routines in precise detail (e.g., insisting on viewing a particular television show regardless of priorities or circumstances)

Exhibits markedly restricted range of interests and a preoccupation with one narrow or specific interest (e.g., interested only in playing with toothpicks and placing them in rows, in gathering facts about astrology, or in discussing characters on favorite television show

Note: It is beyond the scope of this care plan to include every possible specific developmental disorder. Please refer to theory section for further information.

OUTCOME IDENTIFICATION AND EVALUATION

Demonstrates self-care in daily activities within level of cognitive, emotional, and behavioral capabilities

Displays control of angry, impulsive emotions

Demonstrates absence of aggressive acting-out behaviors

Utilizes communication and language skills to express self clearly and get needs met

Verbalizes a variety of feelings in appropriate manner

Exhibits meaningful interactions with staff, peers, and parents consistent with developmental level

Demonstrates ability to perform satisfactory age-appropriate tasks with minimal assistance

Displays significant control of stereotypic, ritualistic behaviors (e.g., hand-flapping, whirling)

Participates appropriately in milieu, group, and individual activities and in classroom setting

Seeks attention appropriately from known persons and refrains from unnecessary interactions with unknown individuals (autistic children often cannot distinguish between strangers and significant others)

Complies with treatment regimen, including medication as needed

Demonstrates increase in self-concept and self-esteem.

Examples:
- Brightened mood, affect
- Increased play, laughter
- Active participation in activities, groups
- Absence of apathy, dysphoria, acting-out behaviors

Note: Include family in outcome criteria as relevant.

PLANNING AND IMPLEMENTATION

Nursing Interventions and Rationale

Mental Retardation

Assess the following: the individual's intellectual function via such tools as the Stanford-Binet Intelligence Scale (IQ) and other assessment tools; gross and fine motor skills; behavior, cognition, mood, affect, language, play, self-care skills (hygiene, toileting, grooming); social communication and interactive capabilities; level of independence; ability to work; ability to solve own problems; adaptation to environment; development of relationships with family, peers, teachers, nurse, therapist, and intimacy with significant person.
Initial assessment of the individual's capabilities and levels of function helps focus on strengths rather than weaknesses and serves as a guide for more accurate, meaningful interventions.

Contrast the client's present developmental tasks with standard age-related tasks as indicated in Erikson's psychosocial stages of man, Piaget's stages of cognition, or Sullivan's interpersonal stages *to identify alterations in growth and development and plan interventions relevant to problem areas.* (Refer to Appendix D for Developmental Theories.)

Approach the client in a calm, nonjudgmental manner rather than an intense, hurried approach *to reduce anxiety, promote trust, and elicit calm responses from the client. Anxiety is transferable.*

Communicate and interact with the client in an age-appropriate manner *to maintain the client's dignity and promote his or her self-esteem. Infantilizing the client increases dependence.*

Accompany the client and family on a tour of the mental health facility *to promote familiarity and comfort and to reduce anxiety.*

Introduce the client to staff members and other clients slowly (no more than three persons per day) *to decrease fear and confusion and to build trust at a pace consistent with the client's tolerance.*

Instruct the client and family slowly in relevant unit rules regarding activities of daily living, safety factors, and behavior toward peers (no more than three rules per day) *to facilitate the client's understanding at a pace consistent with his or her tolerance and ability.*

Supervise the child or adolescent closely for at least 2 days *to assess strengths and capabilities and specific areas that require assistance* (keep in mind that hospitalization or institutionalization can cause the client to regress so that more time may be needed to determine the client's capabilities).

Allow the child or adolescent to be as independent as possible, offering assistance when necessary. *Independence encourages the child or adolescent to maximize his or her developmental potential. Infantilizing the client could foster regression.*

Schedule group activities in a progressive manner and increase as tolerated *to help the client gradually get to know peers and learn to interact with them at a tolerable pace.*

Examples:

- Engage the client in one group activity per day during the first week.
- Ensure that at least one group activity consists of peers in the same age group as the client.
- Allow group activities to last no longer than 20 minutes for the first week.

Engage the client in more structured groups initially (e.g., occupational therapy), and progress to more informal activities (e.g., recreational therapy). *Individuals with developmental disabilities learn more quickly from a structured, individualized activity, which can help prepare them for less-structured groups.*

Establish a routine; schedule meals, naps, medications, and treatments at the same time each day to maintain consistency and structure. *Children and adults with developmental disabilities perform better when they know what to expect. Autistic children especially depend on routine. They constantly exhibit ritualistic behaviors and become agitated if routines and rituals are disrupted.*

Inform the client of each daily activity immediately before the activity, rather than recite the entire daily schedule only once in the morning, *to facilitate attendance, establish a routine, and allay anxiety and confusion. Persons with developmental disabilities need extra reinforcement and reminding.*

Construct activities and groups that will meet the needs of the participants and consist of tasks and strategies that are realistic for the clients' intellectual and social levels of function. *Activities should be modified and planned so that they allow the individual to succeed and thus enhance self-esteem rather than exceed the level of the client's capabilities. Success is the best reinforcement for repetition of positive behaviors.*

Engage the client in activities and exercises *to enhance fine and gross motor skills and promote social interactions with peers and staff.*

Examples:

- Arts and crafts
- Bingo
- Volleyball or "sit down" volleyball
- Ping-Pong
- Simple stretching exercises
- Walking, running

Schedule small group outings with the activity therapist (e.g., a trip to the grocery store or fast-food restaurant, a movie, the zoo, a picnic at the beach, a hike in the park) *to facilitate "normal" recreation and social activities and promote verbal and motor skills.*

Help each client maximize his or her individual developmental potential by offering as many "normal" experiences as possible (supervise as necessary), *to help enhance the client's age-related tasks and build self-esteem.*

Examples:

- Allow the client to make minor purchases in a grocery store or fast-food restaurant
- Assign unit tasks (e.g., setting the table, decorating the unit)
- Engage the client to help set up for activities and clean up afterward
- Assign a different client each day or week to help in the classroom

Provide assistance as needed with personal hygiene, toileting, grooming, and other self-care needs, making certain that nothing is done for the client that he or she can do alone, *to promote the client's comfort, dignity, independence, and self-esteem and to protect the client from the ridicule of peers.*

Engage the client in "normal" experiences (e.g., eat meals in the dining room with other clients, attend all activities) *to promote healthy adjustment to the environment and to promote mental and physical growth, independence, and self-esteem.*

Provide the client with personal space so he or she will have room for personal belongings that can remain visible and accessible to the client. *Belongings that are constantly put away and hidden from view may be forgotten by the client and therefore not used. This may inhibit the client's progress.*

Examples:

- Alphabet board, books, chalkboard
- Blocks with numbers and letters
- Clothing, shoes
- Hairbrush, comb, toothbrush

Help the child or adolescent care for personal belongings and personal, physical environment *to promote independence and increase self-esteem.*

Develop for the child or adolescent and parents a teaching plan in daily living skills based on regular periodic assessments. *Growth and development are continuous and can be enhanced if both client and family agree on basic strategies. Continued assessment is critical because the youngster's physical and emotional state fluctuate and may influence the level of self-care functioning.*

Examples:

- Do not overwhelm child or adolescent with too many tasks at once (e.g., assist with each skill individually until client masters it, then move on to the next skill).
- Repeat skills as often as necessary.
- Praise frequently for efforts and accomplishments.
- Be realistic in expectations and assist the family to be realistic as well.

Provide opportunities for parents to ventilate feelings of frustration without the threat of shame or guilt. *Unresolved feelings could promote hostility and resentment and interfere with the parent-child or parent-adolescent relationship.*

Educate parents in signs and symptoms of physical illness. *Physical illness can be masked by the client's developmental disability or inability to communicate pain or distress. Parents need to be especially alert to signs and symptoms and means of identifying them.*

Examples:

- Sudden change in behavior
- Restlessness
- Facial grimacing
- Diaphoresis
- Change in body temperature, heart rate, skin color
- Loss of appetite, loss of weight
- Change in bowel, bladder function
- Altered sleep patterns
- Vomiting, spitting up blood
- Frequent or sudden crying, moaning
- Holding affected body part (stomach, side, limb)
- Favoring affected body part (not using a hand or limping to avoid use of a leg)
- Bending over in apparent pain or distress
- Seizure activity (may be mistaken for hyperactivity)

Construct a daily behavior rating scale, such as Connor's Behavior Rating Scale, with the parents, teacher, and other multidisciplinary team members *to determine the client's impulse control, attention span, and activity level and to plan appropriate interventions.* (If Connor's Scale is not available, devise a Likert scale with responses such as "never," "some of the time," "most of the time," or "always," which offers a valid rating of the client's observable behaviors.)

Reinforce the client's appropriate behaviors and decrease or defuse unacceptable behaviors, such as temper tantrums or other acting-out responses, by constructing a behavior modification program consistent with the client's age, intellectual and social capabilities, and ability to comply with the program rules. *Children and adolescents with mental retardation need special guidance and direction to help manage impulsive, angry outbursts that interfere with their own growth and progress and with others' rights and physical space. Reinforcement of appropriate behaviors promotes repetition of positive responses.* (See the following interventions for examples of behavior modification.)

Manage lewd or provocative language with a verbal warning initially: "That language is not permitted." *Limit setting is necessary for inappropriate milieu behavior.*

Express a second verbal warning if lewd or provocative behavior continues: "If you do not stop talking like that, you will have to go to your room for 15 minutes." *Consequences should be added to the warning as an additional incentive to stop negative behaviors.*

Initiate a 15-minute time-out if provocative behavior persists *to reinforce verbal warnings with behavior modification technique. Two verbal warnings should be followed by a time-out because the client's inability to stop inappropriate behaviors illustrates the need for external control by staff.*

Help the parents design a behavioral program similar to the one used in the facility and in the child's classroom *to provide consistency and structure for the client.* Behavioral programs are useful in providing structure and setting limits for children with developmental disabilities who have trouble controlling impulses. (Behavioral programs are most effective when combined with other therapies, e.g., psychosocial interventions and/or medication such as Ritalin.)

Administer prescribed medications as needed *to help manage the child's uncontrolled, hyperactive behaviors.* (Refer to Appendix M, Drugs to Treat Mental and Emotional Disorders, and drugs used to treat hyperactivity, e.g., Ritalin.)

Review with the child's teacher, parents, and social worker the therapeutic and nontherapeutic effects of medication. *Knowledge promotes awareness of the role of medication as an adjunct to other therapeutic modalities and thus decreases anxiety.*

Reward and praise the client for genuine efforts to comply with unit rules and regulations (e.g., give verbal praise, points, stickers, or tokens that can be applied toward special privileges or activities) *to reinforce positive behaviors. Children with developmental disabilities need frequent praise and rewards for their efforts as a method of behavior modification:*

"Billy, you picked up all your toys today; you will get 5 points for a treat."

"John, you get 10 points for not talking when others were talking; you can use them for a special activity."

"Kate, you didn't throw anything this afternoon; you will get five tokens to use in the gift shop."

Place a sticker on the child's clothing whenever he or she is actively involved in self-care or other activity of daily living.

Instruct parents and teachers to praise or reward the child or adolescent for paying attention to instruction and progressively increasing his or her attention span in accordance with level of developmental ability *to ensure consistency with behavior modification programs used on the child and adolescent unit.*

Talk to the child or adolescent about the relationship between his or her behaviors and the incidents that preceded them *to increase the patient's understanding of incidents that may provoke overresponsive behaviors.*

Examples:

"You were upset because. . . ."

"When that incident occurred, you became upset."

"This situation happened just before you got upset."

"Just after that incident, you became upset."

Help the client label feelings. *Naming feelings is the first step toward increasing awareness of feelings and connecting them with the behaviors that follow. Naming feelings also enhances language development and gives the client an opportunity to put angry or troubled feelings into words instead of destructive actions.* (Children with autism find it difficult or even impossible to identify feelings and emotions.)

Examples:

"You were angry or mad because. . . ."

"You were feeling bad or sad when. . . ."

Permit the client to express feelings of anger and frustration *to develop an awareness of the source of the client's feelings, help direct his or her energy toward constructive activities, and help the client cope with anger-provoking situations that cannot be changed through relaxation and other techniques.* (Refer to Appendix K for Relaxation Techniques.)

Collaborate with special education teachers to provide opportunities to explain bodily changes, sexual functions, and issues of intimacy to the preadolescent and adolescent client, with specific, concrete examples and simple illustrations as needed. *Individuals with mental retardation often have neither the cognitive ability nor the coping skills to deal with adolescent issues, bodily changes, sexuality, and intimacy. Therefore they may become frightened and confused when normal changes occur (e.g., breast growth, menstruation, sexual arousal, penile erection, orgasm). Feelings and emotions such as sexual attraction and love may cause ambivalence and concern in parents and other caregivers, which could result in fear and guilt within the client, who may sense that he or she is "feeling bad things," "thinking bad thoughts," or "doing something wrong." Special sex education classes are needed to help these individuals develop a positive self-concept and sexual identity and a greater understanding of their bodies and emotions without fear, guilt, embarrassment, or shame.*

Assess the child or adolescent for symptoms of depression, which may be masked by developmental problems such as apathy, dysphoria, acting out, isolation, or a sudden change in usual behavior patterns with no obvious cause, *to prevent self-destructive behaviors.* (Suicide in children and adolescents is generally an impulsive act, often preceded by acting out or apathy.)

(Refer to Appendix J.)

Explore with the client, social worker, parents, and primary therapist plans for group or independent living after assessing the client's readiness for discharge *to facilitate aftercare discharge planning appropriate for the client's needs and consistent with the parents' resources.*

Encourage the client and parents to discuss with the social worker information regarding appropriate facilities for the client *to provide alternative residential facilities from which to choose.* (The social worker may accompany the client and parents on a tour of several facilities for review.)

Explore cultural considerations with the client, parents, and social worker when selecting a permanent residence for the client *to assure the client and parents that cultural issues and preferences will be strongly considered in the decision-making process.*

Consult with the client, teacher, social worker, and occupational therapist to provide the client with a vocation in the community through a program that prepares individuals with developmental disabilities for jobs consistent with their skills and capabilities *to maximize the individual's vocational skills and ability to participate as a productive, independent citizen and to build a positive self-concept and self-worth.*

Autistic Disorder

Utilize a team approach (parents, counselors, special education teachers, nurses, and other significant individuals) to assess the needs of the child with autistic disorder, *to collect baseline information regarding the child's physical, emotional, and social functions and achieve specific, consistent goals and outcomes.*

Examples of roles of multidisciplinary teams.

- Special education teachers—construct a weekly check sheet of child's behavior and progress in the classroom
- Parents—utilize learned strategies consistent with team approach to promote structure in the home and elicit child's cooperation
- Counselors—work with child and family to promote positive interpersonal interactions
- Nurses—utilize the nursing process to collect baseline data such as possible organic disorders (e.g., seizures) that could be masked by behavioral

problems, and coordinate all the multidisciplinary findings within an ongoing treatment plan. (Refer to Chapter 1 for more information on data collection and the nursing process.)

Engage team members, teachers, and parents in frequent meetings *to evaluate the child's progress and outcome attainment and to modify approach and interventions as needed.* (Evaluation of children with long-term developmental disabilities also includes frequent informal assessments and meetings.)

Help the autistic child develop a relationship with a significant person in the facility *to increase socialization skills and build trust. Autistic children often isolate themselves socially and cannot easily discriminate between parents and strangers. They can, however, become attached in an unemotional way to a person who can, with patience and consistent interactions, enhance their developmental skills. Such a significant person can serve as a liaison between the client and others in the environment and help minimize the client's isolation.*

Structure scheduled daily activities to resemble usual routine followed by the child at home or in a residential treatment center to ensure a consistent environment. *Autistic children are especially resistant to change; structured programs that are similar to usual routines allay fear and anxiety.*

Examples of activities that can be structured to fit usual routine:

- Medications (administer at same time, in same manner as usual)
- Meals (serve favorite; usual foods and drinks)
- Naps (plan at usual time; allow client familiar blanket, pillow)
- Play objects (allow favorite toys, objects from home or residential treatment center)
- Routines (continue usual routines, e.g., television shows)

Teach the autistic child one task at a time (e.g., washing hands, putting belongings away, buttoning shirt, zipping up zippers) *to maximize success and minimize failure and frustration.*

Schedule one-to-one times with a primary staff member (e.g., 2 hours per shift at the same time each day). *Consistent staff and meeting times help develop a trusting relationship and maximize the client's language and communication skills.*

Provide a quiet environment (decrease unnecessary sound) *to protect the client from injury and distress. Autistic children may overrespond to sound and behave erratically if there is too much noise.*

Examples:

- Child may cover ears in distress to escape sound
- Child may run from noisy area, injuring self in the process

Place furniture as close to walls as possible, leaving as much open space in client area as feasible. *Autistic children experience disturbances in motility, such as whirling, lunging, darting, rocking, hand-flapping, and head-banging and have a greater chance for injury in a crowded or cluttered area.*

Provide the autistic child of average to above-average intelligence with opportunities and experiences that enhance developmental growth and special interests, such as music, arts, and crafts. *Approximately one quarter to one third of autistic children have average to above-average intelligence but lack the social skills necessary for activities that will promote their special qualities (significant patience is necessary for caregivers).*

Avoid unnecessary or sudden touch. *The autistic child may be unable to accurately interpret or process sensory input such as touch and may overrespond, as if in pain, or panic.*

Ignore the autistic child's temper tantrums only if they are not harmful or life-threatening. *Ignoring tantrums decreases their frequency. Injurious or life-threatening behaviors should be stopped while the tantrum itself is ignored. Even though it is negative, focusing attention on the behavior will reinforce it.*

For the Child Who Impulsively Hits or Strikes Out

Hold the child's hands down and firmly state, "No hitting, [child's name]." If the child persists, utilize time-out for approximately 2 minutes as a behavior modification strategy *to help the client control impulsive behavior and teach the consequences of actions.* (Time-out should take place in a quiet, nonstimulating area.)

For the Child Who Is Easily Distracted and Has Difficulty Attending

Hold the child's head gently between your own hands so that he or she faces you and looks directly into your eyes; establish eye contact and speak to the child slowly, simply, and clearly *to help make the client aware of who is engaging him or her in the interaction and that the interaction is meaningful and requires attention.* (This strategy is useful for all youngsters with attention deficits or who are easily distracted.)

Assess the environment and circumstances in which temper tantrums or overresponses occur *to plan preventive strategies.*

Examples of situations that may promote temper tantrums or rage:

- Sudden change or break in daily routine or activities
- Client is touched inadvertently by another person
- Child is startled or troubled by noise or overstimulation
- A favorite object (e.g., a piece of string, cloth, or article of clothing) is lost or misplaced
- A routine television program is cancelled or interrupted
- Child's ritual is disturbed with no alternative activity to replace it

Speak to the child in short, concise sentences *to enhance the client's understanding and to hold his or her attention.*

For the Child with Psychomotor Rituals

Call the child by name when stereotypic body movements occur (e.g., hand-flapping, spinning) *to distract the client from the activity by gaining his or her attention.*

Redirect the child to a constructive activity *to help the client displace energy in a beneficial, productive way, rather than through exhausting ritualistic behaviors.*

Praise the child immediately for positive behaviors (e.g., attending to verbal instructions by teacher, nurse, parents, therapist; interacting with peers vs. parallel play activities; engaging in constructive activities). *Immediate praise for positive behaviors reinforces appropriate behaviors. Children with autistic disorder especially need instant, frequent reinforcement for work well done.*

Examples of positive feedback:

- Give verbal approval (e.g., "Jimmy, you're doing a good job picking up your toys.")
- Place a "praise sticker" on the child's shirt during an activity in which the child's behavior is appropriate or demonstrates improvement.
- Allow the child to continue with a favorite activity or game for 15 minutes longer because of appropriate behavior.

Provide toys, games, educational supplies, teaching aids, and vocational tools that enhance the client's cognitive, social, and motor skills *to promote the client's interest and enthusiasm for learning while increasing his or her knowledge base, social behaviors, and motor skills.*

Explore with the client, social worker, and parents aftercare facilities *to provide a permanent residence that best fits the client's needs and will maximize his or her strengths and capabilities (if the child cannot reside with the parents).*

Note: Refer to the first part of the intervention section in this care plan for additional interventions relevant to the child with autistic disorder.

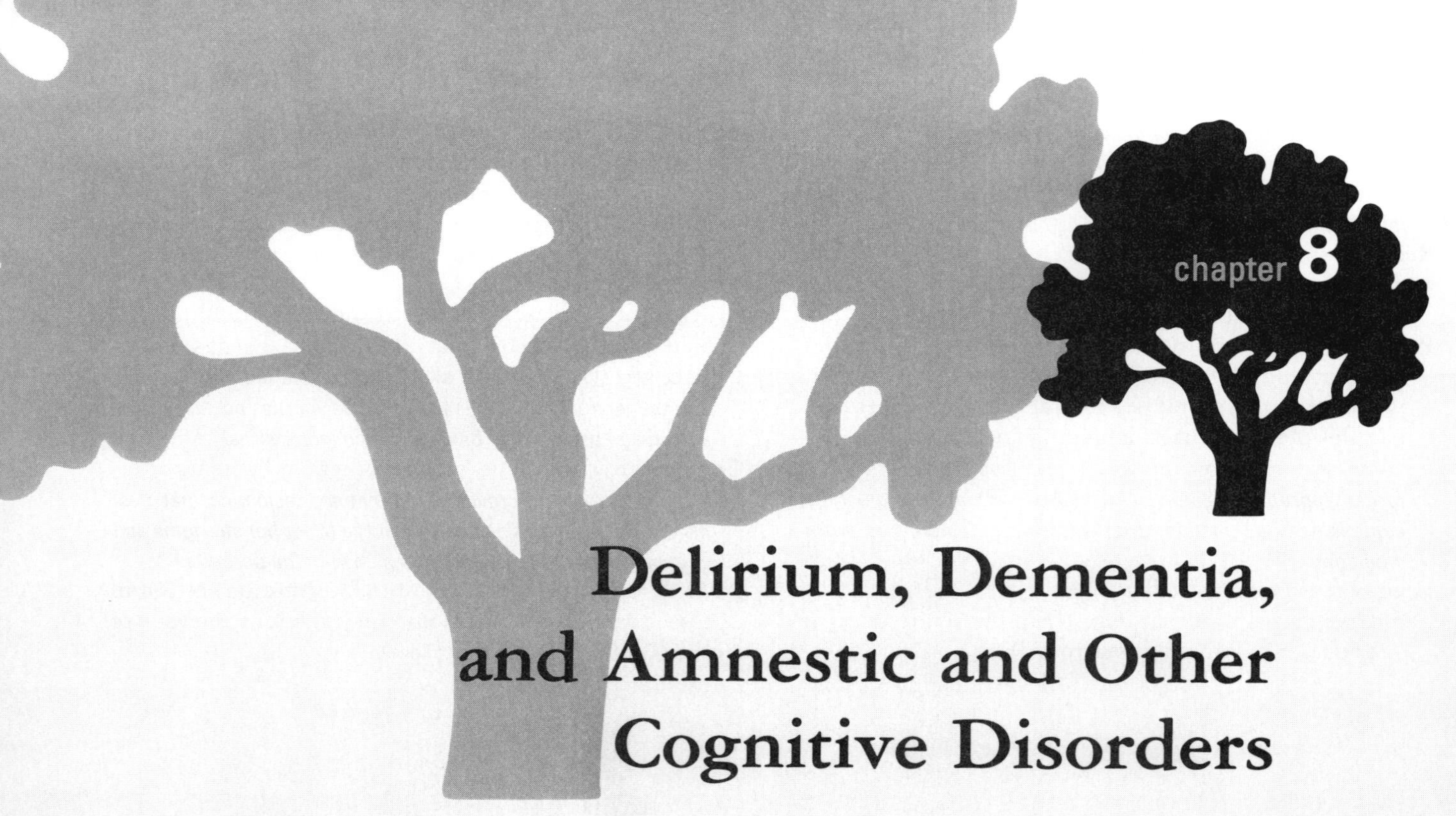

Delirium, Dementia, and Amnestic and Other Cognitive Disorders

The defining characteristics of delirium, dementia, amnestic disorders, and other cognitive disorders are marked impairment of cognition and memory and prominent changes in level of functioning. See Table 8-1.

ETIOLOGY

Etiology is directly attributable in all instances to either (1) a specific medical condition that may or may not be identifiable or (2) a substance in the form of a medication, a drug of abuse, or a toxin. Disorders that originate in the brain are termed *primary* (brain tumor, Alzheimer's disease, cerebral vascular accidents); those resulting from another source are *secondary* (metabolic disturbances, systemic infections, drugs, toxic agents). Box 8-1 provides etiologies for these disorders.

Diagnosis may be difficult because of the often lengthy or complex procedures that are necessary to establish a specific organic causative factor. Sometimes more than one organic disturbance is present in an individual, which further hinders diagnostic accuracy. Another question is whether symptoms occur as a direct result of brain dysfunction or whether they are a reaction to the cognitive, emotional, and behavioral changes resulting from organic disturbances.

EPIDEMIOLOGY

Organic disturbance may occur at any age. For instance, a toddler who adventurously explores his environment may accidentally swallow a poison and develop delirium; a teenager involved in an automobile accident may suffer amnesia; an elderly person may develop dementia from Alzheimer's disease. Generally delirium occurs more commonly in children and in adults over age 60. Intoxication and withdrawal symptoms are more common at ages 18 to 30 but can happen at any age. Dementias are most often seen in the elderly. Box 8-2 provides epidemiology of these disorders.

Specific symptoms relating to each disorder are discussed later in this chapter. Many associated symptoms can appear in conjunction with organic dysfunction and may reflect the type and severity of the abnormality, as well as the individual's personality, life-style, education and interactions with support systems such as family, friends, coworkers, and neighbors.

Anxiety, fear of loss of control, irritability, powerlessness, shame, decreased self-esteem, and depression are only some of the potentially severe emotional effects that accompany organic dysfunction. The individual may become paranoid to the point of being delusional.

Loss of impulse control, insight, and judgment may manifest in socially inappropriate behaviors such as aggressiveness, sexual advances, stealing, exhibitionism, or sloppy eating and hygiene habits. As a result of these changes the person may be avoided or rejected, which leads to social isolation and withdrawal that in turn only exaggerate cognitive difficulties.

Some individuals react to the deficits by becoming compulsively orderly in an attempt to maintain or regain control. Possessions are kept in an exact location, and calendars of events or diaries are meticulously kept as the

Table 8-1

A Comparison of the Clinical Features of Acute Confusion, Dementia, and Depression

Feature	Acute Confusion (Delirium)	Dementia	Depression
Onset	Rapid, often at night	Usually insidious	Coincides with life changes; often abrupt
Course	Fluctuates, worse at night; lucid intervals	Long; symptoms progressive yet relatively stable over time	Diurnal effects, typically worse in the morning; situational fluctuations
Progression	Abrupt	Slow but even	Variable, rapid-slow but uneven
Duration	Hours to less than 1 month	Months to years	At least 2 weeks, but can be several months to years
Awareness	Reduced	Clear	Clear
Alertness	Fluctuates, lethargic or hypervigilant	Generally normal	Normal
Orientation	Fluctuates in severity, generally impaired	May be impaired	Selective disorientation
Memory	Recent and immediate impaired	Recent and remote impaired	Selective or patchy impairment, "islands" of intact memory
Thinking	Disorganized, distorted, fragmented; slow or accelerated incoherent speech	Difficulty with abstraction, thoughts impoverished, judgment impaired, words difficult to find	Intact but with themes of hopelessness, helplessness, or self-deprecation
Perception	Distorted; illusions, delusions, and hallucinations	Misperceptions often present; delusions and hallucinations absent except in severe cases	
Psychomotor behavior	Variable; hypokinetic, hyperkinetic, or mixed	Normal, may have apraxia	Variable; psychomotor retardation or agitation
Sleep-wake cycle	Disturbed, cycle reversed	Fragmented	Disturbed, often early morning awakening
Mental status testing	Distracted from task; poor performance; improves when patient recovers	Frequent "near-miss" answers, struggles with test, great effort to find an appropriate reply; consistently poor performances	Frequent "don't know" answers, little effort, frequently gives up, indifferent

From Lewis S, et al: *Medical-surgical nursing: assessment and management of clinical problems,* ed 4, St Louis, 1996, Mosby.

person attempts to ward off forgetfulness and/or conceal the dysfunction.

Organic disturbances have increased significantly during the past decade, primarily because of the dramatic increase in the elderly population, the largest segment of individuals diagnosed with dementia.

DIAGNOSIS OF DELIRIUM, DEMENTIA, AND AMNESTIC AND OTHER COGNITIVE DISORDERS

Delirium

The onset of delirium is rapid and the duration brief, transient, and usually reversible when treated. Distinguishing characteristics are difficulty maintaining or shifting attention, disorganized thinking, changes in levels of consciousness, sensory misperceptions, disturbances of psychomotor activity and the sleep-wake cycle, memory impairment, and disorientation to time and place, but not usually to person.

Causes of delirium are numerous (see etiology factors). Delirium occurs most often in the very young, the elderly, or those who have a history of delirium, brain damage, or alcohol or drug dependence. The individual is usually confused, disoriented, and unable to test reality. Thought processes are slowed with an inability to think or talk coherently, reason, or problem solve. People often do not know if they are dreaming or awake and frequently misperceive external stimuli in

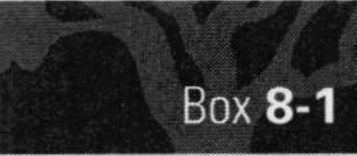
Box 8-1

Etiology of Delirium and Dementia

Delirium

Brain trauma
Brain infections (encephalitis, meningitis)
Systemic infections with fever
Epilepsy
Drugs (psychoactive substances, prescribed medications)
Withdrawal from drugs
Other toxins (heavy metals, carbon monoxide)
Endocrine dysfunction
Organ systems diseases/dysfunctions (liver, cardiovascular, kidney-urinary tract)
Postoperative reaction
Electrolyte imbalance

Dementia (Alzheimer's disease hypotheses)

Genetics—gene for apolipoprotein-E (apo-E) is risk factor for most common form of Alzheimer's
Acetylcholine loss—important for memory and cognition
Aluminum—higher levels in brains of Alzheimer's sufferers on autopsy; no definite causal link found to date
Autoimmune response
Slow-acting virus
Chromosome 19 degenerates with age

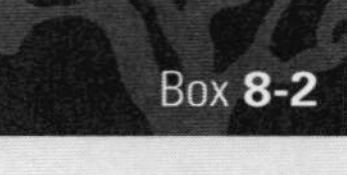
Box 8-2

Epidemiology of Delirium and Dementia

Delirium

Ten to fifteen percent of all hospitalized clients demonstrate symptoms of delirium.
Thirty to forty percent of all intensive care and coronary care clients manifest symptoms.
Twenty percent of all severely burned clients demonstrate symptoms of delirium.

Dementia

Prevalence is age-related.
Sixty percent of people in nursing homes have dementia.
Ten percent of elderly have mild dementia.
Five percent of elderly have severe dementia.
Cost is upward of $15 billion per year to care for people with chronic dementia.
Increase of elderly expected to reach 20% of total population in the next 40 years.

any of the senses, although visual changes are most frequent.

Delirium is usually more pronounced at night or in the early morning and is commonly referred to as *sundowner's syndrome.* This diurnal variation is a prominent diagnostic sign. Clients may become lucid during the day;

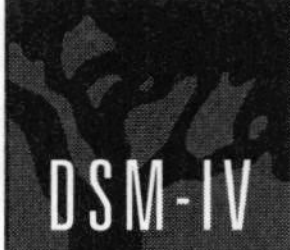
DSM-IV

Delirium

DSM-IV Categories

- Delirium Due to General Medical Condition (Name condition)
- Substance-Induced Delirium
  - Intoxication Delirium
  - Withdrawal Delirium
- Delirium Due to Multiple Etiologies (Example: Cardiac failure and sedative intoxication)

however, the course of delirium is unpredictable, and symptoms can recur at any time, depending on the individual's organic problem, the situation, and the environment. (See care plan for thought processes, altered, in this chapter, for interventions in sundowner's syndrome.)

Emotional disturbances are common and may manifest as fear (which is very common), anxiety, depression, apathy, anger, or euphoria.

Dementia

The distinguishing characteristic of dementia is impaired short- and long-term memory. It is accompanied by multiple cognitive deficits: impairment of intellectual function, reasoning, judgment, abstract thinking. Also, personality and emotional changes interfere with socialization, work, and relationships. Dementia may be permanent or reversible, depending on the underlying pathology, which is usually assumed, although not always specifically identifiable (see Etiology section).

Impaired memory manifests in early stages or milder cases by forgetfulness about things such as names, addresses, phone numbers, directions, and appointments. The affected individual may begin a project but forget to return to it, leave the bathtub water running, or walk out of the house for the day with an iron plugged in or stove left on. In more severe forms or advanced stages, the individual may even forget his or her name or be unable to identify closest significant others.

Reasoning, judgment, and impulse control are compromised and may manifest in many spheres. For example, an individual may begin to neglect hygiene and appearance, demonstrate disregard for the law by stealing or driving the wrong way on a one-way street, make out-of-character lewd gestures or remarks, or withdraw life savings for a foolish investment.

Abstract thinking becomes a problem. The affected individual has trouble acquiring or processing information of an abstract nature. New tasks are avoided and, in some cases, even familiar tasks become impossible because they are too complex.

Aphasia (loss of language), agnosia (inability to recognize objects), and apraxia (loss of purposeful move-

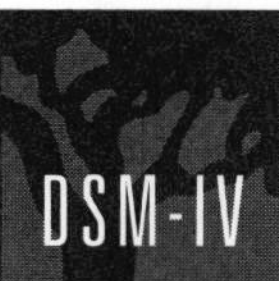

DSM-IV **Dementia**

DSM-IV Categories

Dementia, Alzheimer's type (early onset by age 65)
- Uncomplicated
- With delirium
- With delusions
- With depressed mood

Dementia, Alzheimer's type (late onset after age 65)
- Uncomplicated
- With delirium
- With delusions
- With depressed mood

Vascular Dementia
- Uncomplicated
- With delirium
- With delusions
- With depressed mood

Dementia Due to HIV Disease
Dementia Due to Head Trauma
Dementia Due to Parkinson's Disease
Dementia Due to Huntington's Disease
Dementia Due to Pick's Disease
Dementia Due to Creutzfeldt-Jakob Disease
Substance-Induced Persisting Dementia
Dementia Due to Multiple Etiologies

ment) are other symptoms that can occur. (See Glossary, Box 8-3, and Care Plan for Altered Thought Processes, for additional information and interventions.) Personality changes invariably accompany dementia, and premorbid traits are either accentuated (e.g., a normally quiet, soft-spoken individual may become totally apathetic and socially withdrawn; a friendly, outgoing person may become intrusive, excessively loud, and boisterous) or altered (e.g., a loving, trusting husband or wife may become excessively jealous of the spouse or suspicious about family or friends taking belongings or talking about him or her in a negative way). Loved ones inevitably notice that the individual has "changed." Frequently the person with dementia may become cantankerous and irritable or more compulsive, meticulous, and orderly in an effort to control the deficits. Emotional changes are usually manifested by fear, anxiety, and depression.

By far the most common cause for dementia is Alzheimer's disease, which accounts for 50% to 70% of all cases. Much attention is currently focused on AIDS-related dementias as well as other AIDS-related neuropsychiatric disorders. Primary and secondary causes of dementia appear in Box 8-4.

Pseudodementia is a psychiatric condition that mimics dementia; the mood disorder depression is most often the cause. Many elderly people experience depression, so careful diagnosis must be made to administer specific treatment; effective treatment can result in a good to excellent prognosis. Symptoms that aid in diagnosing appear in Box 8-5.

Box 8-3 **Common Symptoms in Dementia**

Agnosia: Inability to discriminate and comprehend sensory stimuli (can affect any of the senses)
Agraphia: Inability to express thoughts in speech, writing, symbols, or signs
Alexia: Inability to understand and interpret the written word
Alogia: Diminished production of speech
Apraxia: Inability to carry out purposeful, complex movements and to use objects properly
Dysarthria: Difficulty in articulating words

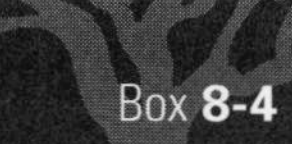

Box 8-4 **Causes of Dementia**

Primary Dementias
Alzheimer's disease
Huntington's chorea
Pick's disease
Creutzfeldt-Jakob disease
Kuru

Secondary Dementias
General paresis (syphilis)
Multiple sclerosis
Brain tumors
Amyotrophic lateral sclerosis (ALS)
Normal pressure hydrocephalus
Korsakoff's disease
Trauma
Metabolic and endocrine disorders
Nutritional disorders
Drugs
Infection

Dementia of the Alzheimer's Type

The distinguishing characteristics of Dementia of the Alzheimer's Type are symptoms of dementia that progressively worsen. The onset is insidious, and all examinations and tests fail to determine another specific etiology. Symptoms include severe loss of intellectual function (memory, judgment, abstract thinking) and changes in personality and behavior.

Although the disorder can occur at any age, it occurs most frequently in people age 65 to 70. At first, changes in personality are subtle; the affected person is usually

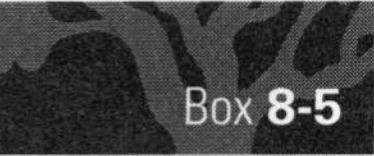

Box 8-5

Symptoms of Pseudodementia and Dementia

Pseudodementia (Depression)

Appears sad, worried

Consistently depressed; may be agitated emotionally

Cognitive deficits follow depressive symptoms

Behavior retarded (slowed); complains of poor memory and intellectual performance; ruminates over problems

Primary cognitive impairment is usually memory disturbance

Dementia

Appears indifferent or apathetic; neglects hygiene, dress, grooming

Superficial or labile emotions

Cognitive deficits precede depression

Denies, conceals, or minimizes cognitive deficits; may become angry when unable to answer questions correctly

Global cognitive and intellectual deficits

not aware of the changes but is reported by relatives and close friends as being different.

Memory impairment manifested as "forgetfulness" in the early stages becomes increasingly more problematic. As the disorder progresses, the individual becomes less spontaneous and appears apathetic and steadily more withdrawn from social activities and contacts. Concentration becomes more difficult as the person struggles to attend to daily tasks and to comprehend fully what is happening around him or her. Disorientation occurs in all these spheres.

Aphasia, apraxia, agnosia, and memory disturbances continue to worsen. Personality changes may be extreme. Although most people remain cooperative, behavior can become unpredictable and include irritable or angry outbursts. Individuals frequently perseverate and display stereotypic, ritualistic behaviors. Appetite may become insatiable, and the person may be prone to hyperorality. Supervision of even the most routine activities is essential with these individuals, requiring caregivers' patience and understanding.

By the last stage of Alzheimer's disease, the affected person has become totally incapable of self-care and is considered terminal. In this stage irritability occurs, all cognitive function is severely disturbed, and psychotic symptoms of hallucinations, delusions, and paranoid thinking and behavior may develop. Eventually, mobility is curtailed; the person becomes bedridden, totally helpless, and dependent on others for fulfillment of all needs. This stage inevitably ends in death from infections, pneumonia, dehydration, or malnutrition. The total course of the disease is approximately 5 to 7 years from onset until death, although the course may last much longer.

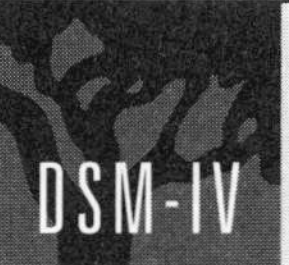

DSM-IV

Amnestic Disorders

DSM-IV Categories

- Amnestic Disorder Due to General Medical Conditions
- Substance-Induced Persisting Amnestic Disorder

The diagnosis of Alzheimer's disease is confirmed by neuropathologic and histologic findings at postmortem examination. Among these findings are general atrophy of the brain, neuritic plaques, neurofibrillary tangles, and neuronal degeneration.

Amnestic Disorders

The distinguishing characteristic of amnestic syndrome is impaired short- and long-term memory. This syndrome differs from delirium and dementia (which also involve memory impairment) in that dysattention is a major symptom accompanying delirium, whereas global cognitive impairment is associated with dementia. Sometimes individuals with amnestic syndrome may have more success in retrieving remote information than they have with recent recall.

One of the most common causes of amnestic syndrome is chronic alcoholism and associated thiamine deficiency (Wernicke-Korsakoff syndrome), but any events or processes that result in bilateral damage to certain brain structures may be etiologic factors.

The retrograde amnesia (loss of memory before onset of illness) and anterograde amnesia (inability to establish new memory after onset of illness) are usually accompanied by lack of insight into the deficit, which the individual may deny or rationalize. A common symptom in clients with amnestic syndrome associated with chronic alcoholism is confabulation, in which the person creates false information to fill in the memory lapses.

INTERVENTIONS FOR DELIRIUM, DEMENTIA, AND AMNESTIC AND OTHER COGNITIVE DISORDERS

A complete history, physical assessment, and diagnostic laboratory workup are essential for proper diagnosis and treatment of organic mental syndromes and disorders.

Success of interventions for these disorders depends primarily on specific identification of the cause and treatment of that cause whenever possible. In addition, treatment is aimed toward alleviation of disorder-related symptoms; relief of stress; prevention of physical, mental, and emotional complications; maintenance of fluid, electrolyte, and nutritional balance; and therapeutic interpersonal support. The last includes empathetic encouragement of optimal independent physical and cognitive function within each individual's capacity, regardless of the deficit. When conditions are irreversible, the caregiver usually offers support without encouraging insight into, or exploration of, problems that defy solutions. When conditions are reversible, teaching and, if warranted, retraining are priorities.

Pharmacotherapy is frequently used to treat organic mental syndromes and disorders. When the cause is, for example, a physiologic disorder such as hypothyroidism, replacement medication is warranted. Symptoms of anxiety, agitation, insomnia, aggression, paranoia, and depression are treated with specific psychotherapeutic medications. (See Appendix M.) Haloperidol, an antipsychotic medication, is frequently used in these disorders. Staff needs to be alert for symptoms of delirium that may develop in clients with dementia as a result of taking any of the psychotropic medications, as well as for other symptoms of idiosyncratic drug effects in the elderly, such as increased sedation, confusion, or paradoxic excitement.

Antidepressants may be used cautiously if depression seems to be exacerbating the dementia, as is often the case. Tranquilizers and sedatives are used sparingly for insomnia, restlessness, or agitation, and those with a short half-life are preferred. Tetrahydroaminoacridine is a recently developed drug treatment for reversal of memory loss and restoration of some cognitive function in early Alzheimer's disease. It is a potent anticholinesterase drug. It and other new medications may offer hope to clients with this devastating disease and their families.

Environment plays a major role in the treatment of individuals with these disorders. A positive, supportive, stable environment is essential for achievement of desired outcome, and clients do best in surroundings that are familiar and stimulating yet not excessively complex or challenging.

Family therapy and support are necessary components in overall client care, as any situation that results in acute symptoms or deficits in the client may be a crisis for the entire family unit. The family whose loved one suffers with a chronic, debilitating, irreversible disorder with increasingly negative personality and behavior changes is in need of continued support as each member struggles with his or her own painful reactions to multiple losses. Many families seek professional counseling to deal with associated issues such as grief, depression, shame, or guilt. (See Appendix E.)

Hospitalization is necessary for acute symptoms that require medical and nursing management; long-term institutionalization in nursing homes may be necessary. It is generally best for each family to decide when members can no longer cope with their loved one's progressive deterioration, resultant dependence, and ultimate need for total care. It is especially important during such emotional times that families of clients with Alzheimer's disease and related organic mental disorders receive the compassion and support they need.

DISCHARGE CRITERIA FOR DELIRIUM, DEMENTIA, AND AMNESTIC AND OTHER COGNITIVE DISORDERS

When symptoms are reversible, retraining and reeducation programs are a priority. Offer hope for the future.

When symptoms are irreversible, avoidance of insightful explorations is imperative to prevent depression, excessive anxiety, irritability, or rage.

Support families in helping clients to maintain their highest possible level of function. Encourage families to seek continued support as needed to maintain their own emotional health and well-being.

Nursing Process for

Delirium, Dementia, and Amnestic and Other Cognitive Disorders

Universal Principles for Interactions and Interventions with Clients with Delirium, Dementia, and Amnestic and Other Cognitive Disorders

- Continue to monitor assessment parameters listed in *Defining Characteristics.*
- Continue to consider the etiologic factors listed in *Etiologic/Related Factors.*
- Utilize principles of the *Therapeutic Nurse-Client Relationship* (Appendix G).
- Address clients' spiritual and cultural needs.

General Principles

- Maintain health and wellness
  Nutrition and hydration
  Bowel and bladder functions
  Sleep (normal day-night pattern)
  Hygiene needs (bathing, grooming)
  Skin integrity
  Infection prevention
  Mobility and exercise
- Ensure a safe environment
- Provide consistency in all spheres of care
- Provide routine schedules and structured environment
- Promote orientation as necessary
- Provide cognitive and sensory stimulation
- Maintain adequate environmental stimulation
- Enhance socialization as tolerated
- Promote recent memory function and reminiscence
- Maintain pleasant, patient, gentle demeanor
- Use humor tactfully
- Refrain from challenge and confrontation
- Medicate when necessary
- Support and educate family and significant others. (When symptoms are reversible, rehabilitate through retraining and reeducation programs and offer hope for recovery; when condition is irreversible, avoid insightful explorations to prevent depression, anxiety, irritability, or rage.)

Care Plans for Delirium, Dementia, and Amnestic and Other Cognitive Disorders Based on Nursing Diagnosis

DSM-IV Diagnosis

Delirium
Dementia (all types)
Amnestic Disorders
Other Cognitive Disorders

NANDA Diagnoses

Thought processes, altered
Social interaction, impaired
Self-care deficit

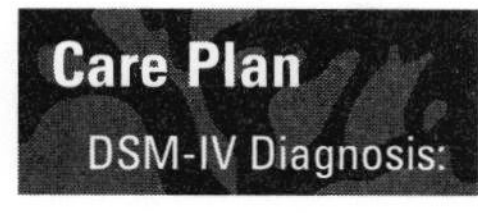

Delirium, Dementia, and Amnestic and Other Cognitive Disorders

NANDA Diagnosis: Thought processes, altered

The state in which the individual experiences a disruption in cognitive operations and activities

Focus:

For the client with dementia, amnestic disorders, and other cognitive disorders (e.g., Alzheimer's disease), who manifests significant disturbances in processing and expressing thoughts in a meaningful way, as a result of histopathologic changes in areas of the brain that control memory and cognition. Consequently, all areas of cognitive and perceptual operations and activities are affected, as the client struggles to retain logic and meaning.

NANDA Taxonomy

Pattern 8—Knowing: A human response pattern involving the meaning associated with information

ETIOLOGIC/RELATED FACTORS (RELATED TO)

Inability to process and synthesize information secondary to pathologic changes in the brain (neuritic plaques, neuronal degeneration, neurofibrillary tangles, brain atrophy)

Recent memory loss that progresses to remote memory loss and eventually extends to global memory loss

Disorientation, decreased concentration, confusional state

Loss of judgment, insight, comprehension, and problem-solving abilities

Impaired abstract thinking

Interruptions in logical stream of thought

Sleep-wake pattern alterations

Difficulty in focusing attention (distractibility)

Cognitive-perceptual alterations (delusions, paranoia)

Sensory perceptual alterations (hallucinations, illusions)

Life-style of dependence

Depressed state (pseudodementia)

Anxiety/apprehension

Fear

Biologic/genetic factors

DEFINING CHARACTERISTICS (AS EVIDENCED BY)

Early Stages

Demonstrates impairment in abstract thinking and reasoning.

Examples:

- Is unable to find similarities and differences between related words or objects (e.g., bus and train; sun and moon; bird and butterfly; dog and goldfish; window and door; pencil and typewriter)
- Has difficulty in defining words and concepts
- Assigns concrete meanings to familiar proverbs (e.g., "people who live in glass houses shouldn't throw stones" or "a rolling stone gathers no moss" are interpreted literally)

Manifests impaired judgment and decision-making skills in typical social situations.

Examples:

- Cannot figure out what to do if a mailman delivered a letter that was not addressed to them; what to do with a stamped, addressed envelope; what action to take if they lost a wallet; how to get help in the middle of the night; what to do if they were in a theater and a fire broke out
- Fails to make realistic or reasonable plans for self or others; cannot meet social or family obligations; is unable to get business affairs in order

Experiences difficulty in calculating simple problems, indicating inability to concentrate and focus on thoughts.

Examples:

- 4×3, 4×6, 42×6, 162×20
- Cannot count backward from 100 in increments of 7

Note: This commonly used test may be influenced by the person's education level.

Exhibits deficiencies in general knowledge, in accordance with educational, sociocultural, and life experiences.

Examples:

- Does not know president of the United States or other well-known world leaders
- Cannot name state capitals or names of oceans
- Cannot state current issues or news events

Note: Information should be based on generally known phenomena.

Demonstrates inability to learn or comprehend new knowledge, which indicates deficits in perception, retention, association, and recent memory function.

Examples:

- Cannot retrieve new content 5 to 10 minutes after it is given (e.g., an address—Apartment 13, Dover Hill Building)
- Cannot repeat a sentence, such as the Babcock sentence, 5 to 10 minutes after it is given (e.g., "one thing a nation must have in order to become rich and great is a large and secure stack of wood")
- Cannot verbalize four unrelated words after 5 to 10 minutes (e.g., boy, window, dog, love)

Note: Persons with dementia have difficulty in recent memory acquisition or learning. This may be a key to early detection of dementia.

Exhibits significant recent memory impairment as indicated by inability to verbalize remembrances after several minutes to an hour.

Examples:

"How long have you been here?"

"What happened just before you came here?"

"What time did you get out of bed today?"

"What did you eat for breakfast today?"

Is able to recall early life events or events from childhood (e.g., place of birth, name of school, vocation or profession, place of work)

Note: The accuracy of past memory may not be readily assessed as early life events cannot be refuted by the examiner.

Demonstrates lack of insight: the ability to perceive self realistically and to understand self.

Example:

- Cannot respond to such questions as "Why did you decide to come to this facility at this time?" or "Have you noticed any change in yourself or in your outlook on life?" or "Have you noticed any change in your feelings?"

Exhibits impairment in semantic or knowledge memory.

Example:

- Is unable to develop a scenario upon request; cannot synthesize and think about events (e.g., unable to describe what he or she did from dinner until bedtime)

Note: Semantic memory is used in language, abstraction, and logic and is generally impaired in persons with Alzheimer's disease.

Advanced Stages

Demonstrates intermittent confusion, disorientation, and poor conceptual boundaries in strange surroundings, as expressed by inappropriate verbal statements

Note: Acute or chronic confusion is more common in delirium than in dementia; nighttime confusion may indicate sedative intoxication or age-related sleeping changes; daytime confusion may indicate a bilateral cerebrovascular accident or lingering hypnotic effects.

Uses confabulation (attempts to fill in the memory gaps with fabricated or made-up responses) when unable to remember or recall events

Note: Confabulation is *not* lying. Often, the person with an amnestic condition in which memory is lost for a time or for certain life events may still be aware of the environment and may use confabulation in an attempt to "cover up" the deficit.

Demonstrates aphasia (loss of language ability); cannot express thoughts through speech, writing, or via symbols; initially has difficulty searching for words and eventually becomes mute as disease progresses

Note: The most common cerebral pathologic condition associated with aphasia is vascular disease.

Manifests agnosia (inability to recognize once-familiar objects because of impaired ability to interpret sensory stimuli): initially the person has trouble recognizing everyday objects; in later stages he or she does not recognize loved ones, self, or own body parts

Note: Aphasia encompasses agnosia and apraxia.

Exhibits apraxia (loss of purposeful movement)

Note: Ideational apraxia means loss of ability to formulate the ideational concepts needed to carry out a skilled motor act; the person cannot conceive or maintain the idea. (Comprehension is normal in apraxia. Ideational apraxia accompanies diffuse cerebral disorders such as arteriosclerosis.

Example:

- A person forgets how to use a once-familiar utensil (e.g., an eggbeater or potato peeler) or cannot recall how to operate a stationary bicycle, although motor function remains intact.

Motor apraxia is decline of kinesthetic motor patterns necessary to perform a skilled motor act, usually related to a precentral gyrus lesion.

The term *ideomotor apraxia* is applied to a person who has lost the skills for a given complex act but may retain conditioned habits and perform them repetitiously (perseveration); may be associated with disease of the supramarginal gyrus.

Demonstrates circumstantiality (digression and extraneous thinking with cumbersome, convoluted detail) volunteered by the person but unnecessary to answer the examiner's questions

Note: This results from excessive associations of an idea that reaches the consciousness and interrupts the stream of logical thinking.

Displays stereotypy (persistently repeats words or phrases) owing to interrupted stream of thought

Manifests perseveration (multiple repetitions of words, phrases, or movements despite efforts to make a new response) related to interrupted stream of thought

Uses circumlocutory phrases (roundabout, non-goal-directed speech patterns); words or phrases seem to avoid meaning or conclusion; may be due to interrupted stream of thought

Demonstrates delusions (thought content disturbance, a fixed belief not changed by logic).

Examples:

- Ideas of reference (object of environmental attention—being watched, spied on, or singled out)
- Alien control (passivity—being guided by external forces)
- Nihilistic (denies reality and existence: "I have no head, no stomach." "I cannot die." "I will live forever.")
- Self-deprecation (feelings of unworthiness, sinfulness, ugliness, or emitting obnoxious odors, generally seen in severe depression)
- Grandeur (elated states, e.g., great wealth, strength, or power, sexual potency, identification with a famous person or God)
- Somatic (organic preoccupations, e.g., having cancer, obstructed bowel, leprosy, or some horrible disease). In severe depression with psychotic features, somatic delusions take on bizarre qualities: a "rotting gut," "heart made of stone," or "brain as a bag of worms." Somatic delusions are to be distinguished from a preoccupation with normal, visceral, or peripheral sensations.

Experiences obsessions and compulsions (thought or impulse disturbance): preoccupation with persistent idea, thought, or impulse that cannot be eliminated by logic, generally followed by an uncontrollable urge to perform an act to relieve anxiety; usually performed in ritualistic fashion according to certain rules held by the individual

Experiences hallucinations, illusions, depersonalization (sensory perceptual alterations). (*Hallucinations* are false perceptions that affect all the senses: sound, sight, touch, taste, smell, and somatic. *Depersonalization* is an alteration in the perception or experience of the self in which the usual sense of one's reality is temporarily lost or changed; feeling as if one is detached from body or mind).

Demonstrates emotional lability (may be due to delusion, hallucination, illusion, depersonalization, fear, anxiety, confusion, disorientation, memory loss)

Example:

- Individual who has been relatively calm and passive suddenly becomes angry and aggressive without apparent provocation.

Manifests depression that may perpetuate altered thought processes or result, in part, from the client's frustration related to progressive dementia.

OUTCOME IDENTIFICATION AND EVALUATION

Demonstrates intellect and judgment to the best of ability based on extent of organic pathology and residual cognitive functions

Reminisces about past life experiences by using long-term memory functions

Responds coherently to simple, concrete statements

Demonstrates absence of overt anxiety, fear, and confusion

Follows repeated, concrete directions

Maintains residual sensory-perceptual functions

Participates in some basic decisions about activities of daily life (e.g., selects favorite foods, chooses clothing to wear)

Oriented to person, place, and time

PLANNING AND IMPLEMENTATION

Nursing Interventions and Rationale

Approach the client gently with an open, friendly, relaxed manner. *Clients with Alzheimer's disease often "mirror'" the affect of those around them. A tense, hurried approach would reflect on the client, who may become anxious and resistant. A gentle, calm approach is comforting and nonthreatening.*

Identify yourself and look directly into the client's eyes, making sure you have his or her attention:

"Mr. Jones, I'm your nurse, Kathy."

Clients with cognitive and memory impairments need to have their nurse's identity constantly reestablished. If you do not have their attention, they could misinterpret your words and actions and become confused and frightened.

Speak to the client in a clear, low-pitched voice. *High-pitched tones create anxiety and tension in clients with Alzheimer's disease.*

Eliminate competing and distracting background stimuli (e.g., radio, television, extraneous talk) when speaking to the client. *Too much stimulation results in sensory overload and confuses the client.*

Ask only one question (or make only one statement) at a time, using short, simple sentences (try not to use more than five or six words at a time), *to decrease confusion, promote concentration, and increase attention span:*

"Are you cold?" "Are you hungry?" "Do you need to urinate?"

"Here is your pill." "Here is your robe."

"That door goes to the bathroom."

Repeat the question if the client does not respond or seem to understand your meaning. Use exactly the same words. *Repetition reinforces comprehension. Changing the words further confuses the client.*

Therapeutic response:

"Do you hurt?" (pause) "Do you hurt?"

Nontherapeutic response:

"Do you hurt?" (pause) "Are you in pain?"

Use "yes" or "no" questions whenever possible, and avoid those that require choices or decision making.

Therapeutic response:

"Would you like to go for a walk?" If the client says, "No," then ask, "Would you like to listen to music?"

Nontherapeutic response:

"Would you like to go for a walk or listen to music?" *Clients with cognitive impairment cannot make complex decisions and feel frustrated when confronted with such a task.*

(In the early stages of the disease, clients may be able to make simple choices.)

Rephrase the question after a few minutes if the client still does not seem to understand the words *to provide another opportunity to enhance understanding, although the client will need time to process new information. (Be patient.)*

Break down task into individual steps and ask the client to do them one at a time:

"Here are your eyeglasses." (pause) "Take them out of the case." (pause) "Put on the eyeglasses." (pause)

Clients cannot attend to more than one task at a time owing to cognitive and memory impairment. Accompany verbal communication with appropriate nonverbal cues or signals (as long as client has your attention) *to enhance client's understanding of your meaning:*

"Do you need to urinate?" (while showing the client the urinal)

"Do you want your sweater?" (while holding the sweater in front of the client)

Use gentle touch when appropriate (e.g., hold the client's hand; place a soothing supportive arm on the client's shoulder) *to communicate the physical expression of caring and empathy.*

(Gentle touch will usually be understood by most clients but may be misinterpreted by a client who is suspicious, paranoid, or delusional. Keen assessment is necessary.)

Use strategies to promote REM (rapid eye movement or dream) sleep.

Examples:

- Allow the client to walk around in a secure area during the day until tired.
- Eliminate or reduce naps during the day.
- Engage the client in an active daily schedule.
- Offer the person a little beer or wine at bedtime (when ordered).
- Offer low-dose sedative or hypnotic medication (with short half-life) if all else fails.
- If restraints are used, remove them when the client falls asleep.

REM sleep promotes rest and avoids confusion, disorientation, and irritability, which may occur as a result of sleep deprivation or disruptions in the client's usual sleep-wake cycle.

Increase stimulation if the client appears restless or confused or attempts to wander during the night (sundowner's syndrome) *to promote sensory stimulation that is missing during the quiet bedtime hours. Clients who are suddenly deprived of their routine daily activities require some stimulation at night to prevent restlessness and promote sleep.*

Examples:

- Place client in a room next to the nurses' station
- Maintain lighting in the room
- Provide some soft music (radio)

Observe the client closely for behavior cues that indicate pain or discomfort *because the client is not able to convey or describe thoughts or feelings.*

Examples:

- Change in posture (bending over)
- Facial grimacing
- Increased restlessness
- Sudden change in behavior

Arrange the unit with a reality-orientation board that includes easy-to-read clock, calendar (with date, day, time, season, weather), menu, name of facility, and city and state, *to enhance optimal memory function, orientation, and thought processes.*

Arrange pictures of familiar objects, utensils, foods, pets, or flowers in key areas on the unit with appropriate identifying labels *to stimulate memory function and cognition.*

Place familiar and cherished objects in the client's room (e.g., family photographs, pet pictures, quilt, statues) *to promote comfort and trust and enhance memory function.*

Use concrete language rather than abstractions or slang verbalizations when interacting with patients.

Therapeutic responses:

"Are you feeling OK?"

"It's time to sleep."

Nontherapeutic responses:

"How is it going?"

"It's time to 'hit the hay.'"

Clients with Alzheimer's disease have lost the ability to comprehend abstract or slang remarks and are confused and frustrated by them.

Maintain routine and structure within the unit rather than submit the client to daily changes in schedule. *The person with Alzheimer's disease has a difficult time coping with changes in routine, owing to short-term memory deficits and emotional lability. A consistent, structured routine supports memory function and orientation and reduces confusion and frustration.*

Use pictures to communicate with clients who demonstrate aphasia, as well as other cognitive and memory deficits, *to enhance the client's understanding of the meaning of the message.*

Redirect the person with a simple task or activity whenever he or she mumbles incoherently, rambles in a confused manner, perseverates on the same topic, or engages in stereotypic behaviors *to reduce confusion, obsessions, and compulsions and to provide a direction for the individual's disorganized thought processes and behaviors (refocus and rechannel anxiety-producing energy).*

Examples:

- Folding towels, pillow cases (familiar tasks are more likely to bring success)
- Stirring cookie or cake mix (familiar smells may have a calming effect)
- Simple exercises (may be done sitting down)
- Sit-down volleyball (use light beach ball)

Note: Repeating a task such as wiping the kitchen counter or folding linen for 20 minutes or more may be comforting. If and when the activity seems to be upsetting for the client, gently redirect him or her toward another activity.

Initiate a pet or plant therapy session with small, nonthreatening, gentle animals and fresh, green plants *to produce a calming effect; promote comfort, love, and affection; enhance the senses; and support memory function.*

Engage the client in frequent reminiscence sessions by reviewing past experiences (look through family photo album together and identify familiar loved ones) *to utilize functional remote memory and promote feelings of enjoyment and belonging—or, conversely, feelings of sadness or anger (client may need to vent extremes of feelings in a safe setting).*

Reassure and comfort a client who seems lost and confused because he or she is in a new or strange place. Inform the client where he or she is, why, and for how long *to decrease fear and anxiety related to feelings of abandonment or confusion and to promote orientation in a simple way:*

Therapeutic responses:

"Mrs. Walker, you are at the day care center for activities today; your son will come to take you home at 4 o'clock; that's 2 hours from now."

"Mrs. Long, this is Mrs. Davis's room. I'll walk you to your room now; it's right down the hall."

"Mr. Campbell, that door leads to the stairs; are you looking for the bathroom? I'll take you there."

(Be sure to pause between each statement.)

Nontherapeutic responses:

"Mrs. Walker, you know you come here 3 days a week; don't worry, your son will pick you up in a while."

This response assumes that the client will remember that she comes regularly to the day care center. There is also some terminology that may be interpreted concretely ("Your son will pick you up"), which may confuse the client.

"Mrs. Long, you're not supposed to be in the other clients' rooms; let's go back to your room and read your name on the door again."

This response scolds the client and thus infantilizes her, then assumes that if she reads the name on the door, she will remember her own room thereafter.

"Mr. Campbell, be careful, that door is the fire exit. What are you looking for, the bathroom again?"

This response assumes that the client knows what a fire exit is and that he can respond to an open-ended question ("What are you looking for?"), when it has been shown that the client is usually searching for the bathroom door and simply needs reminding.

Use colors creatively *to stimulate the client's visual sense, promote identification and direction, and enhance recent memory function:*

Suggest that the facility paint a different color on the door of each client's room, with clients wearing buttons of the same colors as their doors; include color-coded linen and bedspreads.

Initiate painting colored stripes on the floor to serve as codes to different areas in the facility.

(A chart with the various colors and the areas each color represents could be placed on the wall of the main room for continual viewing by the clients.)

Celebrate special events or occasions (e.g., holidays, anniversaries, and birthdays) with client and family (have birthday party with cake and decorations, invite clients and staff who are close to the client, and sing familiar holiday tunes, e.g., "Happy Birthday") *to enhance memory function with familiar traditions and to demonstrate warmth and caring.*

Refrain from confronting or arguing with a suspicious person about the truthfulness of the complaint, *as the client cannot control this behavior; instead, try to deal with the suspicion in the following ways:*

- Respond with empathy and reassurance to the feelings of loss and confusion.
- If the suspicion focuses on "theft," help the person recover the lost item (if feasible).
- Distract the person from the focus of suspiciousness with other tasks or activities, as persistence may lead to agitation and aggression.

Refrain from confronting or arguing with a suspicious or paranoid client; instead, distract the client by redirecting him or her to a more benign task or activity. *Pursuing the client's paranoid ideation may promote agitation or aggression, as the client is unable to respond verbally to logic and reason. Refrain from agreeing with confabulation or made-up stories; instead, gently correct the person rather than try to convince the person that he or she is wrong. This approach decreases anxiety and prevents any embarrassment the person may feel if he or she happens to be aware of his or her progressive decline in mental functions.*

Therapeutic response:

Client to nurse: "I remember you; you're Hilda who lives next door to me in New Jersey."

Nurse to client: "Mrs. Smith, good morning; I'm Karen, a nurse here at Sunnyvale Home in California; you live here now."

Nontherapeutic responses:

"Now, Mrs. Smith, I told you 5 minutes ago; this isn't New Jersey; it's California and I'm Karen. I don't know anyone named Hilda."

This approach attempts to convince the person she is wrong by strongly negating the confabulation, which may increase anxiety and shame and decrease self-esteem. It may also be a futile effort because of the client's short-term memory impairment, which may result in frustration for staff and client.

"Mrs. Smith, if you want this to be New Jersey, that's fine with me. How am I like Hilda?"

This approach agrees with the client, which could further distance her from reality. Asking to be compared with "Hilda" requires the client to process information in a way that may exceed her capabilities and be frustrating and confusing.

Refrain from agreeing or disagreeing with the validity of the client's delusion; instead, respond to the feelings that the client demonstrates *(which are real). Denying or confirming a fixed belief only increases the client's confusion and anxiety because a delusion can be both real and frightening to the client. Addressing the client's feelings and presenting reality in a gentle, nonthreatening manner will promote the client's trust, comfort, and reality.*

Therapeutic responses:

Client to nurse: "Everyone here wants to kill me; they want to see me dead."

Nurse to client: "Mr. Brown, you seem frightened; you won't be harmed here. This is a hospital and these people are nurses."

Nontherapeutic responses:

"Mr. Brown, don't get excited; no one wants to harm you; we all like you."

"Mr. Brown, what makes you think we want to hurt you? This is a hospital; we're your friends."

The first nontherapeutic response challenges the client's delusion by defending the staff and avoiding the client's underlying feelings (fear of being harmed).

The second response implies that the person has no right to his belief unless he can come up with a reason. Because the client may not be capable of such reasoning, he may become more confused.

Therapeutic response:

Client to nurse: "Who are you and what are you doing in my house? You must be a spy."

Nurse to client: "Mr. Jones, I'm Gloria, your nurse; this is your room; it's 5 o'clock and dinner is being served in the dining room."

In this approach the nurse presents reality by identifying herself, the client's room, the time, and the event (dinner) without challenging the delusion, to assuage the client's anxiety and paranoia and promote reality and comfort.

Nontherapeutic response:

"Mr. Jones, I live in this house, too. Remember me, my name is Gloria? Let's have dinner together."

In this approach the nurse validates the delusion by stating that she too lives in "this house." She fails to identify her role as a nurse or to orient the client to time or place, which may further confuse and disorient the client.

Avoid argument or confrontation with a person experiencing a hallucination; instead, listen to the feeling it invokes within the client and respond in a calm, noncommittal manner, without agreeing or disagreeing with the sensory misperception, *to assuage anxiety, reduce confusion, and present a nonthreatening reality.*

Therapeutic responses:

"Mrs. Smith, I don't hear the voices you hear, but it must be upsetting (or frightening) to you."

"Mr. Jones, those people on TV are talking about news events that are going on in the world today."

Nontherapeutic responses:

"Mrs. Smith, there are no voices here; stop worrying about it."

"Mr. Jones, those people on TV are talking to everyone, not just you."

The first nontherapeutic response argues with the client's perception without presenting a nonthreatening reality and fails to acknowledge feelings, which could increase anxiety and confusion. The second nontherapeutic response corroborates the client's perception by suggesting that the TV newspeople are "talking to everyone," which could also increase anxiety and confusion.

Avoid contradicting or challenging the person who is experiencing an illusion (misinterpretation of sensory stimuli); instead, offer a simple explanation of what the individual experiences *to decrease anxiety and promote reality orientation.*

Therapeutic responses:

"That noise is from the pipes under the sink."

"The curtains are being moved by the wind."

"That shadow is from the lamp."

Nontherapeutic responses:

"No, there is not a strange man in the room."

"No one is trying to climb in the window."

"That shadow is not an evil spirit; there are no such things."

Educate the family and significant others about the effects of Alzheimer's disease and other types of organic brain disease on their loved one's short-term memory function and cognitive processes, as well as their struggle to recall past events. *Awareness of the client's capabilities and limitations helps families acquire more realistic expectations and reduces their frustration.*

Teach the family and significant others effective strategies to enhance the client's memory function and decrease confusion *to facilitate communication and interpersonal relationships between clients and families.*

Examples:

- Provide reminiscence sessions
- Maintain structure and routine
- Convey patience and understanding

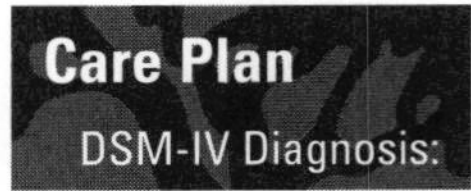

Delirium, Dementia, and Amnestic and Other Cognitive Disorders

NANDA Diagnosis: Social interaction, impaired

The state in which an individual participates in an insufficient or excessive quantity or ineffective quality of social exchange

Focus:

For the client with dementia, amnestic disorders, and other cognitive disorders that reflect deterioration of mental functions owing to response of the brain to disease or damage, resulting in impairment in social skills and inability to relate to others in a healthy, functional manner

NANDA Taxonomy

Pattern 3—Relating: A human response pattern involving establishing bonds

ETIOLOGIC/RELATED FACTORS

Altered thought processes
Confused or disoriented state
Impaired intellect and memory
Sensory/perceptual alterations
Decreased sensorium
Loss of body functions
Self-care deficit
Fear, anxiety, depression
Panic or rage reactions
Self-concept disturbance/powerlessness
Compromised physical ability
Social isolation, apathy
Impaired verbal communication
Emotional lability

DEFINING CHARACTERISTICS

Demonstrates discomfort in social situations with peers, family, and/or others.

Example:

- Restless and agitated during family meals or gatherings (e.g., unable to sit through meals; responds angrily to routine requests such as "pass the salt" or to benign social chitchat)

Exhibits use of unsuccessful social interactions with peers, family, and/or others.

Example:

- Uses confabulation (e.g., conscious attempts to fill in memory gaps with wrong facts or information, not considered intentional lies)

Family reports change of style or pattern of interaction.
Examples:
- Apathy and withdrawal from social interactions and activities (e.g., ceases to attend usual social functions such as bridge club, golf; spends more time in room away from family)
- Lack of spontaneity in interpersonal relations (e.g., hesitates when responding to others, even when topic is familiar to client)

Demonstrates emotional lability (may be due to delusion, hallucination, fear, confusion, anxiety, frustration).
Examples:
- Displays sudden outburst of anger with no obvious provocation when approached by family member, nurse, or another client
- Begins to shout in the middle of an activity such as an exercise class or cooking group
- Expresses fear when nurse or family member attempts to help client into shower or bathtub (may be experiencing an illusion; e.g., shower could be misinterpreted as rain)

Exhibits decreased interest and care in activities of daily living (e.g., basic hygiene, grooming, household chores, business matters).
Examples:
- Forgets to bathe, use deodorant
- Fails to dress completely or appropriately (looks disheveled)
- Wears same soiled clothing repeatedly
- Ceases to do laundry, prepare meals, shop for food, feed family pets
- Stops paying bills, answering mail, attending meetings

Demonstrates diminished regard for social courtesies.
Examples:
- Responds to others with rude or vulgar remarks
- Forgets to thank others or excuse self when appropriate
- Behaves in stubborn or cantankerous manner in presence of others

Wanders aimlessly around facility or home without direction or sense of purpose (may end up in another client's room or bed)
Loses sense of direction in once-familiar surroundings (may be unable to find way home, inciting neighbors or police to search for him or her)
Demonstrates extremely impaired judgment in social behaviors.
Examples:
- Handles own fecal material instead of flushing it in toilet
- Smears feces on walls or furniture
- Disposes of excrement in inappropriate places (e.g., under the bed, in the closet, with no memory of it)

Displays perseveration in the form of compulsive, stereotypic behaviors.
Examples:
- Rubbing hands together until skin is raw
- Licks lips, chews lips or inside of mouth repeatedly
- Explores inedible objects with mouth (hyperorality)
- Taps fingers repeatedly on table top, or feet on floor when seated (irritates others)
- Folds and unfolds sheets, towels, blankets continuously (may be used as therapy as long as it does not irritate or exhaust client)

Demonstrates increased agitation when confronted with new or different situations or unfamiliar people
Exhibits increased restlessness and confusion at bedtime, especially when alone in dark room (sundowner's syndrome, due to sleep pattern disturbances and decreased stimulation)
Loses ability to read, write, connect lines, or draw figures with any depth or detail (agraphia)
Loses ability to carry out purposeful kinesthetic movement (motor apraxia).
Examples:
- Can no longer figure out how to operate once-familiar tools (e.g., eggbeater, hammer)
- Cannot recall how to use simple utensils (e.g., cutting with a knife and fork)

Displays apathy or indifference toward food (stops eating)

OUTCOME IDENTIFICATION AND EVALUATION

Demonstrates increased comfort during social interactions in accordance with capabilities
Exhibits relaxed posture and facial expression
Sits through meals and activities for longer periods of time without agitation or restlessness
Displays decreased emotional lability (angry outbursts, panic, rage reactions) when interacting with others
Responds favorably to reminiscence activities with staff, peers, and family
Interacts successfully when engaged in tasks and activities that are within range of interest and abilities

PLANNING AND IMPLEMENTATION

Nursing Interventions and Rationale

Determine all possible factors that may contribute to the client's decreased sensorium that would lead to cognitive dysfunction and physical and emotional agitation. *Alzheimer's disease is often not the only source of the client's impaired thought processes and interactions. The following problems need to be assessed and treated:*
- Hypoxia
- Electrolyte imbalance (sodium, potassium depletion)
- Renal, hepatic, cardiac, respiratory disorders
- Pain
- Malnutrition, vitamin deficiency
- Drug therapy effects

Initiate treatments necessary to correct the client's dysfunctions as much as possible (e.g., provide adequate fluid, electrolytes, nutrition, vitamins). Administer oxygen as ordered and assess medication effects and restructure medication schedule as necessary *to improve the client's sensorium and cognitive abilities and increase subsequent social interactions.*

Introduce yourself to the client and use eye contact with a calm, reassuring manner and gentle touch while addressing the client by name. *Alzheimer's clients are very sensitive to the moods and emotions of others and can become easily frightened or agitated by an indifferent or negative approach. Conversely, identifying oneself, eye contact, and a calm, gentle approach have a soothing effect on the client and help him or her to focus on subsequent interpersonal interactions. (Refrain from touching a client who is suspicious or paranoid.)*

Use simple, concrete terms and a clear, modulated voice tone to explain procedures to the client *to enhance comprehension, as clients with sensory and cognitive deficits have difficulty understanding abstract terms or vague, unclear generalities. Also, soft, low voice tones may be inaudible if the client has a hearing problem.*

Reduce extraneous environmental stimuli (e.g., loud noise from radio, TV, and unnecessary talk or motion) or accompany client to a quieter area. *Clients are very sensitive to the emotional environment, and reducing distracting stimuli eliminates sensory overload, decreases confusion, prevents agitation, and promotes relaxation.*

Ensure that clients who need dentures, hearing aids, or eyeglasses wear them whenever needed *to enhance the senses and reduce frustration and confusion. Clients who have trouble hearing, seeing, or speaking may misinterpret the environment or be misinterpreted by others, which could further impede social interactions.*

Refrain from challenging or arguing with a client who reacts catastrophically to a situation (rage, aggression); instead, remain calm and remove the client from whatever may be upsetting him or her. *Clients with Alzheimer's disease are sensitive to the behaviors of others and are likely to calm down when distracted by a reassuring nurse. When verbal skills are lost, the client's feelings are generally appropriate, but exaggerated, so that the behavior is socially inappropriate. Distraction, therefore, is more effective than arguing or reasoning.*

Refrain from confronting or arguing with a suspicious, paranoid, or delusional client about the truthfulness of his or her complaint *because the client cannot respond to reason, and challenging the client may result in anger or aggression.*

Refrain from forcing the client to comply with situations that seem to frighten, confuse, or antagonize him or her; instead, wait until the client is more calm and composed. *The client may be experiencing a hallucination or illusion, and the use of force may provoke a panic attack, rage reaction, or aggression and result in harm or injury. Often, the client will calm down after some sleep, rest, or distraction.*

Use strategies and responses that reduce or avoid anger, agitation, and aggression to protect client and others from injury.

Examples:

- Demonstrate empathy and reassurance for the feelings of loss and confusion.
- If the suspicion focuses on "theft," help the person recover the lost item for as long as appropriate (if feasible).
- Distract the person from the focus of suspiciousness with other tasks or activities, rather than pursue the focus of suspicion.

Offer prescribed low-dose medication (haloperidol is a frequently prescribed antipsychotic) if the client's agitation cannot be managed by other means *to reduce the client's agitation and prevent escalation of behaviors that may be harmful. Observe for troubling/untoward effects.* (See Appendix M for a list of medications and effects, and Glossary for *extrapyramidal effects* and *neuroleptic malignant syndrome.*)

Gently restrain the client if he or she cannot be distracted and behavior escalates to an unmanageable level (release the client from restraints as soon as possible) *to protect the client and others from harm or injury.*

(Refer to Guidelines for Seclusion and Restraint, Appendix L.)

Adhere to routine care (whether client is cared for by family or nursing home staff) *to decrease confusion and agitation and avoid regressive behaviors (e.g., acting out, incontinence, smearing feces).*

Redirect the person with a simple task or activity whenever he or she perseverates or engages in stereotypic behaviors (e.g., rubs hands together; taps fingers on tabletop or feet on floor; folds or unfolds sheets, pillowcases, towels) *to redirect anxiety-producing energy toward constructive ends. (Folding towels may be comforting for about 20 minutes. If and when the client seems upset with the activity, redirect him or her toward another activity or interaction.)*

Engage the client in short, routine social interactions throughout the day, using a calm, gentle approach, familiar, simple topics, and concrete language, *to avoid sensory overload, enhance memory function, and support clear thought processes and positive social interactions.*

Demonstrate patience when the client hesitates before initiating conversation or responding to others' requests; attempt to anticipate his or her needs. *Urging the client to speed up his or her remarks or requests only frustrates and confuses the client. Meeting the client's needs prevents adverse effects.*

Use humor when feasible but not at the expense of the client. *Humor is a universal language and an experience that enhances communication and social interactions.*

Ignore crude or vulgar remarks or actions made by the client while assessing the intent behind the client's words or activity. *Clients with Alzheimer's disease occasionally lose their capacity to control socially inappropriate behaviors or expressions. The needs underlying the behaviors should be met by family and/or staff.*

Example:

A client who acts or speaks in a sexually explicit manner may be attempting to get in touch with that part of self that was once sensual and productive. The nurse can engage the client in another rewarding, enjoyable activity such as music, exercise, or preparing a meal.

Assess the client's ability to perform once-familiar motor acts, for example, operating tools, utensils, or instruments (stationary bicycle, eggbeater, using knife and fork together to cut), and offer assistance when necessary. *Clients eventually lose the ability to carry out purposeful, kinesthetic movements (motor apraxia) and need help.*

Assist the client with basic care and personal hygiene needs, such as bathing, dressing, grooming, and cosmetics, *to promote comfort, build self-esteem, and protect the client from rejection or ridicule during social interactions with other clients.*

Allow the client to do as much as possible for himself or herself, as long as the effort does not become frustrating or confusing, *to build self-esteem and promote positive interpersonal relationships.*

Serve the client simple, easy-to-eat meals and drinks *to decrease the amount of time the client is required to sit in one place and to minimize restlessness and agitation.*

Engage the client in interactive therapies (e.g., music therapy, stretching exercises, cooking, sit-down volleyball) *to increase involvement and interpersonal interactions with staff and other clients during the day and to minimize apathy and withdrawal from social situations and activities.*

Arrange schedule so that the client stays awake (avoids naps) during the day. *Sleeping during the day may disrupt or prevent nighttime sleep and result in restlessness and agitation during the night.*

Assess the effectiveness of tranquilizers and any untoward effects they may have (if client is taking them to control agitation). *Drug dosage may need to be reduced or the drug schedule changed if it makes the client sleepy during the day; some tranquilizers may paradoxically increase agitation and confusion and interfere with the client's social interactions.*

(Refer to Appendix M for list of medications.)

Schedule tests and treatments for the morning and afternoon, *so the client can wind down in the late afternoon and evening, which helps to avoid excess stimulation before bedtime.*

Reorient the client in a calm, soothing manner if he or she awakens during the night *to avoid precipitating extreme agitation and loss of control.*

Family Teaching

Inform family members not to be alarmed when the client experiences confusion, anxiety, or rage; instead, calm the client by decreasing stimulation that may be distressing or accompany the client to a less stimulating area, remain with the client, and use stress-reducing strategies that have worked in the past. *Clients with Alzheimer's disease occasionally experience emotional lability, which may result not only from the effects of the disease in areas of the brain that control mood and affect but also from the client's overwhelming frustration and powerlessness. Reducing distracting stimuli helps to calm the client and focus him or her on the task at hand. Stress-reducing strategies decrease anxiety and prevent behavior from escalating to panic or aggressive states.*

(Refer to Appendix K for stress-reducing strategies.)

Educate family members that the client can no longer fully engage in the social conversation that generally accompanies mealtimes and other similar social situations *to increase the family's knowledge of the effects of Alzheimer's disease on the client's social capabilities and decrease their expectations so that they will not make demands that may agitate or anger the client unnecessarily.*

Teach the family that the client may use confabulation in social situations to hide memory deficits, not as an attempt to lie, and that arguing or disagreeing with the client would only antagonize him or her. *Increased knowledge about the behavioral effects of Alzheimer's disease fosters more positive interpersonal relationships between the client and significant others.*

Inform the family that the client reacts best to reminiscences about the past rather than to "here and now" conversations. *The recent memory stores are impaired early in the disease process, whereas clients can still recall many past events. Reminiscing good or bad times is a positive experience as it brings the client in touch with familiar feelings and engages him or her in more meaningful social interactions.*

Encourage the family to enroll clients who live at home in an Alzheimer's day treatment center (if possible), to enhance the client's daily social interactions, educate family members about the disease, and offer families a respite from the arduous care of their loved ones.

Remind families to place an identification band around the wrist of the client with Alzheimer's disease that includes the client's name, address, and other critical information *so that a client who wanders away from home may be returned to the family.*

Arrange for the family to attend Alzheimer's family centers *to learn about the disease and what they can do to help their affected member and to improve social interactions and interpersonal relationships between the client and family members.*

(Refer to Thought processes, altered, in this chapter for additional interventions.)

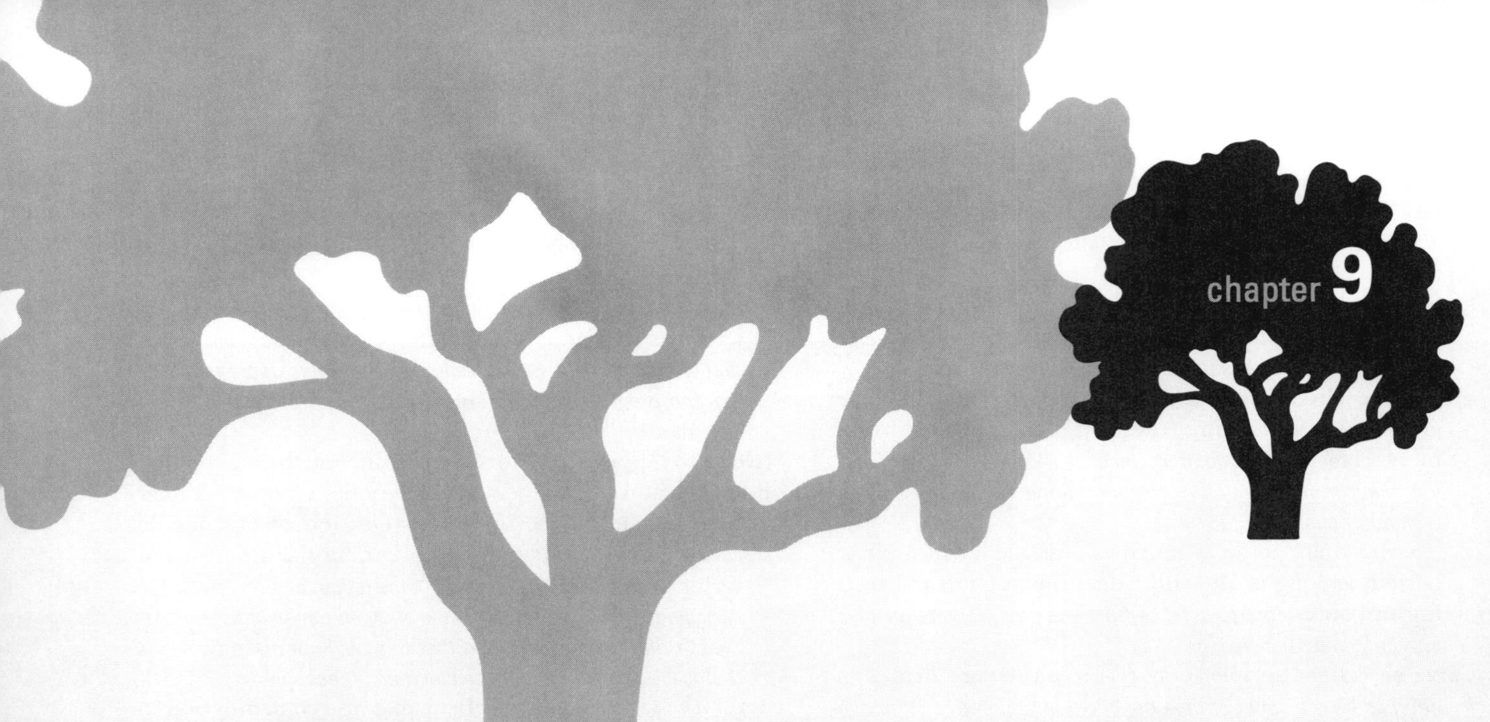

Substance-Related Disorders

Psychoactive substances are drugs or chemicals that, when taken into the body, alter one or several of the following: perception, awareness, consciousness, cognition, thinking, judgment, decision making, insight, mood, affect, and behavior. Substance use has been reported since recorded time began as people sought to alter body, mind, or spirit, and substance use and abuse continue today in increasingly larger numbers and varieties.

Moderate recreational use of certain psychoactive substances (e.g., caffeine, alcohol, tobacco) is accepted in many cultures, and numerous prescribed and over-the-counter substances are used for medicinal purposes (e.g., pain relievers, anxiolytics, sleep aids). Toxic substances (poisons, heavy metals, carbon monoxide, and nerve gases, among others) can also cause substance-related disorders. Regardless of the reason, when the use of substances becomes excessive or uncontrolled, disorders may result. Substance-use disorders and substance dependence are common throughout the world, not only in fast-paced industrialized cultures.

Abuse of, or dependence on, psychoactive substances frequently leads to major complications. In addition to the substance user's feelings of loss of control over choices, impairment of function often leads to inability to attain or maintain satisfying relationships and/or lifework, which contributes to perpetuation of subsequent failures.

Physical complications are common, either from direct drug action on the body or from neglect of nutrition, hygiene, and other aspects of health maintenance. For example, HIV-related diseases such as AIDS are a major complication from sharing needles to inject drugs. Other serious conditions are hepatitis, septicemia, malaria, tetanus, and endocarditis. In addition to being injected, psychoactive substances may be taken orally or intranasally or smoked. The 11 classes of psychoactive substances are listed in Box 9-1.

Substance-specific symptoms and behaviors occur with the use of each drug and are specifically described according to class in the section on diagnosis and in Appendix M. Criteria have been outlined for the general effects of substance use, abuse, and dependence in Box 9-2.

ETIOLOGY

Specific etiologic factors related to substance abuse are listed in Box 9-3.

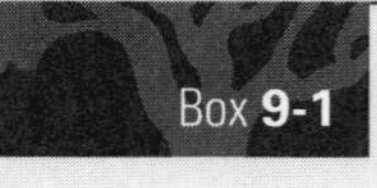

Classes of Psychoactive Substances

Alcohol	Inhalants
Amphetamines	Nicotine
Caffeine	Opioids
Cannabis	Phencyclidine
Cocaine	Sedatives, hypnotics, and anxiolytics
Hallucinogens	

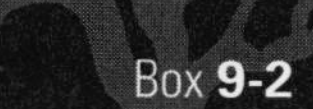

Box 9-2

Criteria for Effects of Substance Use, Abuse, and Dependence

Substance
A drug of abuse, a medication, or a toxin

Intoxication
Development of a reversible substance-specific syndrome following ingestion of or exposure to a substance. Maladaptive behavioral or psychologic changes occur (cognitive impairment, euphoria, labile mood, belligerence) because of direct physiologic effects on CNS.

Substance Abuse
A maladaptive pattern of substance use that results in clinically significant distress or impairment, evidenced by one or more of the following within 1-year period:

1. Role failure at home or work (neglect of family or home, multiple absences, expulsion from school, fired from job)
2. Continued substance use causing hazardous situations (driving vehicle, operating machinery)
3. Related legal problems (arrests for misconduct)
4. Social or interpersonal problems (recurrent arguments with boss or spouse)

Substance Dependence
A maladaptive pattern of substance use that results in clinically significant distress or impairment, evidenced by three or more of the following:

1. Tolerance: progressively increasing need for more of substance to achieve desired effect
2. Withdrawal, evidenced by either
   a. substance-specific withdrawal syndrome
   b. intake of same or related substance to prevent or relieve symptoms
3. Intake of substance exceeds original intention in amount or time (stops for one drink, takes six; plans to "party on weekend," but continues to drink throughout the following week)
4. Continuous desire or unsuccessful effort to control substance use (cut down or quit taking)
5. Much time spent to obtain drug(s), use drug(s), or recover from effects of drug(s)
6. Previously important activities reduced or replaced by drug behavior
7. Continued use despite awareness of physical or psychologic problems (stomach ulcer, drug-induced depression)

Note: Physiologic dependence is evidenced by tolerance or withdrawal.

EPIDEMIOLOGY

General Statistics

Sixty-five percent of the world's drugs are used in America

Box 9-3

Etiologic Factors*

Biologic
Use causes neuroadaptation, leading to dependence
Drug/alcohol dependence is a disease that occurs when a genetically predisposed person abuses the chemical, then finds cessation impossible

Behavioral
Use of psychoactive substances is a learned/conditioned behavior that continues because of reinforcement

Sociocultural
Acceptance/encouragement of use by culture
Excessive psychosocial stressors or deviant subcultures promote drug dependence

Psychoanalytic
Regressed, oral fixation level of psychosexual development; inadequate superego

Psychologic
Personality characteristics: narcissistic, insecure, impulsive, poor tolerance for anxiety

Family Systems
Enmeshed families that discourage individualization; codependency/enabler issues

*Although a specific etiology for these disorders is uncertain, a combination of biologic, psychosocial, and environmental factors contributes to their occurrence. Current research emphasizes biologic factors.

Half of all families in the United States have problems with psychoactive chemicals

Alcohol

Thirty-five percent abstain from alcohol entirely
Fifty-five percent have fewer than three drinks per week
Eleven percent drink 1 ounce or more per day
Ten percent of drinkers consume 50% of the alcohol
Consumption is highest and abstention is lowest between the ages of 21 and 34
Two to 5 times more men than women are heavy drinkers
Approximately 13 million people are diagnosed as alcoholic
Alcoholism is the third leading health problem
Onset in males is usually early (late teens, early twenties); onset in females is generally later
Higher rate of dependence in some cultures (Native Americans)
Affects all ages, cultures, socioeconomic classes
Involved in high percentage of crimes, accidents, and deaths

Marijuana

Marijuana is the most widely abused illegal drug
Ten million people use marijuana regularly
Five percent of high school seniors use marijuana regularly

Known as the "gateway" drug; use leads to use of other drugs, particularly cocaine

Cocaine/CNS Stimulants (Crack, Crystal Methedrine), Over-the-Counter Drugs

Crack (rock cocaine) is the most addicting drug known
Increased number of premature babies of low birth-weight with multiple neurologic problems; subject to becoming victims of child abuse
Incidents of sudden death reported owing to cardiac dysrhythmias

Nicotine

Nicotine is used by 30% of all adult Americans
Number of adults who smoke has decreased, while numbers of female, black, and teenage smokers are rising

Heroin

Heroin is the most widely abused opiate; its abuse has reached epidemic proportions in the United States
Male heroin users outnumber female users 3:1
Hepatitis B and AIDS occur in large numbers of the heroin-injecting population

DIAGNOSIS OF SUBSTANCE-RELATED DISORDERS

Psychoactive substances may alter consciousness, state of mind, mood, or behavior. The defining characteristics of substance-related disorders are (1) substance-specific symptoms and (2) maladaptive behaviors as a result of substance use, abuse, or dependence. Categories under substance-related disorders include the following:

I. (Substance)-Use Disorders
  A) Dependence
  B) Abuse
II. (Substance)-Induced Disorders

Several subcategories may be present under substance-induced disorders, and because the effects of each substance vary, so the subcategories vary. For instance, most of the substances have as subcategories mood, anxiety, and sleep disorder components. The actual symptom manifestations are dependent on the action (i.e., mood becomes depressed or elevated) of each drug and the context within which the symptoms occur (i.e., intoxication or withdrawal). See the DSM-IV categories of substance-related disorders in the DSM-IV box and in Table 9-1.

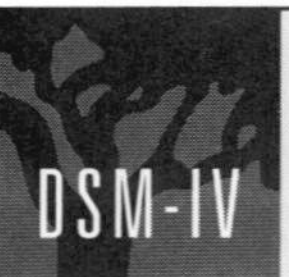

Substance-Related Disorders

DSM-IV Categories

The following specifiers may be applied to Substance Dependence:
With Physiological Dependence/Without Physiological Dependence
Early Full Remission/Early Partial Remission
Sustained Full Remission/Sustained Partial Remission
On Agonist Therapy/In a Controlled Environment

The following specifiers apply to Substance-Induced Disorders as noted:
[I]With Onset During Intoxication/[W]With Onset During Withdrawal

Alcohol-Related Disorders

Alcohol use disorders

Alcohol Dependence[a]
Alcohol Abuse

Alcohol-induced disorders

Alcohol Intoxication
Alcohol Withdrawal
Specify if: With Perceptual Disturbances
Alcohol Intoxication Delirium
Alcohol Withdrawal Delirium
Alcohol-Induced Persisting Dementia
Alcohol-Induced Persisting Amnestic Disorder
Alcohol-Induced Psychotic Disorder
  With Delusions[I,W]
  With Hallucinations[I,W]
Alcohol-Induced Mood Disorder[I,W]
Alcohol-Induced Anxiety Disorder[I,W]
Alcohol-Induced Sexual Dysfunction[I]
Alcohol-Induced Sleep Disorder[I,W]
Alcohol-Related Disorder Not Otherwise Specified

Amphetamine (or Amphetamine-Like)-Related Disorders

Amphetamine use disorders

Amphetamine Dependence[a]
Amphetamine Abuse

Amphetamine-induced disorders

Amphetamine Intoxication
Specify if: With Perceptual Disturbances
Amphetamine Withdrawal
Amphetamine Intoxication Delirium
Amphetamine-Induced Psychotic Disorder
  With Delusions[I]
  With Hallucinations[I]
Amphetamine-Induced Mood Disorder[I,W]
Amphetamine-Induced Anxiety Disorder[I]
Amphetamine-Induced Sexual Dysfunction[I]

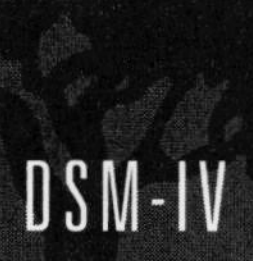

DSM-IV Substance-Related Disorders—cont'd

Amphetamine-Induced Sleep Disorder[I,W]
Amphetamine-Related Disorder Not Otherwise Specified

Caffeine-Related Disorders
Caffeine-induced disorders
Caffeine Intoxication
Caffeine-Induced Anxiety Disorder[I]
Caffeine-Induced Sleep Disorder[I]
Caffeine-Related Disorder Not Otherwise Specified

Cannabis-Related Disorders
Cannabis use disorders
Cannabis Dependence[a]
Cannabis Abuse

Cannabis-induced disorders
Cannabis Intoxication
Specify if: With Perceptual Disturbances
Cannabis Intoxication Delirium
Cannabis-Induced Psychotic Disorder
With Delusions[I]
With Hallucinations[I]
Cannabis-Induced Anxiety Disorder[I]
Cannabis-Related Disorder Not Otherwise Specified

Cocaine-Related Disorders
Cocaine use disorders
Cocaine Dependence[a]
Cocaine Abuse

Cocaine-induced disorders
Cocaine Intoxication
Specify if: With Perceptual Disturbances
Cocaine Withdrawal
Cocaine Intoxication Delirium
Cocaine-Induced Psychotic Disorder
With Delusions[I]
With Hallucinations[I]
Cocaine-Induced Mood Disorder[I,W]
Cocaine-Induced Anxiety Disorder[I,W]
Cocaine-Induced Sexual Dysfunction[I]
Cocaine-Induced Sleep Disorder[I,W]
Cocaine-Related Disorder Not Otherwise Specified

Hallucinogen-Related Disorders
Hallucinogen use disorders
Hallucinogen Dependence[a]
Hallucinogen Abuse

Hallucinogen-induced disorders
Hallucinogen Intoxication
Hallucinogen Persisting Perception Disorder (Flashbacks)
Hallucinogen Intoxication Delirium
Hallucinogen-Induced Psychotic Disorder
With Delusions[I]
With Hallucinations[I]
Hallucinogen-Induced Mood Disorder[I]
Hallucinogen-Induced Anxiety Disorder[I]
Hallucinogen-Related Disorder Not Otherwise Specified

Inhalant-Related Disorders
Inhalant use disorders
Inhalant Dependence[a]
Inhalant Abuse

Inhalant-induced disorders
Inhalant Intoxication
Inhalant Intoxication Delirium
Inhalant-Induced Persisting Dementia
Inhalant-Induced Psychotic Disorder
With Delusions[I]
With Hallucinations[I]
Inhalant-Induced Mood Disorder[I]
Inhalant-Induced Anxiety Disorder[I]
Inhalant-Related Disorder Not Otherwise Specified

Nicotine-Related Disorders
Nicotine use disorder
Nicotine Dependence[a]

Nicotine-induced disorder
Nicotine Withdrawal
Nicotine-Related Disorder Not Otherwise Specified

Opioid-Related Disorders
Opioid use disorders
Opioid Dependence[a]
Opioid Abuse

Opioid-induced disorders
Opioid Intoxication
Specify if: With Perceptual Disturbances
Opioid Withdrawal
Opioid Intoxication Delirium
Opioid-Induced Psychotic Disorder
With Delusions[I]
With Hallucinations[I]
Opioid-Induced Mood Disorder[I]
Opioid-Induced Sexual Dysfunction[I]
Opioid-Induced Sleep Disorder[I,W]
Opioid-Related Disorder Not Otherwise Specified

Phencyclidine (or Phencyclidine-Like)-Related Disorders
Phencyclidine use disorders
Phencyclidine Dependence[a]
Phencyclidine Abuse

Continued.

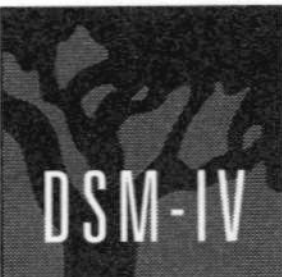

Substance-Related Disorders—cont'd

Phencyclidine-induced disorders
Phencyclidine Intoxication
Specify if: With Perceptual Disturbances
Phencyclidine Intoxication Delirium
Phencyclidine-Induced Psychotic Disorder
With Delusions[I]
With Hallucinations[I]
Phencyclidine-Induced Mood Disorder[I]
Phencyclidine-Induced Anxiety Disorder[I]
Phencyclidine-Related Disorder Not Otherwise Specified

Sedative-, Hypnotic-, or Anxiolytic-Related Disorders
Sedative, hypnotic, or anxiolytic use disorders
Sedative, Hypnotic, or Anxiolytic Dependence[a]
Sedative, Hypnotic, or Anxiolytic Abuse

Sedative-, hypnotic-, or anxiolytic-induced disorders
Sedative, Hypnotic, or Anxiolytic Intoxication
Sedative, Hypnotic, or Anxiolytic Withdrawal
Specify if: With Perceptual Disturbances
Sedative, Hypnotic, or Anxiolytic Intoxication Delirium
Sedative, Hypnotic, or Anxiolytic Withdrawal Delirium
Sedative-, Hypnotic-, or Anxiolytic-Induced Persisting Dementia
Sedative-, Hypnotic-, or Anxiolytic-Induced Persisting Amnestic Disorder
Sedative-, Hypnotic-, or Anxiolytic-Induced Psychotic Disorder
With Delusions[I,W]
With Hallucinations[I,W]
Sedative-, Hypnotic-, or Anxiolytic-Induced Mood Disorder[I,W]
Sedative-, Hypnotic-, or Anxiolytic-Induced Anxiety Disorder[W]
Sedative-, Hypnotic-, or Anxiolytic-Induced Sexual Dysfunction[I]
Sedative-, Hypnotic-, or Anxiolytic-Induced Sleep Disorder[I,W]
Sedative-, Hypnotic-, or Anxiolytic-Related Disorder Not Otherwise Specified

Polysubstance-Related Disorder
Polysubstance Dependence[a]

Other (or Unknown) Substance-Related Disorders
Other (or unknown) substance use disorders
Other (or Unknown) Substance Dependence[a]
Other (or Unknown) Substance Abuse

Other (or unknown) substance-induced disorders
Other (or Unknown) Substance Intoxication
Specify if: With Perceptual Disturbances
Other (or Unknown) Substance Withdrawal
Specify if: With Perceptual Disturbances
Other (or Unknown) Substance-Induced Delirium
Other (or Unknown) Substance-Induced Persisting Dementia
Other (or Unknown) Substance-Induced Persisting Amnestic Disorder
Other (or Unknown) Substance-Induced Psychotic Disorder
With Delusions[I,W]
With Hallucinations[I,W]
Other (or Unknown) Substance-Induced Mood Disorder[I,W]
Other (or Unknown) Substance-Induced Anxiety Disorder[I,W]
Other (or Unknown) Substance-Induced Sexual Dysfunction[I]
Other (or Unknown) Substance-Induced Sleep Disorder[I,W]
Other (or Unknown) Substance-Related Disorder Not Otherwise Specified

THE SUBSTANCES

Alcohol

Alcohol is an orally ingested central nervous system (CNS) depressant that affects every system in the body (see care plan for Injury, risk for, in this chapter).

Physical, psychologic, and interpersonal dysfunction is a by-product of alcohol dependence. Alcoholism is a chronic disease and is the nation's number one drug problem that involves a legal substance.

There are three major patterns of pathologic alcohol use:

1. Need for and consumption of large amounts daily
2. Regular and heavy weekend drinking
3. Long intervals of sobriety with intermittent heavy drinking binges that last weeks or months

Reports indicate an intergenerational familial pattern for alcoholism; that members of an alcoholic family have a higher inborn tolerance for alcohol. Use and abuse of alcohol are often accompanied by use or abuse of additional psychoactive substances (polysubstance abuse). Nicotine dependence is a common accompaniment; other substances frequently used are cocaine, heroin, amphetamines, cannabis, and sedatives, hypnotics, and anxiolytics.

Depression is often a concomitant disorder with alcohol dependence; however, the depression may be secondary

Table 9-1

Diagnoses Associated with Class of Substances

	Dependence	Abuse	Intoxication	Withdrawal	Intoxication delirium	Withdrawal delirium	Dementia	Amnestic disorder	Psychotic disorders	Mood disorders	Anxiety disorders	Sexual dysfunctions	Sleep disorders
Alcohol	X	X	X	X	I	W	P	P	I/W	I/W	I/W	I	I/W
Amphetamines	X	X	X	X	I				I	I/W	I	I	I/W
Caffeine			X								I		I
Cannabis	X	X	X		I				I		I		
Cocaine	X	X	X	X	I				I	I/W	I/W	I	I/W
Hallucinogens	X	X	X		I				I*	I	I		
Inhalants	X	X	X		I		P		I	I	I		
Nicotine	X			X									
Opioids	X	X	X	X	I				I	I		I	I/W
Phencyclidine	X	X	X		I				I	I	I		
Sedatives, hypnotics, or anxiolytics	X	X	X	X	I	W	P	P	I/W	I/W	W	I	I/W
Polysubstance	X												
Other	X	X	X	X	I	W	P	P	I/W	I/W	I/W	I	I/W

*Also hallucinogen persisting perception disorder (flashbacks).

Note: X, I, W, I/W, or P indicates that the category is recognized in DSM-IV. In addition, *I* indicates that the specifier with onset during intoxication may be noted for the category (except for intoxication delirium); *W* indicates that the specifier with onset during withdrawal may be noted for the category (except for withdrawal delirium); and *I/W* indicates that either with onset during intoxication or with onset during withdrawal may be noted for the category. *P* indicates that the disorder is persisting.

From American Psychiatric Association: Diagnostic and Statistical Manual of Mental Disorders, ed 4, Washington, DC, 1994, APA.

Box 9-4 Approximate Caffeine Amounts

Coffee	1 cup	100–150 mg
Tea	1 cup	50–75 mg
Cola	1 cup	30–50 mg
Over-the-counter substances and caffeine prescriptions	1 cup	⅓-½ strength of coffee
Migraine prescriptions	1 tablet	100 mg

to alcohol use, or individuals may drink to "fix" the dysphoria that is already present. Alcoholism and abuse of other substances are often complications in persons with bipolar disorder.

Amphetamines

Amphetamine is a CNS stimulant that is typically taken orally or inhaled, but may also be injected. Use often begins because of the drug's appetite-suppressing effects or the feelings of euphoria the drug produces. Binges may be followed by a period where the individual is exhausted, depressed, irritable, anergic, and withdrawn ("crash"). Paranoia, sexual dysfunction, memory, and attention disturbances are also common with amphetamine dependence. Tolerance to this drug may occur rapidly, resulting in an inability to experience euphoria and an increase of adverse symptoms.

Caffeine

Caffeine consumption in the United States is a common daily occurrence, as a majority of people begin the day with one or more cups of coffee or tea. Many individuals continue throughout the day, evening, and night to drink caffeine-laden beverages that include sodas and cocoa (Box 9-4). Other frequently used products that contain caffeine are chocolate, over-the-counter cold remedies, stimulants, analgesics, and weight loss medications. Symptoms of caffeine intoxication include restlessness, anxiety, insomnia, psychomotor excitement, periods of inexhaustibility, speeded thoughts and speech, increased bowel and bladder activity, tachycardia or cardiac dysrhythmia, muscle twitching, and flushed face. To date, caffeine abuse and dependence have not been clearly defined in DSM-IV; however, a caffeine withdrawal syndrome has been described that includes headache and may include fatigue, drowsiness, anxiety, depression, nausea, and vomiting.

Cannabis

The most common drugs in this group are marijuana, hashish, and purified THC (tetrahydrocannabinol), which are usually smoked but may be ingested orally. Cannabis may produce euphoria, calmness, drowsiness, and oneiroid states (a dreamlike state while awake) or anxiety, paranoia, and, in very high doses or with long-term use, hallucinations.

Dependence on cannabis is sometimes insidious due to the following: the ability of many users to continue to function socially and occupationally; the relative lack of the physical disorders that may accompany other drugs, such as cocaine, alcohol, or heroin. Major problems related to long-term marijuana use are (1) extreme amotivation that renders the individual unable or unwilling to attend to tasks that require persistence, (2) anxiety states, and (3) physical symptoms such as chronic res-piratory diseases, impaired immune responses, and hormonal dysfunction.

Cocaine

Cocaine, legally classified as a narcotic, produces extreme euphoria, so psychologic dependence may occur after the first use. Cocaine can be inhaled, injected, or smoked ("crack" or "freebase"), and in some cultures it is chewed as coca leaves. The clinical effects of cocaine are similar to the effects of amphetamines, and in addition to euphoria the individual may experience increased task performance, both mental and physical, and increased self-esteem. Intoxication occurs rapidly and is followed by a "crash" caused by dramatic depletion of serotonin. Withdrawal brings symptoms of dysphoria, fatigue, irritability, and anxiety; resultant depression is commonly accompanied by suicidal ideation.

"Crack" or "rock" cocaine has been labeled the most addictive drug known and is even more insidious, addictive, and toxic than cocaine. Cardiac dysrhythmias caused by cocaine use in all forms may lead to death. The number of babies born to mothers who use crack is increasing, and they are likely to be born prematurely and have low birthweight and numerous neurologic problems. They are also subject to abuse and neglect, a problem that is currently considered to be of major proportions.

Long term use of cocaine may produce the following:

Inhaled—Stuffy, runny nose; ulcerated or perforated septum

Smoked—Damaged lungs; increased susceptibility to infection

Injected—HIV or other blood-related diseases; infections; embolism

Hallucinogens

Naturally occurring hallucinogens (psychedelics) are found in some species of mushrooms (psilocybin) and cactus (peyote). One of the better-known synthetic hallucinogens is LSD (lysergic acid diethylamide). Hallucinogens are ingested orally and produce physical symptoms of tremors, heart palpitations, tachycardia, blurred vision, and diaphoresis. Psychologic symptoms include extreme perceptual, thought, and mood changes, in which the person may experience separation of self from the environment (depersonalization), heightened sensual stimulation (colors become brilliant; sounds, smells, and tastes are intense; and synesthesia [seeing sounds, hearing visions] may occur), fear of going crazy, labile mood, experiencing two feelings at the same time, or an excessive sense of attachment toward or detachment from others.

"Flashbacks" and "bad trips" are often associated with the use of psychedelics. Flashbacks are a reexperiencing of the drug-induced state that occurs in the absence of recent ingestion of the drug—a reliving of the event. Bad trips refer to a frightening panic reaction to hallucinogen intake. Psychoactive substances may trigger latent psychotic disorders.

Inhalants

Inhalants are volatile substances such as hydrocarbons, esters, ketones, and glycols that are found in paints, glue, gasoline, cleaners, spray can propellants, and typewriter correction fluids. When breathed in through the mouth or nose, these substances act as a CNS depressant, producing dizziness, ataxia, excitement, and euphoria that can lead to aggressiveness and impulsivity. Permanent kidney, liver, and brain damage can result, or death may occur because of depressed respiratory centers.

Nicotine

Nicotine is used most frequently by smoking cigarettes, but nicotine may also be taken by smoking pipes or cigars, chewing tobacco, and inhaling snuff. Cigarette smoking is the most difficult of these habits to break, and in 1989 the surgeon general declared nicotine to be one of the most addicting drugs in the world. The difficulty in stopping nicotine use hinges on several factors, including the reinforcers of repeating the process so many times per day (one pack per day = approximately 7300 cigarettes per year multiplied by numbers of puffs per cigarette!), the availability of cigarettes and the omnipresence of smokers, and the adverse symptoms that occur upon withdrawal from cigarettes. Withdrawal symptoms include anxiety, irritability, nicotine craving, restlessness, increased appetite, and weight gain.

The number of smokers has decreased in the general public but has increased among women, adolescents, and blacks. Cigarette smoking has been implicated in several diseases, including cancer, cardiovascular disease, and emphysema.

Opioids

Opium, the basic substance in this group, occurs naturally in the opium poppy, and several psychoactive substances are derived from it, including morphine, heroin, and codeine. Many synthetic opioids are used in this country, including propoxyphene (Darvon), meperidine (Demerol), and methadone (used in treatment programs to assist in withdrawal from natural opioids, especially heroin).

Opioids may be ingested, smoked, or nasally inhaled. Clinical effects include drowsiness, analgesia, decreased consciousness, mood changes, euphoria, and pleasurable feelings. Heroin, used medically in other countries because of its excellent analgesic properties, is illegal in the United States. Opioids are respiratory depressants and can lead to death through their direct effect on the respiratory centers of the brain. Deaths due to heroin have increased at an alarming rate in the United States because of increased and unexpected purity (potency) of the illegal drugs.

Heroin is the most commonly abused opiate; it is estimated that there are as many as 600,000 heroin addicts in the United States alone. In countries where opiate originates (mainly the Middle and Far East), the incidence per capita is much higher. Once established, opioid dependence dominates the individual's entire life.

Phencyclidine

Phencyclidine (PCP) and similarly acting arylcyclohexylamines such as ketamine or TCP can be taken orally, taken intravenously, smoked, or inhaled. PCP was originally used as a general anesthetic but is now used only by veterinarians because of the severe symptoms that clients experience when emerging from anesthesia.

Users of PCP find the drug effects unpredictable, but many experience feelings of euphoria, warmth, floating sensations, and vivid fantasy in the form of hallucinations and oblivion; users may also experience depersonalization, estrangement, and isolation. PCP psychosis can occur and may be more prevalent than currently recognized because of the unreliability of commonly used drug detection tests. PCP intoxication can lead to convulsions, coma, and death.

Sedatives, Hypnotics, and Anxiolytics

A pattern of use relating to each substance in this category and leading to dependence usually begins through either (1) a prescription given by a physician that eventually fosters prominent drug-seeking behaviors in which the client may subsequently seek several doctors to get an adequate supply of the substance or (2) illegal sources obtained for the purposes of "getting high" with peers or for use with other illicit drugs to enhance, potentiate, or counteract effects. All sedatives, hypnotics, and anxiolytics are cross-tolerant with each other and with alcohol.

Benzodiazepines are among the most widely prescribed and abused legal drugs in the country. Tolerance for remarkably high doses can occur, and, as is true for most other substances in this category, these drugs are capable of producing physical and psychologic dependence. Withdrawal from these substances by addicted individuals can cause death. (See Appendix M for listing of benzodiazepines.)

Polysubstance Dependence

Frequently individuals who use psychoactive substances take several kinds either simultaneously or sequentially. For example, abusers of cocaine may also use alcohol or anxiolytics to contend with anxiety, or marijuana and opioid users may counteract the effects of those drugs by taking amphetamines, anxiolytics, or sympathomimetics.

Repeated use of at least three psychoactive substances (not including caffeine or nicotine) for 6 months or more, without the predominant use of one substance, fulfills the criteria for polysubstance dependence when dependence criteria are met.

INTERVENTIONS FOR SUBSTANCE-RELATED DISORDERS

Individuals with substance-related problems benefit from a multiple treatment approach that includes psychologic and physiologic treatment and support, as well as sociocultural and spiritual counseling when appropriate. If recovery is to be successful, total change in life-style is required by the person who is dependent on substances. Treatment focuses on (1) acute intoxication and withdrawal episodes, (2) chronic health effects of substance abuse, and (3) rehabilitation, which includes changing long-standing self-destructive behavior patterns.

Hospitalization

Overdoses of psychoactive substances can result in medical emergencies or death if intervention is not available. When available, intervention is usually focused on dysfunction or failure of the cardiorespiratory system. Persons may be hospitalized following emergency treatment if the drug user's physical or psychologic dysfunction dictates.

Physical conditions other than an overdose that warrant medical attention include drug toxicity, withdrawal syndrome, infections, and physical debilities such as dehydration, malnutrition, and allergic reactions. Psychologic impairment for which clients may be hospitalized can manifest in one or more of the organic syndromes described earlier, in aggressive behaviors that cause danger to self or others, or in behaviors causing grave disability of the client. Examples include suicidal or homicidal threats, gestures, and attempts and the inability of the client to meet his or her own needs because of compromised mental state.

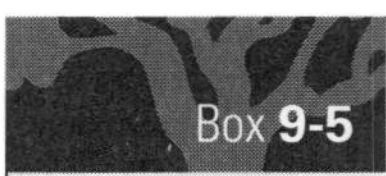

Box 9-5

Medications Used for Withdrawal Symptoms of:

Alcohol
For convulsions, intravenously administered diazepam (Valium); for delirium, orally administered diazepam, vitamin B complex, fluid hydration; for hallucinosis, haloperidol (Haldol); long term, disulfiram (Antabuse)

CNS Stimulants
For agitation, diazepam; for tachycardia, propranolol (Inderal), vitamin C

CNS Depressants
For barbiturates, phenobarbital in divided doses that are decreased daily or diazepam in decreasing doses; for benzodiazepines, gradually reduce doses over 10 days to 2 weeks or more

Hallucinogens
For mild agitation and anxiety, diazepam; for severe episodes, haloperidol. *Note:* Phenothiazines can be used only with LSD and can be fatal when used with other psychedelics.

PCP
Haloperidol; avoid phenothiazines for 1 week following ingestion of PCP

Opioids
For overdose, naloxone (Narcan) and oxygen (keep airway open); for withdrawal, methadone in decreasing doses over 10 or more days

Inhalants
For agitation, haloperidol

Modified from *Desk Reference on Drug Misuse and Abuse.* New York Medical Society, 1984.

Pharmacotherapy

Clients admitted to treatment facilities may receive medications during acute symptom or withdrawal phases from psychoactive substances. Box 9-5 lists some of the pharmacologic substances used.

Antabuse (disulfiram) is a deterrent drug that causes a violent toxic reaction when alcohol is also ingested. It works by inhibiting the enzyme that prevents accumulation of acetaldehyde in the blood. Clients become nauseated, hypotensive, flushed, hot, dizzy, and numb and experience malaise.

Interactive Therapies

Individual therapy. Problems commonly seen in substance abuse and dependence include denial, low self-concept and self-esteem, anger, manipulation, and dependency. Interventions for these problems are located in other chapters in this text. Denial is a major issue with drug abusers, and the client must admit and face the drug problem before recovery is possible. Another priority includes support of the client in his or her journey to wellness; that is best accomplished within a trusting relationship.

The nurse provides a mature nonjudgmental role model, firm and kind limit setting, and realistic encouragement and support as the client learns new ways to tolerate life's inevitable anxieties and to expand his or her social support network to include healthy, sober significant others.

Group therapy. Substance dependence group meetings are an integral part of treatment and provide the individual with support, education, necessary confrontation, coping strategies, and a social network.

Self-help groups. Alcoholics Anonymous (AA) is the model for other self-help groups that provide support for the drug abuser as he or she attains and maintains abstinence. Alanon is a group that provides education and support for spouses or significant others, and Alateen provides support for children of the recovering substance abuser. (See Appendix N.)

Behavior modification. Modification of behavior is a necessary step to recovery from substance dependence, and learning new strategies and techniques provides a method for mastering the environment. Behavior therapy can supply the individual with skills through relaxation training, thought and behavior substitution for self-control, and assertiveness training, to name a few. (See Appendix K.)

Aversion programs in the form of electric shocks or medications that produce vomiting upon drug intake have lost popularity in recent years.

Halfway houses. Transitional living arrangements provide recovering drug abusers interim homes and programs between detoxification and the eventual permanent home. They allow a slow adjustment to the community and ease the client's return home, which may have been a source of difficulty before becoming sober. Family therapy seems to be an essential component of successful recovery.

Employee assistance programs. Many employers have established employee assistance programs to help employees recover from drug or alcohol dependence while retaining their positions; some make participation mandatory if the individual desires continued employment. Statistics for loss of dollars from lost productivity related to substance dependence have risen dramatically in the past decade, and employee assistance programs have proven profitable alternatives to firing trained and skilled personnel.

Family therapy. Family therapy is a critical component in the ongoing recovery of the person who uses alcohol or drugs, as members attempt to eliminate enabling and codependent behaviors that perpetuate the problem. Therapy is directed toward helping the family gain awareness of the negative effects of enabling and codependent behaviors and develop strategies based on more confrontational approaches. (Refer to care plan for Coping, ineffective family: disabling, in this chapter.)

DISCHARGE CRITERIA FOR SUBSTANCE-RELATED DISORDERS

Maintains abstinence
Admits to lifelong dependence on psychoactive substances
Expresses knowledge of continual process of recovery ("one day at a time")
Verbalizes realistic goals
Maintains attendance in support group (Alcoholics Anonymous, Narcotics Anonymous)
Expresses increased self-esteem
Verbalizes decreased guilt, loneliness, shame, despair, anger
Demonstrates methods and strategies for managing anxiety, frustration, and anger
Lists tangible substitutes to replace drug-seeking, drug-taking behaviors (hobbies, school, employment, volunteer work, social functions)
States feeling in control of own life
Expresses hope for future
Attends self-help group (client and family)
Abandons people and situations that influence and contribute to drug-taking behaviors
States consequences of psychoactive substances on biopsychosocial/cultural/spiritual well-being
States names and phone numbers of resources to contact when unable to cope or feeling a need to revert to substance-taking behaviors
Investigates substance abuse assistance programs such as an employee assistance program (EAP)
Continues with Alcoholics Anonymous (AA) if warranted
Supports family and/or significant others to attend Alanon and Alateen

Nursing Process for

Substance-Related Disorders

Universal Principles for Interactions and Interventions for Clients with Substance-Related Disorders

- Continue to monitor assessment parameters listed in *Defining Characteristics.*
- Continue to consider the etiologic factors listed in *Etiologic/Related Factors.*
- Utilize principles of the *Therapeutic Nurse-Client Relationship* (Appendix G).
- Address clients' spiritual and cultural needs.

General Principles

- Maintain health, safety, nutrition, and hygiene for client in crisis because of psychoactive substance use such as overdose, withdrawal, intoxication, and organic mental disorders.
- Examine own awareness, biases, and attitudes regarding substance dependency.
- Establish nonjudgmental, trusting relationship.
- Assess client's level of function/dysfunction.
- Focus on identified strengths.
- Help client build self-esteem.
- Maintain positive, supportive attitude concerning client's recovery.
- Provide mature role modeling.
- Provide feedback to client regarding effects of substance abuse on self and others.
- Engage client in milieu activities and groups.
- Engage client and family in family therapy and self-help groups.
- Encourage client to participate in substance dependency program.
- Assist client to set realistic and attainable goals such as the "one-day-at-a-time" philosophy.
- Assist client to overcome denial.
- Provide client with information that assists him or her to gain intellectual understanding of chemical dependency.
- Provide educational information for client and family.
- Teach effective coping strategies to client and family.
- Praise client and family for initial and continued efforts toward abstinence.
- Teach client how to identify psychosocial stressors and how to recognize, manage, and prevent symptoms associated with potential relapse.
- Identify ongoing sources of support for client and family.

Care Plans for Substance-Related Disorders and Substance-Induced Disorders Based on

DSM-IV Diagnoses

Substance-Related Disorders (all types)
Substance-Induced Disorders
Alcohol-Related Disorders

NANDA Diagnoses

Denial, ineffective
Coping, ineffective family: disabling
Injury, risk for
Violence, risk for: self-directed
Violence, risk for: directed at others

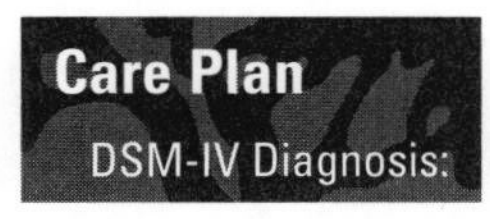

Care Plan

DSM-IV Diagnosis:

Substance-Related Disorders

NANDA Diagnosis: Denial, ineffective

The state in which an individual consciously or unconsciously attempts to disavow the knowledge or meaning of an event to reduce anxiety/fear to the detriment of health

Focus:

For the client who fails to participate in own health care or treatment program to improve health status or prevent illness, injury, or self-destruction, because of prevailing denial of substance abuse or dependency and its deleterious physiologic and psychologic effects on self and emotional effects on family, work, and community.

NANDA Taxonomy

Pattern 5—Choosing: A human response pattern involving the selection of alternatives

ETIOLOGIC/RELATED FACTORS (RELATED TO)

Negative self-concept, low self-esteem, sense of failure or inadequacy
Loss of self-confidence
Guilt, shame, loneliness, boredom, despair
Anxiety, depression, anger, frustration
Ineffective individual coping
A life-style of denial, projection, rationalization
Powerlessness
Hopelessness
Knowledge deficit regarding negative effects of substance abuse or dependency
Culturally permissive attitudes toward alcohol and drug use
Religious sanctions regarding alcohol and drug use
Ineffective problem solving, impaired judgment
Omnipotence (perceives self as indestructible)
Adolescent crisis, peer pressure, feelings of not belonging or being accepted
Adulthood crisis, job stress or loss, spouse or children pressures
Senior citizen crisis, loss of job, spouse, finances, functions; retirement

DEFINING CHARACTERISTICS (AS EVIDENCED BY)

Denies that psychoactive substances such as alcohol or drugs are problematic or destructive to patient or significant others:
"I don't have to give up alcohol/drugs; it's not a problem for me or my family."
"I know alcohol/drugs can be harmful to some people, but I can stop anytime I want to."
"I don't have a problem; I only drink on weekends."
"AIDS is something I don't have to worry about; I'm not the type to contract that kind of disease."

Delays seeking or refuses to accept treatment for substance use–related problems to the detriment of own health:
"I don't need any professional help; I'm feeling fine."
"I'll get help when and if my drinking/drug use gets out of hand."

Cannot admit negative impact of alcohol/drug problem on activities of daily living:
"I'm a good parent; I love my family, and they know it."
"I never miss a day's work; my boss and coworkers have no complaints about me."

Fails to perceive fear of consequences (death or chronic illness) as a result of alcohol/drug use:
"I've never been sick a day in my life, and I plan to keep it that way."
"I'm healthy now and I don't worry about getting ill or dying."
"Longevity runs in my family; I'll live a long, healthy life."
"Alcohol/drugs will never interfere with my health."
"I've never had any symptoms related to alcohol/drugs."

Resorts to self-medication for headaches, gastrointestinal problems, sleep disorders, or tremors related to alcohol/drug use:
"When I occasionally feel bad because alcohol/drugs affect me the wrong way, I get what I need at the drugstore."
"I know exactly what to take to relieve my hangovers; I don't need a doctor."
"I can take care of myself; I have some old family remedies."

Denies potential or actual financial crisis as a result of substance use/abuse:
"No matter what happens, my family will never go without food, clothing, or a home; I'll see to that."
"I'll always make sure that my family is financially secure; I'm not worried about that."
"I'm a good provider; that's all that matters."

Justifies use of alcohol/drugs (rationalization):
"Everyone needs something to lift the spirits; life is rough sometimes."
"The drink/drugs I take during lunch help me get through the rest of the day."
"It's no fun to be the only sober one at a party."
"I get a little shaky at work sometimes; a little drink/pill calms me down so I can do a better job."
"The high feeling I get from alcohol/drugs makes me feel good and doesn't hurt anyone."

Blames others for use of alcohol/drugs (projection):
"I need to take alcohol/drugs; my employer/job is very demanding and stressful."
"My kids are so noisy in the evening; after a day's work I can use a relaxing drink/drug."

"If you think I'm bad, you should see Tim; he puts away a six-pack of beer before lunch, and I don't start drinking until I'm off work."

"Being a wife and mother can be so unfulfilling sometimes; taking a little 'nip/snort' helps me feel more important."

"It's been lonely since my fiancé left me; an occasional drink/pill takes away the pain."

Blames sociocultural permissive attitude toward alcohol:

"Our family always drank wine with meals; I've been drinking since I was young."

"We always had cocktails before dinner at our house; it was a family ritual."

"What good is a picnic or barbecue without beer?"

"Drinking and drugs have always been part of important social gatherings."

Uses religion as a means to sanction substance use:

"Wine has long been used as a symbol during many religious ceremonies."

"There's nothing wrong with drinking a little wine; it's part of our religious ritual."

Reports need for increased amount of alcohol/drugs to reach same effect (increased tolerance; e.g., requires two drinks during lunch instead of one to get the same effect):

"Pour me another drink, dear, the last one seemed so weak; it didn't do anything for me."

Continues to drink/use drugs despite obvious dangers; drinks or takes drugs inappropriately (e.g., driving while intoxicated; drinking/using drugs while at work or school).

Attempts unsuccessfully to abstain from psychoactive substances (going "on the wagon"); individual has recurrent/intermittent periods of abstinence but continually reverts to using substances:

"I try to cut down on alcohol/drugs, but, frankly, I really don't see the need."

Expresses suspiciousness toward others (paranoia):

"I sometimes feel people are out to get me; they're always after me to stop using alcohol/drugs."

"I'm tired of people hounding me about alcohol/drugs; they're all against me."

Verbalizes grandiose, omnipotent feelings:

"I'm practically indestructible. A little alcohol/drugs can never hurt me."

"Alcohol/drugs actually make me feel as if I can rule the world."

Relates underlying low self-esteem:

"I feel more confident when I drink; what's wrong with that?"

"I seem to be able to talk more easily after a few drinks/drugs; people like me better."

Denies that physical problems are associated with alcohol/drug use (e.g., individual continues to drink despite knowledge of enlarged liver, ulcers, cardiac problems, blackouts):

"I actually feel better when I drink; my hands stop shaking." (withdrawal symptoms)

"My wife/husband thinks that alcohol/drugs are causing my sleeping problems. Actually, insomnia runs in my family."

Minimizes alcohol/drug-related symptoms:

"My stomachaches and morning headaches are from stress; I need to learn how to relax more."

"My family and friends tell me I often do things I don't recall later, but I've never been in real trouble during those times." (blackouts)

Displaces source of symptoms to other organs or conditions:

"My physical ailments are not due to alcohol/drugs; I have a little ulcer and it gets irritated once in a while."

"I always get shaky when I drink too much coffee; caffeine really makes my heart beat fast."

Makes dismissive gestures or comments when responding to others' concerns about alcohol/drug use (e.g., shrugs shoulders and changes the topic when confronted; makes jokes to diminish seriousness of problem):

"I'm fine; I know just how much alcohol/drugs I can take; I've never been drunk/stoned to the point that I didn't know what I was doing."

"Don't worry about me; I've never missed a day's work because of booze/drugs."

Seeks doctor's prescription for medication to "calm down" or "get a good night's sleep":

"All I need from my doctor is a tranquilizer to settle my nerves."

"If I can just get my doctor to prescribe a little something to help me sleep, I'll be fine."

OUTCOME IDENTIFICATION AND EVALUATION

Admits to alcohol/drug abuse problem:

"I realize I have a problem with alcohol/drugs."

"I can't control my intake of alcohol/drugs."

"Once I start using alcohol/drugs, I'm not able to stop."

Seeks medical or psychologic treatment for alcohol/drug problem:

"I need professional help for my dependence on alcohol/drugs."

"I admitted myself for treatment because I can't quit using alcohol/drugs by myself."

Describes the negative effects of alcohol/drugs on body systems and emotional health and well-being:

"Alcohol/drugs are ruining my health. If I don't stop, I could develop bleeding ulcers or have a stroke."

"I realize the potential threat of contracting AIDS through the sharing of dirty needles."

"I know about the possibility of fetal alcohol syndrome if I continue to use alcohol during pregnancy."

"I'm aware that smoking cigarettes or marijuana can cause lung cancer or emphysema."

"I've heard that cocaine use has been related to sudden death from heart failure."

"Alcohol/drugs have made me a nervous wreck; I'm agitated, anxious, and suspicious."

"When I use alcohol/drugs, I'm so preoccupied with my habit that I neglect myself emotionally and physically."

Explains the negative effects of alcohol/drugs on family, employment, and social life:

"My alcohol/drug habit has caused my family a lot of heartache. I never have time for my spouse and kids."

"My work is suffering because of my alcohol/drug habit. I can't seem to concentrate the way I used to."

"I'm sure I act peculiar when I use alcohol/drugs, our friends hardly invite us anywhere anymore."

Verbalizes need for continued treatment for alcohol/drug dependency:

"I realize that this is a lifelong problem for which I will always need help."

"I'm going to continue attending alcohol/drug meetings when I leave the hospital."

Attends all therapeutic groups and meetings while in treatment facility

Abstains from alcohol/drug use while in treatment facility

Expresses hope for an alcohol/drug-free future:

"I want to enjoy my family, friends, and work as a sober/clean individual."

"I'm eager to experience life without the effects of alcohol/drugs."

Uses effective coping methods and strategies to reduce stress and anxiety and build self-esteem:

- Engages in favorite sport or hobby (golf, tennis, dance, painting, sculpting)
- Exercises regularly (aerobics, walks, jogs, swims)
- Attends cognitive therapy and assertiveness training classes
- Uses biofeedback, meditation, or relaxation tapes or strategies
- Employs thought-stopping techniques
- Continues to attend alcohol/drug community meetings
- Learns to anticipate stress-producing situations and utilizes strategies to manage or avoid them (see Appendix K).

Reports positive changes in family, job, and social interactions as a result of abstinence from alcohol/drugs:

"I have much more quality time now with my spouse and children. We're all much happier."

"My employer says I'm doing so well that I may be up for a promotion. My coworker and I get along better, too."

"I enjoy myself so much better now at social functions. I know people like me for myself."

Notifies alcohol/drug hotlines, counselors, or support groups (AA/NA) whenever he or she is anxious, fearful, or depressed or craves alcohol/drugs after discharge

Participates in outpatient treatment centers, school programs (adolescents), and employee assistance programs (EAP) after discharge

Abstains from alcohol/drug use after discharge

PLANNING AND IMPLEMENTATION

Nursing Interventions and Rationale

Be aware of your own drinking/drug habits, biases, and attitudes before caring for clients with a diagnosis of alcohol/drug dependency. *Using your own thoughts, feelings, or behaviors about chemical abuse/dependency as guidelines for judging and treating others may sabotage the nurse-client relationship and must be addressed before treatment.*

Discuss your own feelings and biases regarding alcohol/drugs with qualified staff or therapists who can help promote objectivity *to ensure objective, high-quality care for the client with a substance-abuse problem.*

Approach the client in a direct, matter-of-fact, nonjudgmental manner *to gain trust and establish a therapeutic relationship:*

"I'm Kate, your nurse for the day shift. I'm part of the team who will help support you during your stay in the chemical dependency program."

Demonstrate concern and interest for the client as a worthwhile individual who deserves help, rather than use direct confrontation initially.

Therapeutic response:

"Jim, the staff cares about you, and everyone is committed to helping you succeed in the program."

"Joan, you deserve to have things go better in your life; this program will help you with that goal."

Nontherapeutic response:

"Jim, the plain fact is you're an alcoholic, and treatment won't help until you admit it."

"Joan, you're addicted to drugs, and we can only help you when you face your addiction."

Showing concern builds trust and enhances self-esteem. Use of confrontation too early in the client's treatment may result in the client's rejection of your efforts because the chemically dependent person has a low frustration tolerance and low self-esteem. Also, drugs and alcohol alter perceptions and cause memory deficits, especially prevalent in clients with a history of blackouts or sensory perceptual impairment. As the relationship evolves and the client gains more psychologic and physical strength, he or she will be better able to accept the chemical dependency diagnosis.

Continue to demonstrate a positive, supportive attitude toward the client while acknowledging alcohol/drug problem *to increase trust and self-esteem by letting the client know he or she is not alone in the struggle and that staff will help the client gradually overcome denial, confront the problem, and progress toward the goal:*

"Staff realizes it took courage to seek treatment for your alcohol/drug problem; we'll continue to do our part to help you achieve a substance-free life."

"We give you credit for admitting yourself to the chemical dependency program. We'll continue to help you work at eliminating alcohol/drugs from your life."

Assist the client to list the times, amount, and situations related to alcohol/drug use *to help the client overcome denials. (This strategy is especially useful in the early stages of substance abuse and can be done in the form of a chart, log, or journal.)*

Help the client identify critical times in which he or she is vulnerable to alcohol/drug use (e.g., midmorning when the kids are most active; lunchtime in response to stressors at work; evenings after a hard day on the job; before bedtime to get a good night's sleep). *Awareness of key times when the client is prone to drug/alcohol use can assist the client to avoid being alone during these times and to fill those times with learned stress-reducing strategies that replace alcohol/drug use.* (See Strategies, Appendix K.)

Instruct the client to avoid social situations that trigger use of alcohol/drugs (e.g., watching television, attending a sports event, eating in a restaurant that serves alcohol). *Avoidance of situations that may influence the client to use alcohol/drugs is a major factor in maintaining abstinence.*

Help the client to develop an awareness of his or her strengths and abilities *to build self-esteem that will help the client more readily accept his or her vulnerability (chemical dependency) and comply with the treatment plan:*

"John, your coming here for treatment shows real strength of character."

"Pam, you have a real ability to get the group to attend to business; that's a strength."

Assess for nonverbal clues of substance abuse when the client persists in denying problem (e.g., verbal/nonverbal inconsistencies, deterioration of physical appearance, ineffective work performance, impaired social skills) *to help substantiate facts.*

Gently feed back to the client the observed negative effects of drugs and alcohol *to help the client gain clarity and discourage denial:*

"Don, you say you always feel OK, but you also state that your stomach hurts and you have headaches every day."

"Barbara, from your appearance it seems like you haven't felt well enough to care for yourself."

"Jack, you said you haven't been able to go to work for several days. What happened?"

"Joan, just before you were admitted, your family said you were extremely irritable and screamed at everyone."

Assist the client to gain an intellectual understanding that alcohol/drug dependence is an illness and not a moral problem *to eliminate denial and reduce guilt:*

"Chemical dependence is an illness that can be treated."

"Substance abuse is a treatable disorder."

Engage the client in milieu activities that bring success to build the client's confidence in his or her ability to perform successfully. *The client who succeeds in the mental health setting may be able to transfer those same behaviors to attempts to overcome denial and eliminate use of drugs/alcohol.*

Provide the client with educational information about the habitual nature of alcohol/drugs and its deleterious effects on all body systems (include information about HIV-related diseases, fetal alcohol syndrome, lung cancer, and cardiac dysrhythmias), psychologic well-being, and interpersonal relationships. *Increased knowledge and awareness of the negative effects of drugs/alcohol are critical factors in encouraging the client to break through denial and choose to abstain from substance use.*

Examples:

- Films/documentaries
- Pamphlets/books/articles
- Lecture/discussion

(See Appendix M.)

Engage the client in therapeutic groups *to break through ineffective denial and learn new alternative, effective coping strategies through the dynamics and universality of the group process.*

Examples:

- Role play, sociodrama
- Thought-stopping techniques
- Behavioral therapy
- Cognitive therapy
- Assertiveness training
- Process or focus groups
- Alcohol/drug 12-step groups

(See Appendixes K and N and Glossary.)

Communicate staff's ongoing support and expectations that the client will overcome substance abuse problem *to continue to instill in the client confidence and hope for success:*

"Staff knows you can succeed as long as you continue to adhere to the treatment program."

"You can do it; others with chemical dependency problems have succeeded, and we feel positive about you, too."

Engage the client and family in therapy groups with qualified family therapists *to help process the effects of alcohol/drugs on family interactions, devise methods to cope more effectively as a family unit, and assist the client to break through denial.*

Encourage the client to attend several self-help groups (AA/NA) and choose the one he or she is most comfortable with. *Each self-help group is unique, and the client is more likely to succeed with a group he or she can relate to.*

Teach the family the importance of joining companion groups such as Alanon and Alateen *to assist them to understand the concepts of codependency and enabling so they will be better able to change their responses and behaviors and define the boundaries between themselves and the chemically dependent member* (see Glossary).

Demonstrate continued patience with the client's progress and possible relapse. *Treatment of chemical dependence is a long, slow process, and the client may not always be in control. Loss of control and the need to use drugs are primary manifestations of the illness and require patience.*

Assist the client to engage in activities that interest him or her and that promote satisfaction *to replace time that was previously used for alcohol/drugs with rewarding, self-fulfilling activities.*

Assist the client to set short-term, attainable goals (e.g., one-day-at-a-time philosophy) *to prevent the client from becoming overwhelmed with unrealistic expectations and to promote success:*

"Plan to go one day without alcohol/drugs, and you will achieve your goal for today."

"If you're successful in abstaining from alcohol/drugs today, your goal for today will be attained."

"Think about tomorrow when it gets here. Today you successfully abstained from alcohol/drugs."

"Just stop using alcohol/drugs one day at a time rather than insisting you're going to give it all up forever."

Facilitate interactions between the client and other recovering persons *to help instill hope and offer support for continued abstinence.*

Urge the client to avoid previous companions who use alcohol/drugs *to help remove their negative influence on the client and to facilitate an alcohol/drug-free life-style:*

"It's necessary to break away from people who use alcohol and drugs if you want to remain alcohol/drug-free."

"It's best to make friends with people who are also recovering or who have never used alcohol or drugs."

"Recovering alcoholics or drug users can be influenced by persons who drink or use drugs."

"People who have been successful in their recovery are those who have broken away from friends who drink or use drugs."

Help the client replace companions who drink/use drugs with nondrinking/nonusing friends and acquaintances (e.g., introduce the client to members of Alcoholics or Narcotics Anonymous groups). *People who are recovering from alcohol/drugs have more opportunity for success if they associate with other recovering individuals who continually encourage and support them.*

Direct conversations toward realistic concerns and thoughts (e.g., how to reenter the social and work world, how to say no to peers who apply pressure to use alcohol/drugs, how to get through stressful situations) rather than allowing the client to get stuck in denial *to help the client overcome denial and concentrate efforts toward rebuilding a substance-free life.*

Construct situations in which staff and client role play ways to deal with concerns such as socialization, employment, and saying no to peers who use alcohol/drugs. *Role playing during nonstressful, nonthreatening times can help prepare the client to use learned strategies more easily in terms of stress.*

Offer positive feedback to the client whenever he or she socializes with others in the milieu, discusses problems related to drug use with staff and other patients, initiates conversations, and ceases to use ineffective denial, rationalization, projection, or intellectualization. *Praising the client for successful behaviors increases self-esteem and promotes repetition of positive behaviors.*

Praise the client and family for acknowledgment of substance abuse problem and continued participation in self-help groups (AA/NA, Alanon, Alateen, Naranon, Co-dependents Anonymous [CODA], Adult Children of Alcoholics [ACA], school programs, employee assistance program [EAP]). *Positive feedback builds self-esteem, reinforces continued treatment, and promotes abstinence.*

Note: The process of recovery for an individual with the diagnosis of chemical dependence is lifelong.

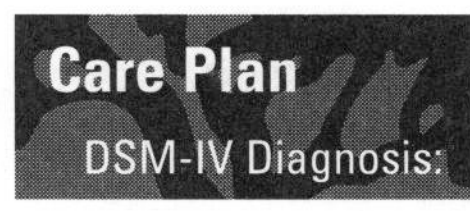

Substance-Related Disorders

NANDA Diagnosis: Coping, ineffective family: disabling

The state in which the behavior of a significant person (family member or other primary person) disables his or her own capacities and the client's capacities to effectively address tasks essential to either person's adaptation to the health challenge

Focus:

For the family that is unable to cope effectively, has a history of destructive overt or covert behaviors, and adapts detrimentally to a stressor such as a substance-dependent member. Differs from the nursing diagnosis Family processes, altered, which describes a family that generally functions well, but whose functions have been altered by a stressor that has exceeded the family's ability to cope

NANDA Taxonomy

Pattern 5—Choosing: A human response pattern involving the selection of alternatives

ETIOLOGIC/RELATED FACTORS (RELATED TO)

Family resistance to treatment for chemically dependent member

Enabling behaviors by family member(s) (See Glossary.)

Inability of family to confront source of problem

Ambivalent family relationships

Codependent family member(s) (See Glossary.)

Knowledge deficit regarding effective coping skills

Ineffective denial

Life-style of impaired family interactions

Destructive family patterns (e.g., domestic violence/abuse)

Self-esteem disturbance

Inadequate psychologic, physical, cognitive, or behavioral resources

Psychosocial stressors that exceed family's ability to cope

Antisocial personality traits demonstrated by family member(s)

Significant family member(s) with unexpressed feelings of guilt, shame, anger, anxiety, or despair

Biologic, genetic, or familial factors (e.g., family history of substance abuse)

DEFINING CHARACTERISTICS (AS EVIDENCED BY)

Distortion of reality regarding the family member's substance-abuse problem, including extreme denial about its existence or severity:

- Family ignores or defends against others' concerns about the member's chemical dependence.
- Family rejects others' attempts to help the chemically dependent member by denying the existence of the problem.
- Family demonstrates inappropriately excessive anger in response to queries about the chemically dependent member.

Demonstration of enabling behaviors toward chemically dependent member:

- Family makes excuses for member's substance abuse.

Examples:

Phones employer to say person is "too sick" to come to work; asks children to go to their rooms to play because parent needs to rest; explains to family and friends that spouse cannot attend a social function owing to a previous commitment

- Assumes other role(s) in addition to own role (e.g., gets a second job to pay bills, runs all errands, makes home repairs, mother coaches son's Little League team)

Nontherapeutic family intervention patterns:

- The chemically dependent member (victim) deceives family member (rescuer) into believing that he or she (rescuer) is therapeutic and that they have a close relationship.
- The victim does not cut down on using alcohol/drugs, but the rescuer avoids telling him or her and becomes a "patsy" because confrontation could endanger their "close" relationship.
- When the victim gets drunk/high, he or she calls the rescuer, who gets angry and assumes the position of "persecutor." The victim then asserts that the rescuer "never really cared" and feels rejected and abandoned.
- The rescuer feels guilty and engages in self-blame.
- The victim feels guilty and repentant and returns to the rescuer, and the pattern continues.

Neglectful care of the chemically dependent person.

Examples:

- Supplies person with alcohol/drugs; keeps liquor/pills in view of person or in unlocked cabinet/cupboard; drinks/uses drugs in presence of person

Decisions are detrimental to family's economic status.

Examples:

- Allows money to be used to supply chemically dependent individual's alcohol/drug habit so other family members go without food or clothing.

Neglectful care of family member's social well-being.

Examples:

- Fails to attend to social needs of individuals (e.g. misses PTA meetings, weddings; refuses invitations to join social clubs; ceases to go shopping or golfing with friends; stops inviting people home, including friends of the children, because of shame or embarrassment

Impaired roles and relationships of family members (holds family together in a paradoxical way); children assume various "roles" in order to survive:

- Hero, caretaker, or "super kid"; takes care of family, becomes little mom or dad; generally is an overachiever; needs approval
- Scapegoat: subject to anger, rage; will do anything for attention; takes the blame for family problem; frequently gets in trouble with the law or school authorities; gets admitted to a psychiatric hospital
- Mascot or "clown": uses humor to lighten up seriousness
- Lost child or "loner": shy, withdrawn, ignored, low achiever

(Refer to previous interventions for examples of enabling, codependent, and rescuer behaviors of spouses/significant adults.)

Note: Roles may overlap or interchange. Children may reverse roles with parent, and cook, clean, shop, remind them of appointments, locate car keys, and care for them when sick.

High rate of alcohol/drug use among family members:

Example:

- Spouse/children begin to abuse substances along with the chemically dependent person.

Frequent loss or change of jobs directly related to substance abuse

Prolonged overconcern for or overprotection of chemically dependent member, which promotes helplessness and dependence.

Examples:

- Drives individual home from bar or party after alcohol/drug binge; attends to member's daily basic needs; contacts family doctor for "medication" to ease physical and psychologic symptoms of substance abuse; hides "family secret" from other relatives, friends, neighbors, and coworkers

Extreme agitation, aggression, or violence among family members in response to frustration and anxiety.

Examples:

- Spousal or child abuse, neglect, or scapegoating

History of chronic anxiety and depression and possible suicide attempts by family members

History of truancy from school or work or other legal problems among family members

OUTCOME IDENTIFICATION AND EVALUATION

Family

Admits alcohol/drug abuse problem of family member to a trusted relative, friend, or professional person (e.g., physician, psychiatrist, nurse, clergy, or members of self-help group)

Attends self-help groups (e.g., Alanon, Alateen, Naranon) to educate self regarding relationship with chemically dependent person.

Examples:

- Does not defend against others' concerns or suspicions about the person's substance abuse
- Seeks or accepts help for chemically dependent individual

- Does not make excuses for alcohol/drug use (e.g., refuses to call employer when person is "sick"); does not hide problem from children, other relatives, friends, neighbors, or coworkers

Refuses to supply or make available alcohol/drugs for the chemically dependent person

Refuses to make finances available to replenish supplies of alcohol/drugs; instead, allocates funds for needed food, clothing, and recreation for other family members' needs

Engages in social functions that benefit nonchemically dependent members rather than hiding or retreating because of fear or shame.

Examples:

- Attends PTA meetings, weddings, and the like; socializes with relatives, friends, coworkers; encourages children to bring friends home

Maintains appropriate family roles and relationships.

Examples:

- Absence of children's roles (e.g., super kid, scapegoat, mascot, lost child); no significant role reversal (e.g., "caretaking")
- Absence of enabling, codependent, or rescuing behavior by spouse/significant adults

Ceases to overprotect the chemically dependent person.

Examples:

- Refuses to complete tasks, attend to daily needs, or hide family "secret"; refrains from contacting physician or emergency room for "medication" to bring "quick relief" of symptoms related to alcohol/drug use

Strongly encourages the chemically dependent member to enter a treatment facility for the survival of the family unit as well as the impaired member:

Examples:

- "John, your alcohol/drug habit is destroying you and the entire family; it's urgent that you get into treatment."
- "Barbara, your continued use of alcohol/drugs has disabled all of us. It's time to get professional help."

Demonstrates significant reduction in anger, aggression, violence, anxiety, or depression; instead manifests calm, stable, cheerful, mature behavior patterns.

Utilizes effective coping strategies to deal with substance abuse problem to vent feelings, share concerns, reduce stress, and decrease isolation.

Examples:

- Phones hotlines
- Seeks supportive individuals (relatives, friends, neighbors, clergy, counselors)
- Engages in positive social interactions and activities
- Attends self-help and other support groups

Replaces disabling behaviors with abling behaviors (begin with assisting chemically dependent member to enter into treatment while family also seeks help) to facilitate a healthy family system.

PLANNING AND IMPLEMENTATION

Nursing Interventions and Rationale

Assess the presence of factors that prevent the family from seeking or accepting help for the chemically dependent member ***to determine the best approach and area of referral.***

Examples:

- Fear for safety of self and children (abuse problems)
- Shame or embarrassment
- Low self-esteem
- Excessive guilt that justifies punishment
- Ineffective denial ("everything is OK")
- Family myth ("this family is no different from any other")
- Knowledge deficit regarding the severity of problem, community resources, legal rights
- Educational deficit regarding alcohol/drug dependence as a disease versus a moral problem
- Lack of finances
- Lack of support system
- Loss of independence
- Health problems

Provide opportunities for the family to discuss disabling effects of substance abuse problem when the family accompanies its member to the treatment facility ***to allow the family to validate their disabling coping methods in response to the stress of substance abuse and to develop an awareness of how those coping patterns perpetuate the problem.***

Examples of questions that elicit key issues:*

"How do you cope with the stress of alcohol/drug use in your family?"

"Is anyone in the family depressed or suicidal?" (If yes, proceed with suicide protocol.) (Refer to Appendix J.)

"What are your thoughts about the disease of alcohol/drug dependency?"

"What are the family's most urgent concerns/fears?"

"How do family members argue?"

"Is there abuse/neglect in the home as a result of alcohol/drugs?" (If yes, notify appropriate authorities, e.g., child protective services, law enforcement agencies, social services.)

"What would the family like to see change?"

"How do you think change can occur?"

"What is the family's source of support?"

"Are you aware of self-help groups such as AA/NA/ACA/CODA?"

"How can staff help you cope more effectively?"

Discuss with the family the importance of regular social contacts with trusted, supportive individuals ***to share concerns, reduce stress, and prevent isolation.***

Provide the family with a list of community services or agencies that offer information, education, and protection ***to ensure continued support that would strengthen the family's coping abilities.***

*Adapted from Carpenito, LJ: Nursing diagnosis: application to clinical practice, ed 5, Philadelphia, 1993, JB Lippincott.

Examples:
- Telephone hotlines
- Counseling agencies
- Legal services
- Family shelters
- Self-help groups
- Child/adult/senior protective services
- Financial aid services

Inform the family that alcoholism and drug dependence have deleterious effects on family systems *to encourage a realistic appraisal of the situation and dispel myths and guilt.*

Educate the family about the dangers of impaired roles and relationships among its members, especially the children, *to promote the knowledge that children from alcohol/drug-dependent families have a greater risk of becoming disabled adults (violent, suicidal, chemically dependent, antisocial, depressed, codependent).*

Teach the family that violence is not normal for most families; violence may stop but usually becomes worse, and the victim is not responsible for violence *to dispel myths and promote impetus for change through education.*

Group Intervention or Confrontation Strategy for Individuals Who Resist Treatment

Facilitate group intervention or confrontation strategy with skilled intervention therapists to privately assist family members, friends, employers, and coworkers to confront the chemically dependent individual by stating facts objectively, in a calm, direct manner, one at a time, without blaming, yelling, or nagging:

"Your speech was slurred when you came home last night, and you didn't respond when I told you our son was injured at school today."

"You've been in your bathrobe all week and haven't made our daughter's school lunches."

"You have alcohol on your breath (or needle tracks on your arms)."

"I found a bottle of whiskey (or pills, or syringe and vial) hidden in the bathroom hamper under the clothes."

"I was so embarrassed when you showed up drunk at my game, Dad."

"We used to have romantic times, but you haven't been able to engage in lovemaking for months."

Calm presentation of facts by significant persons helps the individual overcome denial and resistance by reinforcing awareness of problem and its effects on others, whereas yelling, blaming, or nagging tends to reinforce the denial because the chemically dependent person has a low frustration tolerance and diminished self-esteem.

Proceed with the next step of the group confrontation process by having family, friends, and employer make clear, direct statements of consequences if substance abuse continues *to facilitate the individual's entrance into treatment:*

"Either you enter a treatment program now or you will have to leave your job."

"Either you get help right away or the children and I will move out."

"Either you admit yourself to a treatment program or I will leave your home."

Note: The belief that chemically dependent individuals need to "hit bottom" before they admit their problem and seek help is no longer widely held. In many cases, interventions such as these can take place as soon as the problem is identified.

Teach the family (1) anxiety-reducing techniques *to decrease anxiety to a tolerable level, (2) assertive behaviors to facilitate mature communication responses, and (3) cognitive skills to increase self-esteem* (see Appendix K).

Praise the family for successful attempts to change disabling behaviors and use effective coping methods to manage life stressors. *Positive feedback reinforces positive behaviors and builds confidence and self-esteem.*

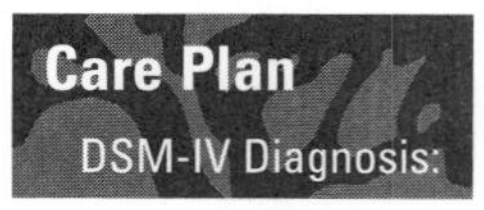

Substance-Related Disorders

NANDA Diagnosis: Injury, risk for

The state in which an individual is at risk for injury as a result of environmental conditions interacting with the individual's adaptive and defense resources

Focus:

For the client who is at risk for injury or disease as a result of potentially damaging effects of alcohol/drugs on physical, physiologic, and psychologic systems, related to psychoactive substance abuse; and potential for injury related to substance withdrawal behaviors

NANDA Taxonomy

Pattern 1—Exchanging: A human response pattern involving mutual giving and receiving

RISK FACTORS

History of injury related to drug/alcohol use.

Examples:
- Car accidents
- Arguments, fights, provocative behavior
- Continues to drive while under influence of alcohol/drugs

Effects of alcohol/drugs on all body systems, organs, and functions, including mental status.

Examples:
- Nutritional, metabolic
- Neurologic
- Cardiorespiratory
- Gastrointestinal

Complications of withdrawal from alcohol/drugs.

Examples:
- Agitation, anxiety, irritability
- Disorientation, hallucinations
- Depression
- Paranoia
- Craving

Organic psychosis:
- Dementia, delusions
- Hallucinations, illusions
- Altered spatial boundaries

Disinhibitor effects of alcohol/drugs on higher cortical centers:
- Impulsive, aggressive behaviors

Sedative or depressive effects of substances on the central nervous system.

Examples:
- Decreased sensorium
- Coma

Ataxia, unsteady gait, incoordination
Amnesia episodes or short-term memory lapses (blackouts)
Psychomotor agitation, hyperactivity, sensitivity, overreactivity
Perception of self as omnipotent, indestructible
Potential for fetal alcohol syndrome
Potential for HIV-related diseases as a result of contaminated needles
Susceptibility of ulcerated or perforated nasal septum related to drug inhalation
Susceptibility for physical disorders (e.g., lung cancer, emphysema, infections, cardiovascular diseases) associated with smoking cigarettes, marijuana

OUTCOME IDENTIFICATION AND EVALUATION

Demonstrates absence of injuries as a result of alcohol/drug use
Demonstrates absence of physical, physiologic, or psychologic symptoms related to alcohol/drug use
Demonstrates absence of substance withdrawal behaviors
Describes negative effects of alcohol/drugs on all body systems, organs, and functions
Explains that driving under the influence of alcohol/drugs can result in accident, injury, chronic disability, or death
Verbalizes potential psychologic effects of alcohol/drugs
Explains damaging effects of alcohol, crack, and other substances on fetal life
Abstains from use of alcohol/drugs
Attends self-help groups and employee assistance programs to maintain substance-free life-style
Explains the danger of contracting HIV-related diseases and their life-threatening consequences
Explains the potential danger of lung cancer and other life-threatening diseases related to nicotine and cannabis
Describes the danger of sudden death because of cardiac dysrhythmias caused by cocaine

PLANNING AND IMPLEMENTATION

Nursing Interventions and Rationale

Alcohol (withdrawal)

Know that the severity of withdrawal symptoms is related to the length and extent of drinking prior to withdrawal, that complete abstinence from alcohol is not necessary for the development of withdrawal symptoms, and that decreased use of alcohol in people who have developed a high tolerance and physical dependence may precipitate withdrawal symptoms. *Knowledge increases awareness and promotes client's safety.*

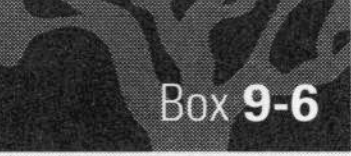

Box 9-6 Stages of Withdrawal From Alcohol

Stage 1: (8 hours or more after abstinence from alcohol): Mild tremors, nausea, nervousness, rapid heart rate, increased blood pressure, diaphoresis
Stage 2: Gross tremors, nervousness, hyperactivity, insomnia, anorexia, generalized weakness, disorientation, illusions, nightmares, hallucinations (mostly visual)
Stage 3: (12 to 48 hours after abstinence): All symptoms described in stages 1 and 2 plus severe hallucinations and grand mal seizures. Stages 2 and 3 are known as delirium tremens.
Stage 4: (3 to 5 days after abstinence): Initial and continuing delirium tremens manifested by confusion, severe psychomotor activity, agitation, sleeplessness, hallucinations, and uncontrolled and unexplained tachycardia.

Assess the client for symptoms of withdrawal as early as 8 hours after abstinence from alcohol; be aware that trauma victims (especially those with a history of head injury) and anyone suddenly admitted to the hospital or drug treatment facility must be observed for withdrawal symptoms *to protect the client from injury, accident, or death.*
Document behaviors and stage of withdrawal *so early symptoms (Stage 1) can be detected, treated, and controlled before client's symptoms progress (Stage 2)* (Box 9-6).
Administer medications at the first sign of withdrawal symptoms *to relieve early symptoms of withdrawal, prevent progression of more serious symptoms (e.g., seizures), and maintain health and safety.*
Stay with the client if he or she is agitated or confused *to ensure the client's safety and reduce fear and anxiety, especially during early phases of withdrawal or detoxification.*
Inform the client that symptoms represent the body's response to alcohol use and are temporary *to reassure the client that control over body functions will be regained.*
Use restraints only if the client loses control and is a danger to self or others *to protect the client and others from injury or destructive behaviors.*
(See Appendix L.)
Inform the client and family that restraints are only temporary and will be removed as soon as the client regains control *to assure client and family that safety is the only reason for restraints.*
Ambulate clients in stages 1 and 2 withdrawal as often as possible *to help the client use the energy of anxiety through goal-directed physical activity.*
Avoid ambulating clients in stages 3 and 4 withdrawal. *Increased activity and stimulation can promote confusion and hallucinations; in addition, the client is prone to convulsions or seizure activity and may sustain an injury.*

Reinforce reality if the client is disoriented, confused, or experiencing hallucinations or illusions *to promote reality orientation and reduce fear and confusion:*

"I'm Kathy, your nurse; you're in the hospital; that shadow is from the curtain on the window."

"Your family is right outside; that noise is coming from people in the waiting room."

Speak to the client in a calm manner with short, concrete statements *to decrease client's anxiety and reinforce understanding. Clients in withdrawal are generally agitated and confused, and calm, concrete responses are helpful.*

Reduce all unnecessary stimulation (lights, noise, movement). *A quiet environment helps to calm the client, promotes orientation, reduces confusion, and diminishes the incidence of illusions from lights, shadows, sounds, and touch.*

Remain with the client, especially during times of restraint, confusion, agitation, disorientation, and hallucinations, *to reduce symptoms, diminish fear, and promote comfort and trust.*

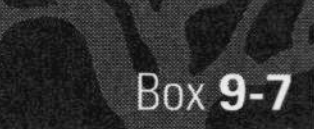

Box 9-7 Levels of Consciousness

- Full consciousness: alert, responsive; oriented to person, time, place; intact recent memory; verbalizes spontaneously, coherently; articulates clearly
- Impaired consciousness: drowsy, lethargic, loss of recent memory, slowed thought processes with appropriate responses
- Confusion/delirium: transient periods of disorientation, restlessness; dazed, uncooperative, easily agitated, irritable, fearful, noisy; responsive to verbal stimuli and light tactile stimuli
- Stupor: responds only to repeated verbal stimuli and continuous, painful tactile stimuli
- Coma: response to intense stimuli is either reflexive or absent

Alcohol (fluid and electrolyte balance)

Monitor intake and output every 8 hours and ensure a daily fluid intake of 2500 ml orally (unless contraindicated); offer juices every 2 hours while awake; discuss intravenous therapy with physician if intake is reduced or dehydration increases, *to ensure fluid and electrolyte balance and meet hydration needs. Dehydration of brain tissue can result in alcoholic "blackouts." Some authors say hypomagnesemia may contribute to blackouts. Hypokalemia is also a danger and can produce cardiac dysrhythmias.*

Drugs

Assess the client's level of consciousness *to intervene early in the process and prevent respiratory failure, cardiac dysrhythmias, irreversible coma, and death due to drug toxicity or overdose* (Box 9-7).

Initiate treatment according to clinical signs and symptoms, the object being to remove the toxic substance from the body as quickly and safely as possible in accordance with hospital protocol and current treatment methods for drug overdose *to prevent physiologic complications of drug toxicity and death.*

Document level of consciousness and report significant changes to physician *to maintain client's safety and prevent progressive decrease in levels of consciousness, coma, and death.*

Check vital signs and neurologic functions every 15 minutes until full consciousness returns *to maintain the client's vital functions and prevent irreversible coma, neurologic dysfunction, and death.*

Assess airway for patency and adequate ventilation; breathing patterns and respiratory tract for obstructions (e.g., mucus plugs, vomitus, tongue); turn head to side and have suction equipment available *to prevent aspiration and facilitate adequate respiratory function.*

Monitor client for symptoms of abnormal respiratory patterns such as wheezes, crowing respiration, apnea, and sternal retractions. Notify physician immediately if they occur *to initiate possible intubation or ventilation therapy as soon as possible.*

Have life-support systems available in accordance with facility's protocol *to sustain and maintain vital functions and prevent death as a result of respiratory failure or cardiovascular collapse.*

Monitor electrocardiography patterns; if necessary, initiate standard emergency life-support systems and notify physician and code team stat (according to hospital protocol) *to prevent cardiovascular collapse and death.*

Catheterize client as indicated; assess intake and output urine analysis, BUN, and other relevant laboratory studies *to determine toxic effects on kidneys due to psychoactive substances and prescription drugs and to evaluate possible need for dialysis.*

Administer appropriate intravenous fluids, progressing to oral fluids when condition permits; continue to monitor intake and output *to maintain fluid and electrolyte balance and to evaluate kidney function.*

Administer appropriate drugs (e.g., sedatives, antipsychotics) as ordered *to treat withdrawal symptoms or to prevent or treat psychosis related to drug toxicity.*

When the client is physically stable, assess for symptoms of organic mental syndrome (e.g., disorientation, aphasia, dementia) *to determine the degree of cognitive-perceptual dysfunction owing to the effects of drugs on the central nervous system and to develop an appropriate treatment plan.*

Communicate with the client in a calm, low-key manner, using low to moderate voice tones and short, simple statements, *to promote orientation, reinforce cognitive-perceptual functions, and decrease anxiety and agitation.*

Avoid using abstractions or proverbs; instead, speak in concrete terms when communicating with the client.

Therapeutic response:

"Jack, you're in the hospital because you have a drug problem; I'm Joan, one of the nurses who will help you."

Nontherapeutic response:

"Susan, you're here to 'get clean'; I'm one of the nurses who will help you beat the drug habit."

Individuals with cognitive-perceptual impairment have difficulty conceptualizing and require clear, concrete statements to enhance understanding and decrease frustration.

Assess the client for behaviors that reflect thought disorders (e.g., delusions, confabulation, ideas of reference, paranoia) *to determine the extent of the client's illogical thinking and develop a treatment plan that promotes logic and trust.*

Avoid challenging the client's delusional system too early in the treatment regimen; instead, try to determine the fears and concerns that may underlie the client's behaviors *to reduce incidents of aggression; clients may become extremely agitated in the early stages of withdrawal because of misinterpretation of the environment. If the client's perceived concerns and threats are addressed, trust and cooperation are more likely to occur.*

Therapeutic response:

"Don, it's not unusual to have uncomfortable thoughts now; what are your concerns when you say nothing can hurt you, and how can staff help you feel more comfortable?"

Nontherapeutic response:

"Barbara, what you're thinking just isn't true; you're not indestructible and you need to trust the staff so we can help you."

This incorrect response strongly negates the person's thoughts, ignores the underlying concerns, and defends the staff (by intimating that the client cannot be helped unless he or she trusts and complies). This type of response may promote the client's self-doubt, diminish self-esteem, and increase perceived threats, which can perpetuate mistrust, resistance, and aggression.

When the client is receptive, reinforce reality with simple, concrete statements in a calm, nonthreatening manner *to promote logical thinking and decrease risk of injury.*

Therapeutic response:

"Paul, you're saying that drugs can't hurt you because you're indestructible; actually you're here because drugs have been harmful to you."

"Sarah, I know you believe the clients acted as if they were all against you in group today; actually they were offering you some honest feedback about your denial."

Nontherapeutic response:

"Paul, why would you be here if drugs can't hurt you?"

"Sarah, it's not going to help you to think everyone's against you; you need to learn to accept the truth."

These incorrect remarks challenge the client in a condescending manner, which may reduce self-esteem and result in more mistrust and denial.

Assess the client for sensory-perceptual alterations (e.g., hallucinations, illusions). *Psychoactive substances are capable of crossing the blood-brain barrier and altering neurotransmitters such as dopamine, which can result in sensory-perceptual disturbances.*

Present a nonthreatening reality to the client who experiences sensory-perceptual disturbances *to correct the distortion without provoking agitation or aggression. Hallucinations or illusions can be very frightening to a client and cause misinterpretation of the environment, which can lead to injury.*

Assess the client (both adolescents and adults) for symptoms of depression and evaluate for suicidal ideation, gestures, attempts, or plans *to interrupt suicide and maintain client safety until he or she no longer demonstrates suicidal behaviors.*

(See Appendix J.)

Facilitate seclusion and/or restraint if the client verbalizes or demonstrates a risk for injury toward others because of the adverse effects of substance use/withdrawal *to protect others in the environment and maintain safety for the client and others.*

(Refer to Guidelines for Seclusion and Restraint, Appendix L.)

Help the client replace drug use with functional, healthy behaviors and activities *to prevent injury, illness, and destruction and maintain a drug-free life-style.*

Examples:

- Develop sports, hobbies, activities of interest.
- Acquire friends who abstain from drugs.
- Avoid situations and friends that encourage drug use.
- Attend therapeutic and self-help groups (Narcotics Anonymous, Cocaine Anonymous, employee assistance programs).

Alcohol/drug education

Teach the client and family about the physical, physiologic, and psychologic effects of alcohol/drugs *to educate the client about the potential for injury, illness, and disability as a result of substance use.*

Educate the client and family about the potential for injury, disability, or death as a result of driving an automobile while under the influence of alcohol/drugs *to deter the client from driving after drinking or using psychoactive substances.*

Explain to the client and family about the potential for injury to and death of a fetus as a result of the ingestion of alcohol or drugs during pregnancy *to discourage client from using psychoactive substances during pregnancy and to educate others.*

Examples:

- Fetal alcohol syndrome
- "Crack" babies

Discuss with the client and family the dangers of impulsive, aggressive behaviors as a result of the disinhibitor effects of alcohol/drugs on the higher cortical centers of the brain *to increase knowledge about potential of injury to self and others as a result of alcohol/drugs.*

Educate the family about the importance of their continued support, encouragement, and attendance at family self-help groups (e.g., Alanon, Naranon) *to promote the individual's continued recovery and prevent injury and illness related to drug use.*

Teach the client and family about the dangers of contracting AIDS and other blood-related diseases, reinforcing that AIDS is a life-threatening illness, *to promote knowledge and information and prevent drug use and related serous diseases.*

Alcohol (nutrition)

Eliminate caffeine from the client's diet (coffee, tea, cocoa, colas, chocolate). *Caffeine is a stimulant that results in tachycardia, which provokes feelings of anxiety and agitation. Withdrawal from any psychoactive substance produces the opposite effect of the drug itself. Because alcohol depresses higher cortical functions and has a disinhibitor, sedative effect on the central nervous system, withdrawal conversely produces anxiety, which would be increased by ingestion of caffeine products.*

Offer the client frequent high-protein foods and snacks and mineral and multivitamin supplements. *The person who craves alcohol is generally uninterested in a well-balanced diet and is therefore nutritionally depleted. Alcohol is an intoxicating by-product of yeast fermentation of carbohydrates (grains, molasses, starch, sugar) with relatively little nutritional value. Protein includes 20 or more amino acids ("building blocks of life") that are necessary to build body tissue, including hemoglobin that carries oxygen to the cells, antibodies for defense against disease, and enzymes for metabolism of nutrients. Vitamin and mineral supplements add to the dietary requirements. The B vitamins are especially critical in that they produce a calming effect on the agitated central nervous system and prevent anemia and peripheral neuropathy. Thiamine deficiency can produce Wernicke-Korsakoff syndrome.**

Teach the client and family about the need for a nutritionally balanced diet that includes foods high in protein and rich in B vitamins *to include the client and family in critical meal-planning that would increase the client's health status and develop a stronger immune system as a defense against disease and disability.*

Alcohol (physical care)

Provide the physical care necessary for clients with diseases, disabilities, or impairment as a result of the deleterious effects of alcohol on all body systems *to maintain health, safety, and comfort and prevent progression of injury and disease.*

Alcohol (depression)

Assess the client for signs of depression that may be experienced as a result of alcoholic life-style (secondary depression) or that may have been present all along and preceded alcohol abuse (primary depression). In either case, symptoms such as loss of energy, anorexia, feelings of worthlessness or hopelessness (adults) or apathy, acting-out behaviors, and trouble with the law (adolescents) must be addressed and treated *to prevent destructive behaviors and maintain health and safety.*

Assess the client for suicidal ideation, gestures, attempts, or plans; seclude and restrain the client, if necessary, *to prevent suicide.* Proceed with the following if the client has no specific suicidal plans but requires close observation:

- Remove all sharp objects from patient areas.
- Initiate other suicidal precautions as indicated by facility protocol.

(See Appendixes J and L.)

Alcohol (education)

Teach the client and family to replace alcohol/drug use with more functional, healthy activities and learning opportunities *to prevent self-destructive behaviors and maintain health and safety and a fulfilling, satisfying life-style.*

Examples:

- Participate in sports, hobbies, recreation
- Attain alcohol/drug-free social life
- Utilize "say no" strategy
- Attend self-help groups, employee treatment programs, and drunk-driving classes and seminars, as needed: Mothers/Students Against Drunk Driving (MADD/SADD); read about potential critical problems (e.g., fetal alcohol syndrome).

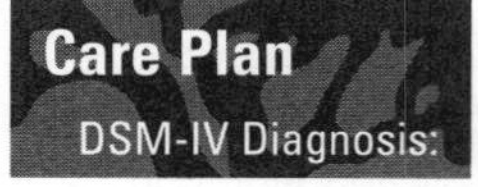

Substance-Related Disorders

NANDA Diagnosis: Violence, risk for: directed at others; Violence, risk for: self-directed

The state in which an individual experiences behaviors that can be physically harmful either to the self or to others

Focus:

For the client whose use/abuse of alcohol/drugs may lead to violent/destructive behaviors as a result of the disinhibitor effects of psychoactive substances, complications of withdrawal (agitation, excitement, irritability), flashbacks, depressed state, and psychoses (hallucinations, illusions, delusions)

NANDA Taxonomy

Pattern 9—Feeling: A human response pattern involving the subjective awareness of information

RISK FACTORS

History of violence related to drug/alcohol use

Complications of withdrawal from alcohol/drugs (e.g., agitation, excitement, suspicion, paranoia, euphoria, mania)

Psychotic symptoms (e.g., hallucinations, illusions, delusions)

Disinhibitor effects on higher cortical centers, leading to impulsive, aggressive, or violent acts

*Wernicke-Korsakoff syndrome is usually associated with alcoholism and characterized by confusion, disorientation, amnesia, and confabulation (thiamine deficiency).

Hyperactivity, extreme sensitivity, overreactivity, psychomotor agitation
Argumentative, provocative, boisterous behavior, verbal threats, threatening gestures (e.g., kicks furniture, slams doors, punches hand with fist)
Panic anxiety
Flashbacks
Low self-esteem
Hopelessness
Depressed state
Suicidal ideation, gestures, plans

OUTCOME IDENTIFICATION AND EVALUATION

Demonstrates absence of suicidal behaviors
Demonstrates absence of violence directed toward others
Abstains from substance use
Explains potential violent effects of alcohol/drug use
Demonstrates no substance-withdrawal behaviors
Manifests no hallucinations, illusions, delusions, paranoia
Demonstrates absence of depressive behaviors
Exhibits increased sense of hope (makes future plans)
Exhibits increased self-esteem
Demonstrates good impulse control
Exhibits no signs of agitation, excitement, irritability
Demonstrates absence of sensitivity, overreactivity, verbal threats
Replaces substance use with functional activities, hobbies
Attends therapeutic groups to maintain substance-free life-style and eliminate potential for violence

PLANNING AND IMPLEMENTATION

Nursing Interventions and Rationale

Assess the client's history for violent or self-destructive behaviors as a result of alcohol or drug use. *A history of violence is the best predictor of violence, and prediction is the most effective means of prevention.*

Assess the client for symptoms of withdrawal from alcohol and drugs *to protect the client and others from destructive behaviors as a result of agitation, irritability, excitement, paranoia, euphoria, or mania.*

(See Injury, risk for, care plan in this chapter for more specific details on withdrawal from alcohol.)

Administer appropriate prn medications to individuals who demonstrate withdrawal behaviors *to relieve symptoms, maintain health and safety, and prevent destructive acts.*

Assess the client for symptoms of organic psychosis (e.g., dementia, hallucinations, illusions, delusions) *to evaluate the extent of the client's reality orientation and intervene to prevent aggression or violence.*

Present a nonthreatening reality to clients who demonstrate psychotic features *to reinforce reality without challenging or angering the client and to prevent violence or aggression.*

(Refer to Injury, risk for, care plan, this chapter, for additional examples and interventions.)

Decrease stimulation when the client's behavior reflects a risk for violence (e.g., reduce noise, movement, lights, TV, radio); accompany the client to a quieter area *to promote a quiet, soothing environment that will calm the client's internal stimulation and reduce or eliminate the risk of aggression or violence.*

Avoid challenging clients who exhibit psychomotor agitation, hypersensitivity, overreactivity, low impulse control, flashbacks, verbal threats, threatening gestures, or pacing and escalating aggression *to prevent violence.*

Administer appropriate prn medications for clients who experience aggressive or destructive behaviors as a result of flashbacks, psychoses, or low impulse control *to protect the client or others from violence or harm. Offering medications during the early stages of agitation often can prevent behaviors from escalating and avoid the need for seclusion and restraint.*

Assess the client for symptoms of hopelessness, despair, or depression and for suicidal thoughts, gestures, or plans *to protect the client from self-destructive behaviors.*

(See Appendix J.)

Seclude and/or restrain clients who are potentially dangerous to themselves or others (e.g., uses verbal threats; exhibits suicidal ideations, gestures, or plans; perceives the environment as hostile and dangerous; demonstrates angry, impulsive outbursts toward others; experiences frightening flashbacks or psychoses) *to protect the client and others from violence or harm when other methods fail.*

(See Appendix L.)

Engage the client in short, simple, concrete interactions during the day, in a calm, low-key manner, *to continually assess the client's potential for destructive behaviors with minimal distraction and stimulation.*

Provide frequent time-outs, especially when the client appears more aggravated, highly sensitive, and overreactive, or following a stimulating experience or intense encounter with staff, group, or psychiatrist, *to calm the client and minimize opportunities for escalating behaviors and violence by providing rest and relaxation.*

Engage the client in activities that involve gross motor movements (e.g., walking, running, stationary bicycles, Ping-Pong, volleyball) *to expend and redirect energy toward functional, rewarding exercises rather than use energy to generate aggressive, violent acts.*

Assign the client to groups in which members discuss with each other concerns and feelings regarding alcohol/drugs *to gain a better understanding of the risk for aggression and violence owing to the disinhibitor and psychoactive effects of alcohol/drugs. People who abuse substances learn best to control themselves by identifying with each other's similar experiences. Dealing with anger in a safe group setting can prepare clients to manage volatile emotions in other situations.*

Examples:

- Focus or process groups
- Relationship groups
- Family and friends
- AA/NA

- Step groups (the 12-step program is discussed in a progressive manner)

Engage the client in groups and strategies that promote relaxation and reduce anxiety and agitation, increase self-esteem and reduce negative self-concept, contrast assertive and aggressive behaviors, and increase the length of time between stimulus and response *to reduce the incidence of impulsive, violent behaviors.*

Examples:

- Deep-breathing exercises
- Relaxation techniques
- Biofeedback
- Behavioral therapy
- Thought stopping
- Visual imagery
- Cognitive therapy
- Assertive responses

(See Appendix K and Glossary.)

Praise the client and family for efforts made toward managing uncontrolled anger and aggression *to reinforce positive behaviors and reduce or eliminate the risk of violence. Reinforcement tends to promote repetition.*

Teach the client the importance of abstaining from alcohol/drugs and the relationship between psychoactive substances and violence *to reinforce abstinence and eliminate risk of violence by teaching cause and effect.*

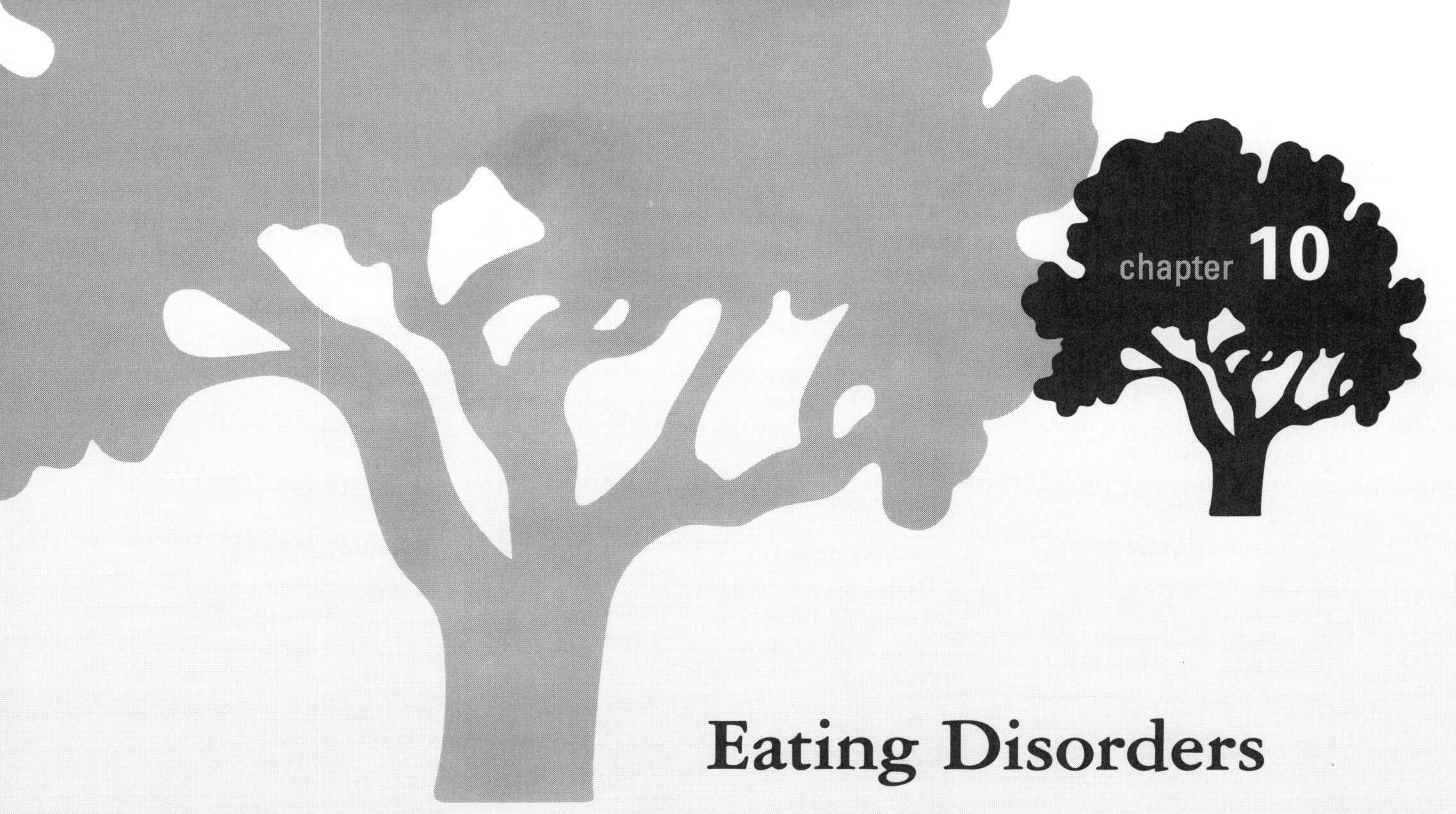

Eating Disorders

Eating behaviors and the issues surrounding them are multiple and complex. Although some people eat to maintain adequate nutrition and sustain life, others (in areas where food is plentiful) partake with great gusto, celebrate food for food's sake, and spend much of their waking time seeking, preparing, and eating food.

Most social gatherings involve eating and drinking, and many business transactions are culminated over a dining table. The food industry—markets, specialty shops, restaurants, and cookbooks, to name a few—has become a multibillion dollar business. For many, eating brings pleasure, but for some people and their significant others, eating problems are a living nightmare. Box 10-1 provides information on the *epidemiology* of eating disorders.

Anorexia Nervosa and Bulimia Nervosa are two eating disorders discussed in this chapter, and Feeding Disorders of Infancy and Childhood are described in Chapter 7. (Obesity is a major factor in the industrialized countries, where there is an abundance of food, but the condition does not appear in DSM-IV because specific psychologic or behavioral criteria have not been established to date.) The *etiologic factors* related to eating disorders are listed in Box 10-2.

DIAGNOSIS OF EATING DISORDERS

Anorexia Nervosa

Defining characteristics of Anorexia Nervosa are (1) refusal to attain or maintain minimal normal body weight for age and height, (2) extreme fear of gaining weight, (3) perceptual disturbance (sees self as "fat," even when grossly underweight, and (4) amenorrhea (after menarche, females miss at least three consecutive menstrual periods; before menarche, menstrual cycle is delayed).

Weight loss is due primarily to food intake reduction, as the diet becomes more and more restricted, eliminating high-caloric foods. The term *anorexia* is a misnomer because there is seldom a loss of appetite until the individual is extremely malnourished and near death. Death occurs in more than 10% of those individuals who require hospitalization and is usually due to starvation, suicide, or results of electrolyte imbalances.

Other methods the individual uses to lose weight are purging (excessive use of diuretics or laxatives and self-induced vomiting) and increased and excessive exercise. Often the voluntary food restriction cannot be maintained, and eating binges occur, followed by the purging. Usually food is constantly thought about, and unusual behaviors may develop, such as passionately collecting recipes and cookbooks, preparing voluminous meals for other people but not eating any of it, and secretly hiding food all over the house.

With the intense fear of weight gain comes a distorted self-image, and a very thin body is still perceived as fat; if the individual perceives self as thin, there remains a perception of "fat parts" (buttocks, thighs, abdomen) where none actually exists. Denial of any accompanying medical disturbances is strong among individuals with Anorexia Nervosa.

Amenorrhea occurs in postmenarcheal females, or menarche is delayed in Anorexia Nervosa because of

Box 10-1 Epidemiology of Eating Disorders

- More prevalent in industrialized countries, where food is plentiful
- Increased incidence in countries where being "thin" is considered attractive
- Virtually nonexistent in countries with inadequate supply of food
- Onset in adolescence most common
- Onset may occur around a stressful life event
- Long-term mortality rate for clients with Anorexia Nervosa who are hospitalized is more than 10% (due to suicide, starvation, or electrolyte imbalance)
- Ninety percent of clients with Anorexia Nervosa are female
- Ninety percent of clients with Bulimia Nervosa are female

Box 10-2 Specific Etiologic Factors Related to Mood Disorders*

Biologic

Increased risk among primary relatives for anorexia and bulimia

Mood disorders common among first-degree relatives of people who have eating disorders

(Substance abuse and dependence high for families of clients with Bulimia Nervosa)

Sociocultural

Early media exposure to values and beliefs about "thinness" as beauty

Psychodynamic

Physical changes in puberty cause sexual and social tensions that trigger phobic avoidance of food

Dependent, seductive relationship with warm or passive father; guilt over aggression toward ambivalently regarded mother

Psychologic

Disturbance of body image or self-perception

Behavioral

Negatively learned experiences cause a sense of ineffectiveness and resultant need for "control" over one's eating

failure of the pituitary to secrete hormones (FSH and LH) that in turn stimulate estrogen production.

Associated disturbances most frequently found with Anorexia Nervosa are (1) symptoms of depression (major depression may be diagnosed, but determinants are necessary regarding depression as a secondary result of physiologic starvation); (2) obsessive-compulsive characteristics both in relation to food and unrelated to food and eating; (3) somatic complaints; and (4) other characteristics such as compulsive stealing, excessive need to control the environment, limited sociability, and feelings of ineffectiveness.

Subtypes assigned to the diagnosis of Anorexia Nervosa are the following:

Restricting Type—weight loss primarily from dieting, fasting, or excessive exercise

Binge-Eating/Purging Type—weight loss results from regular binge eating and purging during the current episode

Bulimia Nervosa

Defining characteristics of Bulimia Nervosa are binge eating coupled with methods to prevent weight gain. Diagnosis is made when binging and associated weight loss methods occur at least twice a week for 3 months.

A binge refers to consumption of an amount of food that is much larger than most individuals can eat, and the eating is done within a time period of usually less than 2 hours. Typically, the type of food is soft, easy to swallow, sweet, and high in calories (ice cream, pastries, cakes), but many individuals eat foods other than sweets. Very often the eating is done inconspicuously or secretively, and the individual feels a lack of control over the behavior. Snacking throughout the day, even though a large volume of food is consumed, is not considered binge eating.

Compensatory techniques are utilized by individuals with bulimia to prevent weight gain after binges. The most common method is self-induced vomiting, which is done by 80% to 90% of the binge eaters. Most often a person sticks fingers down the throat to stimulate a gag reflex, but sometimes implements are used or, rarely, individuals use syrup of ipecac to induce vomiting. Another method of purging the system is through laxatives and diuretics; rarely a person uses enemas for catharsis. Usually the person reaches a point of being able to vomit at will. Vomiting decreases weight gain but also decreases bloating and feelings of being full so that eating can continue. Many individuals describe a sense of relief or release of tension and anxiety after vomiting, but depression follows the episode as the person deals with postbinge remorse or despair.

As with Anorexia Nervosa, individuals with bulimia may employ excessive exercise methods to control weight, but this method is not usually utilized as vigorously as it is in Anorexia Nervosa. Fasting also may be used to control weight.

Control is a major issue in Bulimia Nervosa, and a sense of lack of control predominates. A state of frenzy may exist during the eating binge, or the individual may describe feelings of dissociation during the episode, but in either case affected individuals say they lose an internal locus of control over the situation.

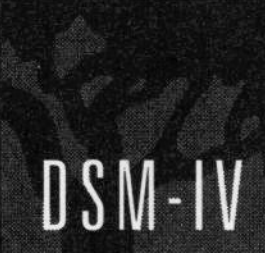

Eating Disorders

DSM-IV Categories

Anorexia Nervosa
 Subtype: Restricting Type
 Binge-Eating/Purging Type
Bulimia Nervosa
 Subtype: Purging Type
 Nonpurging Type

Subtypes of Bulimia Nervosa are the following:

Purging Type—person regularly uses self-induced vomiting; misuses laxatives, diuretics, enemas during episode

Nonpurging Type—uses methods (fasting, excessive exercise) other than purging

PROGNOSIS

The prognosis for eating disorders varies widely. Anorexia Nervosa may spontaneously end without treatment or after multiple treatments, there may be a fluctuating course of weight gain followed by relapses, or the course may be a gradually deteriorating one that ends in death.

The course for Bulimia Nervosa is usually chronic over several years with multiple remissions, or it may be intermittent. Dental caries are a common outcome because stomach acid etches tooth enamel.

INTERVENTIONS

Hospitalization

Individuals may require hospitalization for several reasons related to eating disorders. Medical intervention is required for the person admitted to the hospital when complications of starvation arise. Intravenous fluids may be necessary for dehydration and electrolyte imbalances for the individual with anorexia and for the person who has had prolonged or sustained vomiting. Sometimes, in addition to emergency medical attention, a person may require tube feedings when a strong refusal to eat exists.

Therapies

Pharmacotherapy

Psychiatric hospitals and clinics treat persons who have eating disorders with medications and psychotherapy and provide respite from a potentially troublesome environment. Several types of medications have been utilized for eating disorders, and some of the newer antidepressant drugs have been useful in this area.

Safety

Clients may enter the hospital with suicidal ideation, threats, gestures, or attempts and must be protected from self-harm.

Cognitive-Behavioral

Behavior modification programs and cognitive behavioral therapies, both in individual and group settings, have shown promise. Behavioral interventions focus on interruption of the dysfunctional eating patterns, and psychologic approaches aim at (1) increased insight into the complex dynamics of the disorder and (2) improvement of communication and coping skills.

Family

Dynamics are frequently dysfunctional in families where a member has an eating disorder. Education regarding the disorder and establishing healthy interactions is essential.

DISCHARGE CRITERIA FOR EATING DISORDERS

Maintains adequate nutrition
Maintains weight range as determined by nutritionist
Describes alternative behaviors for disruptive eating patterns.
Maintains attendance in eating disorder support group
Verbalizes realistic goals
Verbalizes sense of self-esteem
Expresses positive body image
Demonstrates internal locus of control
Expresses adequate knowledge about disorder
Demonstrates appropriate family and social relations

Nursing Process for

Eating Disorders

Universal Principles for Interactions and Interventions for Clients with Eating Disorders

- Continue to monitor assessment parameters listed in *Defining Characteristics.*
- Continue to consider the etiologic factors listed in *Etiologic/Related Factors.*
- Utilize principles of the *Therapeutic Nurse-Client Relationship* (Appendix G).
- Address clients' spiritual and cultural needs.

General Principles

- Provide a safe environment to prevent self-harm
- Establish a therapeutic alliance with client
- Provide nutrition to ensure adequate weight
- Monitor eating behaviors
- Set limits in milieu to ensure consistency
- Establish predictable routine
- Encourage client to establish internal locus of control directed at maintaining health
- Assist client to set realistic, attainable goals
- Engage client in all therapeutic modalities to modify behaviors and to gain insight and support
- Provide education for client and family about disorder

Care Plans for Eating Disorders Based on Nursing Diagnosis

DSM-IV Diagnoses

Anorexia Nervosa
Bulimia Nervosa

NANDA Diagnoses

Nutrition, altered: less than body requirements
Body image disturbance

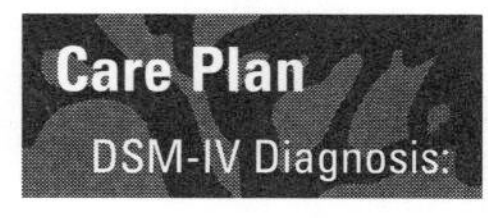

Anorexia Nervosa; Bulimia Nervosa

NANDA Diagnosis: Nutrition, altered: less than body requirements

The state in which the individual experiences an intake of nutrients insufficient to meet metabolic needs

Focus:

For the client whose nutritional state is severely compromised as a result of the diagnosis of Anorexia Nervosa or Bulimia Nervosa, characterized by gross disturbances in eating behaviors (e.g., self-starvation and/or binge-purge cycles).

NANDA Taxonomy

Pattern 1—Exchanging: A human response pattern involving mutual giving and receiving
Level of Assessment—Altered Nutrition

ETIOLOGIC/RELATED FACTORS (RELATED TO)

Anorexia Nervosa

Self-starvation
- Inadequate nutritional intake for age, height, and metabolic need

Body image disturbance
- Inability to perceive body size and shape realistically (e.g., believes self to be overweight, even if emaciated)

Denial of severity or consequences of starvation on the body's physical and psychologic functions
Engages in extreme regimen of physical exercise in an effort to burn unwanted calories
Extreme fear of weight gain, even if obviously underweight or emaciated (fear does not diminish as weight loss progresses)
Enmeshed family patterns (power struggles, overcontrolling mothers, lack of open affection among members)
Multifaceted etiology (biologic, psychologic, developmental, sociocultural, behavioral)
Powerlessness

Bulimia Nervosa

Self-induced vomiting (purging) generally after consuming large amounts of food (binging)
Use of laxatives or diuretics in an effort to lose weight
Engages in strict dieting or fasting to prevent weight gain
Initiates vigorous exercise regimen in an effort to lose weight
Persistent overconcern with body weight and shape (need to be "perfect")
History of depression
Disruptive family behavior patterns (overcontrolling mother; powerful, distant father)
Knowledge deficit regarding possible dire consequences of binge-purge behaviors
Multifaceted etiology (biologic, psychologic, sociocultural, behavioral)
Powerlessness

DEFINING CHARACTERISTICS (AS EVIDENCED BY)

Anorexia Nervosa

Fifteen percent or more under ideal body weight
Refuses to eat nutrients sufficient to maintain body weight for age, height, and stature (self-starvation)
Reports nutritional intake less than recommended daily allowance (RDA)
Verbalizes intense fear of weight gain or becoming fat, even though emaciated or grossly underweight and desirous of food
Expresses disturbance in the way body weight, size, or shape is experienced or viewed; claims to "feel fat" even when emaciated
States that one or more areas of the body are "too fat," even if obviously underweight
Perceives reflection of self in mirror as "fat," although grossly underweight
Absence of three or more menstrual cycles (amenorrhea) not due to any other condition or disorder
Uses laxatives, enemas, suppositories, or diuretics to lose weight (more often done by clients with Bulimia Nervosa)
Hoards, conceals, crumbles, or throws own food away; dawdles over meals
Verbalizes that life is viewed as a "constant struggle with weight"
Prepares elaborate meals for others, often forcing them to eat, yet eats only a narrow selection of low-calorie foods
Demonstrates preoccupation with food, nutrients, food preparation, and serving food to others
Denies thinness, hunger, need for treatment, or probability of illness or death as a result of starvation
Manifests compulsive or bizarre behavior patterns such as frequent hand washing; hoarding food, linen, utensils; calorie counting and preoccupation
Exhibits significantly delayed psychosexual development (in adolescent clients)
Displays marked lack of interest in sex (in adult clients)
Exhibits fluid and electrolyte imbalance
Slow pulse; decrease in body temperature
Marked constipation
Demonstrates hollow face with sunken eyes, growth of lanugo on skin, yellow tinge of skin, and dry hair, which may fall out
Expresses loss of appetite (late stage of Anorexia Nervosa)
Expresses depression and suicidal thoughts and attempts, especially following forced weight gain
Experiences episodes of overeating followed by vomiting (more common in Bulimia Nervosa)

Uses self-starvation as an attempt to strive for control and "perfection"

Bulimia Nervosa

Experiences recurrent episodes of binge eating (rapid consumption of large amounts of food in discrete period of time) with feeling a lack of control during binge episode, followed by self-induced vomiting (purge)

Reports use of laxatives, enemas, or diuretics in an effort to lose weight

Demonstrates vigorous exercise regimen to lose weight

Engages in strict dieting or fasting to prevent weight gain

Verbalizes persistent concern about body shape and weight gain, with frequent fluctuations in weight due to alternating binges and fasts

Exhibits weight that ranges from normal to slightly underweight or slightly overweight

Reports eating sweet-tasting, high-calorie foods with smooth texture that can be rapidly consumed and easily vomited (e.g., ice cream, pastries)

Demonstrates attempts to conceal binge-purge behaviors or to eat as inconspicuously as possible

Expresses frequent disparaging self-criticism, guilt, and depressed mood after binging episodes

Demonstrates dental erosion as a result of acidic gastric secretions from frequent vomiting episodes

Exhibits fluid and electrolyte imbalance (in more serious episodes)

OUTCOME IDENTIFICATION AND EVALUATION

Anorexia Nervosa

Consumes adequate daily calories per kilogram of body weight

Demonstrates and maintains ideal body weight for age, height, and stature

Maintains normal fluid and electrolyte levels

Skin turgor and muscle tone reveal nutritional state commensurate with physiologic and metabolic needs

Perceives ideal body weight and shape as normal, with absence of distorted self-image

Resumes and maintains normal menstrual cycles

Expresses absence of persistent fear of weight gain

Ceases to engage in overly strenuous exercise regimen for the purpose of losing weight

Resumes and maintains psychosexual development commensurate with age (adolescents)

Resumes and maintains sexual interests and behaviors commensurate with age (young adults)

Demonstrates absence of preoccupation with food (e.g., preparing, arranging, and serving food while eating little or none)

Ceases to hoard, conceal, crumble, or throw food away

Verbalizes feeling "in control" of life functions and no longer feels the need to withhold food to feel in control

Resolution or management of family enmeshment issues that perpetuate the disorder

Bulimia Nervosa

Maintains weight that is normal for age, height, and stature

Ceases binge-purge episodes

Demonstrates absence of use of laxatives or diuretics to lose weight

Ceases to exercise vigorously in an effort to lose weight

Stops dieting or fasting to prevent weight gain

Verbalizes feeling comfortable and satisfied with body weight, shape, and image

Demonstrates normal social eating patterns without attempts to conceal food or eat in isolation

Eats nutritionally balanced meals

Maintains normal fluid and electrolyte balance

Verbalizes feeling more "in control" of life functions and no longer needs to control life through binge-purge episodes

Resolution or management of control issues surrounding client and family interactions

PLANNING AND IMPLEMENTATION

Nursing Interventions and Rationale

Anorexia Nervosa

Assess the client's history of menstrual patterns (amenorrhea), diet and nutrition regimen (self-starvation, negative nitrogen balance) weight (15%); skin tone, turgor (triceps skinfold midarm circumference, midarm muscle circumference less than 60% standard measurement); muscle tone (weakness, tenderness); diagnostic studies (abnormal hemoglobin, serum albumin, serum transferrin–iron binding capacity, lymphocytes, thyroid and hormonal function, fluid and electrolytes); cardiac function (tachycardia on minimum exercise, bradycardia at rest); exercise regimen (excessive for weight and condition); mental status (irritability, confusion, anxiety, depression, obsessive-compulsive behaviors); emotional state (negative self-concept, distorted body image); and social and developmental tasks (congruent/incongruent with age and status). *Individuals with Anorexia Nervosa require an in-depth physical, mental, emotional, social, and developmental assessment because this disorder affects multiple systems and dimensions; early assessment and interventions prevent further deterioration and promote restoration of health and function.*

Initiate with the client and family, as indicated, hospitalization for nutritional therapy. *The hospital setting provides a controlled environment in which food and fluid intake and output, medication, and activities and exercise can be monitored. Hospitalization also separates the client from the family (which may be a contributing factor) and provides interactions with others with the same diagnosis so that problems can be shared and discussed. Management of the client's underlying conflicts cannot be addressed until nutritional status is improved and the client is out of danger.*

Weigh daily (or as ordered) at the same time each day, in a hospital gown, with arms at sides, after client voids (clients with phobias related to weighing or scales may choose to be weighed with back to scale) *to ensure accurate weight.*

Provide for weight gain of one-quarter to one-half pound per day or 3 pounds per week (or as ordered). *Slow weight gain is less anxiety-producing and more likely to be maintained.*

Offer the client a choice of food from the hospital menu. *The client experiences more control when given a choice of foods and nutrients.*

or

Provide liquid diets by mouth (1400 to 1800 calories). *Some clients with this disorder have a morbid fear of solid food, especially in the early stage of treatment.*

or

Provide tube feedings of liquid nutrients *if the client has been unable to maintain or increase weight by previous methods*

or

Administer intravenous hyperalimentation *to restore electrolyte, fluid, and nutritional balance compatible with client's physiologic functioning, with slow weight gain.*

Approach the client during administration of fluids, electrolytes, and nutrition in an unhurried, professional, nonjudgmental, nonauthoritarian manner *to allow the client to view replacement therapy as "medication" and minimize guilt the client feels when eating a meal. Hurried, overzealous nutritional restitution may terrify the client who is not psychologically ready to accept body rebuilding and will only be driven to lose more weight. An authoritarian approach may remind the client of old familiar power struggles and other pathologic family patterns, which could promote feelings of anger, frustration, or helplessness in both client and staff. Also, some clients have been known to attempt suicide after rapid or forced weight gain. A slow, calm approach is thus more conducive to therapeutic client-staff relationships and client compliance with therapy. A judgmental attitude may signal the staff member's disapproval and will be counterproductive to promoting the client's self-confidence and faith in his or her own ability to control destiny.*

Help the client maintain weight of at least 90 to 95 pounds. *The client cannot tolerate normal weight initially without feeling "too fat." Ninety to 95 pounds is considered to be the "out of danger" weight for most clients and is usually an acceptable compromise for clients after a brief period of therapy.*

Initiate a structured, supportive environment throughout the day, especially during mealtimes (e.g., establish routine tasks and activities, serve meals at the same time each day). *Clients with this disorder feel out of control and vulnerable. A structured, supportive environment provides external safety and comfort and helps the client establish internal control. The more the client feels in control, the less likely he or she is to use self-starvation as a means of control.*

Sit with the client calmly and consistently during meals initially and present and remove food without persuasion to "eat more" or other similar comments. *Clients detect urgency and react negatively to pressure, a reminder of domineering parents. Consistent behaviors by staff allow the client to trust staff's responses. Food and eating are areas of control for the client, and forcing or coercing the client to eat may evoke guilt. Structuring meals and decreasing discussions about food will minimize power struggles and avoid manipulative games.*

Avoid the use of trickery, bribery, cajoling, force, or threats to get the client to eat. This type of behavior stimulates the client to engage in a power struggle with staff and to be deceitful because it may be reminiscent of family patterns and power struggles.

When There is Evidence That the Client is Inducing Vomiting After Meals:

Remain with the client for at least 2 hours after each meal *to prevent self-induced vomiting.*

Supervise the client's use of the bathroom for at least 2 hours after each meal *to prevent self-induced vomiting.*

Avoid room checks, *which reinforce feelings of powerlessness and perpetuate dysfunctional behaviors.*

Design with the client a behavior modification program (if warranted) that provides rewards for weight gain and does not punish or harass the client for weight loss. *Behavior modification programs provide structured eating situations that allow clients some control in choosing foods. They are generally effective in mild cases of an eating disorder or to facilitate short-term weight gain and should not consist of rigid rules that evoke power plays between staff and clients.*

Administer medications as ordered.

Examples:

Antidepressants: the tricyclics (e.g., amitriptyline [Elavil]) or other types (e.g., fluoxetine [Prozac] or bupropion [Wellbutrin]) *to relieve depression.* Monoamine oxidase inhibitors (MAOIs) are generally avoided because their use requires dietary restrictions that may perpetuate the problem of the client with Anorexia Nervosa. MAOIs may be used, however, if other antidepressants are ineffective.

Antipsychotics: Thioridazine (Mellaril) or chlorpromazine (Thorazine) may be used for *agitation or if there is evidence of an underlying core psychosis, such as paranoia or delusion that "food is poisoned." Antipsychotics relieve psychotic behaviors and help make the client more amenable to the treatment program.* (Antipsychotics are used only when necessary, owing to their extrapyramidal effects.)

Antianxiety medication (e.g., alprazolam [Xanax]) are avoided, *owing to their addictive qualities and the compulsive, addictive nature of clients with Anorexia Nervosa.* Although a few sources list cyproheptadine (Periactin), a serotonin and histamine antagonist that when given in high doses stimulates the appetite, most authorities stipulate that Periactin is not a treatment of choice *because people with Anorexia Nervosa do not experience loss of appetite until very late in the disorder, when more critical measures are taken (e.g., tube feedings).*

Assist the client with electroconvulsive therapy (ECT) by explaining to the client that it is not punishment. *In extremely difficult cases when malnutrition is severe and life-threatening, a short-term series of ECT may help the client begin to eat and become more amenable to psychotherapy and treatment regimen.*

Avoid responding to or focusing on the client's preoccupation with food. *Clients with Anorexia Nervosa are often obsessed with the topic of food and may spend long hours discussing nutrition or preparing and handling food, usually in an effort to stall or avoid actually eating the food. It is not therapeutic to indulge them in this preoccupation, which may give credibility to the topic of food as an issue and perpetuate dysfunctional behaviors.*

Focus on the client's strengths and capabilities, for example, seeking help for problem, attending groups and activities, or participating in treatment program, *to build self-confidence and offer hope for progress and success.*

Have client eventually eat with other clients in the hospital dining room *to promote normal social interactions during mealtimes; to prevent hoarding, concealing, or crumbling food; and to demonstrate trust.*

Collaborate with the hospital nutritionist to prepare a tray with an adequate amount of food *so that the amount of food satisfies nutritional needs but is not overwhelming to the client.*

Engage the client in selecting own foods from various food groups *so he or she has some control in own treatment program. Clients with Anorexia Nervosa withhold food in an effort to control some aspect of their lives. Offering choices gives the client some control in a positive way and builds self-confidence.*

Be alert to the client's choices of low-calorie foods or beverages, hoarding food, and disposing of food in places such as pockets and wastebaskets. *The client will try to avoid taking in what is viewed as excessive calories and may need guidance to select more nutritious foods.*

Praise the client when he or she consumes an adequate amount of food within a prescribed period of time. *Positive reinforcement builds self-esteem and promotes repetition of functional behaviors.*

Teach the client and family about the relationship between self-starvation and a desperate attempt to control one's life *to promote awareness of factors that contribute to the eating disorder and to use the family's support to help the client consider areas in life that he or she can control in a healthy manner.*

Discuss with the client any fears he or she may have about physical development and the association of those fears with self-starvation as a means to slow down the developmental and maturational process and thus avoid adolescent sexuality and independence *to decrease the client's anxiety and fears by bringing them out in the open and to impart information that may help the client problem solve and become aware that self-starvation is a dangerous way to avoid inevitable growth and development.*

Help the client in expressing feelings and fears about his or her sexuality and intimacy *to help the client develop awareness of feelings and fears regarding sexuality and intimacy through discussions with a trusted staff person. Self-starvation is often a dysfunctional attempt to avoid sexuality in clients who are afraid of making the transition from adolescence to intimacy:*

"What are your feelings or concerns about intimacy?"

"Let's talk about your thoughts regarding sexuality."

"How do you associate your fasting behaviors with your fears about intimacy and commitment to others?"

Confront the client with the fact that self-starvation is self-destructive behavior that could lead to death *to help the client realize the serious consequences of the behavior and break through maladaptive denial.*

Respond assertively to clients who use manipulative behaviors to distract from their eating disorder. *Clients benefit from direct communication, as they are often in a state of maladaptive denial regarding their problem and need kind, but firm, confrontation.*

Therapeutic response:

Client: "How can you talk to me about being too thin? You're thin yourself."

Nurse: "While I may be thin, you have an eating disorder problem and we're here to help you with your problem."

Nontherapeutic responses:

Client: "How can you talk to me about being too thin? You're thin yourself."

Nurse: "My thinness is not your concern; I'm not the one with the eating disorder."

Client: "How can you talk to me about being too thin? You're thin yourself."

Nurse: "Let's discuss your feelings about my thinness before we talk about your problem."

The first incorrect response is aggressive rather than assertive, which can put the client on the defensive and block the therapeutic process. The second incorrect response encourages the client to focus on the nurse's thinness, which distracts from the client's problem and is nontherapeutic.

Develop with the client a realistic exercise program *to prevent excessive exercise for the purpose of weight loss and to satisfy the client's need for exercise as an emotional and physical health benefit.*

Discuss with the client unrealistic or irrational perceptions of body shape and size *to challenge the client's belief about his or her body shape and size in a realistic, nonthreatening manner.*

Communicate to the client the staff's expectations of behaviors that are congruent with client's developmental stage *to promote healthy, age-appropriate functioning rather than regression; there is generally a connection between self-starvation and the desire to maintain childlike appearance and behavior.*

Discuss with the client the irrational need to be "perfect" *to give the client permission to talk about possible sources of irrational desires and to convince the client that "perfection" is unattainable for most people and not a prerequisite for success and happiness. Some clients with eating disorders have experienced the need to achieve perfection early in life and thus starve themselves as a way to accomplish a "perfect" image and sense of worth.*

Provide praise for weight gain rather than amount of food consumed *to focus on the results of the client's efforts rather than on food and to reinforce continued positive behaviors in individual and group settings.*

Help the client, in individual and group settings, develop realistic beliefs about food, weight, and physical attractiveness *to break the vicious cycle of Anorexia Nervosa, reduce or eliminate the preoccupation with food and weight, and promote healthy eating habits and a productive life-style:*

- Engage in individual therapeutic interactions.
- Attend cognitive therapy and assertiveness training classes.
- Participate in groups with other clients with Anorexia Nervosa.
- Participate in family therapy sessions.

(Refer to Appendix K, for Cognitive, Assertive, Group, and Family Therapy.)

Engage the client in individual therapy *to help the client understand self and illness and receive continuous feedback regarding progress and behavior from a trusted, knowledgeable, supportive person.*

Provide family therapy in which the concept of *family enmeshment,* a term used to describe families that engage in power struggles, is discussed. Enmeshed families consist of overcontrolling mothers or other significant member or parent-figure and a lack of open affection among family members. *Some clients with Anorexia Nervosa may be members of an "enmeshed family and use self-starvation as a means of gaining control against an overcontrolling mother, member, or family system or to "hold the family together" in a paradoxical sense. In any case, the family of the client with Anorexia Nervosa is concerned with power and control, in addition to massive denial of parental conflicts. Family therapy approaches these conflicts, and parents are asked to focus on their problems and release the client from their persistent control.*

(Refer to Glossary for further explanation of enmeshment.)

Provide cognitive therapy and assertiveness training for client. *Psychodynamic studies reveal that some clients with Anorexia Nervosa were often overly criticized, corrected, or invalidated by dominant, overcontrolling mothers during the formative years. Premorbid personalities of some clients consist of compliance, obedience, passivity, dependence, and the need to be perfect and "make the family proud." Assertive response behaviors can help the client express feelings openly and directly and break the cycle of self-starvation as a means of gaining control of life situations. Cognitive therapy can help the client replace erroneous, self-defeating thoughts with more realistic ones and thus build confidence and self-control.*

(Refer to Appendix K.)

Engage the client in supportive, fact-finding, interpersonal psychotherapy in which the client is primarily responsible for exploring and examining needs, impulses, and feelings that originate from within the self. Avoid a psychoanalytical, interpretive approach that consists of interpreting repressed motives and conflicts. *Fact-finding therapy allows the client, over time, to discover his or her own needs, impulses, and feelings; it can take place through a variety of therapeutic modalities (e.g., individual, group, family, cognitive, assertiveness therapies). (See Appendix K.) As the client learns more about self, cognitive and perceptual difficulties that originate in childhood are better understood and healing can take place. This discovery of thoughts and impulses that originate within the self leads to autonomy, self-assertion, and independence. Conversely, the analytical, interpretive method is not recommended because these clients' lack of identity may lead them to search for clues about their identity from the therapist. They may either incorporate the therapist's interpretations into their own identity or become suspicious of them because the interpretations came from outside the self.*

Participate in daily multidisciplinary team conferences to discuss, evaluate, and support each other *so that staff members give consistent, effective client care with confidence and to avoid splitting of staff by clients.*

Include the client in his or her own care planning process *to elicit the client's approval of, and adherence to, the treatment plan and to promote the client's autonomy and independence.*

Bulimia Nervosa

Assess the client's history of binge-purge patterns; weight fluctuations; use of laxatives, enemas, or diuretics; dieting and fasting behaviors; exercise and activity regimen; fluid and electrolyte status; cardiac and gastrointestinal systems; dental and parotid condition; thyroid function; mood and affect (depressed, suicidal); guilt, shame, or self-contempt, especially following binges; self-esteem/perceptual disturbances; social relationships; abuse of drugs or alcohol; family behavior patterns; life stressors; and background of medical or psychiatric disorders related to self or close family members. *Clients with Bulimia Nervosa require an in-depth, multisystems assessment. This disorder has a multifaceted etiology, and early assessment and interventions will prevent further deterioration and complications by promoting functional healthy eating patterns. Because clients with this disorder generally maintain themselves at or slightly above their ideal weight, many physical and emotional complications can go undiagnosed; for example, extensive dental decay and irreversible perimolysis on lingual surfaces of incisors from frequent contact with gastric secretions from emesis and sugary foods; parotid gland swelling; stomach ulcers; involuntary vomiting; sore throats; esophageal or rectal bleeding; reduced intake of potassium and loss of potassium (in clients who abuse diuretics and laxatives and engage in vomiting); myocardial contractility problems; cardiac dysrhythmias or cardiac arrest because of lowered serum potassium (the most common cause of death in this disorder); low serum phosphate from massive laxative abuse; low serum chloride; low serum potassium and metabolic acidosis (the renal effect of chronic vomiting); muscle weakness and contractility problems owing to hypokalemia; acute gastric dilation and rupture of the stomach; abnormal dexamethasone suppression test (DST) (see Glossary) indicating possibility of major depression; delayed thyroid-stimulating hormone (TSH) response to thyroid-releasing hormone (TRH); preoccupations with food, weight, and body image with faulty perceptions of "feeling fat" even when weight is normal; overwhelming feelings of guilt, shame, and self-contempt following binges; fear of losing control and that a binge may occur even with just a taste of a small amount of favorite food; obsessive-compulsive behaviors (e.g., obsessed with weight and binge eating, or compulsive shoplifting usually involving food, laxatives, or other affordable items); alcohol abuse or addiction; social sensitivity (secretive eating to satisfy binge-purge patterns); major depression, which generally occurs a year prior to the onset of bulimic symptoms; family history of either major depression or bipolar disorder; suicidal behavior; and need to be "perfect" to please controlling mothers and powerful, distant fathers.*

Initiate with the client and family hospitalization for nutritional therapy as indicated, as well as treatment directed toward underlying conflicts that contribute to binge-purge behaviors (e.g., life stressors, need to be "perfect," negative self-concept). *The hospital setting provides a controlled environment in which clients with Bulimia Nervosa can be observed during and after meals to prevent binge-purge behavior. It also exposes the client to a therapeutic environment in which individual, group, and other interactive therapies can take place with others with the same diagnosis. This gives clients the opportunity to share problems and discuss strategies for management of symptoms in a safe, supportive setting.* (Some clients with Bulimia Nervosa may be treated for nutritional, physical, and emotional problems on an outpatient basis if their condition is stable and no emergency exists. In this instance, families should also be counseled with the client to resolve conflicts surrounding the eating disorder.)

(See Appendix K, Group and Family Therapies.)

Weigh the client weekly (or as ordered) in the same amount of attire *to ensure accurate weight.*

Offer structure and support during mealtimes (with an appropriate staff-to-client ratio) by creating a calm, pleasant environment and providing nutritionally balanced, attractive meals *to gain the client's trust and cooperation while providing adequate nutrition and staff guidance and supervision.*

Observe the client for 2 hours after meals *to prevent self-induced vomiting or regurgitation, explaining to the client beforehand that it is part of the therapeutic process. (In some facilities, contracts may stipulate agreed-upon behaviors.)*

Participate in interdisciplinary group meetings *to plan goals and management of client care and ensure consistency among staff members.*

Designate one staff member (whenever possible) each day as the client's primary therapist *to avoid manipulation and possible splitting behaviors.*

Involve the client in his or her own care-planning process (whenever possible) *to promote the client's accountability for own treatment and foster autonomy and self-confidence.*

Have the client avoid laxatives, suppositories, enemas, and diuretics *to prevent potassium loss through urine and stool and serious complications as a result of potassium and other electrolyte depletion.*

Administer fluids and high-fiber foods frequently *to prevent constipation and the resulting temptation to use laxatives and enemas.*

Engage the client in an eclectic therapeutic regimen that includes elements from family therapy, behavior therapy, psychotherapy, drug therapy, and interactive support groups. *There is no consensus as to the appropriate treatment modality for clients with this disorder, but sharing and discussing problems in a variety of therapeutic settings can help clients and their families examine conflicts, define goals for treatment, and use management strategies with input from multidisciplinary therapists and other clients who have had successful experiences.*

(Refer to Therapies, Appendix K, and Family Therapy Intervention in Anorexia Nervosa section of this care plan.)

Act as a role model both in and out of the hospital by practicing good nutrition and weight control. *Prevention of this disorder can be emphasized through role modeling, hopefully before teens reach the age when they are at high risk for Bulimia Nervosa.*

Educate the public through community groups and junior high schools, high schools, and colleges about the importance of well-balanced nutrition for one's physical and mental capacities and the deleterious effects of Bulimia Nervosa. *Increased knowledge prevents dysfunctional eating patterns and promotes healthy nutritional habits in high-risk and future high-risk populations.*

Counsel clients and nonhospitalized persons about the benefits of sensible daily exercise (e.g., walking, running, simple activities, or sports), for a reasonable period of time (20 to 60 minutes a day). *Moderate exercise increases metabolism and produces safe, sensible weight loss. Exercise may also improve the person's mood by activating endorphins and promoting a healthier, more attractive physical appearance, which discourages binge-purge cycles.*

Approach clients with a nonjudgmental, caring attitude *to bolster self-esteem and help moderate the client's usual "perfectionistic" approach to life.*

Administer prescribed antidepressant medications when warranted. *The tricyclic antidepressant imipramine and the monoamine oxidase inhibitors (MAOIs) have been successful in controlling binge episodes, a finding that links Bulimia Nervosa, in some studies, to mood disorders. (Be aware of dietary restrictions required with MAOIs.) Studies reveal that clients with or without positive dexamethasone suppression tests respond equally well to antidepressant therapy.*

(See Appendix M, Drugs to Treat Mental and Emotional Disorders, and Glossary for definition of the *dexamethasone suppression test* [DST].)

Administer metoclopramide (Reglan), as ordered. *Reglan may be used to promote or speed up gastric emptying. Frequent vomiting (purging) decreases the stomach's ability to effectively empty all its contents. When gastric emptying is delayed, the client with bulimia experiences constant sense of "fullness" that promotes more vomiting (purging) and the fear that nothing—not even vomiting—can prevent the feeling of fullness. Reglan empties the stomach's contents more efficiently and reduces or eliminates the sense of fullness, which may discourage vomiting or purge episodes.*

Allow the client to create own menus from a selection of available, nutritious foods. *The client needs to gain confidence in self and feel in control of environment.*

Be alert to the client's choices of sweet, soft, or sugary foods, which can be easily binged and purged, and guide the client toward more balanced nutritional selections *to prevent the temptation to binge and purge.*

Instruct the family to visit the client on a limited basis and to avoid discussions of food. *Food should not be the focal point of family discussions during visiting hours, as it is likely to be a constant issue at home. The client needs to become solely responsible for own food management while in the hospital and continue the behavior on discharge, whether or not he or she returns to the family home.*

Discuss with the client who is over 18 optional living arrangements other than returning to live in the family home (if the family is dysfunctional and/or controlling) *to encourage independence and separation from parental conflicts and domination that perpetuate the binge-purge cycle.*

Confront the client with the information that binge-purge episodes are self-destructive acts and are a dysfunctional attempt to control one's life—and that such behavior could lead to serious physical and emotional complications and even death—*to promote awareness of the harsh realities of life and death and to assist the client to control his or her life in areas of work, play, and love rather than through harmful binge-purge episodes. (The client is better able to deal with confrontation when trust is built and self-esteem is reestablished.)*

Facilitate a behavior modification program that involves the client's input in the program *to provide a structured eating situation while allowing the client some control in the program. Behavior modification may be effective only in mild cases or for short-term weight gain.*

Engage the client in social milieu activities, including meals, *to discourage social sensitivity, minimize secret binge-purge episodes, and increase healthy social interactions in accordance with developmental level.*

Focus on the client's strengths, talents, and capabilities *to build self-esteem and discourage guilt and self-criticism, especially after binge episodes.*

Provide cognitive therapy classes. *Clients learn to replace spontaneous, erroneous thoughts and beliefs about self with more realistic perceptions and to reduce guilty thoughts and perfectionistic desires that lead to binge-purge cycles.*

Engage the client in group therapy sessions with other clients of approximate weight and stature *so the client can compare own normal weight with others with similar weight and stature, gain a healthier perspective of actual physical appearance, and stop "feeling fat."*

Discuss with the client his or her feelings of intimacy and sexuality (if warranted) *to help the client get in touch with developmental needs and to promote interpersonal relationships. Clients with this disorder are generally distracted from social tasks because of their obsession with binge-purge behaviors. The binge-purge behaviors then drive others away, and the resultant loneliness or isolation leads to more binge-purge episodes.*

(Refer to Anorexia Nervosa section for interventions regarding intimacy.)

Discuss with the client irrational beliefs about needing to be "perfect" *to determine sources of irrational beliefs and to give the client permission to be less than "perfect" and still be a worthwhile person.* (Cognitive therapy in appendix K will help to reinforce reality.)

Help the client develop realistic beliefs about food, weight, and attractiveness *to break the binge-purge cycle; lessen obsessions with food, weight, and physical appearance; and promote a healthier, more productive life-style.*

Provide assertiveness training *to help the client learn to ask for what he or she wants and needs directly, thus gaining more control and eliminating the necessity to use binge-purge behaviors to gain control.*

(See Appendix K.)

Explore with the client irrational aspects of this culture's preoccupation with thinness *to encourage the client to think about own values independent of society. (Fashion advertisements tend to prey on the vulnerability of young women, who learn to equate thinness with self-worth.)*

Conduct a suicide assessment if the client expresses thoughts, behaviors, or plans of suicide *to prevent harm or injury and to protect client from uncontrollable impulses.* (Refer to Appendixes J and L.)

Suggest that the client attend self-help groups, especially if the client does not do well on antidepressant therapy, *to expose the client to a source of strength, empathy, support, and encouragement, as well as the social companionship that may be lacking in his or her life.*

Examples:

- Bulimia Nervosa groups (preferred)
- Overeaters Anonymous (if appropriate)
- Chemical dependency groups (if warranted)

Praise the client throughout the treatment program for efforts *to control binge-purge behaviors. Frequent positive feedback, when warranted, increases the client's self-esteem, builds confidence, and reinforces continued successful eating behaviors.*

Praise the client and family for progress made in reducing and finally eliminating conflicts that contribute to the client's binge-purge behaviors. *Positive feedback reinforces continued functional behavior patterns.*

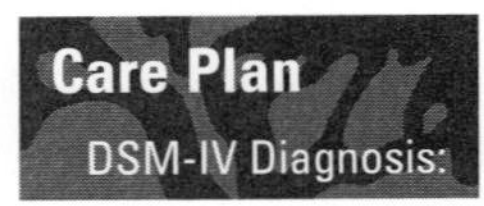

Care Plan
DSM-IV Diagnosis:

Anorexia Nervosa; Bulimia Nervosa

NANDA Diagnosis: Body image disturbance

The state in which an individual experiences a disruption in the perception of one's body image

Focus:
For the client with Anorexia Nervosa who experiences disturbances in body weight, size, or shape (e.g., "feels fat" or perceives physical self as "looking fat' even when emaciated) and for the client with Bulimia Nervosa who is overconcerned with body shape and weight and often "feels fat," even when maintaining ideal weight, but does not experience the severe perceptual distortions of the client with Anorexia Nervosa

NANDA Taxonomy
Pattern 7—Perceiving: A human response pattern involving the reception of information
Level of Assessment—Altered Self-Concept

ETIOLOGIC/RELATED FACTORS (RELATED TO)

Anorexia Nervosa

Cognitive perceptual distortions

Inability to perceive body size, body functions, and physical needs realistically

Maladaptive denial of body image and physical experience of body weight and stature

Bulimia Nervosa

Persistent overconcern with body weight and physical shape

Experiences "feeling fat" even when ideal weight is maintained

OUTCOME IDENTIFICATION AND EVALUATION

Anorexia Nervosa

Demonstrates realistic perceptions of body image, weight, and physical appearance

Experiences realistic feelings about body size, needs, and functions

Demonstrates absence of cognitive-perceptual distortions related to body size, weight, appearance, and physical functions

Exercises within limits of endurance to maintain physical and emotional wellness

Bulimia Nervosa

Demonstrates absence of overconcern or obsessive thoughts regarding body weight, shape, or size

Expresses satisfaction with maintained ideal weight versus "feeling fat"

Maintains reasonable exercise regimen consistent with age, weight, and physical needs

Discusses body size, shape, and appearance in positive terms

PLANNING AND IMPLEMENTATION

Nursing Interventions and Rationale

Anorexia nervosa

Assess the client's degree of body image disturbance (e.g., distortions regarding body size, weight, appearance, body functions, and physical needs) *to determine the extent of the client's denial and cognitive-perceptual disturbance and to plan appropriate interventions.*

Help the client express feelings and concerns about self, body image, body size, weight, body function, and physical needs. *Ventilation of perceptions and distortions helps to clarify areas of conflict and concern that need to be addressed.*

Point out verbalized misperceptions of body image in a calm, direct, nonthreatening manner *to correct the client's distortions without challenging belief system and inciting anger, guilt, or shame:*

Client: "My legs are fat; they're awful."

Client: "Your legs are beginning to look strong and healthy since you're almost at your ideal weight."

Client: "But I'm afraid they look too fat."

Nurse: "Your daily walks will help tone your legs and all your body; let's talk about how your body will change for the better."

Teach the client to visualize and verbalize realistic thoughts and affirmations about body *to replace negative beliefs and distortions with realistic ones:*

Examples:

- "I am healthy when I'm at my ideal weight."
- "I have more energy at my ideal weight."
- "I can choose healthy foods to eat."
- "My body looks healthy when I'm at my ideal weight."

(See Appendix K for Visualization and Cognitive Strategies.)

Have the client create own statements and affirmations to practice and use throughout the day, especially during stressful times such as mealtimes and visiting with family, *to give the client tools to use independently.*

Help the client view self in a full-sized mirror with little clothing and ask the client to describe what she or he sees and how she or he would like to look *to help the client realistically appraise body while progressing throughout the treatment program. In the early stages of anorexia nervosa, clients view their physical image as "fat" even when they are emaciated. A more accurate perception of the body indicates progress.*

Engage the client in exercises that include touch or massage (if not contraindicated) *to help the client get in touch with body boundaries, minimize feelings of depersonalization, and promote realistic perceptions of the physical self (may require an order).*

Advise the client to wear clothing one size larger than current size *to provide motivation for weight gain and a healthier, more appropriate shape for age and stature.*

Verbalize recognition of the client's attempts to communicate perceptions, feelings, and concerns, in individual and group interactions to reinforce the client's continued expressions regarding body image and functions.

Provide support and praise for the client's accurate perceptions of body size, body image, and body functions, as well as for demonstration of more adaptive eating patterns and a reasonable exercise regimen. *Positive feedback reinforces the client's self-esteem and promotes more realistic self-perceptions and healthier eating and exercise behaviors.*

Provide sex educational classes (as necessary). *The major physical and physiologic changes that occur during adolescence can contribute to Anorexia Nervosa. Feelings of powerlessness and loss of control of feelings (particularly sexual), sensations, and physical development often lead to an unconscious effort to desexualize self. The client may try to overcome these fears by taking control of bodily appearance, development, and function. Sex education may help the client confront sexual fears and give up "childlike" physical appearance and image.*

Educate family to relinquish control over and responsibility for the client *to give the client the opportunity to grow and develop and take charge of his or her own life. As the client makes more independent decisions, emotional growth can take place and the client will develop a more positive, mature self-concept.*

Bulimia Nervosa

Discuss with the client feelings and obsessions concerning weight gain, body shape, and size *to clarify the extent of the client's concerns and to allow ventilation of feelings.*

Focus on areas of client's strength and control (e.g., entering hospital to seek help voluntarily, participation in treatment program) *to increase the client's self-esteem and feelings of self-control. Most patients with Bulimia Nervosa have a negative self-concept and feel a lack of control over body, self, and life situations.*

Respond to the client's erroneous statements about body image with realistic, nonjudgmental comments *to correct the individual's perceptions without challenging his or her right to express thoughts and feelings:*

Examples:

Client: "I'm not underweight, so there's nothing really wrong with me."

Nurse: "Your weight is ideal for your height; binging and purging are harmful to your body functions."

Client: "I'm feeling fat and shapeless; I vomit occasionally to control my weight."

Nurse: "Although you feel fat, your weight is ideal for your height; vomiting will not reshape your body, but it will cause other problems."

Discuss with the client irrational beliefs about needing to be "perfect" and resorting to binge-purge behaviors as a means of gaining "perfection" *to determine possible sources of irrational beliefs and give the client permission to be less than perfect and still be a worthwhile individual. Clients with Bulimia Nervosa often judge "perfection" by physical appearance.*

Help the client gain control in areas other than dieting/fasting and binging/purging, such as managing own daily activities, work, leisure time, and social functions. Clients often focus on food, weight, and self-image to control areas in life in which they feel helpless or powerless. *Helping individuals concentrate on other areas of life that have been neglected will increase feelings of control, promote a more positive self-concept, and minimize dysfunctional behaviors.*

Be aware of your own reactions to the client's dysfunctional behaviors. *Feelings of anger, impatience, and irritation are not uncommon because clients with Bulimia Nervosa may continue to see themselves as "fat" and because there are high incidences of depression, social phobias, obsessive-compulsive symptoms, drug abuse, and psychosexual dysfunctions that affect the client's perceptions and may inhibit progress.*

Engage the client in social situations and activities in the milieu *to provide role models of both sexes who can relate to the client and offer approval and positive feedback in a controlled social context. Peer interactions and approval can help increase the client's self-concept and promote more realistic perceptions of body and body image.*

Praise the client for statements that reveal the client's positive feelings about self and body and belief that he or she is attractive and healthy at ideal weight. *Positive feedback reinforces positive self-concept and repetition of functional behaviors.*

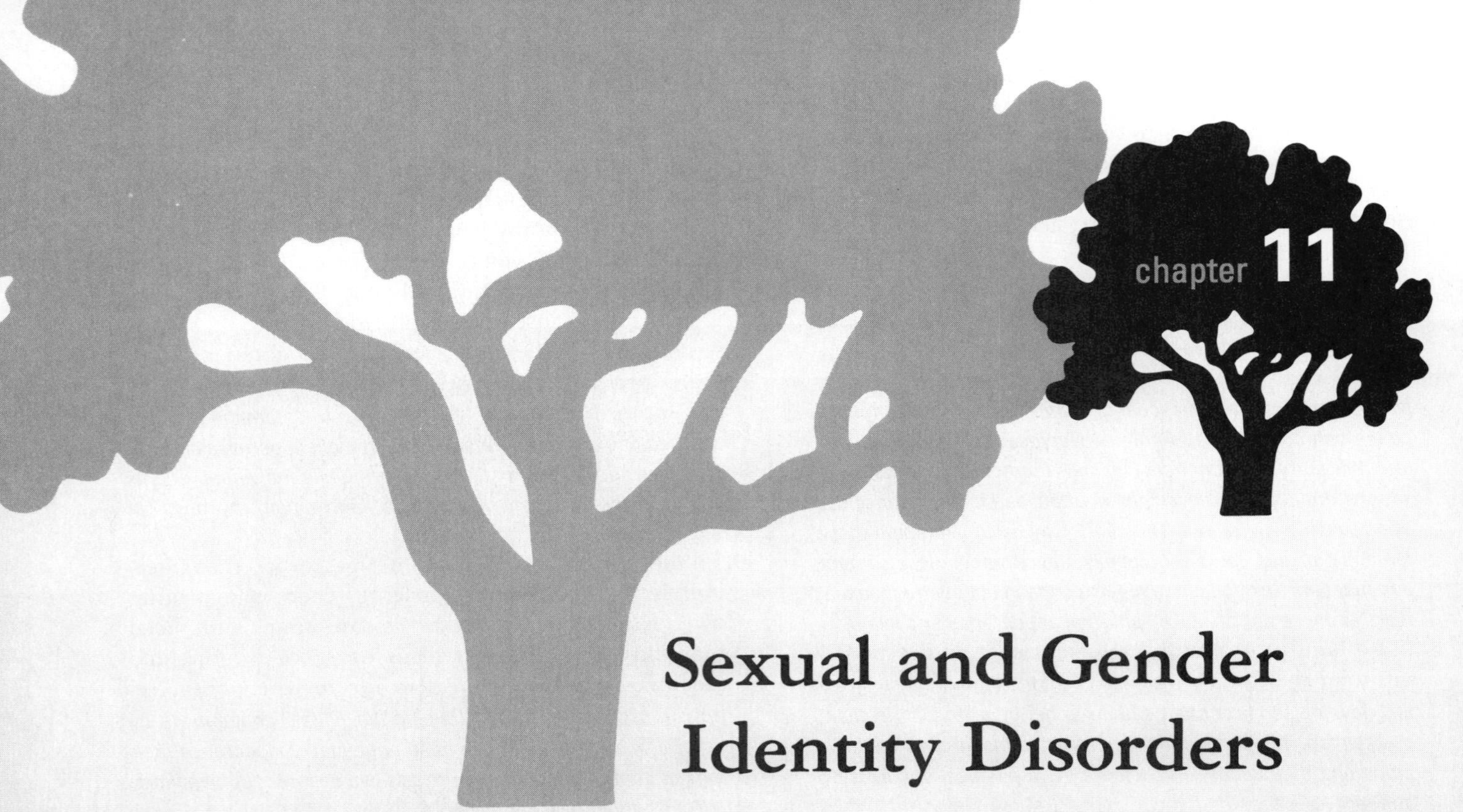

Sexual and Gender Identity Disorders

Most authorities agree that in contemporary society sexual health is defined as the integration of the somatic, emotional, intellectual, and social aspects of a sexual being in ways that are positively enriching and that enhance personality, communication, and love.

Masters and Johnson in 1970 defined and interpreted *sexual dysfunction* as a "sexual problem" or "sexual disorder." More recently (1979) Masters and Johnson and their associates considered sexual apathy and sexual aversion as "nondysfunctions" or problems stemming from a "lack of desire or arousal," differentiating them from organic dysfunctions related to the sex organs themselves. Masters and Johnson thus clarified sexual dysfunction as "those sex problems that appear as difficulties on the physical level, such as problems with orgasms, erections, or penetration." Such physical symptoms have a lesser role in most sexual problems than do psychologic problems.

For the client with mental or emotional problems, however, alterations in healthy sexual expression may result from the following contributing factors, which are the focus of the nursing care plans for this chapter:

- *Nontherapeutic, pharmacologic effects of specific drugs that interfere with sexual energy (libido), sexual function, and performance*

Refer to Appendix M, Drugs to Treat Mental and Emotional Disorders.)

- *Chronic mental and emotional disorders resulting in inability to achieve the age-appropriate developmental task of intimacy necessary for relationships that lead to continued sexual gratification*
- *Long-term continual or intermittent institutionalization that prevents opportunities for healthy socialization, intimacy, and sexual expression*

Nurses and therapists who manage care for clients with sexual and gender identity disorders need to develop awareness of their own sexuality to identify problems and avoid bias.

DIAGNOSIS OF SEXUAL AND GENDER IDENTITY DISORDERS

This section contains information about the three types of sexual and gender identity disorders: sexual dysfunctions, paraphilias, and gender identity disorders.

Sexual Dysfunctions

The defining characteristic of the sexual dysfunctions subclass is inhibition in the appetitive or psychophysiologic changes that characterize the complete sexual response cycle. The diagnosis is not made if the sexual dysfunction is solely attributed to organic factors, such as a physical disorder or medication, or due to another Axis I mental disorder. *Each disorder causes marked distress or difficulty in interpersonal relationships.* In some instances more than one diagnosis may be appropriate, such as Hypoactive Sexual Desire Disorder and Sexual Aversion Disorder.

The complete human sexual response cycle is divided into the following phases:

1. Desire—fantasies about sexual activity and a desire to have sexual activity

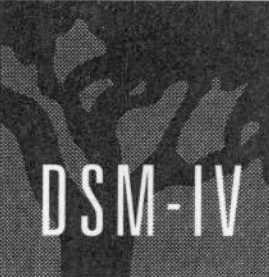

Sexual Dysfunctions

DSM-IV Categories

The following specifiers apply to all primary Sexual Dysfunctions:

Lifelong Type/Acquired Type
Generalized Type/Situational Type
Due to Psychological Factors/Due to Combined Factors

Sexual desire disorders

Hypoactive Sexual Desire Disorder
Sexual Aversion Disorder

Sexual arousal disorders

Female Sexual Arousal Disorder
Male Erectile Disorder

Orgasmic disorders

Female Orgasmic Disorder
Male Orgasmic Disorder
Premature Ejaculation

Sexual pain disorders

Dyspareunia (Not Due to a General Medical Condition)
Vaginismus (Not Due to a General Medical Condition)

Sexual dysfunction due to a general medical condition

Female Hypoactive Sexual Desire Disorder Due to . . .
(Indicate the General Medical Condition)
Male Hypoactive Sexual Desire Disorder Due to . . .
(Indicate the General Medical Condition)
Male Erectile Disorder Due to . . .
(Indicate the General Medical Condition)
Female Dyspareunia Due to . . .
(Indicate the General Medical Condition)
Male Dyspareunia Due to . . .
(Indicate the General Medical Condition)
Other Female Sexual Dysfunction Due to . . .
(Indicate the General Medical Condition)
Other Male Sexual Dysfunction Due to . . .
(Indicate the General Medical Condition)

Substance-induced sexual dysfunction *(refer to substance-related disorders for substance-specific codes)*

Specify if: With Impaired Desire/With Impaired Arousal/With Impaired Orgasm/With Sexual Pain
Specify if: With Onset During Intoxication

Sexual Dysfunction NOS

2. Excitement—subjective sense of sexual pleasure with accompanying physical changes:
   Male–penile tumescence leading to erection and Cowper's gland secretion
   Female—pelvic vasocongestion, vaginal lubrication, and swelling of external genitalia
3. Orgasm—peaking of sexual pleasure with release of sexual tension and rhythmic contraction of perineal muscles and female reproductive organs:
   Male—sensation of ejaculation inevitably followed by semen emission
   Female—contractions of the outer third of vaginal wall not always subjectively experienced
   Both sexes experience generalized muscle tension or contractions such as involuntary pelvic thrusting.
4. Resolution—sense of general relaxation, well-being, and muscle relaxation:
   Male—physiologically refractory to further erection and orgasm for a variable period of time
   Female—may be able to respond immediately to additional stimulation

Inhibitions may occur at one or more of these phases in the response cycle, although inhibition in the resolution phase rarely indicates clinical pathology. In most cases of sexual dysfunction, there is a disturbance in both the subjective sense of pleasure or desire and the objective performance.

Sexual dysfunctions may be only psychogenic, psychogenic and biogenic combined, lifelong or acquired, and generalized or situational. In most cases dysfunctions occur during sexual activity with a partner. In other situations dysfunctions can occur during the act of masturbation.

Age of onset is more commonly early adulthood (late twenties to early thirties). It is stipulated that to meet the diagnostic criteria, most sexual dysfunction disorders should not occur exclusively during the course of another Axis I disorder (other than a sexual dysfunction) such as Major Depression or Obsessive-Compulsive Disorder.

Diagnostic Categories of Sexual Dysfunctions

Sexual desire disorders

Hypoactive sexual desire disorder. Persistent or recurrent absent or deficient sexual fantasies and desire for sexual activity, taking into account age, sex, and the context of the person's life.

Sexual aversion disorder. Persistent or recurrent extreme aversion to and avoidance of all or nearly all genital sexual contact with a sexual partner.

Sexual arousal disorders

Female sexual arousal disorder. Persistent or recurrent partial or complete failure to attain or maintain lubrication-swelling response of sexual excitement until completion of sexual activity

or

persistent or recurrent lack of subjective sense of sexual excitement and pleasure during sexual activity.

Male erectile disorder. Persistent or recurrent partial or complete failure to attain or maintain erection until completion of sexual activity *or*

persistent or recurrent lack of subjective sense of sexual excitement and pleasure during sexual activity.

Orgasmic disorders

Female orgasmic disorder. Persistent or recurrent delay in, or absence of, orgasm following a normal sexual excitement phase. Some females may experience orgasms during noncoital clitoral stimulation but are unable to experience it during coitus in the absence of manual clitoral stimulation. The judgment of whether this condition justifies this diagnosis is made by thorough sexual evaluation and trial of treatment by a qualified expert. Age, experience, and adequacy of stimulation is considered.

Male orgasmic disorder. Persistent or recurrent delay in, or absence of, orgasm following a normal sexual excitement phase, considering the person's age and other factors. Failure to achieve orgasm is generally restricted to an inability to reach orgasm in the vagina, with orgasm possible with other types of stimulation such as masturbation.

Premature ejaculation. Persistent or recurrent ejaculation with minimal sexual stimulation, or before, upon, or shortly after penetration, and before the person wishes it, considering the person's age, newness of the sex partner or situation, and frequency of the sexual activity.

Sexual pain disorders

Dyspareunia. Persistent or recurrent genital pain in either a male or female before, during, or after sexual intercourse, not caused solely by lack of lubrication or vaginismus.

Vaginismus. Persistent or recurrent involuntary spasm of the musculature of the outer third of the vagina, which interferes with coitus.

Substance-induced sexual dysfunction. The defining characteristic of this diagnosis is significant sexual dysfunction causing distress and interference with interpersonal relationships. Symptoms of dysfunction are substance-specific physiologic effects as a result of intake of drugs of abuse, medications, or toxic exposure. Manifestations of dysfunction include the following:

With impaired desire—absent or deficient sexual desire
With impaired arousal—impaired sexual arousal (impaired lubrication, erectile dysfunction)
With impaired orgasm—orgasmic impairment
With sexual pain—pain associated with intercourse

Sexual dysfunction (NOS). Dysfunctions that do not meet criteria for any of the specific sexual dysfunctions listed above.

Examples:

- No erotic sensation or even complete anesthesia, despite normal physiologic component of orgasm
- The female analogue of premature ejaculation
- Genital pain occurring during masturbation

Other sexual disorders

Sexual disorder. Disorders not classified in any of the previous categories. This category rarely may be used concurrently with one of the specific diagnoses when both are necessary to explain or describe the clinical condition.

Examples:

- Marked feelings of inadequacy regarding body habitus, size and shape of sex organs, sexual performance, or other traits related to self-imposed standards of masculinity or femininity
- Distress about a pattern of repeated sexual conquests or other form of nonparaphilic sexual addictions involving a succession of people who exist only as things to be used
- Persistent and marked distress about one's sexual orientation

Individuals who experience sexual disorders as described in the DSM-IV may benefit from intervention with a qualified sex therapist. We have elected to construct a care plan based on common problems related to physiologic and psychologic stressors (e.g., effects of prescribed medication, chronicity of the mental or emotional disorder, and/or long-term institutionalization) that interfere with sexual function, performance, and gratification of the client with a mental or emotional disorder. Thus the care plan that follows is based on these problems experienced by psychiatric clients that are best addressed by nurses.

Paraphilias

The defining characteristics of these disorders is arousal in response to sexual objects or situations that are not considered the normative arousal activity sources; such arousal may in varying degrees interfere with the capacity for reciprocal, affectionate sexual activity.

Examples: Recurrent, intense sexual urges and sexually arousing fantasies involving any of the following:

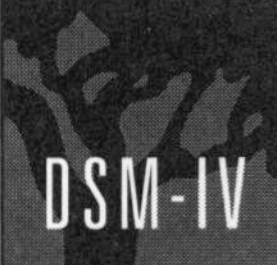

Paraphilias

DSM-IV Categories

Exhibitionism
Fetishism
Frotteurism
Pedophilia
Specify if: Sexually Attracted to Males/Sexually Attracted to Females/Sexually Attracted to Both
Specify if: Limited to Incest
Specify type: Exclusive Type/Nonexclusive Type
Sexual Masochism
Sexual Sadism
Transvestic Fetishism
Specify if: With Gender Dysphoria
Voyeurism
Paraphilia NOS

- Nonhuman objects
- The humiliating or suffering of self or partner
- Children or other nonconsenting individuals

Paraphilic stimuli or fantasies may not always be a prerequisite for erotic arousal in all persons with a paraphilic condition but may occur only in times of stress. Sexual activity may or may not involve a partner. The imagery in a paraphilic fantasy, such as female underclothes, is often the stimulus for sexual arousal in persons without a paraphilic condition. Such fantasies and urges are considered paraphilic only when the individual acts on the urges or is extremely distressed by them.

When the paraphilic imagery (e.g., being humiliated) is not shared with the person's partner, that partner may feel erotically excluded from the sexual interaction. In an extreme situation, paraphilic imagery that is acted out with a nonconsenting partner may injure the partner (sexual sadism) or injure the paraphilic individual (sexual masochism).

People with paraphilias commonly display at least three or four varieties and generally suffer from other mental disorders such as substance-related disorders or personality disorders. They often tend not to think of themselves as ill and may come to the attention of mental health professionals only when their behavior has brought them into conflict with sexual partners, society, or the law. These individuals may often select an occupation, hobby, or volunteer work that brings them into contact with the desired stimulus (e.g., selling women's shoes or lingerie, as in fetishism; working in a child-care setting, as in pedophilia; or driving an ambulance, as in sexual sadism). People without partners may solicit the services of prostitutes or others who provide specialized paraphilic-related services (e.g., bondage and domination or cross-dressing sessions). Others may act out fantasies with unwilling victims, which generally brings them in touch with the legal system. Symptom manifestations need to be present over a 6-month period to meet the diagnostic criteria; age of onset for most paraphilias is generally adolescence.

Diagnostic categories of paraphilias

Exhibitionism. Exposure of one's genitals to unsuspecting stranger(s), followed by sexual arousal.

Fetishism. Use of objects (e.g., female underclothes) or instruments (e.g., vibrators) for purpose of sexual arousal.

Frotteruism. Touching or rubbing against a nonconsenting person, to heighten sexual arousal.

Pedophilia. Sexual activity with a prepubescent child or children 13 years of age or younger. Pedophiliac is generally at least 16 years of age and at least 5 years older than the child/children. May be homosexual, heterosexual, bisexual, limited to incest, exclusive type (attracted only to children), or nonexclusive type (also attracted to adults of either sex).

Sexual masochism. The act of being humiliated, beaten, bound, or otherwise made to suffer by another person.

Sexual sadism. Acts in which physical or psychologic suffering (e.g., humiliation) of the victim is sexually arousing to the perpetrator.

Transvestic fetishism. The act of cross-dressing in a heterosexual male (wears female clothing to achieve sexual arousal) that does not meet the criteria for Gender Identity Disorder, nontranssexual type, or transsexualism.

Voyeurism. The act of observing an unsuspecting person who is naked, in the process of disrobing, or engaging in sexual activity, to achieve sexual arousal.

Paraphilias (NOS). Disorders that do not meet criteria for the specific categories.

Examples:

- Telephone scatologia (lewdness—obscene phone calling, sex line telephoning)
- Necrophilia (sexual activity with corpses)
- Partialism (exclusive focus on body part that generates sexual arousal)
- Zoophilia (sexual activity with animals, also known as *bestiality*)
- Coprophilia (sexual arousal on contact with feces)
- Klismaphilia (sexual arousal generated by the use of enemas)
- Urophilia (sexual arousal on contact with urine)
- Ephebophilia (fondling and/or other types of sexual activities with children who are developing secondary sexual characteristics, such as pubic hair, breasts. Children are generally 13 to 18 years of age.)
- Paraphilic Coercive Disorder (rape; aggressive sexual assault, involving an act of sexual intercourse with a female against her will and without her consent)

Gender Identity Disorder

Defining characteristics of Gender Identity Disorder are (1) the persistent, strong desire to be the opposite sex or insistence that one is the opposite sex (cross-gender identification) and (2) persistent discomfort with own sex (male or female) and feelings of inappropriateness in the gender role of the assigned sex.

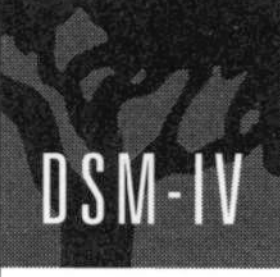

Gender Identity Disorders

DSM-IV Categories

Gender Identity Disorder
 in Children
 in Adolescents or Adults

Specify if: Sexually Attracted to Males/Sexually Attracted to Females/Sexually Attracted to Both/Sexually Attracted to Neither

Gender Identity Disorder NOS

Sexual Disorder NOS

Cross gender identification surpasses merely wanting to be the opposite sex for cultural advantages and instead is manifested as significant preoccupation with activities that are traditionally reserved for the opposite sex. Individuals prefer dressing in clothing of the opposite sex (cross-dressing), have persistent fantasies of being the opposite sex or show preference for cross sex roles in make-believe play, participate in stereotypical games of the other sex, and prefer playmates of the opposite sex.

Discomfort with the individual's own sex or gender role manifests as disgust with his or her genitals, rejection of usual assigned position for urination (boys, standing; girls, sitting), and insistence by the girl that she will not menstruate or have larger breasts and by the boy that he will not have a penis when he grows up.

In both sexes, homosexuality is often an outcome, occurring in one third to two thirds of those who have Gender Identity Disorder, although fewer girls than boys become homosexual. Parents may become alarmed when one of their children displays behaviors they believe are stereotypically associated with the opposite sex, but they need to be reassured in many instances that their child's nonconformity may not represent the profound disturbance of sexual identity defined in this disorder. Marked distress and/or impairment in the affected person must also be present to make a diagnosis.

INTERVENTIONS

Therapy for sexual disorders is usually conducted on an outpatient basis. Diagnostic tests, such as penile plethysmography (to detect and measure erections) or vaginal plethysmography (to determine vaginal blood flow), may take place in institutions. The focus of therapy is multifaceted. It aims at (1) education about normal human sexual function and appropriate education about sexual dysfunction (etiology, symptoms, treatment), (2) enhancement of communication and intimacy skills, (3) relief from anxiety and fear concerning sexuality, (4) self-esteem enhancement, and (5) physical support when necessary (diagnostic and treatment).

DISCHARGE CRITERIA FOR SEXUAL AND GENDER IDENTITY DISORDERS

Verbalizes knowledge regarding sexual disorder, sexual activity, and their relationship to mental disorder, hospitalization, and medication regimen

Verbalizes the desire to engage in a satisfying sexual relationship within capacity

Develops age-appropriate intimacy with significant person within capacity

Demonstrates interest and energy in satisfying sexual activity, with significant reduction in sexual limitations, or dysfunctions, within capacity

Expresses need for ongoing therapy with qualified sex therapist, if necessary or appropriate

Expresses desire for community involvement to enhance socialization, intimacy, and alternate satisfying activities

Nursing Process for

Sexual and Gender Identity Disorders

Universal Principles for Interactions and Interventions for Clients with Sexual Disorders

- Continue to monitor assessment parameters listed in *Defining Characteristics.*
- Continue to consider the etiologic factors listed in *Etiologic/Related Factors.*
- Utilize principles of the *Therapeutic Nurse-Client Relationship* (Appendix G).
- Address clients' spiritual and cultural needs.

General Principles

- Provide for safety, health, and comfort in the milieu.
- Identify client's level of intimacy and its appropriateness to age and development.
- Assess client's ability to engage in age-appropriate social and/or intimate relationships in the milieu.
- Demonstrate acceptance of client without condoning negative sexual behaviors and activities.
- Help the client to verbalize problems, limitations, or dysfunctions related to sexuality or sexual activity.
- Help the client discuss illness, hospitalization, and medication and the effects they may have on sexual dysfunction.
- Provide opportunities for age-appropriate expressions of intimacy and sexuality through milieu and group socialization within the client's capacity.
- Promote self-esteem through verbal praise and therapeutic individual and group exercises (e.g., cognitive and assertive skills). (See Appendix K.)
- Provide alternate, satisfying physical and intellectual activities.
- Facilitate socialization with same-age peers through role modeling and education.
- Educate client, family, and significant others about sexual dysfunctions and disorders with the help of qualified professionals.
- Modify negative sexual behaviors with firm, kind approach, setting limits when necessary.
- Promote opportunities for vocational and recreational activities.
- Facilitate community involvement to meet the needs of the client and family.

Care Plan for Sexual and Gender Identity Disorders Based on Nursing Diagnosis

DSM-IV Diagnosis
Sexual Dysfunction

NANDA Diagnosis
Sexual dysfunction

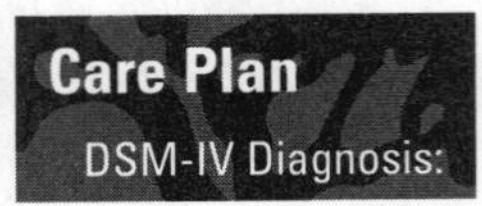

Sexual Dysfunction

NANDA Diagnosis: Sexual dysfunction

The state in which an individual experiences a change in sexual function that is viewed as unsatisfactory, unrewarding, or inadequate

Focus:
For the client who experiences a change in sexual function as a result of the effects of a chronic mental disorder; nontherapeutic effects of psychotropic drugs that may inhibit sexual drive, function, or performance; and institutionalization that interferes with the person's progression toward intimacy and sexual gratification

NANDA Taxonomy
Pattern (3)—Relating: A human response pattern involving establishing bonds

ETIOLOGIC/RELATED FACTORS (RELATED TO)

Biopsychosocial alteration of sexuality:
- Medication effects
- Chronic mental disorder/developmental lag
- Institutionalization

Ineffectual role models:
- Absent or dysfunctional parenting during critical developmental stages

Dependent, ineffective relationships:
- Seeks relations with equally vulnerable clients in mental health facility

Lack of emotionally stable significant other

Inability to attain or maintain a successful intimate relationship

Knowledge deficit regarding sex and sexual practices

DEFINING CHARACTERISTICS (AS EVIDENCED BY)

Verbalizes loss of interest and energy in sexual activity since taking prescribed psychotropic medications:

"I just don't have the stamina or desire for sex since I began taking this medication."

Reports actual or perceived sexual limitations imposed by mental disorder:

"This mental problem has really ruined my sex life."

"No one wants to make love with someone with a mental illness."

Demonstrates alterations in achieving perceived sex role throughout long-term, chronic mental disorder.
- Fails to achieve chronologic developmental task of intimacy
- Unable to engage in sexual activity with another person or significant partner

Expresses lack of knowledge regarding ability to find satisfactory sexual expression or alternate gratifying activities alone or with a partner:

"I just don't know how to have a sexual experience with anyone."

"I wish I could at least find some friend or hobbies to make me happy even if I can't have sex."

OUTCOME IDENTIFICATION AND EVALUATION

Demonstrates ability to attain and maintain ongoing intimate relations with same-age partner

Works with psychiatrist/therapist to adjust prescribed dosage of psychotropic medication to achieve maximum sexual potency and performance

Verbalizes achievement of sexual gratification in accordance with developmental capacity, effects of medication, and mental and emotional functions

Demonstrates ability to engage in alternative satisfying friendships, hobbies, and activities during periods of institutionalization in lieu of sexual activities

PLANNING AND IMPLEMENTATION

Nursing Interventions and Rationale

Assess via interview the client's degree of sexual frustration and dysfunction, beginning with less personal therapeutic statements, and progressing to more personal statements, *to build trust and rapport and determine the extent of the client's sexual problems and to plan relevant interventions.*

Example of interview.

Less personal (to build trust and rapport)
- Reflect client's statements:
  "John, you've expressed concern about your lack of energy and interest lately and you've been avoiding other clients and activities."
- Voice concerns:
  "The staff and I are concerned that you don't seem to want to take your medication. What seems to be the problem?"
- Sit in silence for a while and employ active listening (the client needs an opportunity to vent concerns).
- Elicit feelings with open-ended statement:
  "What is it about your medication and illness that is troubling to you?"
  Allow the client sufficient time to respond.

More personal (to focus on specific problem)
- Offer information when appropriate:
  "John, medication such as yours can affect sexual drive and activity."
- Use direct questioning:
  "Has your illness and/or medication affected your sexual activities and relationships?"

If answer is yes:
- Reassure client that although symptoms are troubling, they are not unique. This will decrease fear or embarrassment.
  "Other clients with mental disorders who take medication similar to yours have experienced some of the same sexual problems."
- Offer suggestions that may bring relief and hope:
  "One suggestion is to discuss your problem with your doctor, who may be able to adjust your med-

ication or provide other ways to relieve your problem."

Note: Modify interview in accordance with each client's developmental stage and cognitive, affective, and social capabilities. Be careful not to offer false hope.

Construct a list of the client's medications that are most likely responsible for altering or decreasing libido, sexual performance, or sexual activity *to reinforce the possibility that the physician's adjustment of the doses of some drugs may correct or ameliorate the problem.*

(Refer to the list of medications and their effects on sexual function and performance, Appendix M.)

Suggest alternative activities to sublimate or substitute overt sexual activity and gratification *so that the client may experience pleasure while he or she is unable to engage in intimate relationships or direct sexual activity during hospitalization:*

- Play a musical instrument (e.g., pound on piano or drums)
- Engage in physical exercise, activity, or sport (e.g., run/walk briskly, pound pillows or batakas, play volleyball)
- Engage in games that require mental energy (e.g., chess or Scrabble)

Note: Supplemental activities should correlate with each client's developmental stage and physical, mental, emotional, and social functioning.

Engage the client in sex-education classes, as needed, *to increase the client's knowledge regarding sexuality and alternative means to enhance interpersonal relationships and increase sexual performance and gratification.*

Enroll the client in an education class with a hospital pharmacologist who teaches the effects of prescribed medications *to increase the client's knowledge regarding the effects of medication on libido, sexual performance, and sexual activity and to give the client an opportunity to voice concerns with other clients who have a similar problem.*

Help the client meet age-appropriate sleep/rest needs *to help him or her preserve energy stores required for interpersonal relationships that could lead to intimacy and healthy sexual expression:*

- Decrease noise and stimulation in the client's immediate environment prior to and at bedtime.
- Provide time for daytime nap(s), if necessary.

Engage the client in appropriate milieu activities with same-age clients *to encourage active socialization as a prelude to intimate relationships and healthy sexual expression compatible with developmental age and preference. (In most psychiatric settings, sexual activity is not encouraged or permitted.)*

Discharge plan

Refer the client to a therapist who specializes in sexual dysfunctions related to mental disorders, institutionalization, developmental lag, and/or medication effects *to ensure that the client receives ongoing qualified help for sexual problem(s).*

Encourage the client to join community groups or organizations and/or use community resources *to help support continuing interpersonal interactions and relationships that could foster intimacy and healthy, satisfying sexual activity and experiences.*

Examples:

- Church group or affiliation
- Youth or adult recreation center

Include family and significant others with client's consent or approval.

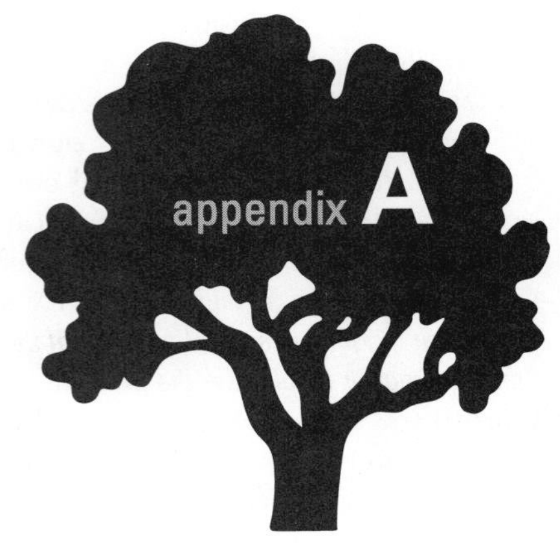

ANA Standards of Psychiatric–Mental Health Clinical Nursing Practice

STANDARDS OF CARE

Standard I. Assessment
The psychiatric–mental health nurse collects client health data.

Standard II. Diagnosis
The psychiatric–mental health nurse analyzes the assessment data in determining diagnosis.

Standard III. Outcome Identification
The psychiatric–mental health nurse identifies expected outcomes individualized to the client.

Standard IV. Planning
The psychiatric–mental health nurse develops a plan of care that prescribes interventions to attain expected outcomes.

Standard V. Implementation
The psychiatric–mental health nurse implements the interventions identified in the plan of care.

Standard Va. Counseling
The psychiatric–mental health nurse uses counseling interventions to assist clients in improving or regaining their previous coping abilities, fostering mental health, and preventing mental illness and disability.

Reprinted with permission from *A Statement on Psychiatric–Mental Health Clinical Nursing Practice and Standards of Psychiatric–Mental Health Clinical Nursing Practice,* Washington, DC, 1994, American Nurses Association.

Standard Vb. Milieu Therapy
The psychiatric-mental health nurse provides, structures, and maintains a therapeutic environment in collaboration with the client and other health-care providers.

Standard Vc. Self-Care Activities
The psychiatric–mental health nurse structures interventions around the client's activities of daily living to foster self-care and mental and physical well-being.

Standard Vd. Psychobiological Interventions
The psychiatric–mental health nurse uses knowledge of psychobiological interventions and applies clinical skills to restore the client's health and prevent further disability.

Standard Ve. Health Teaching
The psychiatric–mental health nurse, through health teaching, assists clients in achieving satisfying, productive, and healthy patterns of living.

Standard Vf. Case Management
The psychiatric–mental health nurse provides case management to coordinate comprehensive health services and ensure continuity of care.

Standard Vg. Health Promotion and Health Maintenance
The psychiatric–mental health nurse employs strategies and interventions to promote and maintain mental health and prevent mental illness.

Standard Vh. Psychotherapy
The certified specialist in psychiatric–mental health nursing uses individual, group, and family psychotherapy, child psychotherapy, and other therapeutic treatments to assist clients in fostering mental health, preventing mental illness and disability, and improving or regaining previous health status and functional abilities.

Standard Vi. Prescription of Pharmacological Agents
The certified specialist uses prescription of pharmacological agents in accordance with the state nursing practice act to treat symptoms of psychiatric illness and improve functional health status.

Standard Vj. Consultation
The certified specialist provides consultation to health-care providers and others to influence the plans of care for clients and to enhance the abilities of others to provide psychiatric and mental health care and effect change in systems.

Standard VI. Evaluation
The psychiatric–mental health nurse evaluates the client's progress in attaining expected outcomes.

STANDARD OF PROFESSIONAL PERFORMANCE

Standard I. Quality of Care
The psychiatric–mental health nurse systematically evaluates the quality of care and effectiveness of psychiatric–mental health nursing practice.

Standard II. Performance Appraisal
The psychiatric–mental health nurse evaluates own psychiatric–mental health nursing practice in relation to professional practice standards and relevant statutes and regulations.

Standard III. Education
The psychiatric–mental health nurse acquires and maintains current knowledge in nursing practice.

Standard IV. Collegiality
The psychiatric–mental health nurse contributes to the professional development of peers, colleagues, and others.

Standard V. Ethics
The psychiatric–mental health nurse's decisions and actions on behalf of clients are determined in an ethical manner.

Standard VI. Collaboration
The psychiatric–mental health nurse collaborates with the client, significant others, and health-care providers in providing care.

Standard VII. Research
The psychiatric–mental health nurse contributes to nursing and mental health through the use of research.

Standard VIII. Resource Utilization
The psychiatric–mental health nurse considers factors related to safety, effectiveness, and cost in planning and delivering client care.

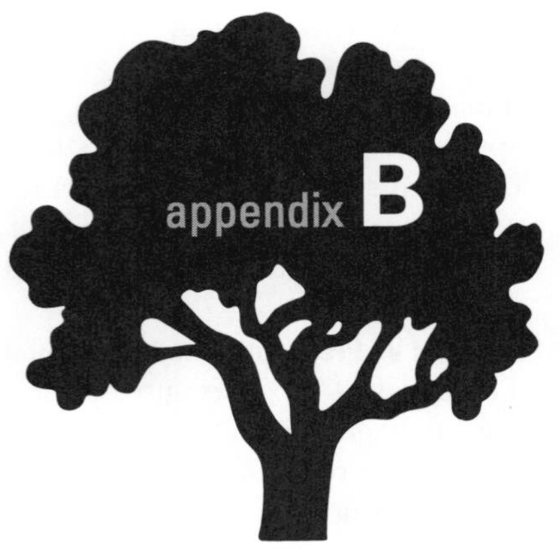

Patients' Rights

ALLOWING FOR GREAT VARIATION AMONG STATES, PATIENTS CURRENTLY HAVE THE FOLLOWING RIGHTS:

Right to communicate with people outside the hospital through correspondence, telephone, and personal visits
Right to keep clothing and personal effects with them in the hospital
Right to religious freedom
Right to be employed if possible
Right to manage and dispose of property
Right to execute wills
Right to enter into contractual relationships
Right to make purchases
Right to education
Right to habeas corpus
Right to independent psychiatric examination
Right to civil service status
Right to retain licenses, privileges, or permits established by law, such as a driver's or professional license
Right to sue or be sued
Right to marry and divorce
Right not to be subject to unnecessary mechanical restraints
Right to periodic review of status
Right to legal representation
Right to privacy
Right of informed consent
Right to treatment
Right to refuse treatment
Right to treatment in the least restrictive setting

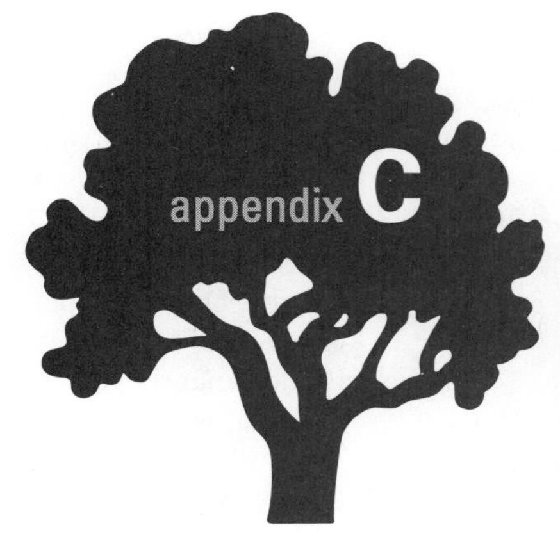

DSM-IV Classification

NOS = Not Otherwise Specified.*

An *x* appearing in a diagnostic code indicates that a specific code number is required.

An ellipsis (. . .) is used in the names of certain disorders to indicate that the name of a specific mental disorder or general medical condition should be inserted when recording the name (e.g., 293.0 Delirium Due to Hypothyroidism).

If criteria are currently met, one of the following severity specifiers may be noted after the diagnosis:

Mild
Moderate
Severe

If criteria are no longer met, one of the following specifiers may be noted:

In Partial Remission
In Full Remission
Prior History

From American Psychiatric Association: *Diagnostic and statistical manual of mental disorders,* ed 4, Washington, DC, 1994, American Psychiatric Association.
*Not Otherwise Specified indicates that symptoms do not clearly fit any particular category in DSM-IV for that disorder (may include symptoms for several categories within the disorder).

DISORDERS USUALLY FIRST DIAGNOSED IN INFANCY, CHILDHOOD, OR ADOLESCENCE

Mental Retardation

Note: *These are coded on Axis II.*

317 Mild Mental Retardation
318.0 Moderate Mental Retardation
318.1 Severe Mental Retardation
318.2 Profound Mental Retardation
319 Mental Retardation, Severity Unspecified

Learning Disorders

315.00 Reading Disorder
315.1 Mathematics Disorder
315.2 Disorder of Written Expression
315.9 Learning Disorder NOS

Motor Skills Disorder

315.4 Developmental Coordination Disorder

Communication Disorders

315.31 Expressive Language Disorder
315.31 Mixed Receptive-Expressive Language Disorder
315.39 Phonological Disorder
307.0 Stuttering
307.9 Communication Disorder NOS

Pervasive Developmental Disorders

299.00 Autistic Disorder

299.80 Rett's Disorder
299.10 Childhood Disintegrative Disorder
299.80 Asperger's Disorder
299.80 Pervasive Developmental Disorder NOS

Attention-Deficit and Disruptive Behavior Disorders

314.xx Attention-Deficit/Hyperactivity Disorder
.01 Combined Type
.00 Predominantly Inattentive Type
.01 Predominantly Hyperactive-Impulsive Type
314.9 Attention-Deficit/Hyperactivity Disorder NOS
312.8 Conduct Disorder
Specify type: Childhood-Onset Type/ Adolescent-Onset Type
313.81 Oppositional Defiant Disorder
312.9 Disruptive Behavior Disorder NOS

Feeding and Eating Disorders of Infancy or Early Childhood

307.52 Pica
307.53 Rumination Disorder
307.59 Feeding Disorder of Infancy or Early Childhood

Tic Disorders

307.23 Tourette's Disorder
307.22 Chronic Motor or Vocal Tic Disorder
307.21 Transient Tic Disorder
Specify if: Single Episode/Recurrent
307.20 Tic Disorder NOS

Elimination Disorders

___._ Encopresis
787.6 With Constipation and Overflow Incontinence
307.7 Without Constipation and Overflow Incontinence
307.6 Enuresis (Not Due to a General Medical Condition)
Specify type: Nocturnal Only/Diurnal Only/Nocturnal and Diurnal

Other Disorders of Infancy, Childhood, or Adolescence

309.21 Separation Anxiety Disorder
Specify if: Early Onset
313.23 Selective Mutism
313.89 Reactive Attachment Disorder of Infancy or Early Childhood
Specify type: Inhibited Type/Disinhibited Type
307.3 Stereotypic Movement Disorder
Specify if: With Self-Injurious Behavior
313.9 Disorder of Infancy, Childhood, or Adolescence NOS

DELIRIUM, DEMENTIA, AND AMNESTIC AND OTHER COGNITIVE DISORDERS

Delirium

293.0 Delirium Due to . . . *{Indicate the General Medical Condition}*
___._ Substance Intoxication Delirium *(refer to Substance-Related Disorders for substance-specific codes)*
___._ Substance Withdrawal Delirium *(refer to Substance-Related Disorders for substance-specific codes)*
___._ Delirium Due to Multiple Etiologies *(code each of the specific etiologies)*
780.09 Delirium NOS

Dementia

290.xx Dementia of the Alzheimer's Type, With Early Onset *(also code 331.0 Alzheimer's disease on Axis III)*
.10 Uncomplicated
.11 With Delirium
.12 With Delusions
.13 With Depressed Mood
Specify if: With Behavioral Disturbance
290.xx Dementia of the Alzheimer's Type, With Late Onset *(also code 331.0 Alzheimer's disease on Axis III)*
.0 Uncomplicated
.3 With Delirium
.20 With Delusions
.21 With Depressed Mood
Specify if: With Behavioral Disturbance
290.xx Vascular Dementia
.40 Uncomplicated
.41 With Delirium
.42 With Delusions
.43 With Depressed Mood
Specify if: With Behavioral Disturbance
294.9 Dementia Due to HIV Disease *(also code 043.1 HIV infection affecting central nervous system on Axis III)*
294.1 Dementia Due to Head Trauma *(also code 854.00 head injury on Axis III)*
294.1 Dementia Due to Parkinson's Disease *(also code 332.0 Parkinson's disease on Axis III)*
294.1 Dementia Due to Huntington's Disease *(also code 333.4 Huntington's disease on Axis III)*
290.10 Dementia Due to Pick's Disease *(also code 331.1 Pick's disease on Axis III)*
290.10 Dementia Due to Creutzfeldt-Jakob Disease *(also code 046.1 Creutzfeldt-Jakob disease on Axis III)*
294.1 Dementia Due to . . . *{Indicate the General Medical Condition not listed above} (also code the general medical condition on Axis III)*

___._	Substance-Induced Persisting Dementia *(refer to Substance-Related Disorders for substance-specific codes)*
___._	Dementia Due to Multiple Etiologies *(code each of the specific etiologies)*
294.8	Dementia NOS

Amnestic Disorders

294.0	Amnestic Disorder Due to . . . *{Indicate the General Medical Condition}* *Specify if:* Transient/Chronic
___._	Substance-Induced Persisting Amnestic Disorder *(refer to Substance-Related Disorders for substance-specific codes)*
294.8	Amnestic Disorder NOS

Other Cognitive Disorders

294.9	Cognitive Disorder NOS

MENTAL DISORDERS DUE TO A GENERAL MEDICAL CONDITION NOT ELSEWHERE CLASSIFIED

293.89	Catatonic Disorder Due to . . . *{Indicate the General Medical Condition}*
310.1	Personality Change Due to . . . *{Indicate the General Medical Condition}* *Specify type:* Labile Type/Disinhibited Type/Aggressive Type/Apathetic Type/Paranoid Type/Other Type/Combined Type/Unspecified Type
293.9	Mental Disorder NOS Due to . . . *{Indicate the General Medical Condition}*

SUBSTANCE-RELATED DISORDERS

[a]*The following specifiers may be applied to Substance Dependence:*

With Physiological Dependence/Without Physiological Dependence

Early Full Remission/Early Partial Remission
Sustained Full Remission/Sustained Partial Remission
On Agonist Therapy/In a Controlled Environment

The following specifiers apply to Substance-Induced Disorders as noted:

[I]With Onset During Intoxication/[W]With Onset During Withdrawal

Alcohol-Related Disorders

Alcohol use disorders

303.90	Alcohol Dependence[a]
305.00	Alcohol Abuse

Alcohol-induced disorders

303.00	Alcohol Intoxication
291.8	Alcohol Withdrawal *Specify if:* With Perceptual Disturbances
291.0	Alcohol Intoxication Delirium
291.0	Alcohol Withdrawal Delirium
291.2	Alcohol-Induced Persisting Dementia
291.1	Alcohol-Induced Persisting Amnestic Disorder
291.x	Alcohol-Induced Psychotic Disorder
.5	With Delusions[I,W]
.3	With Hallucinations[I,W]
291.8	Alcohol-Induced Mood Disorder[I,W]
291.8	Alcohol-Induced Anxiety Disorder[I,W]
291.8	Alcohol-Induced Sexual Dysfunction[I]
291.8	Alcohol-Induced Sleep Disorder[I,W]
291.9	Alcohol-Related Disorder NOS

Amphetamine (or Amphetamine-Like)-Related Disorders

Amphetamine use disorders

304.40	Amphetamine Dependence[a]
305.70	Amphetamine Abuse

Amphetamine-induced disorders

292.89	Amphetamine Intoxication *Specify if:* With Perceptual Disturbances
292.0	Amphetamine Withdrawal
292.81	Amphetamine Intoxication Delirium
292.xx	Amphetamine-Induced Psychotic Disorder
.11	With Delusions[I]
.12	With Hallucinations[I]
292.84	Amphetamine-Induced Mood Disorder[I,W]
292.89	Amphetamine-Induced Anxiety Disorder[I]
292.89	Amphetamine-Induced Sexual Dysfunction[I]
292.89	Amphetamine-Induced Sleep Disorder[I,W]
292.9	Amphetamine-Related Disorder NOS

Caffeine-Related Disorders

Caffeine-induced disorders

305.90	Caffeine-Intoxication
292.89	Caffeine-Induced Anxiety Disorder[I]
292.89	Caffeine-Induced Sleep Disorder[I]
292.9	Caffeine-Related Disorder NOS

Cannabis-Related Disorders

Cannabis use disorders

304.30	Cannabis Dependence[a]
305.20	Cannabis Abuse

Cannabis-induced disorders

292.89	Cannabis Intoxication *Specify if:* With Perceptual Disturbances
292.81	Cannabis Intoxication Delirium
292.xx	Cannabis-Induced Psychotic Disorder
.11	With Delusions[I]
.12	With Hallucinations[I]
292.89	Cannabis-Induced Anxiety Disorder[I]
292.9	Cannabis-Related Disorder NOS

Cocaine-Related Disorders

Cocaine use disorders

304.20 Cocaine Dependence[a]
305.60 Cocaine Abuse

Cocaine-induced disorders

292.89 Cocaine Intoxication
Specify if: With Perceptual Disturbances
292.0 Cocaine Withdrawal
292.81 Cocaine Intoxication Delirium
292.xx Cocaine-Induced Psychotic Disorder
.11 With Delusions[I]
.12 With Hallucinations[I]
292.84 Cocaine-Induced Mood Disorder[I,W]
292.89 Cocaine-Induced Anxiety Disorder[I,W]
292.89 Cocaine-Induced Sexual Dysfunction[I]
292.89 Cocaine-Induced Sleep Disorder[I,W]
292.9 Cocaine-Related Disorder NOS

Hallucinogen-Related Disorders

Hallucinogen use disorders

304.50 Hallucinogen Dependence[a]
305.30 Hallucinogen Abuse

Hallucinogen-induced disorders

292.89 Hallucinogen Intoxication
292.89 Hallucinogen Persisting Perception Disorder (Flashbacks)
292.81 Hallucinogen Intoxication Delirium
292.xx Hallucinogen-Induced Psychotic Disorder
.11 With Delusions[I]
.12 With Hallucinations[I]
292.84 Hallucinogen-Induced Mood Disorder[I]
292.89 Hallucinogen-Induced Anxiety Disorder[I]
292.9 Hallucinogen-Related Disorder NOS

Inhalant-Related Disorders

Inhalant use disorders

304.60 Inhalant Dependence[a]
305.90 Inhalant Abuse

Inhalant-induced disorders

292.89 Inhalant Intoxication
292.81 Inhalant Intoxication Delirium
292.82 Inhalant-Induced Persisting Dementia
292.xx Inhalant-Induced Psychotic Disorder
.11 With Delusions[I]
.12 With Hallucinations[I]
292.84 Inhalant-Induced Mood Disorder[I]
292.89 Inhalant-Induced Anxiety Disorder[I]
292.9 Inhalant-Related Disorder NOS

Nicotine-Related Disorders

Nicotine use disorder

305.10 Nicotine Dependence[a]

Nicotine-induced disorder

292.0 Nicotine Withdrawal
292.9 Nicotine-Related Disorder NOS

Opioid-Related Disorders

Opioid use disorders

304.00 Opioid Dependence[a]
305.50 Opioid Abuse

Opioid-induced disorders

292.89 Opioid Intoxication
Specify if: With Perceptual Disturbances
292.0 Opioid Withdrawal
292.81 Opioid Intoxication Delirium
292.xx Opioid-Induced Psychotic Disorder
.11 With Delusions[I]
.12 With Hallucinations[I]
292.84 Opioid-Induced Mood Disorder[I]
292.89 Opioid-Induced Sexual Dysfunction[I]
292.89 Opioid-Induced Sleep Disorder[I,W]
292.9 Opioid-Related Disorder NOS

Phencyclidine (or Phencyclidine-Like)-Related Disorders

Phencyclidine use disorders

304.90 Phencyclidine Dependence[a]
305.90 Phencyclidine Abuse

Phencyclidine-induced disorders

292.89 Phencyclidine Intoxication
Specify if: With Perceptual Disturbances
292.81 Phencyclidine Intoxication Delirium
292.xx Phencyclidine-Induced Psychotic Disorder
.11 With Delusions[I]
.12 With Hallucinations[I]
292.84 Phencyclidine-Induced Mood Disorder[I]
292.89 Phencyclidine-Induced Anxiety Disorder[I]
292.9 Phencyclidine-Related Disorder NOS

Sedative-, Hypnotic-, or Anxiolytic-Related Disorders

Sedative, hypnotic, or anxiolytic use disorders

304.10 Sedative, Hypnotic, or Anxiolytic Dependence[a]
305.40 Sedative, Hypnotic, or Anxiolytic Abuse

Sedative-, hypnotic-, or anxiolytic-induced disorders

292.89 Sedative, Hypnotic, or Anxiolytic Intoxication
292.0 Sedative, Hypnotic, or Anxiolytic Withdrawal
Specify if: With Perceptual Disturbances
292.81 Sedative, Hypnotic, or Anxiolytic Intoxication Delirium
292.81 Sedative, Hypnotic, or Anxiolytic Withdrawal Delirium
292.82 Sedative-, Hypnotic-, or Anxiolytic-Induced Persisting Dementia
292.83 Sedative-, Hypnotic-, or Anxiolytic-Induced Persisting Amnestic Disorder
292.xx Sedative-, Hypnotic-, or Anxiolytic-Induced Psychotic Disorder

.11 With Delusions[I,W]
.12 With Hallucinations[I,W]
292.84 Sedative-, Hypnotic-, or Anxiolytic-Induced Mood Disorder[I,W]
292.89 Sedative-, Hypnotic-, or Anxiolytic-Induced Anxiety Disorder[W]
292.89 Sedative-, Hypnotic-, or Anxiolytic-Induced Sexual Dysfunction[I]
292.89 Sedative-, Hypnotic-, or Anxiolytic-Induced Sleep Disorder[I,W]
292.9 Sedative-, Hypnotic-, or Anxiolytic-Related Disorder NOS

Polysubstance-Related Disorder

304.80 Polysubstance Dependence[a]

Other (or Unknown) Substance-Related Disorders

Other (or unknown) substance use disorders

304.90 Other (or Unknown) Substance Dependence[a]
305.90 Other (or Unknown) Substance Abuse

Other (or unknown) substance-induced disorders

292.89 Other (or Unknown) Substance Intoxication
Specify if: With Perceptual Disturbances
292.0 Other (or Unknown) Substance Withdrawal
Specify if: With Perceptual Disturbances
292.81 Other (or Unknown) Substance-Induced Delirium
292.82 Other (or Unknown) Substance-Induced Persisting Dementia
292.83 Other (or Unknown) Substance-Induced Persisting Amnestic Disorder
292.xx Other (or Unknown) Substance-Induced Psychotic Disorder
.11 With Delusions[I,W]
.12 With Hallucinations[I,W]
292.84 Other (or Unknown) Substance-Induced Mood Disorder[I,W]
292.89 Other (or Unknown) Substance-Induced Anxiety Disorder[I,W]
292.89 Other (or Unknown) Substance-Induced Sexual Dysfunction[I]
292.89 Other (or Unknown) Substance-Induced Sleep Disorder[I,W]
292.9 Other (or Unknown) Substance-Related Disorder NOS

SCHIZOPHRENIA AND OTHER PSYCHOTIC DISORDERS

295.xx Schizophrenia
The following Classification of Longitudinal Course applies to all subtypes of Schizophrenia:

Episodic With Interepisode Residual Symptoms (*Specify if:* With Prominent Negative Symptoms)/Episodic With No Interepisode Residual Symptoms
Continuous (*specify if:* With Prominent Negative Symptoms)
Single Episode In Partial Remission (*specify if:* With Prominent Negative Symptoms)/Single Episode In Full Remission
Other or Unspecified Pattern
.30 Paranoid Type
.10 Disorganized Type
.20 Catatonic Type
.90 Undifferentiated Type
.60 Residual Type
295.40 Schizophreniform Disorder
Specify if: Without Good Prognostic Features/With Good Prognostic Features
295.70 Schizoaffective Disorder
Specify type: Bipolar Type/Depressive Type
297.1 Delusional Disorder
Specify type: Erotomanic Type/Grandiose Type/Jealous Type/Persecutory Type/Somatic Type/Mixed Type/Unspecified Type
298.8 Brief Psychotic Disorder
Specify if: With Marked Stressor(s)/Without Marked Stressor(s)/With Postpartum Onset
297.3 Shared Psychotic Disorder
293.xx Psychotic Disorder Due to . . . *{Indicate the General Medical Condition}*
.81 With Delusions
.82 With Hallucinations
___.__ Substance-Induced Psychotic Disorder *(refer to Substance-Related Disorders for substance-specific codes)*
Specify if: With Onset During Intoxication/With Onset During Withdrawal
298.9 Psychotic Disorder NOS

MOOD DISORDERS

Code current state of Major Depressive Disorder or Bipolar I Disorder in fifth digit:

1 = Mild
2 = Moderate
3 = Severe Without Psychotic Features
4 = Severe With Psychotic Features
Specify: Mood-Congruent Psychotic Features/Mood-Incongruent Psychotic Features
5 = In Partial Remission
6 = In Full Remission
0 = Unspecified

The following specifiers apply (for current or most recent episode) to Mood Disorders as noted:

[a]Severity/Psychotic/Remission Specifiers/[b]Chronic/[c]With Catatonic Features/[d]With Melancholic Features/[e]With Atypical Features/[f]With Postpartum Onset

The following specifiers apply to Mood Disorders as noted:

[g]With or Without Full Interepisode Recovery/[h]With Seasonal pattern/[i]With Rapid Cycling

Appendix C

Depressive Disorders

296.xx Major Depressive Disorder
.2x Single Episode[a,b,c,d,e,f]
.3x Recurrent[a,b,c,d,e,f,g,h]
300.4 Dysthymic Disorder
Specify if: Early Onset/Late Onset
Specify if: With Atypical Features
311 Depressive Disorder NOS

Bipolar Disorders

296.xx Bipolar I Disorder
.0x Single Manic Episode[a,c,f]
Specify if: Mixed
.40 Most Recent Episode Hypomanic[g,h,i]
.4x Most Recent Episode Manic[a,c,f,g,h,i]
.6x Most Recent Episode Mixed[a,c,f,g,h,i]
.5x Most Recent Episode Depressed[a,b,c,d,e,f,g,h,i]
.7 Most Recent Episode Unspecified[g,h,i]
296.89 Bipolar II Disorder[a,b,c,d,e,f,g,h,i]
Specify (current or most recent episode): Hypomanic/Depressed
301.13 Cyclothymic Disorder
296.80 Bipolar Disorder NOS
293.83 Mood Disorder Due to . . . *{Indicate the General Medical Condition}*
Specify type: With Depressive Features/With Major Depressive–Like Episode/With Manic Features/With Mixed Features
___.__ Substance-Induced Mood Disorder *(refer to Substance-Related Disorders for substance-specific codes)*
Specify type: With Depressive Features/With Manic Features/With Mixed Features
Specify if: With Onset During Intoxication/With Onset During Withdrawal
296.90 Mood Disorder NOS

ANXIETY DISORDERS

300.01 Panic Disorder Without Agoraphobia
300.21 Panic Disorder With Agoraphobia
300.22 Agoraphobia Without History of Panic Disorder
300.29 Specific Phobia
Specify type: Animal Type/Natural Environment Type/Blood-Injection-Injury Type/Situational Type/Other Type
300.23 Social Phobia
Specify if: Generalized
300.3 Obsessive-Compulsive Disorder
Specify if: With Poor Insight
309.81 Posttraumatic Stress Disorder
Specify if: Acute/Chronic
Specify if: With Delayed Onset
308.3 Acute Stress Disorder
300.02 Generalized Anxiety Disorder
293.89 Anxiety Disorder Due to . . . *{Indicate the General Medical Condition}*
Specify if: With Generalized Anxiety/With Panic Attacks/With Obsessive-Compulsive Symptoms
___.__ Substance-Induced Anxiety Disorder *(refer to Substance-Related Disorders for substance-specific codes)*
Specify if: With Generalized Anxiety/With Panic Attacks/With Obsessive-Compulsive Symptoms/With Phobic Symptoms
Specify if: With Onset During Intoxication/With Onset During Withdrawal
300.00 Anxiety Disorder NOS

SOMATOFORM DISORDERS

300.81 Somatization Disorder
300.81 Undifferentiated Somatoform Disorder
300.11 Conversion Disorder
Specify type: With Motor Symptom or Deficit/With Sensory Symptom or Deficit/With Seizures or Convulsions/With Mixed Presentation
307.xx Pain Disorder
.80 Associated With Psychological Factors
.89 Associated With Both Psychological Factors and a General Medical Condition
Specify if: Acute/Chronic
300.7 Hypochondriasis
Specify if: With Poor Insight
300.7 Body Dysmorphic Disorder
300.81 Somatoform Disorder NOS

FACTITIOUS DISORDERS

300.xx Factitious Disorder
.16 With Predominantly Psychological Signs and Symptoms
.19 With Predominantly Physical Signs and Symptoms
.19 With Combined Psychological and Physical Signs and Symptoms
300.19 Factitious Disorder NOS

DISSOCIATIVE DISORDERS

300.12 Dissociative Amnesia
300.13 Dissociative Fugue
300.14 Dissociative Identity Disorder
300.6 Depersonalization Disorder
300.15 Dissociative Disorder NOS

SEXUAL AND GENDER IDENTITY DISORDERS

Sexual Dysfunctions

The following specifiers apply to all primary Sexual Dysfunctions:

Lifelong Type/Acquired Type
Generalized Type/Situational Type
Due to Psychological Factors/Due to Combined Factors

Sexual desire disorders

302.71 Hypoactive Sexual Desire Disorder
302.79 Sexual Aversion Disorder

Sexual arousal disorders

302.72 Female Sexual Arousal Disorder
302.72 Male Erectile Disorder

Orgasmic disorders

302.73 Female Orgasmic Disorder
302.74 Male Orgasmic Disorder
302.75 Premature Ejaculation

Sexual pain disorders

302.76 Dyspareunia (Not Due to a General Medical Condition)
306.51 Vaginismus (Not Due to a General Medical Condition)

Sexual dysfunction due to a general medical condition

625.8 Female Hypoactive Sexual Desire Disorder Due to . . . *{Indicate the General Medical Condition}*
608.89 Male Hypoactive Sexual Desire Disorder Due to . . . *{Indicate the General Medical Condition}*
607.84 Male Erectile Disorder Due to . . . *{Indicate the General Medical Condition}*
625.0 Female Dyspareunia Due to . . . *{Indicate the General Medical Condition}*
608.89 Male Dyspareunia Due to . . . *{Indicate the General Medical Condition}*
625.8 Other Female Sexual Dysfunction Due to . . . *{Indicate the General Medical Condition}*
608.89 Other Male Sexual Dysfunction Due to . . . *{Indicate the General Medical Condition}*
___.__ Substance-Induced Sexual Dysfunction *(refer to Substance-Related Disorders for substance-specific codes)*
Specify if: With Impaired Desire/With Impaired Arousal/With Impaired Orgasm/With Sexual Pain
Specify if: With Onset During Intoxication
302.70 Sexual Dysfunction NOS

Paraphilias

302.4 Exhibitionism
302.81 Fetishism
302.89 Frotteurism
302.2 Pedophilia
Specify if: Sexually Attracted to Males/Sexually Attracted to Females/Sexually Attracted to Both
Specify if: Limited to Incest
Specify type: Exclusive Type/Nonexclusive Type
302.83 Sexual Masochism
302.84 Sexual Sadism
302.3 Transvestic Fetishism
Specify if: With Gender Dysphoria
302.82 Voyeurism
302.9 Paraphilia NOS

Gender Identity Disorders

302.xx Gender Identity Disorder
.6 in Children
.85 in Adolescents or Adults
Specify if: Sexually Attracted to Males/Sexually Attracted to Females/Sexually Attracted to Both/Sexually Attracted to Neither
302.6 Gender to Identity Disorder NOS
302.9 Sexual Disorder NOS

EATING DISORDERS

307.1 Anorexia Nervosa
Specify type: Restricting Type; Binge-Eating/Purging Type
307.51 Bulimia Nervosa
Specify type: Purging Type/Nonpurging Type
307.50 Eating Disorder NOS

SLEEP DISORDERS

Primary Sleep Disorders

Dyssomnias

307.42 Primary Insomnia
307.44 Primary Hypersomnia
Specify if: Recurrent
347 Narcolepsy
780.59 Breathing-Related Sleep Disorder
307.45 Circadian Rhythm Sleep Disorder
Specify type: Delayed Sleep Phase Type/Jet Lag Type/Shift Work Type/Unspecified Type
307.47 Dyssomnia NOS

Parasomnias

307.47 Nightmare Disorder
307.46 Sleep Terror Disorder
307.46 Sleepwalking Disorder
307.47 Parasomnia NOS

Sleep Disorders Related to Another Mental Disorder

307.42 Insomnia Related to . . . *{Indicate the Axis I or Axis II Disorder}*
307.44 Hypersomnia Related to . . . *{Indicate the Axis I or Axis II Disorder}*

Appendix C

Other Sleep Disorders

780.xx Sleep Disorder Due to . . . *{Indicate the General Medical Condition}*
- .52 Insomnia type
- .54 Hypersomnia Type
- .59 Parasomnia Type
- .59 Mixed Type

___.__ Substance-Induced Sleep Disorder *(refer to Substance-Related Disorders for substance-specific codes)*
Specify type: Insomnia Type/Hypersomnia Type/Parasomnia Type/Mixed Type
Specify if: With Onset During Intoxication/With Onset During Withdrawal

IMPULSE-CONTROL DISORDERS NOT ELSEWHERE CLASSIFIED

312.34 Intermittent Explosive Disorder
312.32 Kleptomania
312.33 Pyromania
312.31 Pathological Gambling
312.39 Trichotillomania
312.30 Impulse-Control Disorder NOS

ADJUSTMENT DISORDERS

309.xx Adjustment Disorder
- .0 With Depressed Mood
- .24 With Anxiety
- .28 With Mixed Anxiety and Depressed Mood
- .3 With Disturbance of Conduct
- .4 With Mixed Disturbance of Emotions and Conduct
- .9 Unspecified

Specify if: Acute/Chronic

PERSONALITY DISORDERS

Note: *These are coded on Axis II.*

301.0 Paranoid Personality Disorder
301.20 Schizoid Personality Disorder
301.22 Schizotypal Personality Disorder
301.7 Antisocial Personality Disorder
301.83 Borderline Personality Disorder
301.50 Histrionic Personality Disorder
301.81 Narcissistic Personality Disorder
301.82 Avoidant Personality Disorder
301.6 Dependent Personality Disorder
301.4 Obsessive-Compulsive Personality Disorder
301.9 Personality Disorder NOS

OTHER CONDITIONS THAT MAY BE A FOCUS OF CLINICAL ATTENTION

Psychological Factors Affecting Medical Condition

316 . . . *{Specified Psychological Factor}* Affecting . . . *{Indicate the General Medical Condition}*
Choose name based on nature of factors:
Mental Disorder Affecting Medical Condition
Psychological Symptoms Affecting Medical Condition
Personality Traits or Coping Style Affecting Medical Condition
Maladaptive Health Behaviors Affecting Medical Condition
Stress-Related Physiological Response Affecting Medical Condition
Other or Unspecified Psychological Factors Affecting Medical Condition

Medication-Induced Movement Disorders

332.1 Neuroleptic-Induced Parkinsonism
333.92 Neuroleptic Malignant Syndrome
333.7 Neuroleptic-Induced Acute Dystonia
333.99 Neuroleptic-Induced Acute Akathisia
333.82 Neuroleptic-Induced Tardive Dyskinesia
333.1 Medication-Induced Postural Tremor
333.90 Medication-Induced Movement Disorder NOS

Other Medication-Induced Disorder

995.2 Adverse Effects of Medication NOS

Relational Problems

V61.9 Relational Problem Related to a Mental Disorder or General Medical Condition
V61.20 Parent-Child Relational Problem
V61.1 Partner Relational Problem
V61.8 Sibling Relational Problem
V62.81 Relational Problem NOS

Problem Related to Abuse Or Neglect

V61.21 Physical Abuse of Child *(code 995.5 if focus of attention is on victim)*
V61.21 Sexual Abuse of Child *(code 995.5 if focus of attention is on victim)*
V61.21 Neglect of Child *(code 995.5 if focus of attention is on victim)*
V61.1 Physical Abuse of Adult *(code 995.81 if focus of attention is on victim)*
V61.1 Sexual Abuse of Adult *(code 995.81 if focus of attention is on victim)*

Additional Conditions That May Be a Focus of Clinical Attention

V15.81	Noncompliance With Treatment
V65.2	Malingering
V71.01	Adult Antisocial Behavior
V71.02	Child or Adolescent Antisocial Behavior
B62.89	Borderline Intellectual Functioning *Note: This is coded on Axis II.*
780.9	Age-Related Cognitive Decline
V62.82	Bereavement
V62.3	Academic Problem
V62.2	Occupational Problem
313.82	Identity Problem
V62.89	Religious or Spiritual Problem
V62.4	Acculturation Problem
V62.89	Phase of Life Problem

ADDITIONAL CODES

300.9	Unspecified Mental Disorder (nonpsychotic)
V71.09	No Diagnosis or Condition on Axis I
799.9	Diagnosis or Condition Deferred on Axis I
V71.09	No Diagnosis on Axis II
799.9	Diagnosis Deferred on Axis II

MULTIAXIAL SYSTEM

Axis I	Clinical Disorders Other Conditions That May Be a Focus of Clinical Attention
Axis II	Personality Disorders Mental Retardation
Axis III	General Medical Conditions
Axis IV	Psychosocial and Environmental Problems
Axis V	Global Assessment of Functioning

AXIS IV PSYCHOSOCIAL AND ENVIRONMENTAL PROBLEMS

Axis IV designates psychosocial and environmental stressors that may influence and affect diagnosis, treatment, and prognosis of mental disorders. Problems may be negative (e.g., loss, family stress, or deficiency) or positive (e.g., job promotion). Problems are categorized as follows:

- Problems with primary support group
- Problems related to the social environment
- Educational problems
- Occupational problems
- Housing problems
- Economic problems
- Problems with access to health care services
- Problems related to interaction with the legal system/crime
- Other psychosocial and environmental problems

AXIS V GLOBAL ASSESSMENT OF FUNCTIONING (GAF) SCALE

Consider psychological, social, and occupational functioning on a hypothetical continuum of mental health–illness. Do not include impairment in functioning due to physical (or environmental) limitations.

Code	(**Note:** Use intermediate codes when appropriate, e.g., 45, 68, 72.)
100–91	**Superior functioning in a wide range of activities, life's problems never seem to get out of hand, is sought out by others because of his or her many positive qualities. No symptoms.**
90–81	**Absent or minimal symptoms** (e.g., mild anxiety before an exam), **good functioning in all areas, interested and involved in a wide range of activities, socially effective, generally satisfied with life, no more than every day problems or concerns** (e.g., an occasional argument with family members).
80–71	**If symptoms are present, they are transient and expectable reactions to psychosocial stressors** (e.g., difficulty concentrating after family argument); **no more than slight impairment in social, occupational, or school functioning** (e.g., temporarily falling behind in schoolwork).
70–61	**Some mild symptoms** (e.g., depressed mood and mild insomnia) **OR some difficulty in social, occupational, or school functioning** (e.g., occasional truancy, or theft within the household), **but generally functioning pretty well, has some meaningful interpersonal relationships.**
60–51	**Moderate symptoms** (e.g., flat affect and circumstantial speech, occasional panic attacks) **OR moderate difficulty in social, occupational, or school functioning** (e.g., few friends, conflicts with peers or co-workers)

The rating of overall psychological functioning on a scale of 0-100 was operationalized by Luborsky in the Health-Sickness Rating Scale (Luborsky L: "Clinicians' Judgments of Mental Health." *Archives of General Psychiatry* 7:407-417, 1962). Spitzer and colleagues developed a revision of the Health-Sickness Rating Scale called the Global Assessment Scale (GAS) (Endicott J, Spitzer RL, Fleiss JL, Cohen J: "The Global Assessment Scale: A Procedure for Measuring Overall Severity of Psychiatric Disturbance." *Archives of General Psychiatry* 33: 766-771, 1976). A modified version of the GAS was included in DSM-III-R as the Global Assessment of Functioning (GAF) Scale. DSM-IV also adds a global assessment of relational functioning (GARF) scale.

50 **Serious symptoms** (e.g., suicidal ideation, severe obsessional rituals, frequent shoplifting) **OR any serious impairment in social, occupational, or school functioning** (e.g., no
41 friends, unable to keep a job).

40 **Some impairment in reality testing or communication** (e.g., speech is at times illogical, obscure, or irrelevant) **OR major impairment in several areas, such as work or school, family relations, judgment, thinking, or mood** (e.g., depressed man avoids friends, neglects family, and is unable to work; child frequently beats up younger children, is defiant
31 at home, and is failing at school).

30 **Behavior is considerably influenced by delusions or hallucinations OR serious impairment in communication or judgment** (e.g., sometimes incoherent, acts grossly inappropriately, suicidal preoccupation) **OR inability to function in almost all areas** (e.g., stays
21 in bed all day; no job, home, or friends).

20 **Some danger of hurting self or others** (e.g., suicide attempts without clear expectation of death; frequently violent; manic excitement) **OR occasionally fails to maintain minimal personal hygiene** (e.g., smears feces) **OR gross impairment in communication** (e.g., largely
11 incoherent or mute).

10 **Persistent danger of severely hurting self or others** (e.g., recurrent violence) **OR persistent inability to maintain minimal personal hygiene OR serious suicidal act with clear
1 expectation of death.**

0 Inadequate information.

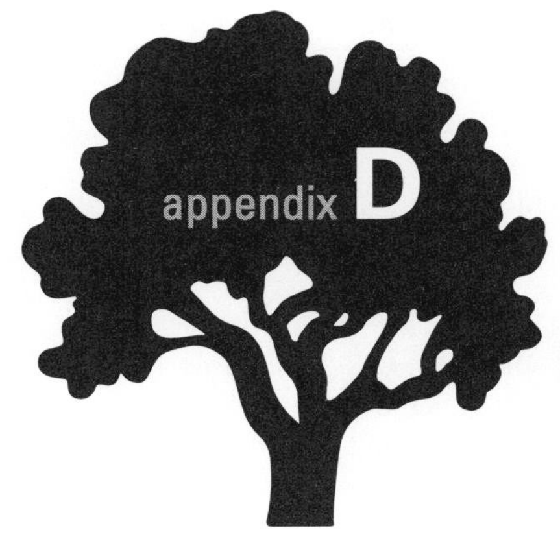

Comparison of Developmental Theories

Stages and Ages	Characteristics of Stages	Theory Addendum
Freud's psychosexual theory		
Oral-sensory (birth to 12-18 mo) (infancy)	Activities involving mouth such as sucking, biting, and chewing are chief source of pleasure.	Child deprived of sufficient sucking might attempt to satisfy this need later in life through activities such as gum chewing, smoking, and overeating.
Anal-muscular (12-18 mo to 3 yr) (toddlerhood)	Sensual gratification is derived from retention and expulsion of feces. Smearing is common activity.	External conflicts may be encountered when toilet training is attempted and later result in behaviors such as constipation, tardiness, or stinginess.
Phallic-locomotion (3-6 yr) (preschool)	Manipulation of genitalia results in pleasurable sensations. Masturbation begins and sexual curiosity becomes evident.	Emergence of Oedipus and Electra complexes for males and females, respectively, occurs. Brashness, bashfulness, and timidity may be expressions of fixation at this stage.
Latency (6 yr to puberty) (school-age)	This is tranquil period when Freud believed sexual drives were dormant; however, child may engage in erogenous activities with same-sex peers.	Child's use of coping and defense mechanisms emerge at this time; any sexual interest may be sublimated through vigorous play and skill acquisition.
Genital (puberty through adulthood) (adolescence and adulthood)	Genitalia become center of sexual tension and pleasure. Sexual hormone production stimulates development of heterosexual relationships.	This is time of biological upheaval, when immature emotional interactions often occur in early phase. In time, ability to give and receive mature love develops.

From Potter P, Perry A: *Fundamentals of nursing: concepts, process, and practice,* ed 4, St Louis, Mosby, 1997.

Stages and Ages	Characteristics of Stages	Theory Addendum
Erikson's Psychosocial Theory		
Trust vs. mistrust (birth to 1 yr) (infancy) Mode: taking in and getting Virtue: hope	Caregiver's satisfaction of infant's basic needs for food and sucking, warmth and comfort, and love and security in consistent and sensitive manner results in trust.	When basic needs of infant are not met or are met inadequately, infant becomes suspicious, fearful, and mistrusting. This is evidenced by poor eating, sleeping, and elimination behaviors.
Autonomy vs. doubt and shame (1-3 yr) (toddlerhood) Mode: holding on and letting go Virtue: will	Child develops beginning independence while gaining control over bodily functions of undressing and dressing, walking, talking, feeding self, and toileting. Self-control begins.	If toddler's developing independence is discouraged by parents, child may doubt personal abilities; if child is made to feel bad when attempts to be autonomous fail, child develops shame.
Initiative vs. guilt (3-6 yr) (preschool) Mode: intrusive attack and conquest Virtue: purpose	Child develops initiative when planning and trying out new things. Behavior of child is characterized as vigorous, imaginative, and intrusive. Conscience and identification with same-sex parent develop.	Parental restrictiveness may prevent child from developing initiative. Guilt may arise when child undertakes activities in conflict with those of parents. Child must learn to initiate activities without infringing on rights of others.
Industry vs. inferiority (6-12 yr to puberty) (school-age) Mode: doing and producing Virtue: competence	Child wins recognition by demonstration of skill and production of things and develops self-esteem through achievements. Child is greatly influenced by teacher and school.	Feelings of inferiority may occur when adults perceive child's attempt to learn how things work through manipulation to be silly or troublesome. Lack of success in school, development of physical skills, and making of friends also contribute to inferiority.
Identity vs. role confusion or diffusion (puberty to 18-21 yr) (adolescence) Virtue: fidelity	Individual develops integrated sense of "self." Peers have major influence over behavior. Major decision is to determine vocational goal.	Failure to develop sense of personal identity may lead to role confusion, which often results in feelings of inadequacy, isolation, and indecisiveness. Psychosocial moratorium provides extra time for making vocational decision.
Intimacy vs. isolation (18-21 to 40 yr) (young adulthood) Mode: loving Virtue: love	Task is to develop close and sharing relationships with others, which may include sexual partner.	Individual unsure of self-identity will have difficulty developing intimacy. Person unwilling or unable to share self will be lonely.
Generativity vs. self-absorption or stagnation (40-65 yr) (middle adulthood) Mode: nurturing Virtue: care	Mature adult is concerned with establishing and guiding next generation. Adult looks beyond self and expresses concern for future of world in general.	Self-absorbed adult will be preoccupied with personal well-being and material gains. Preoccupation with self leads to stagnation of life.
Ego integrity vs. despair (65 yr to death) (older adulthood) Mode: acceptance Virtue: wisdom	Older adult can look back with sense of satisfaction and acceptance of life and death.	Unsuccessful resolution of this crisis may result in sense of despair in which individual views life as series of misfortunes, disappointments, and failures.
Maslow's Theory of Human Need		
Physiological needs	Physiological needs include food, beverages, and sleep.	Theory of motivation depicts individual driven to fulfill potential, capacities, and talents to become unique being. Person moves up and down hierarchy as life situations change.
Safety needs	Satisfying safety needs allows individual to feel safe and secure.	

Stages and Ages	Characteristics of Stages	Theory Addendum
Maslow's Theory of Human Need—cont'd		
Belongingness and love needs	Belongingness allows individual to affiliate with and be accepted by others.	
Esteem needs	Esteem allows individual to gain approval of others.	
Self-actualization	Self-fulfillment potential is recognized.	
Piaget's Theory of Cognitive Development		
Sensorimotor (birth to 2 yr)	Child learns about world through sensory and motor activities.	Child slowly develops concept that people and objects have permanence, even though they are no longer visible.
Reflex activities (birth to 1 mo)	Child exercises inborn reflexes and gains some control over them.	Modified reflexes become more efficient. Sucking is more effective and selective.
Primary circular reactions (1-4 mo)	Infant repeats pleasurable actions that first occur by chance. Activities focus on body of infant; coordination begins.	Eye, eye-ear, and hand-mouth coordination develop, and activities such as thumb sucking and bottle sucking become more intentional and proficient.
Secondary circular reactions (4-8 mo)	Child attempts to reproduce interesting, pleasant events in environment. Interest goes beyond body.	Infant searches for object dropped and recognizes partially hidden object. Child begins to associate two behaviors such as cradle position and feeding.
Coordination of secondary schemes (8-12 mo)	Child puts together skills used earlier to reach goal in new situation.	Child will crawl across room to get desired toy and search for hidden objects where they were previously hidden.
Tertiary circular reactions (12-18 mo) ("trial and error")	Child actively explores world and varies actions to see novelty of object, event, or situation. Trial and error are used to problem solve.	Child might try to get toy out of small opening of container with hand first and then turn it upside down and hit it so that toy falls out. Child comprehends series of object displacements if visible.
Invention of new means through mental combinations (18-24 mo) ("representation")	Toddler begins creating mental images and thus can devise new ways to deal with environment. Child begins to think about events without resorting to action.	Child attains true object permanence and will search for objects they have not seen hidden; for example, toddler will look many places for bottle. Insight is demonstrated by looking for bottle in refrigerator.
Preoperational (2-7 yr)	Child develops representational system and uses symbols such as words to represent people, places, and objects.	Preoperational concepts are limited by ability to focus on only one aspect at time (centration), and thought often seems illogical because child reasons from one specific to another (e.g., car hit dog because boy was mad at it).
Preconceptual (2-4 yr)	Child is primarily egocentric. Perceptual-bound and transductive thinking begin; child is animistic.	Deferred imitation (imitation of observed action after time has passed) demonstrates use of symbolism.
Intuitive (4-7 yr)	Child begins to figure things out but cannot explain them rationally. Child is unable to consider parts as composing whole.	Intuitive concepts allow classification of items by one attribute, usually color or shape (e.g., inability to focus on more than one characteristic at a time).

Stages and Ages	Characteristics of Stages	Theory Addendum
Piaget's Theory of Cognitive Development—cont'd		
Concrete operations (7-11 yr)	Ability to understand law of conservation results in logical thought patterns and mental operations such as reversibility, decentering, seriation, transformation, classification of two or more attributes, and inductive and deductive reasoning.	Limitations are inability of child to understand abstractions. Child's thinking is restricted to immediate and physical. School-age child can reason about what is but cannot hypothesize about what may be and thus cannot think about future problems (e.g., ability to play game of checkers).
Formal operations (develops 11-15 yr, used throughout life)	Ability to think in abstract manner develops, and scientific reasoning emerges. Initially, thought is rigid, but it becomes adaptable and flexible.	Adolescent may confuse ideal with practical but, when confronted with problem (real or hypothetical), can suggest number of solutions. Ability to consider moral and political issues from variety of perspectives is present.
Kohlberg's Theory of Moral Reasoning		
Premoral level (birth to 9 yr)	There is little awareness, which is socially acceptable moral behavior. Control is external.	Infant defers to power and authority. Life is valued for number and power of possessions.
Punishment and obedience orientation (birth to 6 yr)	Rules of others are followed to avoid punishment.	Child integrates labels of *good* and *bad* and *right* and *wrong* into behavior in terms of the consequences of actions.
Naively egoistic orientation (6-9 yr)	Child conforms to rules out of self-interest; child reasons that reward or favor will be earned.	Elements of bargaining, equal sharing, and fairness are evident. Life is valued for how child can satisfy needs of others.
Conventional morality (9-13 yr)	Efforts are made to please other persons. Control is becoming internal.	Child is loyal and concerned with maintaining family expectations regardless of consequences.
"Good boy, nice girl" (9-10 yr)	Desire to please and help others is foremost. Child conforms to avoid rejection.	Life is valued for how good interpersonal relationships are (identify with emotionally important persons).
Authority maintaining morality	Child does duty to avoid criticism by authorities.	Identification shifts to religious or social institutions such as school.
Postconventional level of morality (13 yr to death)	Individual attains true morality. Conduct control is internal.	Attainment of true morality occurs after formal operations have been reached. Not everyone reaches this level.
Contractual and legalistic orientation	Individual selects moral principles by which to live and obeys laws.	Individual is careful not to violate rights and wills of others. Moral and legal views conflict. Person will work to change laws.
Universal ethical-principle orientation	Individual behaves in way that respects dignity of all.	This stage is rarely attained. If internal set of ideas are violated, guilt results.

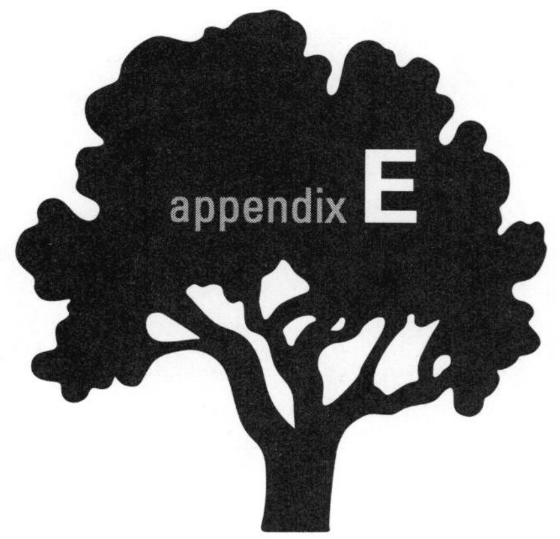

Grief and Loss: Caregivers, Patients, and Families

GRIEF

Grief is a painful experience with lifelong consequences in response to real or perceived loss. It is a personal experience with commonly shared symptoms. Grief is not an illness that needs to be cured. It is a normal response to loss and must be experienced rather than suppressed so that healing can take place. Grief work is the means by which survivors move through the phases of grief. It is a struggle to avoid despair and a willingness to confront the reality of despair. The grieving person strives to move forward with the business of life while expressing and coping with the deeply painful emotions of grieving. The literature reports a clear link between grief and increased vulnerability to physical and mental dysfunction.

Although grief is most often associated with the death of a loved one or even the loss of a treasured pet, it can also occur as a result of other types of losses.

Losses Resulting in Grief

- Loss of a valued job or position
- Loss of a business; financial reverses
- Loss of self-esteem or self-worth
- Loss of family or friends to mental illness
- Loss of a helpful therapist or caregiver
- Loss of a body part or function
- Loss of experience, such as inability to have a child

Grief is not reserved solely for survivors of elderly patients who die from age-related illnesses. Grief can descend on anyone.

People Experiencing Grief

- A young mother diagnosed with cancer
- A middle-aged husband who gambled the family savings
- A family whose only child is sent to prison
- A parent whose newborn infant is severely retarded
- An elderly woman caring for her husband who has Alzheimer's disease
- A war veteran struggling to cope with traumatic memories

Physiologic Responses

- Crying or sobbing
- Sighing respirations
- Shortness of breath and palpitations
- Fatigue, weakness, and exhaustion
- Insomnia
- Loss of appetite
- Choking sensation
- Tightness in chest
- Gastrointestinal disturbances

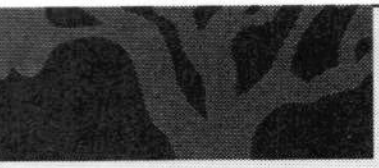

Psychologic Responses

- Intense loneliness and sadness
- Anxiety or panic episodes
- Difficulty concentrating and focusing
- Disorientation
- Anger or rage (directed inward or toward others)
- Ambivalence and low self-esteem (may be warning of possible suicidality and need for professional help)

Grief also manifests myriad physiologic and psychologic responses.

PHASES OF GRIEF

Phase I (1 to 3 weeks): Shock, Numbness, Denial

- Well organized, quiet, polite, immobilized
- Flat, isolated affect with intermittent periods of sobbing
- Responds with simple statements: "I have to go home soon and feed the dog." "I must pick up the clothes from the cleaners." "I need to water the plants and prepare dinner."
- Lack of connection between the loss and its full meaning.

Important tasks of mourning: Phase I

- Ritual of the funeral ceremony
- Planning and preparation for family and friends
- Seeking comfort and support from family and friends
- Feeding the mourners (an important part of the mourning ritual in many cultures)

Interventions: Phase I

- Acknowledge the grief; give permission to vent: "This is a bad time for you. It's OK to talk about it, it's OK to cry, and it's OK even to be angry at your loss."
- Assure the survivor that she or he won't be alone at this time: "I'd like to be with you and stay with you for a while." "Ann and Joe want to spend time with you, too." "We'll all make sure someone is with you every day."
- Be calm, warm, and caring; accept his or her anguish even if it is difficult.
- Offer to help with family tasks: kids, meals, phone calls.
- Involve person in brief familiar tasks.
- Engage chaplain or person's clergy as needed or requested.

There is a higher than normal death rate in survivors during the first year of loss. Survivors won't ask for help; they need stimulation, involvement, and company.

Phase II (3 weeks to 4 months): Yearning and Protest, Anger, Confrontation

- Intensity of grief heightens.
- Person experiences full impact of distress and has no peace.
- Headaches and restlessness or agitation may occur.
- Person bargains with God or fates: "If only I had another chance" (may be part of Phase I also).
- Person expresses feelings of "going crazy" or "losing mind."
- Somatic complaints (can't eat, sleep) are common.
- Person is preoccupied with the dead.
- Person is unable to concentrate or focus on work or school.
- Anger expressed over the loss: "Why did this have to happen?"
- Self-pity expressed: "Why did this happen to me?"
- Regret expressed: "I should have been a better sister."
- Person searches for the deceased and revisits places often visited by deceased.

Interventions: Phase II

- Be direct: "How are you sleeping?"
- Focus on person's feelings; show acceptance.
- Determine person's ability to function, eat, and perform ADLS.
- Assess person's ambivalence; suicide ideation.
- Establish your availability.
- Make appointments to visit person on a regular basis: "I'll be visiting you every day just to talk or listen or have a meal with you." "I'll phone you regularly; so will Jim or Alice."

Phase III (4 to 14 months): Apathy, Aimlessness, Disorganization, Despair

Difficulty getting back into the swing of things. Preoccupation, dreams, or hallucinations may prevail.

Normal

- Perceiving deceased as dead (reinforcing reality and finality of death)
- Smelling perfume or shaving lotion of deceased
- Discussing deceased as being *both good and bad*
- Talking about *good and bad times* together
- Laughing about the good times shared
- Sleeping and eating better
- Displays more energy and interest in usual activities

Dysfunctional

- Seeing or hearing deceased as still living; unable to let go
- Experiencing scary, vivid, threatening hallucinations
- Idealizing deceased as perfect, not deserving to die
- Sleep disturbances with nightmares about deceased
- Suggesting he or she should have died instead of the deceased
- Expresses desire to join deceased because "life is not worth living" (suicidal ideation)
- Demonstrates significant weight loss (6 to 10 lb)
- States has no energy or interest in usual activities
- Exhibits symptoms of depression (DSM-IV criteria)

Nearly two-thirds of persons in a major study continue to experience this phase a year after the death or other loss.

Phase IV (14 months throughout rest of life): Recovery, Resolution, Acceptance

- Survivor is slowly but surely getting more involved in life.
- Reorganization of life evolves out of the chaos of grief (e.g., a camping trip is planned with the kids; old habits resume, such as little irritations, glimpses of the old sense of humor). Affect still reverts to sadness with talk of the deceased, but there are moments of tenderness, too.
- Energy is more plentiful and directed toward life.
- Scents of the deceased are gone; survivor may wish for them back on occasion.
- Life seems tolerable, although it may never reach the heights of joy before the loss.
- There may still be bouts of immense sadness and even panic, but they will go away.
- Dreams are more pleasant and may occasionally include the deceased, but there are no more dreams of seeing the deceased dead or threatening.
- Memories are warm, with intellectual integration of the loss.
- Reestablishment of the old life is evident.

Interventions: Phase IV

- Contact the survivor, especially at key times.
- Share memories of the deceased.
- Acknowledge the long, painful process of grieving.
- Continue to assess for signs of hidden depression or suicidality.
- Assess for ambivalence, low self-esteem, or internalized rage: "Life is not worth living." "Deceased was so good; I'm so bad."

ANTICIPATORY GRIEF: PREMOURNING, PREDEATH

Anticipatory grief is associated with the anticipation of a predicted death or loss. Examples include grieving for persons with long term or life-threatening illness, or grieving for elderly relatives whose life functions are deteriorating.

Positive aspects of anticipatory grief include the opportunity to resolve relationships, to prepare survivors for the loss, and to work on spiritual reconciliation.

Negative aspects of anticipatory grief include increased stress on caregivers, resentment and anger caused by ambivalent relationship, hopelessness or powerlessness, and depression.

Interventions in Anticipatory Grief

- Allow caregivers time to come to terms with the inevitable loss.
- Offer empathy and information about the illness when person is ready.
- Identify sources of support such as grief groups.
- Be available to listen and assess signs of depression.

The anguish that caregivers feel during anticipatory grief does not substitute for postdeath grief.

CHRONIC SORROW

Chronic sorrow is a form of grief that is a response to ongoing loss, such as chronic mental or physical illness. It includes characteristics of other types of grief as well.

Interventions in Chronic Sorrow

- Acknowledge the demands of the illness on caregivers.
- Recognize caregiver behavior patterns as ongoing grief responses.
- Assess the phases of grief and intervene accordingly.
- Discuss the diagnosis and expected outcomes with family and caregiver.
- Dispel the myth that it is the family's fault (to avoid blame and guilt).
- Promote adaptive coping skills among family members.
- Enhance communication among family, caregiver, and client (to prevent burnout, exhaustion, depression).
- Help family and caregiver develop realistic expectations (to avoid despair and promote hope).

SUMMARY OF THEORIES OF GRIEF

Lindemann

Grief is manifested by predictable psychologic and somatic symptomatology. Acute mourning (feeling or expressing grief or sorrow) is characterized by somatic distress, preoccupation with the deceased person's image, guilt, hostile reactions, and loss of patterns of conduct. Dysfunctional or "morbid" grief reactions are distortions of some aspect of "normal grief." The duration of grief and the development of dysfunctional grief depend on the success of grief work.

Kubler-Ross

Elisabeth Kubler-Ross's stages of dying (denial, anger, bargaining, depression, and acceptance) are often applied to grief (Table E-1). The initial response to loss may include denial, anger, and bargaining. Denial is characterized by refusal to accept loss. Anger may initially be directed at health care staff and, later, at the person who died. Bargaining and denial are often mixed in a futile attempt to reverse reality. Depression tends to be the longest phase and, in dysfunctional grief, may become chronic and meet criteria for major depression. Acceptance of the loss is a gradual process that includes aspects of previous stages. Grieving individuals may not reach acceptance.

Table E-1

Kubler-Ross's Stages of Grieving

Stage	Behavioral Responses	Nursing Implications
Denial	Refuses to believe that loss is happening With death or trauma, one may actually block the memory of the incident or momentarily believe it has not occurred Is unready to deal with practical problems, such as prosthesis after loss of leg May assume artificial cheerfulness to prolong denial	Verbally support client's denial for its protective function Examine your own behavior to ensure that you do not share in client's denial
Anger	Client or family may direct anger at nurse or hospital staff about matters that normally would not bother them There may be an acute sense of unfairness, fear, anger, and even rage. Questions may arise such as "Why me?" or "How could you die and leave me alone?"	Help client understand that anger is a normal response to feelings of loss and powerlessness Avoid withdrawal or retaliation with anger; do not take anger personally Deal with needs underlying any angry reaction Provide structure and continuity to promote feelings of security Allow client as much control as possible over his or her life
Bargaining	Seeks to bargain to avoid loss The bargain may be struck with God, the deceased, or oneself May express feelings of guilt or fear of punishment for past sins, real or imagined	Listen attentively and encourage client to talk to relieve guilt and irrational fears If appropriate, offer spiritual support
Depression	Grieves over what has happened and what cannot be May talk freely (e.g., reviewing past losses such as money or job) or may withdraw An important stage in which one acknowledges feelings, allows nurturing by self or others, and moves forward in the process	Allow client to express sadness Communicate nonverbally by sitting quietly without expecting conversation Convey caring by touch Help support persons understand importance of being with the client in silence
Acceptance	Comes to terms with loss Depression has been lifted; loss is acknowledged May have decreased interest in surroundings and support persons as loss is no longer focal point May wish to begin making plans (e.g., will, prosthesis, altered living arrangements) Now free to move forward	Help family and friends understand client's decreased need to socialize and need for short, quiet visits Encourage client to participate as much as possible in the treatment program

Bowlby

Grief and loss are characterized first by numbness, during which the loss is recognized but not necessarily felt as real. Numbness is followed by yearning and searching, in which the individual yearns for the loved one and protests the loss. In the third phase, disorganization and despair, the loss is real, and intense emotional pain and cognitive disorganization occur. Reorganization, the final phase, is characterized by a gradual adjustment to life without the deceased.

Engel

The initial response to loss is shock and disbelief. Awareness and meaning of the loss develop during the first year of mourning. Eventually the relationship is resolved and put into perspective (Table E-2).

Shneidman

Conceptualizing less structure and fewer stages than other theorists of grief, Shneidman views the expression of grief as dependent primarily on an individual's personality or style of living. An individual who goes through life feeling depressed and guilty is likely to grieve similarly. One who avoids emotional investments with others also tends to try to avoid grief.

Theory synthesis

Grief tends to occur in several phases. The initial response to loss may be shock, numbness, denial, or other attempts to defend against the reality and pain of loss. This initial phase is followed by painful psychologic and physical disequilibrium, which, in the case of dysfunc-

Table E-2
Engel's Stages of Grieving

Stage	Behavioral Responses
Shock and disbelief	Refusal to accept loss Stunned feelings Intellectual acceptance but emotional denial
Developing awareness	Reality of loss begins to penetrate consciousness Anger may be directed at hospital, nurses, etc. Crying and self-blame
Restitution	Rituals of mourning (e.g., funeral)
Resolving the loss	Attempts to deal with painful void Still unable to accept new love object to replace lost person May accept more dependent relationship with support person Thinks over and talks about memories of the dead person
Idealization	Produces images of dead person that are almost devoid of undesirable features Represses all negative and hostile feelings toward deceased May feel guilty and remorseful about past inconsiderate or unkind acts to deceased Unconsciously internalizes admired qualities of deceased Reminders of deceased evoke fewer feelings of sadness Reinvests feelings in others
Outcome	Behavior influenced by several factors, such as importance of lost object as source of support, degree of dependence on relationship, degree of ambivalence toward deceased, number and nature of other relationships, and number and nature of previous grief experiences (which tend to be cumulative)

tional grief, may last indefinitely. The third phase of resolution or recovery is a gradual process in which the good days begin to outnumber the bad. Ultimately, although not forgotten, the relationship with the deceased is resolved and put into perspective.

TIPS FOR HELPING SURVIVORS

- Listen; say little.
- Avoid clichés such as "Everything will be fine" or "I know how you must feel."
- Be there for the long haul, not just for the funeral or memorial service.
- Include them in the first holiday after the loss.
- Remember the anniversary of the death in a special way (a call, card, flower).
- Love them and accept them.

References

Adams JP and others: Accumulated loss phenomenon among hospice caregivers, *American Journal of Hospice and Palliative Care* 8(3):29-37, 1992.

Atkins S: Grieving and loss in parents with a schizophrenic child, *Am J Psychiatry* 151(8):1137-1139, 1994.

Bodnar J and Kiecolt-Glaser J: Caregiver depression after bereavement: chronic stress isn't over when it's over, Journal of the American Psychological Association 9(3) 1994.

Bowlby J: Loss: *Sadness and depression, vol 3, attachment and loss,* New York, 1980, Basic Books.

Burke ML and others: Current knowledge and research on chronic sorrow: a foundation for inquiry, *Death Studies* 16:231-245, 1992.

Cowles KV and Rodgers BL: The concept of grief: a foundation for nursing research and practice, *Res Nurs Health* 14(2):119-127, 1991.

Engel G: Grief and grieving, *Am J Nurs* 64:93-98, 1964.

Freud S: Mourning and melancholia. In Strachey J, editor: *The standard edition of the complete psychological works of Sigmund Freud,* vol 14, London, 1917, Hogarth.

Goodman M and others: Cultural differences among elderly women in coping with the death of an adult child, *J Gerontol* 46(6): 321-329, 1991.

Kemp C: Grief and loss. In Fortinash K and Holoday-Worret P, editors: *Psychiatric mental health nursing,* St Louis, 1996, Mosby.

Kubler-Ross E: *On death and dying,* New York, 1969, Macmillan.

Levy LH: Anticipatory grief: Its measurement and proposed reconceptualization, *Hospital Journal* 7(4): 1-28, 1991.

Liken J and Collins C: Grieving: facilitating the process for dementia caregivers, *J Psychosoc Nurs Ment Health Serv* 31:21-26, 1993.

Lindemann E: Symptomatology and management of acute grief, *Am J Psychiatry* 101:141-148, 1994.

McFarland GK and Gerety EK: Grieving. In Kim MJ and others, editors: *Pocket guide to nursing diagnoses,* ed 5, St Louis, 1993, Mosby.

Nuss WS and Zumenko GS: Correlates of persistent depressive symptoms in widows, *Am J Psychiatry* 149(3):346-351, 1992.

Rando TA: *Grieving,* Lexington, Mass, 1988, Lexington Books.

Research Mental Health Service. *When a loved one dies: coping with loss.* Kansas City, Mo, 1989, Research Mental Health Services.

Schneidman ES: *Deaths of man,* New York, 1973, Quadrangle.

Schneidman ES: *Voices of death,* New York, 1980, Harper & Row.

Titleman D: Grief, guilt and identification in siblings of schizophrenic individuals, *Bull Menninger Clin* 55(1):72-81, 1991 (abstract).

Wolfelt AD: Toward an understanding of complicated grief: a comprehensive overview, *American Journal of Hospice and Palliative Care* 8(2):28-30, 1991.

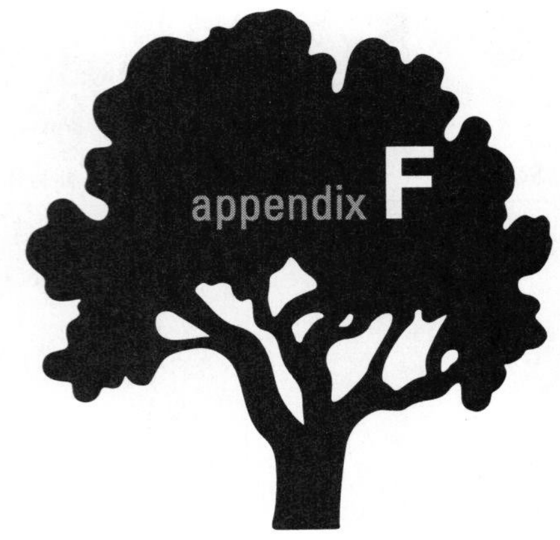

Spirituality as a Dimension of the Person

People are composed of multidimensional facets that include physical, cognitive, affective, relational, and spiritual. To ignore any of these components eliminates a critical part of a person's humanness, with significant consequences to the total life experience. Although everyone has a spiritual dimension, spirituality is expressed in many ways, both formally and informally. Spirituality is an integral part of the person's identity. It is a critical thread that connects people together, binds cultures, and gives meaning to nature and the universe. Through the spiritual dimension, one can make sense of powerful life experiences that might otherwise be confusing or devastating and use them in life-sustaining ways. Spirituality addresses some of the core images and beliefs a person holds regarding humanity, the divine, and the relationship between them.

DESCRIPTIONS OF TERMS

Spirituality

- The search for the sacred and the holy
- The need to experience the divine or higher power
- The desire to find meaning in the universe that transcends a physical or finite existence

Spirituality may be expressed through religion and religious rituals, but it is not limited to those things. It may also be expressed in music, art, poetry, dance, and storytelling.

Religion

- A formal, organized system that utilizes a set of rituals, practices, and ceremonies, through which a specific community can express spiritual beliefs
- A less formal, less organized system that enables a more diverse community to express individualized spiritual beliefs and practices

Religious expression may also include music, art, literature, and dance, as well as religious rituals, practices, and ceremonies, or regular participation in a congregation with a specific understanding of religious history and future.

Major Types of Formal Religions

- Christianity
- Judaism
- Buddhism
- Islam
- Taoism

Goals of Spirituality

- Provide an image of the divine
- Provide an image of humanity
- Provide understanding of the relationship between the divine and humanity
- Examine thoughts of divine punishment, reward, or neutrality
- Give belief and meaning to life
- Give a sense of duty, vocation, calling, or moral obligation
- Examine one's experience of the divine and sacred
- Cope with situations that conflict with spiritual understanding
- Provide spiritual rituals and practices
- Provide a community of faith
- Provide authority and guidance for a system of belief, meaning, and ritual

New Age religions or *spirituality* refer to a collection of individual practices that are largely unconnected to formal communities but nonetheless offer meaning and enlightenment to some individuals.

Faith

- The ability to draw on spiritual resources without physical or empirical proof
- An internal certainty that comes from one's own experiences with the divine

Faith, although only a part of spirituality, is an essential component. Through faith, a deep, individual spirituality can be mobilized to assist in the challenges and celebrations of life.

SPIRITUALITY IN MENTAL HEALTH

In the treatment of mental disorders, it is imperative to address the spiritual dimension of a person. For many individuals with mental disorders, spirituality offers a powerful sense of hope in the face of devastating, chronic illness.

For those who experience rejection by family and friends because of the impact of the diagnosis on their relationships, spirituality can help maintain a sense of connection and belonging. A healthy spirituality can provide a sense of love and acceptance in the face of loneliness and abandonment. Spirituality can also evoke a sense of peace and calm in individuals whose illnesses create feelings of internal chaos and confusion. The spiritual images and beliefs that can be healing and sustaining for some individuals may also seem punitive and threatening to others because of the nature of their mental disorder. These people may be troubled and tormented by a distorted or negative view of religion and spirituality, as a result of severe anxiety, irrational guilt, deep depression, or psychosis. Some individuals who experience mental illness may become hyperreligious and preoccupied with religious rituals and practice. They may spend inordinate amounts of time praying, chanting, or reading religious doctrine. Others may believe that they are so evil they deserve to be punished by God or the devil and may even require suicide precautions. Left unattended, these individuals may harm themselves or, at the very least, be unable to comply with treatment, which could delay the therapeutic healing process.

THE ROLE OF THE CHAPLAIN IN MENTAL HEALTH

As a result of the obvious need for spiritual guidance, the chaplain role is becoming more common in the mental health arena. These ministers of spirituality are generally multidenominational, which allows them to address the spiritual needs of many individuals who request or require their services. Chaplains who work in the mental health setting recognize the boundaries between the need for spiritual guidance and the mental disorder, which may provoke a negative view of religion or an unhealthy preoccupation. They collaborate closely with the psychiatric staff as a critical part of the therapeutic team. They may be involved in patient groups, provide individual counseling, facilitate in-services, or offer nondenominational spiritual services for those patients who are interested.

STAGES OF FAITH IN SPIRITUAL PRACTICE AND INTERVENTIONS

The Impartial Individual

The religiously impartial (30% of the population) generally are not involved or minimally involved in faith communities and have only a casual acquaintance with faith community practices. They tend to do only things that interest them.

Interventions. Appropriate interventions are well-known scripture, hymns, psalms, or readings such as Psalm 23, the poem "Footprints," the Serenity Prayer, the Lord's Prayer, "Amazing Grace," and "Beautiful Savior." Alcoholics Anonymous, Narcotics Anonymous, or other materials may also be helpful.

The Institutional Individual

Regular church attendees (40% of the population) who adhere to institutional rules largely adopt a "good person/bad person" concept in their view of spirituality.

Interventions. Include the previous interventions as well as visits from the minister and members of their local spiritual community. Normal use of prayer, anointing, and laying on of hands is also acceptable. Prayer books and music specific to the denomination, congregation, or faith are also appropriate.

Individual Seeker

Some people (20% of the population) challenge the formal religious community and many of their beliefs and tenets. They seek new or personal answers to questions, problems, or crises. On the surface, they seem to be impartial in regard to faith.

Interventions. Individualized, creative, and varied approaches may encompass historic elements from Eastern and Western spiritual traditions, including meditation, healing touch, devotional readings, communal prayer, and a variety of music. The individual is the best guide in selecting the spiritual resources at this stage.

Integrated Individuals

Faith is internalized, and the rules of religion and spirituality are accepted and obeyed (10% of the population). They may not belong to formal faith communities and can often be seen as teachers or mystics.

Interventions. Many of the traditional rituals, rites, and expressions of formal spirituality noted for institutional people are appropriate, but with an increased internal meaning. They may have the need to leave a spiritual legacy.

SUMMARY OF SPIRITUALITY

Spirituality helps individuals cope with major common issues such as fear, death, and other losses by providing a sense of hope and meaning to experiences that would otherwise be devastating. Having a spiritual understanding that one's connection with the universe is more than physical may help to ease the fear and pain of loss. Feeling connected to the divine eases loneliness, grief, abandonment, and alienation and offers a feeling of unconditional acceptance for one's unique place in life. Spirituality allows people to make sense of the mystery of life and death and of other phenomena that are not within human control. It offers the hope and strength to celebrate life, while consciously acknowledging the reality of illness and tragedy. Spirituality is a key component of the human experience that can ease the pain of mental and physical illness, enhance treatment, and speed the healing process.

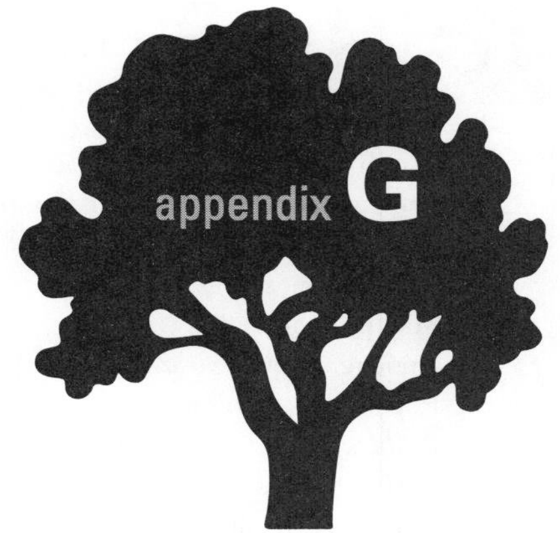

Therapeutic Nurse-Client Relationship

ESSENTIAL QUALITIES FOR A THERAPEUTIC RELATIONSHIP

1. *Genuineness* Sincerity, verbal and behavioral congruence, authenticity; does not mean confessing all truths; able to meet the client's needs versus his or her wants.
2. *Respect* Unconditional positive regard; nonpossessive warmth; consistency and active listening convey respect.
3. *Empathy* Viewing the world through the client's eyes yet remaining objective; not identifying or agreeing with the client but able to zero in on his or her feelings.
4. *Concreteness/Specificity* Speak in realistic, literal terms versus vague, theoretic concepts; identify client's feelings through skillful listening, not with expectations of client as a stereotypical, textbook picture.
5. *Self-Disclosure* Appropriate disclosure of a view of one's attitudes, feelings, and beliefs; role-modeling some shared experiences helps the client to reveal self, become more open, and feel more secure; share feelings only when it is clear client will profit from them.
6. *Confrontation* Expression of nurse's perceived discrepancies in the client's behavior; to help client develop an awareness that he or she does not always say what he or she means; must be done in an accepting manner after rapport is established.
7. *Immediacy of Relationship* Focusing on the nurse-client interaction as a prototype of the way the client may relate in other relationships; being careful not to share too many spontaneous feelings all at once; divulging too many negative or personal experiences can be detrimental to the relationship, especially at the beginning.
8. *Self-Exploration* Helping the client to explore his or her feelings and to vent them during appropriate intervals throughout the interaction; catharsis.
9. *Role Playing* The acting out of a particular event, situation, or problem to help the client gain understanding; may also be cathartic.

PRINCIPLES OF A THERAPEUTIC NURSE-CLIENT RELATIONSHIP

1. Continually evaluate client's potential for suicide using principles of suicide assessment (see Appendix J).
2. Engage in active listening, utilizing a warm, accepting, empathetic approach.
3. Develop an awareness of own feelings, fears, and biases regarding clients with mental disorders (autodiagnosis or self-diagnosis).
4. Discuss own fears and concerns with qualified peers.
5. Speak in a moderate voice tone, utilizing a calm "matter-of-fact" approach and nonjudgmental

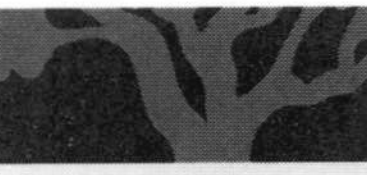

Client Responses to Orientation Phase

1. May willingly engage in therapeutic relationship.
2. May test you and the limits of the relationship:
   a. May be late for meetings.
   b. May end meetings early.
   c. May play nurse (you) against the staff.
3. May not remember your name or appointment time:
   a. Put information on a card and give this to client.
   b. Reinforce contract in early meetings and restate limits if necessary.
4. May attempt to shock you:
   a. May use profane words.
   b. May share an experience that client feels will shock or frighten you.
   c. May use bizarre behavior.
5. May focus on nurse in an attempt to see if nurse is competent. Refocus on client.

attitude (refrain from extremes of expression or responses that indicate surprise or disbelief).

6. Continue to develop trust and rapport through shared time and support throughout the day (brief one-to-one contacts rather than lengthy, drawn-out conversations).
7. Remain quietly with depressed or withdrawn clients who are unable to engage in conversation at first.
8. Allow sufficient time for client to respond, while assessing client's ability to tolerate silence and presence of nurse. (Do not prolong the contact if the client is obviously uncomfortable or resistant, unless the client is troubled or suicidal and cannot be left alone.)
9. Individualize client's needs throughout contact, to acknowledge client's value and worth.

THE NURSE-CLIENT RELATIONSHIP

The nurse-client relationship is *therapeutic,* not social in nature. It is always *client-centered* and *goal-directed.* It is *objective* rather than subjective. The intent of a professional relationship is for client behavior to change. It is a limited relationship, with the goal of helping the client find more satisfying behavior patterns and coping strategies and increase his or her self-worth. It is *not* for mutual satisfaction.

Some texts include the *preorientation phase,* in which the nurse gathers data about the client and his or her situation and condition (chart, staff, physician). The nurse also utilizes the process of *autodiagnosis* to determine his or her own perceptions, possible biases, and attitudes concerning the client. A commitment to nonjudgmentalism and avoidance of stereotyping is imperative.

Questions nurse asks self during autodiagnosis

1. "Do I label clients with the stereotype as a group?"
2. "Is my need to be liked so great that I become angry or hurt when a client is rude, hostile, or uncooperative?"
3. "Am I afraid of the responsibility I must assume in this relationship?" (This fear may decrease the nurse's independent functions.)
4. "Do I cover feelings of inferiority with an air of superiority?"
5. "Do I require sympathy and protection so much myself that I drown my clients with it also?"
6. "Do I fear closeness or identifying myself with the client to the extent of being cold and indifferent?"
7. "Do I need to feel important and keep clients dependent on me?"

Orientation phase. The purpose of the orientation phase is to become acquainted, gain rapport, demonstrate genuine caring and understanding, and establish trust. The orientation phase usually lasts from 2 to 10 sessions but with some clients can take many months.

1. Build trust and security (first level of any interpersonal experience):
   a. Establish contract.
   b. Be dependable—follow contract, keep appointments.
   c. Allow client to be responsible for contract.
   d. Convey honesty.
   e. Show caring and interest.
   f. When client is unable to control behavior, nurse sets limits and/or provides appropriate alternative outlets.
2. Discuss the contract: dates, times, and place of meetings; duration of each meeting; purpose of meetings; roles of both client and nurse; use of information obtained; arrangements for notifying client/nurse if unable to keep appointment.
3. Facilitate the client's ability to verbalize his or her problem.
4. Be aware of themes:
   a. Content (what the client is saying).
   b. Process (how the client interacts).
   c. Mood (hopeless, anxious).
   d. Interaction (did the client ignore you, was he or she submissive, did he or she dominate conversation?).
5. Observe and assess the client's strengths, limitations, and problem areas. Build on client's strengths and positive aspects of his or her personality. Include the client in identification of his or her own attributes.
6. Identify client problems, nursing diagnoses, outcome criteria, and nursing interventions; formulate nursing care plan.

Working phase. This phase begins when the client assumes responsibility to uphold the limits of the relationship. Focus is on the "here and now." The purpose of the work-

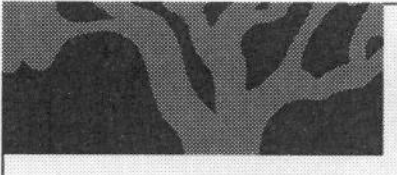

Client Responses to Working Phase

1. May use less testing, less focusing on nurse, fewer attempts to shock nurse.
2. May remember and anticipate appointment with nurse.
3. May use more description and clarification to facilitate understanding; wants you to know how he or she feels.
4. May be more responsive in interactions.
5. May improve appearance.
6. May bring up topic he or she wishes to discuss.
7. May confide more confidential material. The working phase is painful for the client and is reached when change occurs as problems are analyzed and discussed by client and nurse.

ing phase is to bring about positive changes in the client's behavior.

1. Set priorities when determining client needs:
   a. Preserve life and safety: is client suicidal, not eating, smoking in bed while medicated, acting out behavior harmful to others?
   b. Modify behavior that is unacceptable to others (e.g., acting out or hostile verbalization, bizarre behavior, withdrawal, poor hygiene, inadequate social skills).
   c. Identify with client those behaviors he or she is willing to change; set realistic goals. Make goals testable and attainable for successful experiences. This will increase sense of self worth and help client accept need for growth.

Termination phase. The purpose of this phase is to dissolve the relationship and assure the client that he or she can be independent in some or all of his or her functioning.

Ideally, the termination phase begins during the orientation phase. The more dependent and involved relationships require longer time for termination. Termination normally occurs when the client has improved sufficiently for the relationship to end, but it may occur if a client is transferred or you as a nurse leave the agency.

Methods of Decreasing Involvement

1. Space your contacts further apart (not usually necessary in student clinical experience).
2. Reduce the usual length of time you spend with client.
3. Change the emotional tone of the interactions by:
   a. Not responding to or following up clues that lead to new areas to investigate.
   b. Focusing on future-oriented material.
4. Some clients may want to work up to the last meeting; use your judgment.

What to Discuss with Client About Termination

1. Help client to discuss his or her feelings about it.

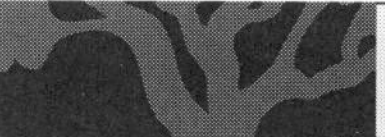

Client Responses to Termination

1. May deny separation.
2. May deny significance of relationship and/or separation.
3. May express anger or hostility (overtly or covertly). Anger, openly expressed to nurse, may be a natural and healthy response to event. Client feels secure enough to show anger. Nurse responds in accepting, neutral manner.
4. May display marked change in attitude toward nurse/therapist; may make critical remarks about nurse or be hostile because of pending break of emotional ties. If the nurse does not understand the reason for the client's reaction, he or she may react with anger or defensiveness and block the termination process.
5. May display a type of grief reaction. It takes time to get over the loss, which is why it is important to start the termination process early.
6. May feel rejected and experience increased negative self-concept.
7. May terminate relationship prematurely.
8. May regress to exhibition of old symptoms.
9. May request premature discharge.
10. May make a suicide attempt.
11. May be accepting but still express regret or feel momentary resentment. This is a healthy response. Make a clean break, or you may hinder the client's realization that relationships often must, *and do,* terminate.

2. Have client talk about gains he or she has made (include negative aspects of sessions also).
3. Share with client the growth you see in him or her.
4. Express benefits you have gained from the experience.
5. Express your feelings regarding leaving client.
6. Never give client your address or telephone number.

Impasses that Obstruct a Therapeutic Relationship

1. *Resistance* Client is reluctant to divulge information about self as he or she doubts ability to be helped; unconditional acceptance and persistence by the nurse is critical
2. *Transference* Client views the nurse as a significant person in his or her life and transfers feelings, emotions, and attitudes felt for that person onto the nurse; the nurse may need assistance to deal with transference issues; clarification of the nurse-client relationship is imperative during this time.
3. *Countertransference* Nurse views the client as a significant person in her or his life and transfers feelings for that person onto the client; assistance by qualified health care personnel is imperative to help the relationship regain its objective, therapeutic core.

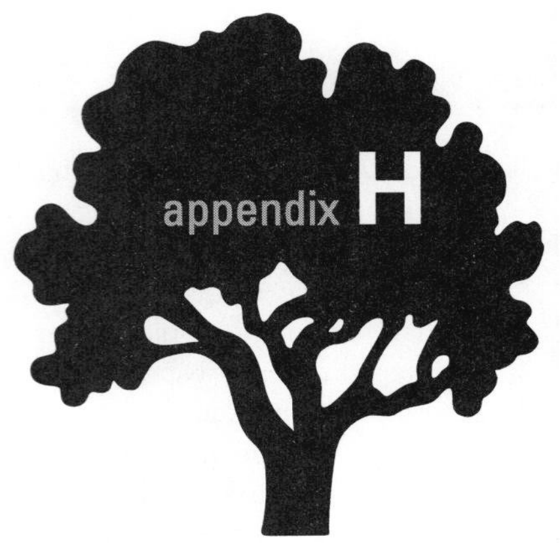

Interpersonal Techniques

Therapeutic Techniques	Examples
Using silence	Yes, that must have been difficult for you.
Giving recognition or acknowledging	I noticed that you've made your bed.
Offering self	I'll walk with you.
Giving board openings or asking open-ended questions	Is there something you'd like to do? How do you feel about that?
Offering general leads or door-openers	Go on. You were saying . . . .
Placing the event in time or in sequence	When did your nervousness begin? What happened just before you came to the hospital?
Making observations	I notice that you're trembling. You appear to be angry.
Encouraging description of perceptions	What does the voice that you hear seem to be saying? How do you feel when you take your medication?
Encouraging comparison	Has this ever happened before? What does this resemble?
Restating	*Client:* I can't sleep. I stay awake all night. *Nurse:* You can't sleep at night.
Reflecting	*Client:* I think I should take my medication. *Nurse:* You think you should take your medication?
Focusing on specifics	This topic seems worth discussing in more depth. Give me an example of what you mean.
Exploring	Tell me more about your job. Would you describe your responsibilities?
Giving information or informing	His name is . . . . I'm going with you on the field trip.
Seeking clarification or clarifying	I'm not sure that I understand what you are trying to say. Please give me more information.
Presenting reality or confrontation	I see no elephant in the room. This is a hospital, not a hotel.
Voicing doubt	I find that hard to believe. Did it happen just as you said?

Therapeutic Techniques—cont'd	Examples
Encouraging evaluation or evaluating	Describe how you feel about taking your medication. Does participating in group therapy enable you to discuss your feelings?
Attempting to translate into feelings or verbalizing the implied	*Client:* I'm empty. *Nurse:* Are you suggesting that you feel useless?
Suggesting collaboration	Perhaps you and your doctor can work together to determine living arrangements for you after your discharge.
Summarizing	During the past hour we talked about your plans for the future. They include . . . .
Encouraging formulation of a plan of action	If this situation occurs again, what options would you have?
Asking direct questions	How do you feel about your hospitalization? How do you view your progress?

Nontherapeutic Techniques	Examples
Reassuring (falsely)	I wouldn't worry about . . . . Everything will be all right. You're coming along fine.
Giving approval	That's good. I'm glad that you . . . .
Rejecting	Let's not discuss . . . . I don't want to hear about. . . . .
Disapproving	That's bad. I'd rather you wouldn't.
Agreeing	That's right. I agree.
Disagreeing	That's wrong. I definitely disagree with . . . . I don't believe that.
Advising	I think you should . . . . Why don't you . . . ?
Probing	Now tell me about . . . . Tell me your life history.
Challenging	But how can you be president of the United States? If you're dead, why is your heart beating?
Testing	What day is this? Do you know what kind of a hospital this is? Do you still have the idea that . . . ?
Defending	This hospital has a fine reputation. No one here would lie to you. But Dr. B. is a very able psychiatrist. I'm sure that he has your welfare in mind when he . . . .
Requesting an explanation	Why do you think that? Why do you feel this way? Why did you do that?
Indicating the existence of an external source	What makes you say that? Who told you that you were Jesus? What made you do that?
Belittling expressed feelings	*Client:* I have nothing to live for. . . . I wish I was dead. *Nurse:* Everybody gets down in the dumps *(or)* I've felt that way sometimes.
Making stereotyped comments	Nice weather we're having. I'm fine, and how are you? It's for your own good. Keep your chin up. Just listen to your doctor and take part in activities—you'll be home in no time.

Nontherapeutic Techniques—cont'd	Examples
Giving literal responses	*Client:* I'm an Easter egg. *Nurse:* What shade? *or* You don't look like one. *Client:* They're looking in my head with television. *Nurse:* Try not to watch television *(or)* With what channel?
Using denial	*Client:* I'm nothing. *Nurse:* Of course you're something. Everybody is somebody. *Client:* I'm, dead. *Nurse:* Don't be silly.
Interpreting	What you really mean is . . . . Unconsciously you're saying . . . .
Introducing an unrelated topic	*Client:* I'd like to die. *Nurse:* Did you have visitors this weekend?

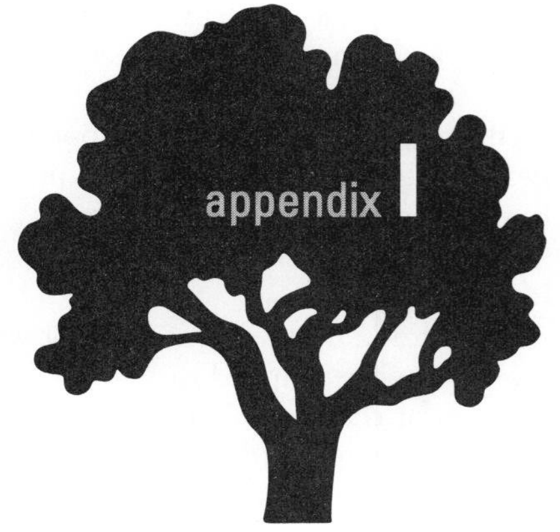

Defense Mechanisms

Defense mechanisms, also called *ego-defense mechanisms* or *mental mechanisms,* are put into play by the ego to protect the personality from anxiety associated with the conflicts of internal drives and desires. All of the defense mechanisms except suppression are unconscious. Defense mechanisms are an important part of the adaptive process that allow the individual to continue with the daily tasks of living in the face of internal and external conflicts. However obvious another person's methods of coping may appear, they are not that obvious to the individual using them. Everyone uses defense mechanisms to obtain relief from emotional conflict and anxiety. Healthy individuals may use many of them throughout their lives in times of stress. For example, many people commonly use rationalization to justify ideas, actions, or feelings; reduce guilt; and maintain respect and social approval. But as long as the individual is growing and progressing emotionally and able to solve most problems in a manner congruent with his or her stage of development, then the person is most likely not in danger of maladaptive use of defense mechanisms.

Problems arise when an individual uses the same defense mechanism repeatedly, to the exclusion of reality, probably because the individual perceives most situations as threatening even though they may not be viewed as such by others. For example, the person who constantly projects his or her own negative feelings, attitudes, or beliefs onto another person is demonstrating a rigid, maladaptive use of a defense mechanism. One of the reasons people develop psychiatric problems is because the ego loses its ability to use defense mechanisms in a way that relieves the person's psychic pain. Put another way, their psychic stress is greater than the ego's ability to relieve it through healthy use of defense mechanisms.

A major task for nursing, then, is not to remove the client's defense mechanisms through exposure and confrontation but rather to help the client develop greater ego strength through the development of a strong, therapeutic alliance. As the client develops trust, builds self-esteem, and learns to accept failure without fear of consequences, he or she may be able to let go of rigid, maladaptive defenses and begin to use healthy, flexible, adaptive defense mechanisms.

DEFENSE MECHANISMS

Repression

In repression unacceptable feelings or thoughts are automatically pushed into one's unconsciousness. They may be painful, traumatic conflicts involving such things as sexual molestation or rape or the feelings experienced during a life-threatening accident or illness. Repression is an operative force in the use of all defense mechanisms and is necessary for the survival of the organism. It is believed, however, that if important conflicts are not resolved during critical stages of growth and development, repressed material can result in disordered or maladaptive behavior later in life.

Introjection

Introjection begins in infancy and involves the incorporation of characteristic traits, attitudes, and ideas of significant persons. The early introjects are the most important because they are influential in the formation of morals, values, and conscience. Introjection has been called an intense form of identification. In the area of psychiatry and mental health, the client has opportunities to introject healthy, desirable qualities from nurses and other health care professionals.

Identification

Identification involves the desire or wish to emulate or be like another person and to assume the mannerisms, style, or dress of that individual. Most notable during adolescence, when one's identification with peers is a critical part of healthy growth and development, it promotes acceptance and security that provide the adolescent with the strong sense of self-esteem necessary for the difficult tasks of adulthood. It actually begins in early childhood (ages 3 to 6) when identification with the parent of the same sex is a critical developmental task.

Projection

In projection an individual projects onto others unwanted or undesirable feelings, thoughts, and attitudes related to self. He or she may blame others for faults, maladaptive behaviors, and other negative qualities that are unacceptable to the self. Projection begins in early childhood, when the child realizes that consequences are less threatening if he or she assigns the blame to a sibling for spilling a glass of milk or breaking a valued object, for example.

Projection is noted in people with substance use disorders, who find it easier to blame everyone else for their habit rather than seek help. It is used to a pathologic degree in clients with paranoid disorders, who project toward others their own unhealthy feelings of mistrust, suspiciousness, and hostility. Paranoid and persecutory delusions reflect projectile patterns, in that the client assigns his or her own lack of self-trust to others in the environment.

Displacement

In displacement an individual discharges or displaces feelings and emotions (such as frustration, hostility, or anxiety) onto another person, object, or situation that is less threatening than the actual source. Simple, adaptive forms of displacement include slamming a door or kicking the wall after the boss refuses a request for a pay increase. Such innocuous acts release pent-up emotions without fear of negative consequences. An example of a more intense use of displacement is noted, according to psychoanalytic theory, in some forms of phobic behavior. The feared object or event is believed to be a symbol of an early childhood conflict that has been successfully repressed, such as sexual molestation or abuse. The feelings experienced when the person is confronted with the feared object or event are *displaced* from the early conflict (the actual source), which cannot be recalled.

Reaction Formation

In reaction formation, an individual expresses toward another person or situation feelings, attitudes, or behaviors that are the opposite of what would normally be expected under the circumstances, while unacceptable feelings are repressed. It begins in early childhood, when a child, for example, may hug and squeeze the new baby in the family just a bit too hard while smiling and saying, "I love you." Another example is when a person acts cold, aloof, and uncaring toward the spouse of a best friend toward whom strong sexual feelings are felt. Reaction formation can be adaptive when it prevents the person from responding to significant individuals in ways that would be hurtful, inconsiderate, or unacceptable.

Regression

In regression an individual retreats to past levels of behavior and seeks a dependent role in an effort to reduce anxiety. It may be simple (an adult who behaves like an adolescent when invited out on a rare date), or it may be complex (as in schizophrenia, when the individual regresses to early stages of growth and development and is unable to care for his or her own basic needs).

Undoing (Restitution)

In undoing (restitution) a previous, consciously intolerable action or experience is negated, generally to relieve feelings of guilt. It may be a simple act, such as sending a gift after embarrassing someone in front of friends, or a complex ritual, such as the repetitive hand washing, cleaning, or checking of clients with obsessive-compulsive disorder, who are attempting to undo the painful anxiety evoked by their troubling thoughts.

Compensation

In compensation an individual attempts to make up for a real or imagined physical or emotional deficit or inability with a specific behavior or skill, to maintain self-respect or self-esteem. A person who is compensating strives to become proficient in another area; for example, the short, thin young man who did not make the football team becomes the class wizard in mathematics, or the tall young woman who rarely gets a date because she stands head and shoulders above her male classmates selects the latest styles in clothes and becomes the class fashion expert. Compensation is most often an adaptive defense mechanism; however, it can divert people from developing talents in other areas as it forces them to focus all their creative energies toward one goal.

Denial

Denial is characterized by avoidance of disagreeable realities and unconscious refusal to face intolerable thoughts, feelings, needs, or desires. Denial may be adaptive when it helps the individual get through a difficult, traumatic experience until he or she is better able to cope with reality (e.g., during the early stages of grief or when first diagnosed with a life-threatening illness). It can also be maladaptive when a person persistently denies a serious disorder (e.g., alcoholism or drug abuse or the failure to seek medical attention for a lump in the breast that may be cancer).

Suppression

The only conscious mental mechanism, suppression is characterized by the willful or deliberate refusal to acknowledge a thought, feeling, or event. The individual intentionally excludes the unwanted material from the conscious mind but, unlike repression, is able to retrieve it at will. Suppression is adaptive when a person is overloaded with stimuli and information and needs to prioritize by postponing less important matters for those that are more urgent. However, suppression can also lead to procrastination and result in even more anxiety for the individual who ultimately has to deal with the "forgotten" material.

Dissociation

Dissociation is a defense mechanism that protects the self from the awareness of feelings related to an emotionally charged conflict by separating and detaching the conflict from the consciousness. Dissociation has been noted in people who have been assaulted or raped and are later found wandering around in public, dazed and disheveled. On questioning by a physician or a police officer, these individuals generally cannot recall the traumatic event.

Rationalization

The most commonly used defense mechanism is rationalization, in which a person justifies ideas, actions, or feelings with seemingly acceptable reasons or explanations. Rationalization is often used to preserve self-respect, reduce guilt feelings, or obtain social approval or acceptance. An example of rationalization is the student who insists she or he received a poor grade on an exam because the teacher never explained the class content sufficiently but actually the student was not adequately prepared for the exam. Rationalization is maladaptive when the person uses it continuously and refuses to take responsibility for actions or feelings.

Intellectualization

In intellectualization an individual transfers emotions and feelings into the intellectual domain. The person uses reasoning and logic, often with sophisticated words or jargon, to distance the self from painful feelings and emotions. Intellectualization is often demonstrated by survivors in the early stages of grief who give funeral instructions in a calm, logical manner to avoid the devastating pain of reality. Another example is that of a person who has recently been the victim of a broken love relationship and tries to figure out what went wrong through lengthy, involved explanations instead of demonstrating the appropriate emotions of sadness, disappointment, and anger. It may be adaptive if used for a short period but maladaptive if it prevents healthy emotions from being expressed for the better part of one's lifetime.

Sublimation

Sublimation involves the rechanneling of consciously intolerable or socially unacceptable impulses or behaviors into activities that are personally and socially acceptable. For example, an aggressive high school student joins the football team and rechannels angry impulses on the football field, or a middle-aged woman who craves love rechannels her emotions to catering to a pet. The most common drives used in sublimation are sexuality and aggression.

Isolation of Affect

Isolation of affect is characterized by the separation of an unacceptable feeling, idea, or impulse from one's thought processes. For example, a nurse working in a busy emergency department is able to care for seriously injured accident victims by separating or isolating feelings and emotions related to the clients' pain, injuries, or death. The nurse focuses on the care and treatment rather than the pain, suffering, or outcome of the clients. Isolation of affect, also known as *emotional isolation,* may be adaptive for short periods when people need to perform rather than react. It may become maladaptive, however, if used for a long time without healthy release of emotions.

Symbolization

In symbolization an object, idea, or act represents another through some common aspect and carries the emotions and feelings that are associated with it. Common examples of symbols are the flags that represent the different nations of the world. Many symbols are culture-specific, but suffice it to say, every culture has its own unique symbols for love, patriotism, and other ideals. Clients who are experiencing psychosis sometimes use symbolism in an idiosyncratic manner; for example, the color red may represent blood or death, or blue-eyed people may symbolize purity.

Fantasy

In fantasy imagined events or mental images, such as daydreams, are used to express unconscious conflicts, satisfy desires, or prepare for future events. A person may fantasize to resolve an emotional conflict or as a means of mental rehearsal. Fantasy may be adaptive and even beneficial at any age as long as developmental tasks are being met and the person functions in a manner that reveals he or she is able to distinguish between fantasy and reality.

Conversion

In conversion an individual transfers a mental conflict into a physical symptom to reduce anxiety. For example, an individual experiences sudden blindness after witnessing an accident in which several people were injured, or an elderly person loses function in the lower extremities when told a close friend has died.

Splitting

In splitting, a person is unable to integrate the good and bad aspects of oneself or of one's image of another individual. The person views self and others as either all good or all bad at any given time and acts accordingly. For example, a client compliments a staff nurse in the morning, and in the afternoon the client confronts the same nurse with anger and contempt, or a client expresses admiration for the daytime staff and extreme dislike for the nighttime staff. Splitting is a frequently used defense mechanism of clients with borderline personality disorder.

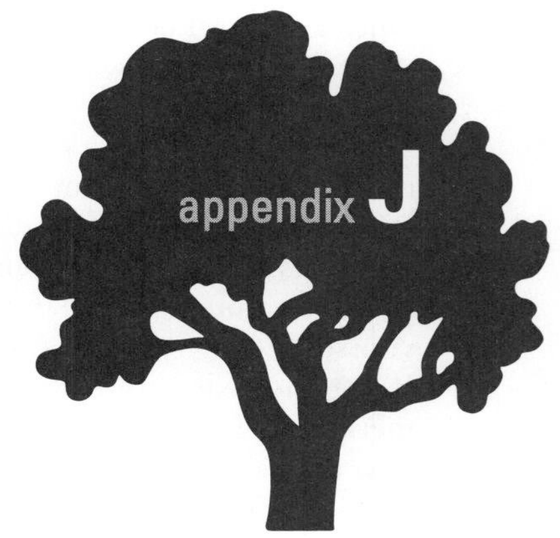

Suicide Assessment and Intervention Guidelines

Appendix J

PRINCIPLES

1. Continually evaluate the client's risk for suicide by assessing the following:
   a. Has history of suicide attempts.
   b. Talks about death, suicide, wanting to be dead; appears morose, overly contemplative.
   c. Asks questions that suggest thoughts or plans of suicide, for example, "How much time alone can clients have without staff around?" "How many pills like these would it take to kill someone?" "If someone jumped from this window, would he or she be killed instantly?"
   d. Fears being unable to sleep and fears nighttime.
   e. Appears depressed and cries often.
   f. Isolates self from others (self-imposed), especially in secluded area or behind locked doors.
   g. Is tense, worried, and conveys a hopeless, helpless attitude.
   h. Imagines he or she has a serious physical illness, such as cancer or AIDS, and may want to end suffering for self and loved ones.
   i. Expresses extreme guilt about a real or imagined incident or situation and feels that he or she is not worthy of living.
   j. Ruminates about being punished, tortured, or persecuted.
   k. Listens to voices (may be telling him or her to kill self).
   l. Suddenly seems very happy or relieved without any apparent reason, after a long period of depression (may be a signal that ambivalence about whether to take own life is relieved by decision to do it).
   m. Collects objects that may be used to inflict injury, such as soda cans, pieces of string or shoelaces, pieces of glass, or a knife from the kitchen.
   n. Acts aggressively or impulsively, suddenly and unexpectedly.
   o. Displays an unusual amount of interest in settling personal affairs.
   p. Gives away personal possessions.

Nursing Interventions

1. Ensure the safety of the client and the physical environment.
2. Establish contact with the client.
3. Determine the degree of suicidal intent or risk by noting if there is a history of suicide attempts. (Previous attempts are the most accurate risk factors.)
4. Establish a therapeutic relationship based on trust, respect, acceptance, empathy, and support.
5. Conduct a suicide assessment based on criteria identified previously.
6. Assess for biologic or organic causes of depression, such as substance use, organic brain disease, or other medical problems.

7. Once a suicidal client is identified, evaluate the person's intent with a direct question that clarifies the meaning: "You're saying you feel so bad you don't want to live; do you mean that you intend to harm yourself?"
8. If the response to the previous question is yes, assess for plans with another direct question: "Do you have a plan for harming yourself?"
9. If the client describes a plan, ask for the method and determine how lethal it is and how accessible the weapons, equipment, or pills are. (The most common methods of self-destruction involve guns and poisoning, generally through prescription drugs, which are readily accessible. Clients have been known to use strangulation as a method with socks, towels, pieces of string, or shoelaces that are easily available. Other methods include hanging, jumping, cutting, piercing, or drowning. Men tend to choose more violent methods; women seem to prefer less aggressive means.)
10. Express your concern for the client while explaining that this information will be shared with other qualified personnel for the protection of the client: "Bill, I'm very concerned that you're feeling troubled enough now to want to harm yourself. I need to share this with the staff so we can keep you safe until you no longer feel this way."
11. Offer hope for the future: "Bill, you're feeling badly now, but you won't always feel this way. Therapy and medication have been known to help people who feel as troubled as you do now."
12. Remain with the client, or get qualified personnel to remain with the client, until safety is secured. (A suicidal client should continually be observed.)
13. Initiate suicide precautions or hold procedures according to the protocol of the mental health facility.

Psychiatric/Psychosocial Therapies

Behavior therapy A type of therapy that focuses on modifying observable behavior, emotions, and verbalizations, by manipulating the environment, the behavior, or the consequences of the behavior. In contrast to psychoanalytic therapy, which focuses on repressed, intrapsychic conflicts, behavioral approaches focus on the effects rather than the cause. They include the works of Ivan Pavlov (classical conditioning) and B.F. Skinner (operant conditioning) but have also been applied to many other types of therapies, including rational-emotive therapy, a type of cognitive therapy developed by Ellis, and the cognitive therapy developed later by Beck, both listed separately. Behavioral strategies are also used in behavioral contracts to reinforce positive behaviors and diminish maladaptive behaviors.

Cognitive therapy A form of therapy (developed by Aaron Beck) most often used in depression and currently being used for other nonpsychotic disorders that stem from the individual's negative self-concept or exaggerated, prolonged guilt and the consequent automatic thoughts of self-deprecation.

The goal of cognitive therapy is to diminish depressive symptoms by helping the individual recognize, challenge, and invalidate distorted automatic thoughts through a series of mental exercises and ultimately to replace them with appropriate, realistic thoughts, based on more accurate evaluations. In practice cognitive and behavioral therapeutic concepts are often used in conjunction.

Beck, however, places much more importance on the internal or mental experiences of his clients than does behaviorism. He emphasizes that behavioral techniques are used to supplement the cognitive work. One of the main reasons for using a behavioral technique is to demonstrate to the client that the negative assumptions and conclusions are incorrect and thus pave the way for improved performance in those aspects of life that are important to the client.

Thought stopping A cognitive strategy used to treat individuals with depression characterized by irrational, anxiety-provoking, and brooding behaviors. The goal of thought stopping is to inhibit these maladaptive behaviors by instructing the client to shout "stop" after he or she expresses the illogical behavior. In this way, the client learns to control the thoughts and thus control the maladaptive behavior. Thought stopping has been reported to be useful in the treatment of obsessive-compulsive disorders. In these cases, the word *stop* is initiated by the nurse-therapist, followed by an exaggerated stimulus, such as a loud noise, or by the client loudly echoing the work *stop.* Consequently, the troublesome thought is interrupted or blocked by principles of counterconditioning, and the behavior is inhibited as well.

Thought substitution A cognitive approach (developed by Wolpe) in which the client is instructed to substitute a positive or rational thought for a negative, distorted thought.

Reframing/relabeling A cognitive technique in which the nurse-therapist renames or relabels seemingly dysfunctional behavior as reasonable and understandable behavior to take away the negative motive for the act. The goal of renaming or relabeling is to emphasize the positive aspects of interpersonal feelings and behaviors. For example, a client who is scheduled to lead the morning community meeting may repeatedly refer to herself as "anxious." The nurse, knowing the client is well prepared, relabels "anxious" as "enthusiastic." In another example, a client may continually refer to a nurse's actions as "hovering." The nurse, realizing the client needs to be closely watched, renames "hovering" as "caring."

Rational-emotive therapy (RET) A type of cognitive therapy (developed by Albert Ellis) that preceded Beck's work, based on the premise that an individual's values and beliefs control his or her behavior. Many beliefs and assumptions are irrational and self-defeating, and people often evaluate their behavior by using these faulty thoughts. Some false assumptions include the following:

1. A person should be loved and approved of by everyone.
2. A person should be competent and talented to prove he or she is adequate.
3. A person has little control over his or her life, and pressures make one feel angry, hostile, and depressed.
4. Past experiences are the most important influence on present behavior and cannot be changed.
5. Order and understanding of the world are necessary for happiness and well-being.
6. One should not question society's beliefs or one may be punished.

RET helps individuals or groups examine irrational thoughts and behaviors thorough verbal discussions and written assignments, followed by activities that allow individuals to challenge their faulty beliefs by directly confronting the feared situations and noting that the results are not devastating. Individuals can thus rid themselves of irrational thoughts and self-defeating behaviors and replace them with rational beliefs and healthy behaviors. RET is especially useful in mild to moderate anxiety states, when insight and reasoning can overcome the physiologic symptoms of anxiety. This form of therapy is useful for high-functioning individuals.

Deep-breathing exercises A simple, adaptive therapeutic technique for reducing anxiety in individuals with mild to moderate levels of anxiety. It may be used in conjunction with relaxation exercises.

The person is instructed as follows:

1. Sit in a quiet place.
2. Breathe slowly and deeply through the nose (may close eyes).
3. Allow the breathing to become natural and set its own pace.
4. Concentrate on the breathing—the air coming in, slowly filling the lungs with oxygen, expanding the chest cavity, and slowly being exhaled.
5. Count silently during inhalations, and then exhale.
6. Disregard distracting thoughts or stimuli and focus back on the slow, rhythmic breathing patterns.
7. Accept whatever thoughts, feelings, or sensations arise, and redirect attention back to the breathing.

Deep-breathing exercises reduce the physiologic effects of anxiety by slowing the heart rate, which positively influences the person's emotional status.

Benson's relaxation response A simple, basic procedure (developed by M. Benson) for eliciting relaxation in persons experiencing tension and mild to moderate levels of anxiety. The person is instructed as follows:

1. Sit in a quiet place in a position of comfort.
2. Close eyes.
3. Relax all muscles as deeply as possible, beginning at the feet and progressing slowly up to the face.
4. Keep all the muscles relaxed.
5. Breathe through the nose with awareness of the breathing.
6. Say the word *one* silently, when breathing out.
7. Breathe easily and naturally, not forcefully.
8. Continue the exercise for 10 to 20 minutes, opening eyes to check time periodically; do not use alarm clock.
9. Sit quietly for several minutes on completion of exercise, first with eyes closed, then with eyes open.
10. Do not stand up for several minutes after exercise.

Do not be concerned about achieving total relaxation. Maintain a passive, matter-of-fact attitude and allow relaxation to occur at its own pace. Try to ignore distracting thoughts or stimuli by not concentrating on them; simply return to repeating "one." Practice relaxation techniques once or twice a day but not within 2 hours after meals because digestion seems to interfere with the relaxation response.

Progressive relaxation technique Another form of relaxation therapy (developed by Jacobson) in which the person alternately tenses and relaxes all voluntary muscle groups progressively from toes to head to elicit a response opposite to that of anxiety.

Visualization (visual or guided imagery) An effective means of deepening relaxation and desensitizing a real-life situation that is generally met with stress and tension (e.g., taking an exam). The individual is instructed to imagine with all the senses a mental picture or image of the feared or troubling situation, based on past memory of the event. The person is then instructed as follows:

1. Relax self in own usual manner.
2. Breathe slowly and deeply several times, concentrating on the feeling of the body as it relaxes.
3. Experience the tension draining from every part of the body, beginning with the feet and working its way upward.
4. Take the time to enjoy the feeling of being totally relaxed (e.g., the warm, tingling sensations).
5. Now, picture self in a favorite place, one that brings peace, joy, or tranquility, and visualize the details. (For example, for an ocean, imagine the waves and foamy whitecaps, smell the sea air, feel the breeze on your face and the warm sand under your feet, etc.)

Visual imagery combines positive experiences with actual or perceived negative events or situations in an effort to desensitize the trauma of the negative event and/or correct cognitive distortions surrounding the event. It is often combined with relaxation techniques to enhance its effectiveness.

Strategic therapy Part of the communication theory, strategic therapy is a unique departure from medical model–based approaches. It is based on the approach of one of its founders, Gregory Bateson, an anthropologist whose position is that behavior makes sense in the context in which it occurs and that behavior is continually being shaped and reinforced by the person's support system (significant others) and vice versa (the interactive context of behavior). A strategic therapist always examines the problem behavior in the context of the surrounding behaviors. There are variations of strategic therapy (e.g., solution-focused therapy and brief therapy), and all trace their beginnings to the ground-breaking work of Gregory Bateson, Don Jackson, Paul Watzlawick, John Weakland, and Richard Fisch at the Mental Research Institute in Palo Alto, California, in the 1950s and 1960s. The Palo Alto group attempted to reduce treatment time. They studied the change process and examined problem formulation and maintenance in human systems and how best to promote change in those systems.

Assertiveness training Assertiveness training, a component of behavior therapy, is a process by which an individual learns to communicate needs, refuse requests, and express both positive and negative feelings in an open, honest, direct, and appropriate manner. Individuals who use assertive responses stand up for their own rights and also respect the rights and dignity of others. A major focus in assertiveness training is the right to choose one's responses in any given situation, which allows the individual to experience control over his or her behavior. Acquisition of power over one's behavior decreases anxiety.

The following is a comparison of assertive, aggressive, and acquiescent behaviors:

Assertive: Stands up for rights and respects those of others. Uses expressive, directive, self-enhancing speech. Chooses appropriate words and actions.

Aggressive: Stands up for rights but abuses those of others. Speaks in demeaning or attacking manner. Fails to monitor or control words or actions.

Acquiescent: Does not stand up for own rights and accepts the domination and bullying of others. Performs unwanted tasks and feels victimized.

Examples of Assertive Behaviors

1. "I" messages: "I need," "I feel," "I will."
2. Eye contact: looking directly into the eyes of the person while making or refusing a request.
3. Congruent verbal and facial expressions: making certain that the facial expression matches the intent of the spoken message. A serious message accompanied by laughter could negate the credibility of the message.

Example of Assertive Plan for Change

1. Target the behavior that one desires to change, for example, how to say no and mean it.
2. List approximately 10 situations in which it is difficult to say no, and order them from least to most difficult.
3. Practice saying no, using the least threatening method first and working up to more challenging situations: imagery, tape recorder, feedback, role playing, and practice in actual situations.
4. Say no as the first word in the practice response, as it is a clear message without excuses or apologies.
5. Follow with a clear, concise, declarative statement, such as "I will not rearrange my schedule. I need my day off."
6. Use eye contact appropriate to the intent of the verbal message.

Assertiveness training is most often done in small group sessions and has been described in detail in a variety of textbooks.

Desensitization The object of desensitization is to lessen the negative impact of a frightening or troubling object, thought, or event by exposing the individual to the object, thought, or event in a progressive, least to most threatening manner. The following is an example of desensitization in a student with text anxiety:

1. Instruct student to write down all the thoughts surrounding the test-taking event.
2. Request student to isolate the irrational thoughts, for example, "I'm sure to fail"; "All tests are tricky"; "I can never find enough time to study."
3. Inform student that irrational thoughts set up conflicts that result in anxiety.

4. Engage student in a discussion that helps transform irrational thoughts into rational ones, such as "You cannot predict failure; you can choose to study, which will increase your chances for success." "All tests are not tricky; why would a teacher put effort into devising trick questions that would result in mass failure?" "You have to make time to study; time is not found, it is structured; and it is time worth spending because it has to do with a career goal."
5. Instruct the student to write down three or four rational thoughts and commit them to memory, for example, "I will pass this exam because I will make the time to study for it"; "I cannot control the content of the exam, but I can control my choice of answers"; "My career is important to me, and I will make the time to study"; "Studying will enhance my chances of passing the test."
6. Practice a test-taking scenario with the individual, using the following steps:
   a. Visualize the usual routine on the morning of the exam.
   b. Experience the examination scene in a relaxed state.
   c. Repeat learned rational thoughts to self, in a calm, optimistic manner.
   d. Experience the incidents that generally cause tension (e.g., being late, confronting tense classmates) and envision self reacting to them in a calm, accepting manner.
   e. Focus on relaxed feeling state and optimistic thoughts of doing the best to pass the exam.
   f. Continue to envision going in to take the exam.
   g. Imagine sitting down and holding onto the pencil, and experience the "feel" of the chair and pencil.
   h. Experience relaxation and mental alertness.
   i. Practice going through the exam questions, beginning with question number 1, taking time to read the question calmly and respond to it. Look at the distractors, feeling confident that the choice made was the correct one.
   j. Concentrate totally on the exam, as question number 2 is read. This time, experience the situation of not being able to find the correct answer, even after reviewing the distractors. Mark question number 2 in the margin and calmly proceed to question number 3. After responding to number 3, return to number 2 and answer it. Proceed in this manner, in a relaxed and confident state.

Desensitization is best performed after experiencing the relaxation response (see Benson's relaxation response). The scenario may be taped for convenience. Desensitization techniques may be used with clients who are able to tolerate such exercises, during times of tension or mild to moderate anxiety. Behavioral therapists use systematic desensitization strategies to help clients with phobic disorders and obsessive compulsive disorders.

Psychoanalytic therapy A type of therapy (developed by Sigmund Freud and his followers) that focuses on repressed, intrapsychic conflicts that are produced through interactions among three theoretic constructs of the mind: the id (the storehouse of all unconscious material), the ego (problem solver or mediator, which lies mostly in the conscious), and the superego (conscience or moral system, which lies in both the conscious and unconscious). Psychoanalysis employs insight-oriented techniques such as free association and dream analysis to explore the meanings behind behaviors. Childhood experiences are discussed in depth, as they are believed to be at the root of adult "neuroses." The goal of psychoanalytic therapy is to help the client clarify the psychologic meaning of events, feelings, and behavior and to gain insight into why one behaves or feels a certain way. This type of therapy is a lengthy process that may take as long as 10 years for some individuals.

Gestalt therapy Gestalt, which means "the whole," is based on gestalt psychology. The therapist helps the individual become aware of his or her "total self" and "the world" that surrounds him or her. Gestalt theory (developed by Fritz Perls) explains the "here and now" in that it emphasizes self-expression, self-exploration, and self-awareness in the present. Awareness of feelings is the major focus of therapy, and this awareness renders the individual capable of change, which leads to problem-solving and problem resolution. One Gestalt technique is to have the person vent feelings toward an empty chair in which an imagined significant person sits. Gestalt techniques can be applied to individuals and groups and are used with high-functioning persons.

Client-centered therapy A humanistic approach developed by Carl Rogers in which the therapist encourages expression of feelings through reflection and clarification. Some transference and countertransference are allowed in this approach, as the therapist demonstrates unconditional acceptance of client and their feelings in a nonjudgmental manner. The goals for the individual are (1) acceptance of own feelings, (2) to gain a positive self-regard, and (3) self-acceptance. Inherent in this theory is the belief that growth and change can take place at any time. This type of therapy can be done with individuals or in groups. The group approach is called Rogerian group therapy.

Family therapy; family systems therapy A specific mode of intervention for the purpose of establishing open communication and healthy family interactions.

Family therapy, based on the family systems theory, is built on the premise that the family (whole) is more than the sum of its parts (the individual family members). Family therapy is most often warranted when the member with the presenting symptom (identified client) signals the presence of pain or dysfunction within the whole family. The therapist works to help family members identify and express their thoughts and feelings, define family roles and rules, experiment with more productive styles of relating, and restore strength to the family system.

Group therapy The facilitation of psychotherapy with several clients at the same time, in the same session. It may emphasize examination of the interpersonal relationships between group members. Groups may be homogeneous (e.g., people with similar problems, or of the same sex or age) or heterogeneous (e.g., people with different problems or of both sexes or various ages). Ten curative factors of group therapy, as described by I.D. Yalom, are (1) imparting of information, (2) instillation of hope, (3) universality, (4) altruism, (5) the corrective recapitulation of the primary family group, (6) development of socializing techniques, (7) imitative behavior, (8) interpersonal learning, (9) group cohesiveness, and (10) catharsis. There are many types of group therapies, and many types of therapies can be accomplished in group situations.

Transactional Analysis (TA) A type of therapy (developed by Eric Berne) in which it is theorized that individuals are capable of responding from three distinct ego states (parent, child, and adult) and that successful interpersonal transactions depend on the use of an appropriate combination of these ego states between the communicators.

Parent Ego State Incorporates feelings and behaviors that are learned from parents or authority figures. May be nurturing or critical.

Child Ego State Unrefined, childlike emotions or responses that stem from early developmental life experiences. May be adaptive (conforming) or free-spirited (nonconforming).

Adult Ego State Responsible for objective, mature appraisal of reality and the problem-solving capacity to process data.

A *Complementary Transaction* Occurs when the transactional stimulus and transactional response originate from identical ego states—that is, parent to parent, child to child, adult to adult. A *crossed transaction* occurs when the transactional stimulus and transactional response originate from different ego states, such as parent to child, adult to parent, child to adult. Complementary and crossed transactions may be either successful or unsuccessful, depending on the responses of the individuals and the situation.

A major goal of TA groups is to enable members to communicate from the ego state that is appropriate to the situation and the responses of the individuals, thereby decreasing conflict and promoting mature interpersonal relationships.

Psychodrama A method of group psychotherapy (developed by Jacob Moreno) in which the truth is explored via improvised dramatizations of emotionally charged situations and conflicts. During psychodrama, the subject (or client) produces a topic to be explored. The director (or therapist) guides the subject through a series of role-playing scenes related to the topic. The use of auxiliary egos (or therapeutic aides) is incorporated in the action and may represent significant people relevant to the subject and the chosen topic. The audience closely relates to the drama that takes place on the stage, and a catharsis occurs for the subject and the audience. Psychodrama is not a mainstream therapy and is performed with select, high-functioning groups.

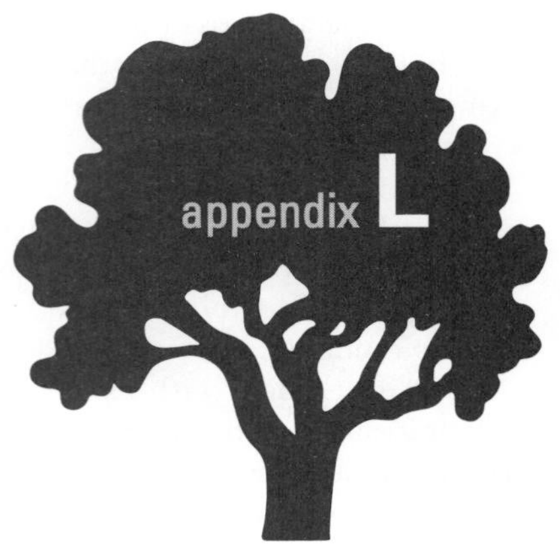

Guidelines for Seclusion and Restraint

Rationale: To prevent injury or death to aggressive clients, other clients, and staff and to prevent the destruction of property and the environment. Knowledge of the client's history of violence and awareness of behaviors that indicate risk for violence are critical factors in the prevention of violence.

NURSING ASSESSMENT

Client demonstrates behaviors that are aggressive and or potentially destructive to self or others. Behaviors may be subtle or obvious, verbal or nonverbal.

Examples of verbal behaviors:

- Shouting obscenities
- Threats to self or others

Examples of nonverbal behaviors:

Sudden changes in behavior, such as a client who has been reasonably calm suddenly becomes agitated or a client who has been reasonably active suddenly becomes quiet or withdrawn; psychomotor agitation that increases in intensity; clenched fists; hand-to-fist pounding; angry, wild-eyed facial expression; clenched jaw; pacing back and forth in an agitated manner; bumping carelessly into walls, furniture, or people in the environment.

Plan of Action and Rationale

Immediately inform key staff of client's aggressive behavior *to prevent harm or injury to client, other clients, and staff.* (Never leave an aggressive client unattended or attempt to control a potentially dangerous client without qualified help.)

Plan to approach the client on a continuum, using the least restrictive to most restrictive measures as a model for intervention.

Model for Intervention

Verbalize methods to help client maintain control and dignity.

Medicate client as necessary.

Seclude.

Restrain.

Interventions and Rationale

Intervene as soon as the client begins to act in an aggressive manner, and attempt to identify sources leading to aggressive behavior, if possible, *to resolve volatile issues and prevent escalation of behaviors.*

Verbal Interaction

Approach client in a calm, direct, nonchallenging manner *to assure client that staff is in control to increase client's control and trust in staff.*

Offer client the opportunity to control self, indicating that if this is not possible, staff will assist in helping to control client until he or she can regain control, *to ensure security and safety of client and others in the environment.*

Inform client that his or her concerns will be addressed as soon as client regains control *to rein-*

force staff's expectations that client will regain control and to promote trust.

If client calms down at any time during the verbal interaction, quietly accompany client to an area of decreased stimulation *to decrease anxiety and exert least restrictive measures whenever possible.*

If client's behavior fails to respond to verbal intervention, prescribed medication may be required *to continue to use least restrictive measures.*

INTERVENTIONS AND RATIONALE IN THE USE OF SECLUSION POLICY

On determining the necessity for the use of a seclusion room, obtain the physician's written order or, in an emergency, obtain the written order from the charge nurse and secure the order from the attending physician within a reasonable period of time. (All orders for the use of a seclusion room must comply with individual state laws.)

The charge nurse documents the justification for use of the seclusion room, which includes the following:

- Events leading up to the need for seclusion
- Other interventions used prior to seclusion
- Purpose for the use of seclusion
- Clinical justification for length of seclusion time

Procedure

Explain procedure and purpose of seclusion to client before placement in the seclusion room *to inform and support the client and reduce anxiety.*

Escort the client into the seclusion room in a calm, direct manner that does not cause discomfort, harm, or pain *to ensure the client's safety and preserve his or her dignity.* (The charge nurse should be present to observe the procedure.)

Check the client every 15 minutes with a qualified staff person *to ensure safety and provide support, reassurance, and opportunities for the client to vent feelings.*

Supervise the client's nutrition, hygiene, grooming, and elimination needs *to ensure the client's comfort and safety.* (Bathroom privileges should be offered at least every 2 hours.)

Clear the seclusion room of all articles or utensils that the client might use to harm self or others *to ensure safety of client and others.* (Food should be served in plastic dishes.)

Regulate number of people who enter the seclusion room *to reduce stimulation and provide consistent, therapeutic relationships.* (Only the physician, nurses, and primary therapist should have access to the seclusion room.)

Ensure safe exit of client in case of emergency (fire, disaster) *to ensure client's safety.* (The seclusion room door should open automatically when the alarm is sounded.)

Provide Continual Documentation

Nursing documentation includes the following:

- Factors, events, and client behaviors prior to seclusion
- Other interventions used prior to seclusion
- Time the physician and/or charge nurse was notified and time the client was seen for purpose of seclusion order
- Name of nurse who accompanied client to seclusion room
- Name of staff person who supervised and checked client
- Client's response to seclusion room
- Time that client is removed from seclusion room

Notify physician, medical director, and all appropriate administrative personnel *to inform key people of the client's status.*

Approach the client and offer him or her the opportunity to talk *to allow ventilation of feelings about seclusion.*

RESTRAINT

Rationale: To provide temporary external controls for clients who cannot provide their own internal controls on the unit or in the seclusion room and whose behavior may result in injury to the client or others. Restraints are applied only after less restrictive measures have failed.

Policy

Obtain a physician's written order or, in an emergency situation, a registered nurse's order after he or she has observed and assessed client *to provide adequate justification for use of (leather) restraints and comply with state laws.*

Documentation (Mandatory for Restraint Order)

Events leading up to restraint

Rationale for use of restraint

Length of time client is to be restrained

Justification for length of time

Notification of attending physician and others in accordance with state mental health laws *to ensure adequate documentation of restraint order, provide ongoing communication, and comply with laws that protect client's rights.*

Procedure (Supervised by Qualified Charge Nurse)

Provide an adequate number of trained staff members *to prevent injury to clients and staff.*

Use a minimum amount of restraints *to ensure client's safety with least amount of control.*

Explain to client briefly and simply the reason for use of restraints *to assure client that staff is in control.*

Set up restraints on bed in seclusion room (should be done in advance, although restraints are never left unattended) *to ensure organized application of restraints and promote safety.*

Apply (leather) restraints to all four extremities in a manner that will control client but will not cause undue physical or emotional discomfort *to control client, prevent injury to client or staff, and maintain client's dignity as much as possible.*

Inform client as simply as possible, in a matter-of-fact way, what is happening and why *to facilitate client's understanding without offering own biases and interpretation:*

"You are being restrained so you will have time to control your behavior."

"We're concerned that your behavior will harm you or others."

Refrain from unnecessary authoritative or condescending remarks *to prevent undue anger or shame.*

Examples of nontherapeutic statements:

"We warned you this would happen."

"This is for your own good."

Check the client every 15 minutes with a qualified staff person *to prevent isolation and assure client of staff concerns.*

Provide relief from restraints at least every 2 hours *to promote comfort and maintain muscle tone.*

Examples:

- Allow client to perform active range-of-motion exercises (if safe to remove restraints)

or

- Provide passive range-of-motion exercises on each extremity every 2 hours (if unsafe to remove restraints).

Offer circulation and skin condition as often as necessary *to maintain circulatory function and prevent skin breakdown.*

Offer fluids and nutrition *to maintain dietary and hydration needs.*

Document the following by registered nurse:

- Events leading up to need for restraints
- Least restrictive measures attempted (including medication) prior to restraints
- Response of client to least restrictive measures
- Statement that registered nurse was present when client was placed in restraints
- Specific individual who ordered use of restraints
- Whether the client was examined prior to being placed in restraints
- Exact time restraints were applied
- Exact time client was removed from restraints for relief periods
- Summary of client's response to restraints and relief periods
- Exact time client was removed from restraints and client's behavior at that time.

Postrestraint Procedures

Notify those individuals required by law *to comply with state laws.*

Notify attending physician *to inform physician and plan subsequent care.*

Release client from restraints immediately in case of fire or other disaster *to ensure client's safety.*

Approach client and provide opportunity to talk (registered nurse). *Clients who have just been released from restraints may need to discuss their thoughts and feelings.*

Discuss procedure and feelings about procedure with staff members involved in restraint of the clients *to clarify own and other's perceptions and vent feelings among trusted colleagues.*

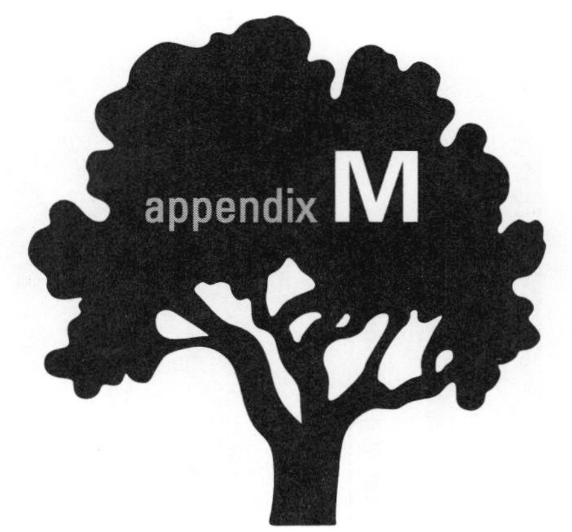

Drugs to Treat Mental and Emotional Disorders

Appendix M

Sedative-Hypnotic and Antianxiety Drugs: Benzodiazepines

Generic name/Trade name	Administration/Dosage/Mechanism of Action	Adverse Effects	Nursing Considerations
alprazolam/Xanax*	Oral: *Adults*—0.25 to 0.5 mg 3 times daily. Maximum daily dose: 4 mg. *Elderly*—0.25 mg 2 or 3 times daily. Potentiates inhibitory transmitters and depresses limbic system and reticular activating activity system.	*CNS:* Drowsiness, dizziness, confusion, headache, anxiety, tremor, stimulation, fatigue, depression, insomnia, paradoxic agitation can occur. *Peripheral:* Photophobia due to mydriasis, blurred vision due to cycloplegia; sleep-like slowing of respirations with therapeutic doses; cough; orthostatic hypotension; tachycardia; hypotension; constipation, dry mouth.	Used to treat anxiety. Schedule IV substance (can promote drug dependence). Pregnancy Category D. Teach patient about abuse and drug dependence; avoid alcohol and OTC CNS depressants that potentiate action.
chlordiazepoxide/Libritabs Librium* Medilium† Novopoxide† Various others	Oral: *Adults*—for anxiety, 15 to 100 mg divided in 3 or 4 doses or in 1 dose at bedtime. *Elderly*—5 mg 2 to 4 times daily. Children—0.5 mg/kg of body weight daily in 3 to 4 doses. May be given intramuscularly. Intravenous: *Adults*—for alcohol withdrawal, 50 to 100 mg slowly over at least 1 min, then 25 to 50 mg every 6 to 8 hr, with the total dose not more than 300 mg. Potentiates inhibitory transmitters and depresses limbic system and reticular activating system	*CNS:* Drowsiness, dizziness, confusion, headache, anxiety, tremor, stimulation, fatigue, depression, and insomnia. *Peripheral:* Photophobia due to mydriasis, blurred vision due to cycloplegia; sleep-like slowing of respirations with therapeutic doses; cough; orthostatic hypotension; tachycardia; hypotension; constipation, dry mouth.	Used to treat anxiety and alcohol withdrawal. Schedule IV substance. Teaching: see alprazolam
clonazepam/Klonopin	Oral: *Adults*—initially, 0.5 mg 3 times daily. Increase in increments of 0.5 mg to 1 mg every 3 days, if necessary. Inhibits spike, wave formation in absence seizures (petit mal); decreases amplitude, frequency, duration, and spread of discharge in minor motor seizures.	*CNS:* Drowsiness (50%), ataxia (30%), dizziness, confusion, behavioral changes, tremor, insomnia, headache, and suicidal tendencies. *Peripheral:* Nausea, constipation, polyphagia, anorexia, xerostomia, diarrhea, rash, alopecia, hirsutism, increased salivation, nystagmus, diplopia, abnormal eye movements, sore gums, respiratory depression, dyspnea, congestion (from increased salivation), palpitations, bradycardia, thrombocytopenia, leukocytosis, eosinophilia.	Primarily used as an anticonvulsant. Use to treat panic disorders is under investigation. Schedule IV substance.

diazepam/Valium[*] E-PAM† Various others	Oral: *Adults*—4 to 40 mg divided into 2 to 4 doses or a single dose of 2.5 to 10 mg at bedtime. *Elderly*—2 to 2.5 mg once to twice daily. *Children*—0.12 to 0.8 mg/kg daily in 3 to 4 doses. Intravenous: Administer no more than 5 mg/min. For severe anxiety, severe muscle spasm, status epilepticus, or recurrent seizures. Potentiates inhibitory transmitters and depresses limbic system and reticular activating systems.	*CNS:* Drowsiness, dizziness, confusion, headache, anxiety, tremor, stimulation, fatigue, depression, and insomnia. *Peripheral:* Photophobia due to mydriasis, blurred vision due to cycloplegia; sleep-like slowing of respirations with therapeutic doses; cough; orthostatic hypotension; tachycardia; hypotension; constipation, dry mouth.	Used to treat anxiety, severe muscle spasm, status epilepticus, and acute alcohol withdrawal symptoms and to provide sedation. Teaching: see alprazolam.
flurazepam/Dalmane[*] Various others	Oral: *Adults*—as hypnotic, 15 to 30 mg at bedtime. *Elderly*—15 mg. Onset: 20 to 45 min. Duration: 7 to 8 hr. Produces CNS depression.	*CNS:* Lethargy, drowsiness, daytime sedation, dizziness, confusion, light-headedness, headache, anxiety, and irritability. *Peripheral:* Nausea, vomiting, diarrhea, heartburn, abdominal pain, constipation, chest pain, pulse change, palpitations.	Used as a hypnotic only. Schedule IV substance.
lorazepam Ativan[*] Various others	Oral: *Adults*—for anxiety, 1 to 2 mg 2 to 3 times daily, may increase dose to 10 mg maximum daily; as hypnotic, 2 to 4 mg at bedtime. *Elderly*—½ adult dose. Potentiates inhibitory transmitters and depresses limbic system and reticular activating systems.	*CNS:* Drowsiness, dizziness, confusion, headache, anxiety, tremor, stimulation, fatigue, depression, and insomnia. *Peripheral:* Photophobia due to mydriasis, blurred vision due to cycloplegia; sleep-like slowing of respirations with therapeutic doses; cough; orthostatic hypotension; tachycardia; hypotension; constipation, dry mouth.	Used to treat anxiety and insomnia. Repeated use for insomnia can cause rebound insomnia. Schedule IV substance. FDA Pregnancy Category D. Teaching: see alprazolam.
temazepam Restoril[*]	Oral: *Adults*—30 mg at bedtime. *Elderly*—reduce dose to 15 mg. Produces CNS depression.	*CNS:* Euphoria, drowsiness, daytime sedation, dizziness, confusion, light-headedness, headache, depression, and irritability. *Peripheral:* Nausea, vomiting, diarrhea, heartburn, abdominal pain, constipation, chest pain, palpitations.	Used as a hypnotic only. Slowly absorbed. Schedule IV substance. FDA Pregnancy Category X.
triazolam/Halcion*	Oral: *Adults*—0.25 to 0.5 mg at bedtime. *Elderly*—reduce dose to 0.25 mg. Produces CNS depression.	*CNS:* Anterograde amnesia, drowsiness, daytime sedation, dizziness, confusion, light-headedness, headache, and irritability. *Peripheral:* Nausea, vomiting, diarrhea, heartburn, abdominal pain, constipation, chest pain, palpitations.	Used as a hypnotic. May also be used as an antianxiety drug and an anticonvulsant. Schedule IV substance.

*Available in Canada and United States.
†Available in Canada only.

Miscellaneous Sedative-Hypnotic and Antianxiety Drugs

Generic name/Trade name	Administration/Dosage/Mechanism of Action	Adverse Effects	Nursing Considerations
buspirone/BuSpar	Oral: *Adults*—initially, 5 mg 3 times daily. May increase by 5 mg daily every 2 to 3 days until desired response is obtained. Maximum daily dose: 60 mg. Unknown; not related to benzodiazepines; may act by binding to serotonin receptors in brain.	*CNS:* Dizziness, headache, depression, stimulation, insomnia, nervousness, light-headedness, numbness, paresthesia, incoordination, tremor, excitement, involuntary movements, confusion, and akathisia. *Peripheral:* Nausea, dry mouth, diarrhea, constipation; tachycardia, palpitations; hypotension; sore throat, tinnitus, blurred vision, nasal congestion; frequency, hesitancy; muscle cramps; hyperventilation, chest congestion; shortness of breath; rash, edema, pruritis, alopecia, dry skin.	Less sedation than older antianxiety drugs. Does not react with alcohol or antidepressants. FDA Pregnancy Category B.
hydroxyzine hydrochloride/ Atarax* hydroxyzine pamoate/ Vistaril Various others	Oral: *Adults*—for anxiety, 75 to 400 mg daily in 4 divided doses. For allergic skin reactions: Oral: *Adults*—25 mg 3 or 4 times daily. *Children under 6 yr*—50 mg daily in 3 or 4 divided doses. Intramuscular: *Adults*—for anxiety, 50 to 100 mg q4–6h. Depresses subcortical CNS (i.e., limbic and reticular areas)	*CNS:* Drowsiness (transient); rarely reported: tremor and seizures. *Peripheral:* Dry mouth; respiratory problems have occurred.	An antihistamine that has antiemetic and antianxiety properties. It is used in treating allergic skin rashes and motion sickness and as a preanesthetic medication. The usual doses of barbiturates or narcotics must be cut 50% if given concurrently.

*Available in Canada and United States.

Antipsychotic Drugs

Antipsychotic drugs produce a neuroleptic effect characterized by sedation, emotional quieting, psychomotor slowing, and affective indifference; exact mode of action is not fully understood; antipsychotics block dopamine receptors

Generic Name/Trade Name	Administration/Dosage/Mechanism of Action	Adverse Effects	Nursing Considerations
Benzisoxazole derivative			
risperidone/Risperdal	Oral: *Adults*—1 mg bid, with incremental increases of 1 mg bid on days 2 and 3 to a dose of 3 mg bid by day 3; then do not increase dose for at least 1 week.	Note: Less incidence of *extrapyramidal symptoms with this medication* *CNS: Extrapyramidal symptoms (pseudoparkinsonism, akathisia, dystonia, tardive dyskinesia) drowsiness, insomnia, agitation, anxiety, headache, seizures, neuroleptic malignant syndrome.* CV: Orthostatic hypotension, tachycardia. *EENT:* Blurred vision. *GI:* Nausea, vomiting, anorexia, constipation, jaundice, weight gain. *RESP:* Rhinitis.	*Atypical antipsychotic.* Unknown; may be mediated through both dopamine type 2 (D_2) and serotonin type 2 ($5\text{-}HT_2$) antagonism; more effective for negative symptoms.
Butyrophenone			
haloperidol/Haldol* Peridol† Novoperidol† haloperidol decanoate/ Haloperidol Decanoate 50 *Decanoate is an injectable form of slow-release medication for noncompliant patients.	Acute psychotic management: Oral: *Adults and children over 12 yr*—1 to 15 mg in divided doses initially, which can be increased gradually up to 100 mg to bring symptoms under control. Dosage is then gradually reduced. Maintenance dose, usually 2 to 8 mg daily. *Elderly clients and children under 12 yr*—0.5 to 1.5 mg daily initially. Dosage increased by 0.5-mg increments if necessary. Usual maintenance dose, 2 to 4 mg daily. Intramuscular: *Adults and children over 12 yr*—2 to 5 mg q4-8h or every hour if acute state requires. Acute symptoms are usually under control in 72 h, and 15 mg daily is usually sufficient. Decanoate: Initial dose IM is 10-15 times daily oral dose at 4-wk interval.	*CNS:* Extrapyramidal symptoms: pseudoparkinsonism, akathisia, dystonia, tardive dyskinesia; seizures, *neuroleptic malignant syndrome,* confusion, drowsiness, headache. *RESP:* Laryngospasm, dyspnea, respiratory depression. *INTEG:* Rash, photosensitivity, dermatitis. *EENT:* Blurred vision, glaucoma, dry eyes. *GI:* Dry mouth, nausea, vomiting, anorexia, constipation, diarrhea, jaundice, weight gain, ileus, hepatitis. *GU:* Urinary retention, urinary frequency, enuresis, impotence, amenorrhea, gynecomastia. *CV:* Orthostatic hypotension, hypertension, cardiac arrest, ECG changes, tachycardia.	Management of psychotic disorders. Likely to produce extrapyramidal reactions in clients prone to neurologic reactions. In severe cases of hyperkinetic, retarded clients, large doses may bring improvement in social behavior and concentration. Drug of choice for the treatment of Tourette's syndrome. Spectrum of side effects is similar to that of the piperazine phenothiazines: low incidence of sedation and autonomic effects, but high incidence of extrapyramidal reactions. FDA Pregnancy Category C.

*Available in Canada and United States.
†Available in Canada only.

Continued.

Antipsychotic Drugs—cont'd

Generic name/Trade name	Administration/Dosage/Mechanism of Action	Adverse Effects	Nursing Considerations
	Tourette's syndrome: Initial dosages to achieve control are same as for chronic schizophrenia. Maintenance dosages: *Adults and children over 12 yr*—9 mg daily; *children under 12 yr*—1.5 mg daily.		
Dibenzoxazepine clozapine/Clozaril	Oral: *Adults*—initially, 25 mg 1 to 2 times/day, increasing in increments of 25 to 60 mg/day, as tolerated, to achieve a dose of 300 to 450 mg/day by the end of 2 weeks. Subsequent dosage increments should not exceed 100 mg 1 or 2 times a week. Interferes with binding of dopamine at D_1 and D_2 receptors; preferentially more active at limbic than at striatal dopamine receptors, probably accounting for the *relative lack of extrapyramidal side effects.*	*CNS: Has relatively few extrapyramidal side effects;* other symptoms include drowsiness, dizziness or vertigo, headache, tremor, syncope, disturbed sleep or nightmares, restlessness, akinesia, agitation, dose-related seizures, rigidity, akathisia, and confusion. *Peripheral:* Salivation, sweating, dry mouth, visual disturbances, tachycardia, hypotension, hypertension, constipation, nausea, fever, agranulocytosis; fatalities have occurred often enough to necessitate a special monitoring system.	*Atypical antipsychotic,* indicated in the management of severely ill schizophrenic clients who fail to respond to other drugs. *Monitor for agranulocytosis and seizures;* more effective for negative symptoms.
Phenothiazines *Aliphatic* chlorpromazine hydrochloride/Thorazine CPZ Chlor-Promanyl† Largactil† Novo-Chlorpromazine†	Psychiatric outpatients: Oral: *Adults*—12 to 40 yr, average dose 400 to 800 mg daily; over 40, a limit of 300 mg daily is suggested. Acutely psychotic, hospitalized clients: Intramuscular: *Adults*—25 to 100 mg q1-4h until symptoms are controlled. *Elderly or debilitated clients*—10 mg q6-8h to control acute symptoms. *Children*—0.5 mg/kg of body weight q6-8h, gradually increasing dose to a maximum of 40 mg for children under 5 yr and 75 mg for those aged 5 to 12. Intravenous: Not recommended because it is highly irritating. Drug must be diluted to at least 1 mg/ml, and no more than 1 mg/min given.	*CNS: Parkinsonism, akathisias, dystonias, tardive dyskinesias, extrapyramidal side effects.* *Peripheral:* Blurred vision (cycloplegia or paralysis of accommodation); ocular pain, photophobia, mydriasis, impaired vision; intolerance of extreme heat or cold, possible heat stroke or fatal hyperthermia; nasal congestion, wheezing, dyspnea; hypotension, especially orthostatic, leading to dizziness, syncope; tachycardia, irregular pulse, arrhythmias; dry mouth, constipation, jaundice, abdominal pain; urinary retention, urinary hesitancy, galactorrhea, gynecomastia, impaired ejaculation, amenorrhea.	Control of initial acute psychotic episodes is achieved with high doses, which are then tapered to the lowest maintenance dose when the client's condition stabilizes. Best tolerated by clients under 40 years old and those hospitalized less than 10 years. Sedation is pronounced at the start of therapy, which may be desired for highly agitated clients. Incidence of hypotension, ophthalmic changes, and dyskinesias is high in older clients. Antiadrenergic and anticholinergic side effects usually diminish after first week. Not for seizure-prone clients.

	Oral: *Adults*—200 to 600 mg daily in divided doses, increased every 2 to 3 days by 100 mg, up to 2 g if needed. *Elderly or debilitated clients*—⅓ to ½ of adult dose with 20- to 25-mg increments. *Children*—0.5 mg/kg q4-6h. To control nausea and vomiting: Oral: 10 to 25 mg q4-6h. Intramuscular: 25 mg initially, then 25 to 50 mg q3-4h to stop vomiting. Other uses: Oral: *Adults*—25 to 50 mg 3 or 4 times daily.		Severe nausea and vomiting can be controlled by low doses. Other uses include intractable hiccups, tetanus, acute intermittent porphyria.
***Piperazine*††**			
fluphenazine decanoate/ Prolixin Decanoate (injectable slow-release form, for noncompliant patients)	Intramuscular, Subcutaneous: *Adults* under 50 yr–12.5 mg initially, then 25 mg every 2 wk. Increase by 12.5-mg amounts if needed.	*CNS:* Parkinsonism, akathisias, dystonias, tardive dyskinesias, oculogyric crisis; neuroleptic malignant syndrome. *Peripheral:* Blurred vision (cycloplegia or paralysis of accommodation); ocular pain, photophobia, mydriasis, impaired vision; intolerance of extreme heat or cold, possible heat stroke or fatal hyperthermia; nasal congestion, wheezing, dyspnea; hypotension, especially orthostatic, leading to dizziness, syncope; tachycardia, irregular pulse, arrhythmias; dry mouth, constipation, jaundice, abdominal pain; urinary retention, urinary hesitancy, galactorrhea, gynecomastia, impaired ejaculation, amenorrhea.	Long-acting depot forms lasting at least 2 weeks. Dosage should be stabilized in the hospital because severe episodes of parkinsonism can appear. Not recommended for elderly clients or clients who have had difficulty with extrapyramidal reactions.
fluphenazine hydrochloride/ Moditen† Prolixin Permitil	Oral: *Adults*—2.5 to 10 mg initially, reduced to 1 to 5 mg daily for maintenance. *Elderly clients*—⅓ to ½ of adult dose. Intramuscular: *Adults*—1.25 mg increased gradually to 2.5 to 10 mg daily in 3 to 4 doses. *Elderly clients*—⅓ to ½ of adult dose.	*CNS:* Parkinsonism, akathisias, dystonias, tardive dyskinesias, oculogyric crisis; neuroleptic malignant syndrome. *peripheral:* blurred vision (cycloplegia or paralysis of accommodation); ocular pain, photophobia, mydriasis, impaired vision; intolerance of extreme heat or cold, possible heat stroke or fatal hyperthermia; nasal congestion, wheezing,	Most potent of the phenothiazines used for the management of psychotic disorders.

Continued.

†Available in Canada only.

††The piperazine phenothiazines are less effective and have fewer autonomic side effects than other phenothiazine classes. Extrapyramidal reactions are more common, particularly in large doses in clients over age 40. Piperazine phenothiazines are less likely to produce allergic reactions and do not change ECG tracings.

Antipsychotic Drugs—cont'd

Generic name/Trade name	Administration/Dosage/Mechanism of Action	Adverse Effects	Nursing Considerations
		dyspnea; hypotension, especially orthostatic, leading to dizziness, syncope; tachycardia, irregular pulse, arrhythmias; dry mouth, constipation, jaundice, abdominal pain; urinary retention, urinary hesitancy, galactorrhea, gynecomastia, impaired ejaculation, amenorrhea.	
perphenazine/Phenazine† Trilafon	Oral: *Adults*—16 to 64 mg daily in divided doses. *Elderly clients*—1/3 to 1/2 of adult dose. *Children over 12 yr*—6 to 12 mg daily. Intramuscular: *Adults*—5 to 10 mg initially, then 5 mg q6h with 15 mg maximum daily in ambulatory and 30 mg daily in hospitalized clients. *Elderly clients*—1/3 to 1/2 of adult dose. *Children over 12 yr*—lowest adult dose. Antipsychotic drugs produce a neuroleptic effect characterized by sedation, emotional quieting, psychomotor slowing, and affective indifference; exact mode of action is not fully understood; antipsychotics block dopamine receptors in the basal ganglia, hypothalamus, limbic system, brain stem, and medulla; antipsychotics are also thought to depress certain components of the reticular activating system that partially control body temperature, wakefulness, vasomotor tone, emesis, and hormonal balance; additionally, antipsychotics have significant anticholinergic and α-adrenergic blocking effects; antiemetic effect r/t inhibition of chemoreceptor trigger zone.	*CNS:* Parkinsonism, akathisias, dystonias, tardive dyskinesias, oculogyric crisis. *Peripheral:* Blurred vision (cycloplegia or paralysis of accommodation); ocular pain, photophobia, mydriasis, impaired vision; intolerance of extreme heat or cold, possible heat stroke or fatal hyperthermia; nasal congestion, wheezing, dyspnea; hypotension, especially orthostatic, leading to dizziness, syncope; tachycardia, irregular pulse, arrhythmias; dry mouth, constipation, jaundice, abdominal pain; urinary retention, urinary hesitancy, galactorrhea, gynecomastia, impaired ejaculation, amenorrhea.	For acute psychotic disorders. Lower doses needed when used as an antiemetic.
prochlorperazine/Compazine prochlorperazine edisylate/ Compazine edisylate	Psychiatric disorders: Oral: *Adult*—5 to 10 mg 3 to 4 times daily. Raise dosage every 2 to 3 days as	*CNS:* Euphoria, depression, extrapyramidal symptoms, restlessness, tremor, and dizziness.	More widely used to control severe nausea and vomiting than for psychiatric treatment. Hypotension is

prochlorperazine maleate/ Compazine maleate Stemetil†	required. From 50 to 75 mg daily is common range for mild cases and 100 to 150 mg for severe cases. *Elderly clients*—⅓ to ½ of adult dosage. *Children over 2 yr*—2.5 mg 2 to 3 times daily up to a total dose of 20 to 25 mg. Same dosage used rectally. Intramuscular: *Adults*—10 to 20 mg in buttock; repeat q2-4h up to 80 mg total. *Elderly clients*—⅓ to ½ of adult dose. *Children over 2 yr*—0.13 mg/kg of body weight initial dose only, then switch to oral. Nausea and vomiting: Oral: *Adults*—5 to 10 mg 3 or 4 times daily. *Children*—20 to 29 lb, 2.5 mg 1 to 2 times daily; 30 to 39 lb, 2.5 mg 2 to 3 times daily; 40 to 85 lb, 2.5 mg 3 times daily or 5 mg 2 times daily. Intramuscular: *Adults*—5 to 10 mg q3-4h. *Children*—0.06 mg/lb. Rectal: *Adults*—25 mg twice daily. *Children*—same as oral dosage. Acts centrally by blocking chemoreceptor trigger zone, which in turn acts on vomiting center.	*GI:* Nausea, vomiting, anorexia, dry mouth, diarrhea, constipation, weight loss, metallic taste, cramps. *CV:* Circulatory failure, tachycardia. *RESP:* Respiratory depression.	seen when given intravenously for surgery.
Piperidine			
mesoridazine besylate/Serentil*	Oral: *Adults*—150 mg daily initially, increased by 50-mg increments until symptoms controlled. *Elderly clients*—⅓ to ½ of adult dose. Intramuscular: *Adults and children over 12 yr*—25 to 175 mg daily in divided doses (irritating). Depresses cerebral cortex, hypothalamus, limbic system, which control activity, aggression; blocks neurotransmission produced by dopamine at synapse; exhibits strong α-adrenergic, anticholinergic blocking action; mechanism for antipsychotic effects is unclear.	*CNS:* Extrapyramidal symptoms: pseudoparkinsonism, akathisia, dystonia, tardive dyskinesias, drowsiness, and headache. *HEMA:* Anemia, leukopenia, leukocytosis, agranulocytosis. *INTEG:* Rash, photosensitivity, dermatitis. *EENT:* Blurred vision, glaucoma. *GI:* Dry mouth, nausea. vomiting, anorexia, constipation, diarrhea, jaundice, weight gain. *GU:* Urinary retention, urinary frequency, enuresis, impotence, amenorrhea, gynecomastia. *CV:* Orthostatic hypotension, hypertension, cardiac arrest, ECG changes, tachycardia.	Management of psychotic disorders. This is a metabolite of thioridazine with antiemetic activity and no reported retinopathy.

*Available in Canada and United States.
†Available in Canada only.

Continued.

Antipsychotic Drugs—cont'd

Generic name/Trade name	Administration/Dosage/Mechanism of Action	Adverse Effects	Nursing Considerations
thioridazine hydrochloride/ Mellaril Novoridazine†	Psychotic disorders: Oral: *Adults*—50 to 100 mg 3 times daily, increasing up to 800 mg. *Elderly clients*—⅓ to ½ of adult dose. *Children over 2 yr*—1 mg/kg of body weight in divided doses. Depressive neurosis, alcohol withdrawal syndrome, intractable pain, senility. Oral: 10 to 50 mg 2 to 4 times daily.	*CNS:* Parkinsonism, akathisias, dystonias, tardive dyskinesias, oculogyric crisis. *Peripheral:* Blurred vision (cycloplegia or paralysis of accommodation); ocular pain, photophobia, mydriasis, impaired vision; intolerance of extreme heat or cold, possible heat stroke or fatal hyperthermia; nasal congestion, wheezing, dyspnea; hypotension, especially orthostatic, leading to dizziness, syncope; tachycardia, irregular pulse, arrhythmias; dry mouth, constipation, jaundice, abdominal pain; urinary retention, urinary hesitancy, galactorrhea, gynecomastia, impaired ejaculation, amenorrhea.	Management of psychotic disorders. Little antiemetic activity. Safe for clients with epilepsy. "Possibly effective" in alcohol withdrawal syndrome, intractable pain, senility. Pronounced sedative and hypotensive side effects initially. One of the least likely of the antipsychotic drugs to cause extrapyramidal reactions because of the pronounced anticholinergic action. Photosensitivity has not been reported. Doses over 800 mg daily have produced serious pigmentary retinopathy.
Dibenzothiazepine			
Quetiapine fumerate/ Seroquel	Oral: 25 mg/100 mg/200 mg Acts as antagonist to multiple neurotransmittors.	*CNS:* Extrapyramidal symptoms (dystonias, parkinsonian symptoms, akathisia, tardive dyskinesia. Neuroleptic malignant syndrome, although rare, has been reported (1%); somnolence; orthostatic hypotension; cataracts may develop.	Caution for use in patients with impaired cardiac, hepatic, or renal function.
Thienbenzodiazepine			
olanzapine/Zyprexia	Oral: 5 to 10 mg initially, qd. May increase dosage by 5 mg at 1 week.	*CNS:* EPS *CV:* Orthostatic hypotension, tachycardia, chest pain *EENT:* Blurred vision *GI:* Dry mouth, nausea, vomiting, constipation *GU:* Urinary retention, urinary frequency, enuresis *INTEG:* Rash *RESP:* Dyspnea, rhinitis, cough, pharyngitis	Monitor bilirubin, CBC, liver function studies monthly. Assess dizziness, faintness, palpitations, tachycardia on rising. Monitor skin turgor daily. Monitor constipation, urinary retention daily; increase bulk and water in diet.

†Available in Canada only.

Antidepressant Drugs

Generic Name/Trade Name	Administration/Dosage/Mechanism of Action	Adverse Effects	Nursing Considerations
First-Generation Antidepressants *Tricyclic Antidepressants (TCAs)*			
amitripthyline hydrochloride/ Elavil* Endep Levate† Novotriptyn†	Oral: *Adults*—begin with 50 mg at bedtime, increasing dosage by 25 to 50 mg if necessary to 150 mg. Alternatively, start with 25 mg 3 times daily, increase to 50 mg 3 times daily. Total dosage should not exceed 300 mg daily. Maintenance doses are usually 50 to 100 mg at bedtime. These are outpatient dosages; inpatient dosages may be twice as much. *Adolescents and elderly*—10 mg 3 times daily plus 20 mg at bedtime (50 mg total) is usually sufficient. Intramuscular: 20 to 30 mg 4 times daily. Blocks reuptake of norepinephrine, serotonin into nerve endings, increasing action of norepinephrine, serotonin in nerve cells; also r/t changes in receptor sensitivity; therapeutic plasma levels 110 to 250 ng/ml.	*CNS:* Sedation, ataxia; confusion, delirium. *Peripheral:* Blurred vision, photophobia, increased intraocular pressure, decreased tearing, orthostatic hypotension, arrhythmias, tachycardia, palpitations, dry mouth, constipation, diarrhea, decreased sweating, urinary retention, hesitancy.	Bedtime administration is preferred to lessen the discomfort of the sedation and anticholinergic effects prominent with this drug. FDA Pregnancy Category C.
clomipramine/Anafranil	Oral: *Adults*—initially, 25 mg 3 times daily, then up to 200 mg for outpatients, 300 mg for inpatients. *Geriatric clients*—20 to 30 mg daily in divided doses. Blocks serotonin reuptake while the active metabolite desmethylclomipramine blocks norepinephrine reuptake; therapeutic plasma levels 150 to 300 ng/ml.	*CNS:* Sedation, headache, insomnia, libido change, nervousness, myoclonus, increased appetite, ataxia; confusion, delirium. *Peripheral:* Blurred vision, photophobia, increased intraocular pressure; decreased tearing, orthostatic hypotension; arrhythmias, tachycardia, palpitations; dry mouth, constipation, diarrhea, increased sweating; urinary retention, hesitancy, ejaculation failure, impotence, fatigue, weight gain.	Used for obsessive compulsive disorders, for blocking panic attacks, and to treat cataplexy associated with narcolepsy.

*Available in Canada and United States.
†Available in Canada only.

Continued.

Antidepressant Drugs—cont'd

Generic name/Trade name	Administration/Dosage/Mechanism of Action	Adverse Effects	Nursing Considerations
doxepin hydrochloride/Adapin Sinequan* Triadapin†	Oral: *Adults*—75 mg, increased to 150 mg in divided doses or at bedtime; maintenance dose usually 25 to 150 mg daily and should not exceed 300 mg daily. Blocks reuptake of norepinephrine, serotonin in nerve endings; increasing action of norepinephrine, serotonin in nerve cells; also r/t changes in receptor sensitivity; therapeutic plasma levels 100 to 200 ng/ml.	*CNS:* Sedation, ataxia, confusion, and delirium. *Peripheral:* Blurred vision, photophobia, increased intraocular pressure; decreased tearing, orthostatic hypotension; arrhythmias, tachycardia, palpitations; dry mouth, constipation, diarrhea, decreased sweating, urinary retention, hesitancy.	Bedtime administration is preferred to lessen the discomfort of the sedation and anticholinergic effects prominent with this drug. Doxepin is reported to have much less effect on the heart than the other tricyclic antidepressants.
imipramine hydrochloride/ Tofranil* Janimine Impril† umipramine pamoate/ Tofranil-PM	Oral: *Adults*—75 mg daily in divided doses or at bedtime. Dose may be increased up to 200 mg daily if required. These are outpatient doses; inpatient doses are ⅓ higher. *Adolescents and elderly*—30 to 40 mg daily, increased to a maximum of 100 mg/day. *Children over 6 yr*—for bed-wetting, 25 mg, 1 hr before bedtime; if no response in 1 week, increase to 50 mg; *over 12 yr*—may receive up to 75 mg. Blocks reuptake of norepinephrine, serotonin in nerve endings; increasing action of norepinephrine, serotonin in nerve cells; also r/t changes in receptor sensitivity; therapeutic plasma levels 100 to 200 ng/ml.	*CNS:* Sedation, ataxia, confusion, and delirium. *Peripheral:* Blurred vision, photophobia, increased intraocular pressure; decreased tearing, orthostatic hypotension; arrhythmias, tachycardia, palpitations; dry mouth, constipation, diarrhea, decreased sweating, urinary retention, hesitancy.	Imipramine is the prototype tricyclic antidepressant. Sedative and anticholinergic effects are moderate. Can be taken at bedtime.
Monoamine Oxidase Inhibitors (MAOIs)			
phenelzine sulfate/Nardil*	Oral: *Adults*—45 to 75 mg daily in 3 doses or 1 mg/kg of body weight in divided doses. Daily dosage should not exceed 90 mg. Inhibits monoamine oxidase (responsible for breakdown of tyramine), resulting in increased neurotransmitters that may place client at risk for *hypertensive crisis*	*CNS:* Dizziness, drowsiness, confusion, headache, anxiety, tremor, stimulation, weakness, hyperreflexia, mania, insomnia, fatigue, and weight gain. *Peripheral:* Change in libido; constipation, dry mouth, nausea and vomiting, anorexia, diarrhea, rash, flushing, increased perspiration, jaundice, orthostatic	Client should be instructed about food and drug interactions with MAOI and be given lists of tyramine-rich foods and OTC drugs that may cause hypertensive crisis, such as aged, fermented foods and beverages and OTC diet and cold remedies.

	when MAOIs are ingested with tyramine-rich foods. Also avoid several over-the-counter drugs.	hypotension, hypertension, arrhythmias, hypertensive crisis, blurred vision.	Assess for occipital headaches, nosebleeds, nausea, and vomiting.
New-Generation Antidepressants			
amoxapine/Asendin*	Oral: *Adults*—75 mg initially; increase to 200 mg daily in divided doses. If no improvement in 3 wk, increase dosage 50 mg daily every other week to maximum of 400 mg for outpatients, 600 mg for inpatients. Blocks reuptake of norepinephrine, serotonin in nerve endings; increasing action of norepinephrine, serotonin in nerve cells; also blocks dopamine receptors and can produce EPSEs; therapeutic plasma levels 200 to 500 ng/ml.	*CNS:* Sedation, ataxia, confusion, delirium, tardive dyskinesia, and NMS. *Peripheral:* Blurred vision, photophobia, increased intraocular pressure; decreased tearing, orthostatic hypotension; arrhythmias, tachycardia, palpitations; dry mouth, constipation, diarrhea, decreased sweating, urinary retention, hesitancy, nausea.	Related to TCAs. Low incidence of anticholinergic, sedative, and cardiovascular effects. May be taken at bedtime to lessen daytime sedation or to treat insomnia. FDA Pregnancy Category C.
bupropion/Wellbutrin	Oral: *Adults*—initially, 100 mg 2 times/day, the dosage being increased gradually after 3 days of therapy to 100 mg 3 times/day as needed and tolerated. Not clear; does not block reuptake of serotonin or norepinephrine well; does not inhibit monoamine oxidase.	*CNS:* Seizures that are dose-related (doses below 450 mg/day reduce risk of seizures); agitation, confusion, insomnia, headache, sedation, and tremor. *Peripheral:* Blurred vision, dizziness, tachycardia, arrhythmias, dry mouth, constipation, weight loss or gain, nausea and vomiting, anorexia; excessive sweating, menstrual complaints, rash, impotence, upper respiratory tract complaints.	Seizures may occur at high doses.
trazodone/Desyrel*	Oral: *Adults*—75 mg initially, increased by 50 mg daily every 3 or 4 days to 300 mg if necessary. If no improvements in 3 wk, increase dosage 50 mg daily every other week to maximum of 300 mg. Selectively inhibits serotonin uptake in brain; therapeutic plasma levels 800 to 1600 ng/ml.	*CNS:* Anger, ataxia, confusion, delirium. *Peripheral:* Blurred vision, photophobia, increased intraocular pressure, decreased tearing, orthostatic hypotension, arrhythmias, tachycardia, palpitations, dry mouth, constipation, diarrhea, decreased sweating, priapism.	Sedation may be noted. Low incidence of anticholinergic and cardiovascular effects. May be taken at bedtime to lessen daytime sedation or to treat insomnia. FDA Pregnancy Category C.
fluoxetine/Prozac	Oral: *Adults*—PO 20 mg daily in AM; after 4 wk if no clinical improvement is noted, dose may be increased to 20 mg bid AM, afternoon, not to exceed 80 mg/day.	*CNS:* Headache, nervousness, insomnia, drowsiness, anxiety, tremor, dizziness, fatigue, sedation, poor concentration, abnormal dreams, agitation, convul-	Inhibits CNS neuron reuptake of serotonin, but not of norepinephrine.

*Available in Canada and United States.
†Available in Canada only.

Continued.

Antidepressant Drugs—cont'd

Generic name/Trade name	Administration/Dosage/Mechanism of Action	Adverse Effects	Nursing Considerations
		sions, apathy, euphoria, hallucinations, delusions, psychosis. *GI:* Nausea, diarrhea, dry mouth, anorexia, dyspepsia, constipation, cramps, vomiting, taste changes, flatulence, decreased appetite. *INTEG:* Sweating, rash, pruritis, acne, alopecia, urticaria. *RESP:* Infection, pharyngitis, nasal congestion, sinus headache, sinusitis, cough, dyspnea, bronchitis, asthma, hyperventilation, pneumonia. *CV:* Hot flashes, palpitations, angina pectoris, hemorrhage, hypertension, tachycardia, first-degree AV block, bradycardia, MI, thrombophlebitis. *MS:* Pain, arthritis, twitching. *GU:* Dysmenorrhea, decreased libido, urinary frequency, urinary tract infection, amenorrhea, cystitis, impotence. *EENT:* Visual changes, ear/eye pain, photophobia, tinnitus. *SYST:* Asthenia, viral infection, fever, allergy, chills.	
paroxetine/Paxil	Oral: *Adults*—PO 20 mg daily in AM; after 4 wk if no clinical improvement is noted, dose may be increased by 10 mg/day qwk to desired response, not to exceed 50 mg/day.	*CNS:* Headache, nervousness, insomnia, drowsiness, anxiety, tremor, dizziness, fatigue, sedation, poor concentration, abnormal dreams, agitation, convulsions, apathy, euphoria, hallucinations, delusions, psychosis. *GI:* Nausea, diarrhea, dry mouth, anorexia, dyspepsia, constipation, cramps, vomiting, taste changes, flatulence, decreased appetite. *INTEG:* Sweating, rash. *RESP:* Infection, pharyngitis, nasal congestion, sinus headache, sinusitis, cough, dyspnea.	Inhibits CNS neuron reuptake of serotonin, but not of norepinephrine.

		CV: Vasodilation, postural hypotension, palpitations. *MS:* Pain, arthritis, twitching, myalgia, myopathy, myasthenia. *GU:* Dysmenorrhea, decreased libido, urinary frequency, urinary tract infection, amenorrhea, cystitis, impotence, abnormal ejaculation. *EENT:* Visual changes. *SYST:* Asthenia, fever.	
sertraline/Zoloft	Oral: *Adults*—PO 50 mg daily; may increase to a maximum of 200 mg/day; do not change dose at intervals of <1 wk; administer in AM, PM.	*CNS:* Insomnia, agitation, somnolence, dizziness, headache, tremor, fatigue, paresthesia, twitching, confusion, ataxia. *GU:* Male sexual dysfunction, micturition disorder. *GI:* Diarrhea, nausea, constipation, anorexia, dry mouth, dyspepsia, vomiting, disorder. *CV:* Palpitations, chest pain, hypotension. *EENT:* Vision abnormalities.	Inhibits serotonin reuptake.
venlafaxine hydrochloride/ Effexor	Oral: *Adults*—PO 75 mg/day in 2 or 3 divided doses; taken with food, may be increased to 150 mg/day; if needed, may be further increased to 225 mg/day; increments of 75 mg/day should be made at intervals of no less than 4 days; some hospitalized clients may require up to 375 mg/day in 3 divided doses.	*CNS:* Emotional lability, vertigo, apathy, ataxia, CNS stimulation, euphoria, hallucinations, hostility, increased libido, hypertonia, hypotonia, psychosis. *CV:* Migraine, angina pectoris, extrasystole, hypotension, syncope, thrombophlebitis. *EENT:* Abnormal vision, ear pain, cataract, conjunctivitis, corneal lesions, dry eyes, otitis media, photophobia. *GI:* Dysphagia, eructation, colitis, gastritis, gingivitis, rectal hemorrhage, stomatitis, stomach and mouth ulceration. *GU:* Anorgasmia, dysuria, hematuria, metrorrhagia, vaginitis, impaired urination, albuminuria, amenorrhea, kidney calculus, cystitis, nocturia, breast and bladder pain, polyuria, uterine hemorrhage, vaginal hemorrhage, moniliasis. *INTEG:* Ecchymosis, acne, alopecia, brittle nails, dry skin, photosensitivity.	Potent inhibitor of neuronal serotonin and norepinephrine reuptake, weak inhibitor of dopamine; no muscarinic, histaminergic, or α-adrenergic receptors in vitro.

Continued.

Antidepressant Drugs—cont'd

Generic name/Trade name	Administration/Dosage/Mechanism of Action	Adverse Effects	Nursing Considerations
		META: Peripheral edema, weight gain, diabetes mellitus, edema, glycosuria, hyperlipemia, hypokalemia. *MS:* Arthritis, bone pain, bursitis, myasthenia tenosynovitis. *RESP:* Bronchitis, dyspnea, asthma, chest congestion, epistaxis, hyperventilation, laryngitis. *SYST:* Accidental injury, malaise, neck pain, enlarged abdomen, cyst, facial edema, hangover effect, hernia.	
fluvoxamine maleate/Luvox	Oral: 50 to 300 mg. Also marketed for Obsessive-Compulsive Disorder; reduces anxiety and agitation.	Fever, chills, rash, dry mouth; excessive sweating and thirst; GI disturbance; drowsiness; changes in sexual function (abnormal ejaculation, impotence); suicide ideation.	Monitor for safety and physiologic dysfunction.
mirtazapine/Remeron	Oral: 15-45 mg gradual increase. Peak plasma level in 2 hrs; half-life 20-40 hr.	Sedation, fatigue, insomnia, agitation, restlessness, weight gain; usual anticholinergic effects; hypotension, dizziness.	Monitor WBC if client has signs of infection; *caution* with liver or renal dysfunction.
nefazodone/Serzone	Oral: 200 to 600 mg. Do not discontinue abruptly.	*CV:* Postural hypotension. *GI:* Nausea, constipation, dry mouth. *EENT:* Blurred vision. *GU:* Urinary frequency, retention, UTI. *RESP:* Pharyngitis, cough.	Monitor blood and hepatic studies. Monitor urinary retention, constipation; constipation is more likely to occur in the elderly. Identify alcohol consumption; if alcohol is consumed, hold dose until A.M.

Lithium (Antimanic)

Generic Name/Trade Name	Administration/Dosage/Mechanism of Action	Adverse Effects	Nursing Considerations
lithium carbonate/Eskalith Lithane* Lithizine† Lithonate Lithotabs	Oral: *Adults*—initially 0.6 to 2.1 g daily divided into 3 doses. Increase or decrease dose by 0.3 g/day to obtain a blood level of 0.8 to 1.5 mEq/L. Alters sodium ion transport in nerve, muscle cells; effects norepinephrine reuptake and increases serotonin receptor sensitivity.	*CNS:* Headache, drowsiness, dizziness, tremor, twitching, ataxia, seizure, slurred speech, restlessness, confusion, stupor, memory loss, and clonic movements. *Peripheral:* Dry mouth, anorexia, nausea, vomiting, diarrhea, hypotension, leukocytosis, blurred vision, hypothyroidism, hyponatremia, muscle weakness.	Antimanic. Blood should not be drawn for determination of lithium levels earlier than 8 h after the last dose. Concentrations above 2 mEq/L are toxic. Clients should be instructed not to "make up" a missed dose of lithium. FDA Pregnancy Category D.
lithium citrate/Cibalith-S	Maintenance dose usually 0.9 to 1.2 g daily in divided doses.	*CNS:* Headache, drowsiness, dizziness, tremor, twitching, ataxia, seizure, slurred speech, restlessness, confusion, stupor, memory loss, and clonic movements. *Peripheral:* Dry mouth, anorexia, nausea, vomiting, diarrhea, hypotension, leukocytosis, blurred vision, hypothyroidism, hyponatremia, muscle weakness.	Antimanic. Blood should not be drawn for determination of lithium levels earlier than 8 h after the last dose. Concentrations above 2 mEq/L are toxic. Clients should be instructed not to "make up" a missed dose of lithium. FDA Pregnancy Category D.

*Available in Canada and United States.
†Available in Canada only.

Appendix M

Anticonvulsant Drugs

Generic Name/Trade Name	Administration/Dosage/Mechanism of Action	Adverse Effects	Nursing Considerations
valproic acid/Depakene Sodium Depakote/ divalproex	Oral: *Adults and children*—PO 15 mg/kg/day divided in 2 to 3 doses; may increase by 5 to 10 mg/kg/day qwk, not to exceed 30 mg/kg/day in 2 to 3 divided doses.	*CNS:* Sedation, drowsiness, dizziness, headache, incoordination, paresthesia, depression, hallucinations, behavioral changes, tremors, aggression, weakness. *HEMA:* Thrombocytopenia, leukopenia, lymphocytosis, increase prothrombin. *GI:* Nausea, vomiting, constipation, diarrhea, heartburn, anorexia, cramps, hepatic failure, pancreatitis, toxic hepatitis, stomatitis. *INTEG:* Rash, alopecia, bruising. *GU:* Enuresis, irregular menses.	Antimanic drug. Increases levels of γ-aminobutyric acid (GABA) in brain.
carbamazepine/Tegretol	Oral: *Adults and children over 12 yr*—PO 200 mg bid; may be increased by 200 mg/day in divided doses q6-8h; maintenance 800-1200 mg/day, maximum 1200 mg/day; adjustment is needed to minimum dose to control seizures. *Children under 12 yr*—PO 10 to 20 mg/kg/day in 2 to 3 divided doses.	*CNS:* Drowsiness, dizziness, confusion, fatigue, paralysis, headache, hallucinations. *GI:* Nausea, constipation, diarrhea, anorexia, vomiting, abdominal pain, stomatitis, glossitis, increased liver enzymes, hepatitis. *INTEG:* Rash, Stevens-Johnson syndrome, urticaria. *EENT:* Tinnitus, dry mouth, blurred vision, diplopia, nystagmus, conjunctivitis. *CV:* Hypertension, CHF, hypotension, aggravation of cardiac artery disease. *RESP:* Pulmonary hypersensitivity (fever, dyspnea, pneumonitis). *GU:* Frequency, retention, albuminuria, glycosuria, impotence.	Antimanic drug. Inhibits nerve impulses by limiting influx of sodium ions across cell membrane in motor cortex.

Central Nervous System Stimulants for Hyperkinesis

Generic Name/Trade Name	Administration/Dosage/Mechanism of Action	Adverse Effects	Nursing Considerations
methylphenidate hydrochloride/ Methidate† Ritalin	Attention deficit disorder: Oral: *Children 6 yr and older*—5 mg before breakfast and lunch; increase by 5 to 10 mg at weekly intervals up to 0.3 to 0.5 mg/kg of body weight. Maximum daily doses should not exceed 60 mg. Mild CNS stimulant, mechanism unknown.	*CNS:* Hyperactivity, insomnia, restlessness, talkativeness, dizziness, headache, chills, stimulation, dysphoria, irritability, and aggressiveness. *Peripheral:* Nausea, vomiting, anorexia, dry mouth, diarrhea, constipation, weight loss, metallic taste, cramps, impotence, change in libido, palpitations, tachycardia, hypertension, hypotension.	Drug of choice for most hyperkinetic children. Schedule II substance (United States). Class C (Canada).
	Narcolepsy: Oral: *Adults*—10 to 60 mg daily. Common dose is 10 mg 2 or 3 times daily.		May be used with imipramine to treat narcolepsy.
pemoline/Cylert*	Attention deficit disorder: Oral: *Children 6 yr and older*—37.5 mg daily in a single dose; increase weekly by 18.75-mg increments until response is obtained. Effective dosage range usually 56 to 75 mg daily. Do not exceed 112.5 mg daily. Exact mechanism not known; may work through dopaminergic pathways.	*CNS:* Hyperactivity, insomnia, restlessness, dizziness, depression, headache, stimulation, irritability, aggressiveness, hallucinations, and seizures. *Peripheral:* Nausea, anorexia, diarrhea, abdominal pain, increased liver enzyme levels, hepatitis, growth suppression in children, rashes.	Clinical effects develop over 3 to 4 wk. Schedule IV substance (United States).

*Available in Canada and United States.
†Available in Canada only.

Cholinesterase Inhibitors

Generic Name/Trade Name	Administration/Dosage/Mechanism of Action	Adverse Effects	Nursing Considerations
tachrine hydrochloride/Cognex	Oral: 10-40 mg progressive dosing to maximum of 160 mg daily.	GI disturbance; confusion, depression, restlessness, agitation; ataxia; suicide ideation. Not recommended for people with kidney, bladder, or prostate problems.	Monitor for safety and physiologic effects, specifically liver function tests. *Caution:* Do not stop drug abruptly.
donepeziz/Aricept	Oral: 5-10 mg daily; maximum of 10 mg daily.	GI disturbance; confusion; cardiovascular effects; kidney problems.	Monitor for safety and physiologic effects. *Caution:* Do not stop drug abruptly.

Antiparkinson/Anticholinergic

Generic Name/Trade Name	Administration/Dosage/Mechanism of Action	Adverse Effects	Nursing Considerations
Trihexyphenidyl hydrochloride/Artane	Oral: 1-10 mg progressive dosing (also extended-release capsules). Used to treat extrapyramidal symptoms resulting from use of antipsychotics.	Anticholinergic effects, such as dry mouth, GI disturbance; urinary disturbance; CNS effects. *Caution:* Do not administer within 14 days of MAOI use.	Observe for agitation, anxiety, depression, suicide ideation, confusion, and disorientation.
benztropine mesylate/Cogentin	Oral: 0.5-4 mg progressive dosing. Injectable: 1 mg IM, 1 ml IV to treat extrapyramidal symptoms from antipsychotic medications.		See trihexyphenidyl.

Antihistamine

Generic Name/Trade Name	Administration/Dosage/Mechanism of Action	Adverse Effects	Nursing Considerations
diphenhydramine/Benadryl	Oral: 25-50 mg. Treats extrapyramidal symptoms. Antihistamine with anticholinergic effects.	*CNS:* Sedation, ataxia. *GI:* Nausea, vomiting. Skin rash, urticaria.	Teach client not to drive while taking drug. *Caution:* No use with glaucoma, ulcers, or prostate hypertrophy.

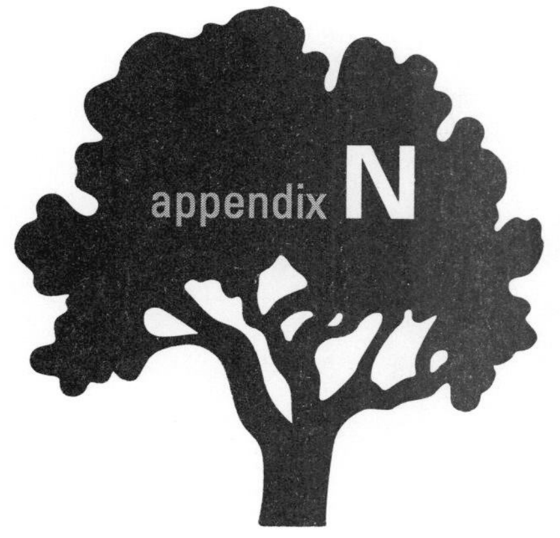

Twelve Steps of Alcoholics Anonymous

1. We admitted we were powerless over alcohol—that our lives had become unmanageable.
2. Came to believe that a Power greater than ourselves could restore us to sanity.
3. Made a decision to turn our will and our lives over to the care of God, as we understood Him.
4. Made a searching and fearless moral inventory of ourselves.
5. Admitted to God, to ourselves, and to another human being the exact nature of our wrongs.
6. Were entirely ready to have God remove all these defects of character.
7. Humbly asked Him to remove our shortcomings.
8. Made a list of all persons we had harmed, and became willing to make amends to them all.
9. Made direct amends to such people wherever possible, except when to do so would injure them or others.
10. Continued to take personal inventory and when we were wrong promptly admitted it.
11. Sought through prayer and meditation to improve our conscious contact with God, as we understood Him, praying only for knowledge of His will for us and the power to carry that out.
12. Having had a spiritual awakening as the result of these steps, we tried to carry this message to alcoholics, and to practice these principles in all our affairs.

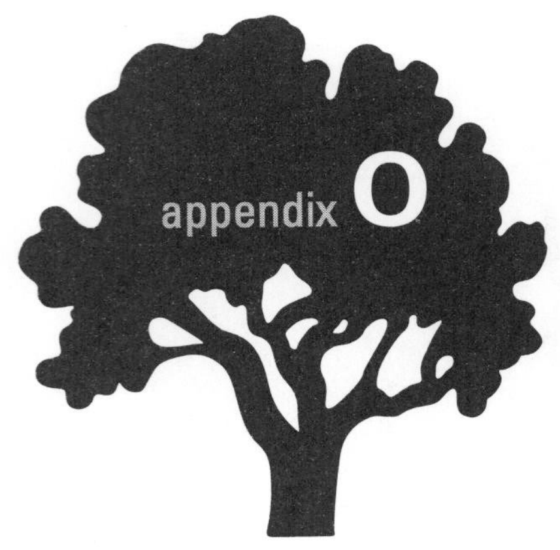

Crisis and Crisis Intervention

Crisis has been defined in many ways, but regardless of the definition it can be viewed as a turning point. From a psychiatric–mental health nursing view, *crisis* can be defined as "a state of psychologic disequilibrium that results from an individual's inability to problem solve a situation or event (real or perceived) that involves change, loss, or threat (psychologic, biologic, social, cultural, spiritual)." Inherent in a state of crisis is the individual's failure to resolve the problem after using previously learned coping strategies and techniques and/or automatic defense mechanisms (denial, repression, suppression).

As a further result of the crisis state, the person's behavior, affect, and cognitive ability are disrupted. Symptoms include anxiety, powerlessness, helplessness, depression, and varying degrees of mental, emotional, and behavioral disorganization and acting out.

TYPES OF CRISIS

Developmental

Sometimes referred to as *maturational* or *internal* types of crisis, developmental crises represent events that are built into normal periods of human growth and development.

- The birth of a normal baby
- Graduation from school
- Marriage
- Timely death of an elderly parent

These events can usually be anticipated. Crisis can occur around the events if a person is unprepared for the amount of change that is required to complete role responsibilities associated with the event or situation or if the person perceives that the event represents a major loss. Symptoms, as described previously, may result.

Situational

Situational crises are usually unanticipated events in the process of everyday life and have external rather than internal sources. The unexpected events usually require immediate change and response, and often the person is unable to negotiate the event, resulting in crisis.

- Divorce
- Job change
- Rape, robbery, other victimization
- Death of loved one by accident

INFLUENCING FACTORS

The resolution of a crisis may be affected by several factors.

- Individual's perception of the event
- Past experience with similar events
- Capacity to accept the need to change
- Cognitive abilities
- Control of mood or affect
- Coping style
- Personality traits
- External support system (availability, genuine concern)
- Person's ability to engage support systems

CRISIS INTERVENTION

Crisis intervention is an effective, short-term therapy that focuses only on immediate problems to be resolved.

The primary goal of intervention is to return the individual to either the precrisis level of function or, ideally, to a higher level of function because of new skills that were learned in the process of resolving the crisis.

Therapist's Role

The therapist must remember that crisis has a dual nature. It is, according to ancient Chinese teachings, both a time of danger and threat and a time of opportunity. This belief holds today. Because a person in crisis cannot solve the problem by previously known and used methods, at this vulnerable time she or he is open to suggestions and willing to learn new skills that provide an opportunity for growth and change.

A crisis counselor is an active participant rather than a passive listener during the crisis intervention process. Working through a step-by-step methodology, the client is assisted out of the seeming maze. Although crisis will resolve without intervention, the result of an unsuccessful resolution can be diminished levels of function and possible disorder in the form of mental, emotional, physical, spiritual, or social disruption. The client usually benefits from a caring and educated guide.

Active Intervention Process

- Stay focused in the present. Do not allow digressions or unrelated material to interfere. For example, redirect the client who discusses past problems that are not directly related. (Client may need additional therapy for other problems later.)
- Discuss client's positive actions and strengths during the crisis. For example, reinforce all positive attempts the client made to resolve the problem. A strength to always reinforce is that the client looked for help!
- Direct client when necessary. For example, a disorganized client has taken alcohol to alter mood before the therapy session and is getting ready to drive home. The nurse tells the client to call a family member for a ride to home to avoid accident or arrest.
- Allow and encourage client to express feelings for relief.
- Encourage client to express thoughts. While verbalizing, the client will begin to formalize thoughts. Guide the client in the problem-solving process. (Use nursing process.)
- Help the client name techniques that were tried and discuss new options and alternative approaches for solving the problem. For example, "What else could you have done instead?" "Did you try . . . ?" "Some people have done . . . in similar situations. Is that something you could do?" "What has worked in the past for some people is . . . ."
- Assist client to identify and connect with support people and agencies.

Although crisis intervention is traditionally completed within 6 weeks, clinicians today are sometimes pressured by managed care organizations to complete the process in a much briefer time frame. If necessary, clients who have other psychiatric issues are referred to subsequent therapies after the brief crisis therapy has ended. Before crisis therapy with a client ends, the therapist does the following:

- *Summarize:* Review, with client participation, the components of the client's crisis. Summarize all action taken and action proposed by the client in the near future. Review learned skills.
- *Anticipatory planning:* Evaluate the client's understanding of the process and content of this crisis and his or her readiness and ability to manage future similar events.
- *Praise:* Genuinely praise the client's efforts to engage in resolution of this crisis, and offer hope without giving any false reassurance.

Glossary

aberrant Departing from the right, usual, or normal course; deviating from the ordinary; exceptional or abnormal; as in aberrant behavior.

abuse A maladaptive pattern of substance use leading to problems in psychosocial, biologic, cognitive, perceptual, or spiritual/belief dimensions of life.

acrophobia Abnormal fear of heights.

acting out A reaction of the client's life experiences, relationships with significant others, and resultant unresolved conflicts. Acting out may include, but is not limited to, destructive actions.

active listening A communication skill in which the nurse or therapist illustrates active vs. passive listening responses toward the client. Incorporates such behaviors as appropriate eye contact, general leads (e.g., "I hear you," "please go on," "uh-huh"), and/or occasional nodding of the head. Active listening demonstrates respect, interest, and caring toward the client. Techniques should be used with discretion rather than in a continuous, exaggerated manner.

acute dystonic reaction Irregular, involuntary spastic muscle movement, e.g., wryneck (the neck twists to one side in a distorted, abnormal fashion), facial grimacing, abnormal eye movements, or backward rolling of the eyes in their sockets. May occur any time after the first dose of an antipsychotic drug.

adaptation The result of an interchange between a human being (or any organism) and the environment that involves a modification of the organism that enhances its ability for further interchange; involves assimilation and accommodation, e.g., adaptive behavior vs. maladaptive behavior.

addiction (Known today as *chemical dependence.*) A cluster of cognitive, behavioral, and physiologic symptoms characterized by physical dependence, tolerance, and psychologic dependence on a drug or substance. The addicted person is emotionally dependent on the drug or substance, is able to obtain a desired effect from a specific dosage, and experiences withdrawal symptoms when he or she ceases to take the drug or substance. The person is generally in a state of chronic or recurrent intoxication.

adjustment disorder A maladaptive reaction in response to an identifiable event or situation that is stress producing and not the result or part of a mental disorder. Reaction occurs within approximately 3 months of the stressor event and is manifested by impaired social or occupational functioning that is more intense than the "normal" expected response. Reduction of the reaction generally occurs when the identified stressor diminishes or is no longer present.

adolescence A stage of growth and development ranging from 11 or 12 years to 16 or 17 years in which major physiologic, cognitive, and behavioral changes take place. According to prominent theorists, there are specific tasks to be met, such as identification and conceptualization. (See Appendix D.)

adult children of alcoholics (ACA) A self-help group concerned with helping members cope with the residual, ongoing problems of adults who were children of alcoholic parent(s).

adult ego state In transactional analysis theory, the ego state responsible for the objective, mature appraisal of reality and the problem-solving capacity to process data.

affect Emotional range attached to ideas, outwardly manifested. *Appropriate affect:* emotional tone in harmony with the accompanying idea, thought, or verbalization. *Blunted affect:* a disturbance manifested by a severe reduction in the intensity of affect. *Flat affect:* absence or near absence of any signs of affective expression. *Inappropriate affect:* incongruence between the emotional feeling tone and the idea, thought, or speech accompanying it. *Labile affect:* rapid changes in emotional feeling tone, unrelated to external stimuli.

affective disorders A specific group of psychiatric diagnoses that are predominantly characterized by disturbances in mood, accompanied by a full or partial manic or depressive syndrome. Known as mood disorders in DSM-IV.

aggression Overt or suppressed hostility, either innate or resulting from continued frustration, and directed outward or against oneself (self-directed).

agitation Restlessness; inability to concentrate or remain motionless.

agnosia Inability to discriminate sensory stimuli. *Acoustic* or *auditory agnosia:* impaired ability to recognize familiar sounds. *Tactile agnosia:* impaired ability to recognize familiar objects by touch or feel. *Visual agnosia:* impaired ability to recognize familiar objects by sight. *Somatagnosia:* disturbance in recognition of own body parts.

agoraphobia Marked fear of being in places or situations from which escape might be difficult or embarrassing; fear of being out of control or fear of losing control when in a public place, e.g., a restaurant, shopping mall, or classroom. Fear of being in a place or situation in which help might not be available in the event of a panic attack.

agraphia Total or partial inability to write owing to organic cerebral pathology.

AIDS-related complex (ARC) The condition of having some clinical symptoms diagnosed as AIDS-related but without formal indicators of AIDS as defined by the Centers for Disease Control.

akathisia One of the classes of nontherapeutic effects caused by neuroleptic drugs; thought to be a result of the blockade effect of these drugs on the neurotransmitter dopamine. Signs of this condition include motor restlessness, a subjective sense of anxiety, and the inability to lie down or sit still. Classified as an extrapyramidal symptom.

akinesia Delay or slowness in beginning and carrying through voluntary motor movements and sudden or unexpected stops in motion. Akinesia is an extrapyramidal symptom and is often seen in clients with Parkinson's disease.

akinesthesia Inability to sense movement.

Al-Anon An organization concerned with helping spouses and partners of alcoholics cope with the disorder.

Alateen An organization concerned with helping teenage children of alcoholics cope with the disorder.

alcoholic One whose continued or excessive drinking results in impairment of personal health, disruption of family and social relationships, and loss of economic security.

Alcoholics Anonymous (AA) A self-help organization that uses a 12-step program to assist alcoholics in achieving and maintaining sobriety. Acknowledgment of loss of control over alcohol and willingness to seek help through a "higher power" is a major part of the organization's program.

alcoholism A chronic disorder characterized by dependence on alcohol, repeated excessive use of alcoholic beverages, the development of withdrawal symptoms on reducing or ceasing alcohol intake, morbidity that may include cirrhosis of the liver, and decreased ability to function socially and vocationally. Currently believed by many to be a disease with strong genetic links.

alert A state of complete awareness and attentiveness. In physical and mental health assessment, often used in conjunction with the term *oriented,* as in "alert and oriented."

alexia Inability to understand and interpret the written word.

alexithymia Inability or difficulty in describing or naming feelings or in being aware of one's emotions or moods.

algophobia Fear or dread of pain.

alienation Inability to identify with family, peer group, society, or culture; commonly associated with schizophrenia.

alogia Inability to express language in a logical manner.

Alzheimer's disease A progressive condition of atrophy of the brain and degeneration of the neurons, generally fatal within a few years; may be known as *senile dementia* or *presenile dementia.* Usually occurs in late middle-age. As the condition progresses, there is often memory and judgment impairment, loss of interest, and carelessness. Symptoms worsen until disorientation, epileptiform attacks, and contractures occur. Diagnosis is made on autopsy, based on histopathologic changes in the brain, including plaques and neurofibrillary tangles. The cause is unknown. Treatment trials are ongoing.

ambivalence The coexistence of two opposing feelings, impulses, or attitudes directed toward the same person, object, or situation, at the same time.

American Nurses' Association (ANA) A professional organization whose function is to establish and maintain guidelines and social policies for the practice of nursing. (Refer to Appendix A for ANA Standards of Practice.)

American Psychiatric Association (APA) A professional organization responsible for the classification and revision of mental health disorders as listed in their publication *Diagnostic and Statistical Manual of Mental Disorders,* fourth edition (DSM-IV), which is part of the International Classification of Diseases (ICD).

amnestic syndrome A category of an organic mental syndrome in which relatively selective areas of cognition, such as short- and long-term memory, are impaired as a result of a specific organic factor.

anger A strong feeling of displeasure, wrath, fury, or rage that is provoked within an individual as a result of a perceived wrongdoing, injustice, injury, frustration, or exasperation. Anger-producing stimuli may or may not be obvious.

anger rape Rape distinguished by physical violence and cruelty to the victim. The ability to injure, traumatize, and shame the victim provides the rapist with an outlet for the rage and concomitant relief.

anhedonia The inability to experience pleasure. In major depression, anhedonia is commonly noted as loss of pleasure in activities or experiences that the client deemed as pleasurable or enjoyable prior to the onset of the depressed episode.

anorexia Loss of appetite or without appetite.

anorexia nervosa An eating disorder primarily affecting adolescent girls and young adult women, characterized by a pathologic fear of becoming fat, distorted body image, excessive dieting, and emaciation. No loss of appetite occurs until the late stages of the disease.

anorexic A person without an appetite or, more commonly, a person suffering from anorexia nervosa.

Antabuse (disulfiram) A drug given to alcoholics that produces adverse effects such as nausea, vomiting, dizziness, flushing, and tachycardia if alcohol is consumed. The drug's effectiveness is largely due to its role as a deterrent.

anterograde amnesia Amnesia for short-term memories. Long-term memories remain intact. It is seen in alcoholic blackouts and in organic mental disorder.

anticholinergic effects Nontherapeutic effects in specific areas of the autonomic nervous system caused by the use of neuroleptic medications. Symptoms may include dry mouth, constipation, blurred vision, and dry mucous membranes. Effects may be temporary and relieved by adjustment of prescribed medication.

antidepressant medication Psychopharmacologic preparations used to treat symptoms of depression, whether or not the client's primary diagnosis is that of a mood disorder. Antidepressants derive from classes such as tricyclic and monoamine oxidase inhibitors.

antiparkinsonism drugs Drugs used to treat the extrapyramidal effects of antipsychotic drugs. Anticholinergic agents are generally the drugs of choice. (See Appendix M.)

antipsychotic medication Psychopharmacologic preparations used to treat the symptoms of psychosis, such as disintegrated thought processes, perception, and affect. Also called *neuroleptics* or *major tranquilizers,* they include the following classes: phenothiazine, thioxanthene, butyrophenone, dihydroindolone, and dibenzoxazepine.

antisocial Behavior that is counterproductive or hostile to the well-being of society as a whole.

antisocial personality disorder A personality disorder with the essential feature of a pattern of irresponsible and antisocial behavior. Individuals diagnosed with this disorder do not appear to recognize the consequences of their actions. Common belief is that, in some cases, the individual may be devoid of a conscience (underdeveloped superego; Freudian).

anxiety Nonspecific, unpleasant feeling of apprehension, discomfort, and, in some cases, dread and impending doom that is manifested physically by such symptoms as motor tension, autonomic hyperactivity, or hyperattentiveness. Symptoms prompt the person to take some action to seek relief. Anxiety can be communicated interpersonally.

anxiety disorders Patterns of symptoms and behaviors in which anxiety is either the primary disturbance or a secondary problem that is recognized when the primary symptoms are removed.

anxiety syndrome Anxiety of at least 1 month's duration.

apathy Lack of interest and blunting of affect in conditions that would normally stimulate interest or elicit feeling or emotion.

anxiolytic medications Psychopharmacologic preparations used to relieve anxiety-related symptoms and behaviors. Classes of drugs used for this effect include benzodiazepines, β-blockers, antihistamine sedatives, sedatives with hypnotic effects, and propanidids.

aphasia Dysfunction or loss of ability to express thoughts by speech, writing, symbols, or signs. *Fluent aphasia:* ability to produce words but with frequent errors in the appropriate choice of words or in the creation of words. *Nonfluent aphasia:* inability to produce words, either in spoken or written form.

apparel Clothing, attire, and garments, especially outerwear. In conducting a mental health assessment, the client's apparel is evaluated in terms of its appropriateness to age, culture, individual taste, and contemporary style. May include jewelry.

appearance The state, condition, manner, or style in which a person or object manifests itself outwardly. In the context of conducting a mental health assessment, the client's appearance involves such things as hygiene, grooming, posture, and general behavior. May include cosmetics.

apperception Perception that is modified by a person's own emotions or thoughts.

appropriate Suitable or fitting for a particular person, purpose, or occasion, as in "appropriate dress" or "appropriate behavior." In conducting a mental health assessment, a client's affect would be considered appropriate if his or her emotions were congruent with the thought, idea, or speech accompanying it.

appropriate death Maintaining as high a level of function as possible, being as pain-free as possible, and being able to make choices, resolve conflicts, and fulfill wishes within capacity, until the end of life.

apraxia Impairment in the ability to carry out purposeful movement, although muscle and sensory apparatus are intact; e.g., the inability to draw or construct forms or figures in two or three dimensions.

assaultive behavior The act of being physically aggressive toward another person; a violent attack on another individual that may lead to harm or injury (may be an attempt to do violence with or without battery).

assertiveness The art of asking for what one needs and wants in a way that respects the person being asked and retains the dignity of the person doing the asking.

assertiveness training A type of therapy that is usually accomplished in groups to assist individuals who tend to act passively or aggressively, by practicing assertive behaviors in a controlled setting. Assertive techniques are designed to teach persons to ask for what they want in a clear, direct manner and to refuse requests from others without guilt or frustration. The right to choose one's response is a major point in assertiveness training.

ataxia Impairment of coordination of muscular activity, as in ataxic gait.

attention deficit–hyperactivity disorder A disorder that most commonly develops in childhood in which the individual demonstrates developmentally inappropriate inattention, impulsiveness, and hyperactivity, often leading to disruptive behaviors in a classroom or group setting.

autistic A term relating to private, individual thoughts, ideas, and affects that are derived from internal drives, wishes, and hopes. Most commonly seen in persons diagnosed with schizophrenia who, in the course of their disorder, may experience a private reality rather than the shared reality of the external world.

autistic disorder A severe, pervasive developmental disorder, with onset in infancy or childhood, characterized by impaired social interactions, severe communication deficits, and a markedly restricted repertoire of activities and interests.

autogenic training A training program consisting of systematic, structured exercises designed to reduce or eliminate stress-induced conditions or disorders and to modify pain.

automatic thoughts In cognitive therapy theory, thoughts that are unwilled, spontaneous, irrational, and self-deprecating. Cognitive therapy techniques help the individual replace automatic thoughts with rational beliefs based on exercises that challenge their validity.

avoidant personality disorder A personality disorder in which the essential feature is a pervasive pattern of discomfort in social situations related to the individual's marked timidity and fear of negative evaluation.

aware A state of alertness and consciousness; being cognizant, knowledgeable, or informed, especially in matters relevant to the individual and his or her environment.

Beck's depression inventory A 21-item multiple-choice questionnaire used by individuals to rate themselves on selected variables related to depression, such as sadness, guilt, suicidal ideation, fatigue, weight loss, loss of appetite, insomnia, and social withdrawal.

behavior Any observable, recordable, and measurable move, response, or verbal or nonverbal act demonstrated by an individual.

behavior contract An agreement between client and staff that clearly delineates expected client behaviors and outcomes.

behavior modification A method of treatment, deconditioning, or reeducation based on the principles of Ivan Pavlov and developed further by B. F. Skinner, the goal of which is to change an individual's behavior patterns and responses through techniques that manipulate stimuli.

behavior therapy Treatment that focuses on modifying observable behavior by manipulating the environment or the behavior. Focuses on the effects rather than the cause. Derived from Pavlovian conditioning and useful in the treatment of phobic and obsessive-compulsive disorders. Systematic desensitization is an example of behavioral therapy.

behavioral psychiatry A model of psychiatric practice based on the research of Ivan Pavlov and J. B. Watson that is also known as *stimulus-response learning* or *behavioral conditioning.* It implies that psychiatric symptoms are clusters of learned behaviors that persist because they are inherently rewarding to the individual.

bestiality See *zoophilia.*

bioenergetics Strategies for reducing muscle tension by releasing feelings through physical exercises and verbal techniques.

biofeedback A therapeutic technique used to gain conscious control over unconscious body functions, such as blood pressure and heart rate, to achieve relaxation or relief of stress-related physical symptoms. Self-monitoring equipment is used to measure body functions.

bipolar disorder An affective or mood disorder characterized by episodes of mania and periods of depression, with normal mood intervals occurring between the manic and depressive states.

bizarre delusion A fixed belief held by the individual that involves a phenomenon that the individual's culture would regard as totally implausible, such as being controlled by a dead person.

blackouts Anterograde amnesia, most commonly experienced by alcoholics and those with an organic brain syndrome. Some believe blackouts are a result of dehydration of brain tissue. The individual retains consciousness with the memory loss.

blaming Behavior in which an individual accuses others for thoughts or deeds that are rightfully attributed to the person doing the blaming; projecting one's own responsibility for behavior to others.

blocking or thought deprivation A sudden pause in the train or stream of one's thoughts, most likely caused by unconscious emotional conflicts. Noted in persons with schizophrenia.

blunted affect An extreme restriction in emotional expression in which only minimal degrees of emotions are evident. Restrictions are not as severe as in flattened affect.

body dysmorphic disorder A disorder characterized by a preoccupation with an imagined defect in one's appearance or excessive concern over a slight, actual physical anomaly.

body image An individual's concept of the size, shape, and physical mass of his or her body and its parts; the internalized perception that one has of the physical appearance of one's body.

borderline personality disorder A personality disorder with the essential feature being a pervasive pattern of unstable self-image, mood, and interpersonal relationships. Persons diagnosed with this disorder frequently display mood shifts directed outwardly toward staff and others, sometimes in an effort to divide staff to meet their own needs, a mechanism commonly referred to as *splitting.*

bulimia nervosa An eating disorder characterized by recurrent cycles of binge eating followed by episodes of purging. The individual suffers from persistent overconcern with body shape and weight but lacks the body image distortion and degree of weight loss experienced by the person with anorexia nervosa.

catalepsy State of unconsciousness in which an immobile position is constantly maintained.

catatonia A disturbance in psychomotor behavior that can be demonstrated either by a stuporous state, in which the client seems unaware of the environment, or by rigidity, in which the person may maintain a rigid posture and resist efforts to be moved.

catatonic An unusual behavior state in which the dysfunctional person assumes a fixed position and may remain in that state for hours. Commonly described in a form of schizophrenia.

catatonic excitement A disturbance in psychomotor behavior characterized by excitement demonstrated by the individual without apparent external stimuli or provocation.

catatonic posturing A voluntary assumption of a bizarre or inappropriate posture that may be maintained for a long period.

catatonic waxy-flexibility A condition in which the individual's body posture and limbs may be manipulated and repositioned by others and remain in the positions in which they are placed. During this state, the person's limbs have been described by examiners as feeling like "pliable wax."

checking perceptions A therapeutic communication technique in which the nurse-therapist shares how he or she perceives the information communicated by the client. Facilitates understanding.

child ego state A term used in transactional analysis theory to describe childlike, unrefined emotions or responses that stem from early developmental life experiences.

chronic mentally ill A population whose persistent dysfunctional behavior may be attributed to a psychiatric disorder, regardless of specific diagnosis or living situation.

circular thinking A pattern of thinking in which the individual persistently repeats the same thoughts in a circular fashion. May be caused by depletion of the energy necessary for assimilation and processing of new thoughts.

circumlocutory speech A roundabout or indirect way of speaking; the use of more words than necessary to express an idea. Noted in various degrees in organic mental disorders.

circumstantiality Interruption in the stream of thought caused by excessive associations of an idea reaching the conscious level. Characterized by extraneous thinking in which the individual digresses into unnecessary details and inappropriate thoughts before communicating a central idea. In some cases it may serve to avoid an emotionally charged area.

clanging A speech pattern in which sounds govern the choice of words, as in rhyming or punning. Words often simulate a "clanging" tone. Noted most often in persons with schizophrenia, mania, or autism.

clarifying A therapeutic communication skill in which the nurse-therapist asks the client to give an example of what the client stated in order to clarify the client's meaning and enhance the nurse's understanding.

clinical specialist in psychiatric nursing A graduate of a master's program that provides specialization in the clinical area of psychiatric–mental health nursing and that qualifies graduates to obtain certification (by examination) by the American Nurses' Association.

closed-ended questions Questions that generally elicit yes or no responses. Useful in gathering factual data and in situations in which short responses are warranted, such as anxiety, confusion, or disorientation.

codependence Behaviors that characterize an individual's reliance on the impaired behavior of a spouse or partner as a way to meet his or her own needs for survival, security, and/or control. A common example is a person's codependence on his or her partner's alcoholism or drug abuse. Codependence can result in enabling, in which the partner engages in behaviors that perpetuate the affected person's impairment.

cognition Pertaining to the mental processes that include knowing, thinking, learning, judging, and problem solving.

complementary transactions A term used in transactional analysis theory in which the transactional stimulus and transactional response occur at identical ego levels: adult to adult, child to child, or parent to parent. Complementary transactions are not always beneficial.

comprehension The ability to perceive, understand, and grasp knowledge, ideas, and logic in accordance with one's chronologic age and developmental capacity.

compulsion An uncontrollable impulse to perform an act or ritual repeatedly; may be in response to an obsession (unwilled, persistent thought) as in obsessive-compulsive disorder. The compulsive behavior serves to decrease anxiety. Some examples of rituals are hand washing, cleaning, and checking.

concepts Abstractions that generalize and categorize observations based on likenesses and differences. Persons with schizophrenia often find it difficult to conceptualize.

conceptual framework A preliminary stage in theory building in which interrelated concepts are used as a model to conduct research or to categorize data. For example, the NANDA Taxonomy is a conceptual framework used to categorize nursing diagnoses.

concrete communication Literal interpretation of meanings; inability to think or communicate in an abstract or conceptual manner. May be a sign of departure from reality or preoccupation with a delusion.

conduct disorder A disorder of childhood that is characterized by a persistent pattern of conduct in which the basic rights of others and the rules of society are disrupted or violated.

confabulation Fabrication of facts or events in response to questions regarding situations that are not recalled by the individual because of memory impairment. Most notable in organic mental disorder, in which the person attempts to fill in the memory gaps with unrelated information. It is *not* lying.

confidentiality Treating as private information divulged by a client unless it reveals the client's intent to harm self or others. In such a case, only persons qualified to help the client may be notified, with the client's knowledge of the purpose and intent. Confidentiality conveys respect.

conflict A clash of wills between two opposing forces. It may be unconscious or conscious, intrapersonal or interpersonal. Psychotherapeutic interventions are often directed toward helping clients cope with or resolve conflicts.

confrontation A process by which a client is told something about himself or herself by a nurse-therapist that encourages self-examination. Also used to clarify an inconsistency or incongruence between what the client says and does.

confused state Bewildered, perplexed, or unclear. The type and degree of confusion need to be specified.

congruent Accordant states. For example, "mood-congruent" means that the person's visible emotional state correlates with his or her mood or feeling state.

consciousness State of awareness.

constricted Narrowed or restricted range, as in emotion. For example, a "constricted affect."

consultation The provision of psychiatric–mental health expertise to assist with a client or problem at the request of another health provider. Some examples of consultants are psychiatrists, clinical nurse specialists, social workers, and occupational therapists.

conversion disorder Loss or alteration in physical functioning that suggests a physical disorder. The symptom allows the individual to avoid an activity or situation that is perceived as threatening and anxiety-provoking and allows the person to gain support from the environment, which they feel may not be otherwise forthcoming. The symptom may be related in time to a psychologic conflict or need. Diagnosis may be supported by the client's inappropriate lack of concern regarding the physical symptom, a condition known as *la belle indifference* (beautiful indifference). Two examples of conversion disorders are "blindness" and "paralysis."

coping behavior Behaviors used by persons under stress to reduce anxiety. They may be innocuous, such as going on a shopping spree, driving a car, or having a good cry, or may be bizarre, such as the rituals of hand washing, cleaning, and checking seen in obsessive-compulsive disorder. When the coping behavior renders the person dysfunctional, he or she needs help to learn to cope in a more adaptive, satisfying manner.

coping mechanisms See *defense mechanisms.*

coping strategy Learned techniques used by individuals to reduce tension, stress, and anxiety. Some examples are deep-breathing techniques, relaxation exercises, visual imagery, and thought substitution. (See Appendix K).

cotherapy The sharing of responsibility for the therapeutic process, usually facilitated in groups or with families.

countertransference An irrational attitude taken by an analyst, therapist, nurse toward his or her client. The therapist views the client as a significant person in his or her life rather than as a client and may lose objectivity, which could create problems in the therapeutic work. Therapists need to be aware of countertransference and seek supervision when it occurs.

crisis A sudden change in a person's life situation or status in which customary methods of coping or problem solving fail or are inadequate; also called a *state of disequilibrium* for which a person needs outside help. It may be a developmental crisis and may be a turning point in one's life.

crisis counseling Brief counseling sessions (5 to 6 weeks) in which specific strategies focus on the issues surrounding the crisis. May be individual, group, or family oriented.

crossed transaction In transactional analysis theory a transaction in which the response of the individual stems from an ego state other than the one addressed, which terminates the complementary relationship. Some crossed transactions are healthy. Some examples of crossed transactions are child to parent, adult to child, and parent to adult.

culture The learned values, beliefs, perceptions, and behaviors of specific groups of people. Nurse-therapists value cultural differences and recognize mental disorders within the context of their individual cultures.

cyclothymic disorder A chronic mood disturbance of at least 2 years' duration categorized by periods of depression alternating with episodes of hypomania, with normal mood states in between. Neither the depressed nor manic state is as severe or intense as the depression seen in major depression or the mania noted in bipolar disorder. Clients are often treated on an outpatient basis.

daydreaming A process of musing in a dreamlike state, or fantasizing, while awake. Problematic if it occurs to such an extent that it interferes with reality-based activities.

decanoate A long-acting, injectable form of neuroleptic (e.g, Prolixin decanoate) that is released into the body over a period of approximately 2 weeks. It is useful for clients who cannot be relied on to take medication or are unable to ingest oral medication. Nurses must examine injection sites for swelling and inflammation, which could indicate a sterile abscess.

decompensate The decline or deterioration of areas of mental or physical functioning. A loss of ability to maintain adequate or appropriate psychologic defenses that may result in anxiety, depression, or psychosis.

deep-breathing technique A stress-reduction technique in which the act of deep, slow inhalations moves the diaphragm downward and fills the lungs with air, followed by slow exhalations. Oxygen slows the heart rate, which reduces the individual's physiologic and psychologic symptoms of anxiety. (See Appendix K).

defense mechanisms (ego-defense mechanisms) The psychoanalytic term for coping mechanisms, also called *mental mechanisms*. Operations that are put into play at an unconscious level by the ego to protect the organism from anxiety by preventing conscious exposure of a noxious, threatening conflict. Defense mechanisms may be used adaptively or maladaptively and should not be challenged until the person demonstrates that he or she can function without them. (See Appendix I for a list of defense mechanisms.)

déjà vu Illusion of visual recognition in which a new situation is incorrectly regarded as a repetition of a previous memory.

delirium A clouded state of consciousness; decreased sensorium; reduction in clarity of awareness of the environment, accompanied by a reduced capacity to shift, focus, and sustain attention to environmental stimuli. May be reversible, depending on the underlying disease process.

delirium tremens (DTs) An acute, psychotic state usually occurring during reduction or cessation of alcohol intake after a prolonged or copious intake of alcohol; characterized by symptoms such as tremors, hallucinations, or seizures. Requires immediate treatment; may be life-threatening.

delusion A fixed belief unrelated to the client's cultural and educational background, improbable in nature, and not influenced or changed by reason or contrary experience. Categorized as a thought disorder. *Bizarre delusion:* an absurd belief, such as being controlled by a dead person. *Mood-congruent delusion:* a delusion whose content is mood-appropriate. *Mood-incongruent delusion:* a delusion whose content is mood-inappropriate. *Somatic delusion:* false belief involving a body's parts of functions. *Delusion of grandeur:* exaggerated conception of importance. *Delusion of persecution:* false belief that one is being persecuted. *Delusion of reference:* false belief that the behavior of others in the environment refers to oneself; derived from ideas of reference in which one falsely feels he or she is being discussed. *Delusion of control:* false feeling that one is being controlled by others. *Paranoid delusion:* oversuspiciousness, leading to persecutory delusions. *Delusion of nihilism:* false feeling that self, others, or the world is nonexistent. *Delusion of poverty:* false belief that one lacks material possessions.

dementia An organic mental syndrome characterized by impairment of cognitive abilities of sufficient magnitude to interfere with social or occupational functioning. There is a progression of impairments, beginning with loss of recent memory, personality changes, and inability to think in an abstract manner or make judgments, leading to loss of remote memory. There is no clouding of consciousness in dementia, but delirium may occur in the final stages of the disease.

denial A defense mechanism that is demonstrated by avoidance of disagreeable realities by the mind's refusal to acknowledge them at a conscious level. May or may not be adaptive, depending on the information being denied.

dependent personality disorder A personality disorder with the essential feature being a pervasive pattern of dependency on others and/or submissiveness.

depersonalization An alteration in the perception or experience of the self in which one's usual sense of reality is temporarily lost or changed. Feeling as if one is detached, in a dreamlike state, or an outside observer of one's mind and body, rather than a participant. May lead to withdrawal.

depersonalization disorder A dissociative disorder characterized by a persistent or recurrent feeling of being detached from one's mental processes or body accompanied by intact reality testing. Not to be confused with the depersonalization state that may occur in other disorders such as schizophrenia, panic disorder, acute stress disorder, or another type of dissociative disorder.

depression A term used to define (1) a mood, (2) a syndrome, or (3) an illness (i.e., major depression). The *mood* of depression is a feeling of dejection and sadness with a concomitant lowering of functional activity. It can be a normal state that may be a response to frustration and loss. The *syndrome* of depression includes a depressed mood in combination with one or more of the following symptoms: inability to concentrate, anorexia, weight loss, loss of self-esteem, and suicidal ideation. The *illness* of depression is similar to the syndrome of depression but longer in duration. Functional impairment may include inability to carry on daily activities, particularly work.

depressive disorder One or more episodes of major depression without a history of a manic or hypomanic episode.

derailment Gradual or sudden deviation in train of thought without blocking.

derealization A feeling of being disconnected from the environment, that the world around one is not real. It may be manifested by a feeling that the environment has changed and may be associated with depersonalization. Distortion of spatial relationships occurs so that the environment becomes unfamiliar.

dereistic thinking Thought processes that are not based in an external, commonly accepted reality. Dereism generally means a disconnection with reality and logic and occurs just prior to autistic thinking, when the person then engages in private, idiosyncratic thoughts and ideas that are derived from internal drives and desires. Dereism is seen in clients with schizophrenia. The terms *dereistic thinking* and *autistic thinking* are often used interchangeably.

desensitization A method or technique used most often by behaviorists to countercondition individuals who experience irrational fears or phobias by gradually exposing them to anxiety-producing stimuli in a controlled environment. In phobic disorder, the technique is called *systematic desensitization.*

devaluation Sustained, persistent criticism some individuals use to defend against their own feelings of inadequacy. Noted in persons with personality disorders, such as borderline personality disorder.

developmental stages or phases Universal experiences that are based on a chronologic timetable, including biologic, social, and psychologic stages and events. Includes specific tasks and challenges to be met at each stage. (See Appendix D.)

dexamethasone suppression test (DST) A test used to diagnose endogenous depression (chronic depression not caused by external factors such as grief or loss). Involves administration of a single dose of dexamethasone at a specific time, followed by monitoring of blood and/or urine cortisol levels. In depressed persons, the dexamethasone does not suppress adrenocortical functioning. The DST is judged within the context of other methods of client evaluation and diagnostic criteria.

Diagnostic and Statistical Manual of Mental Disorders, Fourth Edition, 1994 A classification of mental disorders that defines and describes criteria for diagnoses based on specific behaviors and categorizes the disorders on a multiaxial scale (Axes I through V). Abbreviated as DSM-IV, it includes several modifications and additions since the previous DSM-III revised edition of 1987, one of which is a section on culture.

disinhibition A condition noted following the ingestion of alcohol or benzodiazepines, in which a person experiences less control over basic emotions and demonstrates irritability, verbal hostility, and violent outbursts.

disorientation Lack of awareness of time, place, or person.

displacement A defense mechanism in which an individual discharges or displaces pent-up feelings and emotions on persons or objects that are less threatening than the source. May or may not be adaptive, depending on the situation.

dissociation A defense mechanism that protects the self from awareness of feelings that threaten to produce overwhelming anxiety by denying the existence of those feelings.

dissociative disorders Disorders that are characterized by disturbances or alterations in consciousness, memory, or identity. Dissociative identity disorder and certain types of amnesia and fugue states are among the dissociative disorders.

dissociative identity disorder The existence of two or more distinct personalities or personality states within one person that recurrently take control of the person's behavior. Formerly known as *multiple personality disorder.*

distractibility Inability to concentrate or attend to the task at hand; inattentiveness.

dopamine hypothesis The biochemical hypothesis that schizophrenia may be related to overactive neuronal activity that is dependent on the neurotransmitter dopamine. Increased dopamine activity is associated with increased schizophrenic symptoms, which explains the decrease in symptoms following treatment with antipsychotic medications that block dopamine activity.

double-bind communication Paradoxic or contradictory message that demands an incongruent response, thus placing the receiver of the message in a "double-bind" situation. For example, "You don't mind if I sit here and talk with you, do you?" "You really didn't feel like going on the field trip with the group, did you?" The receiver who is a client may be unable to comment on the incongruity or not know how to escape from it and may therefore succumb to the will of the message sender.

DRGs (diagnosis-related groups) A list of medical conditions that are grouped in categories on which prospective hospital costs and payments are calculated. DRGs are intended to predict use of resources.

drug holidays Carefully planned and managed withdrawal from psychotropic medications; may be executed to reduce nontherapeutic effects; most often done with neuroleptic medications.

dual diagnosis The coexistence of a medical diagnosis and a mental disorder; for example, substance use disorder and major depression.

dysfunctional family See *family patterns.*

dysfunctional grief Grief or mourning that is not resolved within an appropriate time period and/or demonstration of behaviors that are dysfunctional or inappropriate in accordance with the stages of the grieving process. May result in depression.

dyskinesia Difficulty of movement. (See *tardive dyskinesia.)*

dysphasia Disturbance in speech manifested by lack of coordination in speech patterns and inability to express words in their proper order.

dysphoria A sense of restlessness, agitation, or malaise. People with depression are noted to experience dysphoria.

dysprosody Difficulty in speech in which inflection, pronunciation, pitch, and rhythm are impaired.

dysthymia A chronic disturbance in mood involving depressed mood for at least 2 years. Less intense than major depression. Characterized by a depletion of usual coping strategies and the tendency to feel worse as the day progresses, most likely because of inability to cope with accumulated stressors.

echolalia Repetition of words that are addressed to the client by others; may also be repetition of the client's own thoughts. Generally noted in schizophrenia and organic mental disorders.

echopraxia A disturbance of motor behavior (conation) characterized by the pathologic imitation of movements of one person by another.

ecstasy A feeling of intense rapture or exhilaration, often described by clients experiencing a manic episode.

ego A (Freudian) conceptual construct of the mind that is considered to be the organized part of the personality, which screens stimuli from the external world and controls internal demands. Considered in psychoanalytic theory to be the intermediary or "referee" between the superego (conscience) and id (primitive impulses), the ego puts the defense mechanisms into play whenever repressed, anxiety-provoking material threatens to come into conscious awareness and expose the individual. Although consciousness resides in the ego, some of its operations are out of the person's awareness.

ego-dystonic Feelings or actions that are distressing to the individual or not congruent with his or her self-image (e.g., "ego-dystonic" homosexuality).

ego-syntonic Feelings or actions that are congruent with the individual's self-image even if they are not consistent with the mainstream of society (e.g., "ego-syntonic" homosexuality).

elation Elevation of mood; emotional excitement. May be a temporary response to an exciting event in a mentally healthy individual or may be characteristic of the mania seen in bipolar disorder. Also seen in schizophrenia.

Electra complex In psychoanalytic (Freudian) theory, an incestuous attachment of girls to their fathers during the phallic or genital stage of growth and development (ages 3 to 6), when the child's task is to identify with the parent of the same sex. Parallels the Oedipus complex for boys.

electroconvulsive therapy (ECT) The treatment of inducing convulsive seizures via the passage of an electric current through electrodes applied to temporal areas of the head (unilaterally or bilaterally). Used most frequently in the treatment of severe depression. Also known as *electroshock therapy.*

elopement The departure or flight from a mental health facility by an inpatient, against medical advice (AMA).

emotion A complex feeling state with psychic, somatic, and behavioral components that is related to mood and affect.

empathy The ability to understand the feelings of others, especially clients, as if they were one's own feelings, without losing objectivity, and to accept others' experiences on their terms. Differs from sympathy by its lack of condolence, pity, or agreement.

enabler Family member or significant person in an alcoholic or drug addict's life who contributes to the afflicted person's continued use and abuse of the substance. Examples of enabling include making excuses for the afflicted person and/or supplying the person with the alcohol or drug.

enmeshment A family pattern characterized by overcontrol, intrusiveness, and interference, usually from parent to child. Noted in families of clients with anorexia nervosa.

euphoria A false sense of elation of well-being; pathologic elevation of mood. Most notable in clients experiencing the manic phase of bipolar disorder.

euthymic mood A normal range of mood.

excitement Excited motor activity.

expansive mood Expression of one's feelings without the willful capacity to stop; often noted in manic episodes.

extrapyramidal side effects (EPSEs) Side effects caused by neuroleptic medications that include three separate classes of effects: parkinsonism, dystonias, and akathisia.

extrapyramidal system A system of descending motor tracts that originate from various regions of the cerebral cortex and subcortical areas. Because these tracts do not travel through the pyramids of the medulla oblongata, they are called extrapyramidal (outside the pyramids).

eye contact 1. A skill in which a staff member looks into the eyes of a client during the communication process for the purpose of demonstrating interest, caring, and respect. It is recommended that eye contact be intermittent and accompanied by a calm, interested facial expression, rather than constant, tense, glaring, or staring. 2. An assertive, nonverbal response from one person to another (generally peers) for the purpose of sending a clear, congruent message. In this instance, the eye contact would be more constant and accompanied by a facial expression that is congruent with the person's verbal message.

facial tic Spasmodic, repetitive motor movements of the face. Tics can occur in other parts of the body as well.

facies A term that refers to the expression of the facial structure. In specific conditions, such as Parkinson's disease or parkinsonian syndrome, which may be related to neuroleptic effects, facies may be described as "masked" or "masklike," meaning there is infrequent blinking noted.

factitious disorder Physical or psychologic symptoms that the individual does not voluntarily or consciously produce.

family patterns A family's unique methods of coping with the outside world; biased perceptions by a group of people who cohabit; the lifestyle a family presents to others. In the area of mental health, the identified client frequently acts out the symptoms of a dysfunctional family unit, indicating that the family as well as the client needs help.

family therapy The treatment of family members for the purpose of establishing open communication and healthy family interactions. Also known as *family systems therapy.*

fantasy Often cited as a defense mechanism, fantasy involves a sequence of mental images that can be likened to a daydream. It may be conscious or unconscious. A person may fantasize to help resolve an emotional conflict or as a means of mental rehearsal. Fantasizing may be adaptive and even beneficial at any age, as long as developmental tasks are being met and the person functions in a manner that reveals the ability to distinguish between fantasy and reality consistent with his or her age-appropriate level.

fasciculation Rapid, fine, twitching movements that result from contraction of a fasciculus (bundle of nerve fibers) controlled by a single anterior horn cell. Generally does not cause joint movement.

fear A response that is the same as anxiety but caused by consciously recognized and realistic danger.

feedback In communication, a method by which one person checks out the verbal or nonverbal communication of another. Also a process by which one offers commentary on another's performance. Useful in the therapeutic process.

female sexual arousal disorder Inability to attain or maintain adequate lubrication during sexual activity and/or lack of a subjective sense of sexual excitement during sexual activity.

fetal alcohol syndrome (FAS) Physical or mental defects noted in infants of mothers who used or abused alcohol during their pregnancies.

fetishism The requirement of the presence of a nonviable object, such as shoes, hair, or underclothing, for sexual arousal.

fight or flight The response to stress of aggression (fight) or withdrawal (flight), provoked in part by the effects of the autonomic nervous system.

flat affect A lack of emotional range or expression, also referred to as *flattened affect.*

flight of ideas A nearly continuous flow of rapid speech with abrupt changes from topic to topic. Most often observed during manic episodes of bipolar disorder in which the person's thoughts and ideas accelerate to an unintelligible degree. Flight of ideas is distinguished from the looseness of associations observed in people with schizophrenia in that flight of ideas is generally more based in reality than the internally stimulated thoughts revealed in the fragmented pattern of loose associations. However, flight of ideas may reach a level of psychosis in the form of grandiose or paranoid delusions. Flight of ideas may be perpetuated by stressful stimuli.

frotteurism Intense sexual arousal associated with acts or fantasies of rubbing against a nonconsenting person.

fugue A period of memory loss in which an individual recalls nothing of the lost time and may start a new life while in the fugue state.

functional encopresis Repeated involuntary or intentional passage of feces in inappropriate places.

functional enuresis Repeated involuntary or intentional urination into bed or clothing past the age at which urinary continence is expected.

gait The manner of progression in walking. *Ataxic gait:* foot raised high with sole striking down in sudden movement. *Parkinsonism gait:* a shuffling gait with absent arm swing and rigid posture. Clients who are taking neuroleptics may demonstrate restless movements (akathisia) and some rigidity in their gait, most likely related to dopamine blockade.

gender identity The sex role assigned at birth as either male, female, or ambivalent, generally based on external genitalia.

gender role The socialization and demonstration of the sexual behaviors expected of an assigned sex.

general adaptation syndrome (GAS) The objectively measurable structural and chemical changes produced in the body when stress affects the whole organism. The GAS occurs in three stages: alarm, resistance, and exhaustion.

general systems theory A conceptual framework that can be applied to living systems or people and that integrates the biologic and social sciences logically with the physical sciences. The theory views individuals as open systems that can influence and be influenced by all other systems.

generalized anxiety disorder A disorder characterized by free-floating, unrealistic, excessive anxiety, manifested by autonomic hyperactivity (diaphoresis, dizziness), irritability, and musculoskeletal tension. Symptoms may progress to panic state at any given time if stressors in the individual's environment exceed his or her ability to cope. People with this disorder benefit from learned coping strategies because adaptive use of defense mechanisms seems to elude them.

goal-directed thinking A flow of ideas and associations initiated by a problem or task that leads toward a reality-based conclusion. According to Kaplan and Sadock, thinking is "normal" when a logical sequence of events occurs.

grief or mourning Sadness appropriate to an actual loss, characterized by specific behaviors that occur in stages of the grieving process, in an acceptable time period. In functional grief, the individual is able to perform activities of daily living in a progression congruent with the stages of the grieving process.

grimace Distorted facial expression.

grooming A term used in mental health assessment, meaning a client's overall appearance, including neatness, cleanliness, condition and tidiness of hair, clothing, and so on, consistent with age and sociocultural preference. Lack of grooming may be an indicator of mental or emotional illness.

hallucination A perceptual disorder involving any of the five senses that occurs in the absence of external stimuli; a subjective experience in an individual whose sensorium is clear. The most common hallucinations are auditory and involve hearing voices that originate from the person's internal world. The client may perceive that the voices are coming from a transmitter, such as a radio, television set, or computer. Visual hallucinations are the second most common type and are likely to take the shape of threatening or frightening monsters or scenarios. Less common are hallucinations that involve the other three senses: olfactory, a false perception of smell; gustatory, a false perception of taste; and tactile, a false perception of movement or sensation. Other types of hallucinations are hypnagogic (a false sensory perception while falling asleep) and hypnopompic (a false sensory perception while awakening from sleep). A hallucination is considered mood-congruent when its content is mood-appropriate and mood-incongruent when its content is mood-inappropriate.

health assessment A comprehensive collection of data derived from examination of the current and past health status of an individual. Information can be obtained from various other qualified sources and includes mental, physical, social, environmental, and occupational functions.

here-and-now interactions Interpersonal communications that deal with current problems and issues that are either "on the spot" or recent enough to affect the individual's present situation.

heterosexuality Preference for sexual activity with a partner of the opposite sex.

histrionic personality disorder A personality disorder with the essential feature being a pervasive pattern of excessive emotional display and attention-seeking behaviors.

HIV seropositive Having blood serum that tests positive for the HIV antibody but not necessarily having a diagnosis of ARC or AIDS.

holistic Pertaining to totality or the whole; for example, the health profession subscribes to the philosophy of holism, in that it views the individual as an integrated whole whose parts share an organic and functional relationship.

homelessness Absence of housing that may involve movement from one temporary shelter to another because of financial crisis or emergency or, in the more extreme form, that refers to street dwellers (the homeless).

homeostasis The principle that all living organisms struggle to maintain a relatively constant internal environment in response to changing conditions; maintaining a balance or equilibrium.

homicidal A state characterized by one person's verbal or behavioral threats to harm or kill another person. Requires immediate intervention. (See Appendix L).

homophobia The irrational fear of homosexuals and homosexuality, generally stemming from myths and stereotypes.

homosexual panic Extreme anxiety and agitation as a result of emerging repressed homosexual impulses.

homosexuality Preference for sexual activity with a partner of the same sex.

hot line A telephone crisis counseling service frequently used in crisis intervention centers to provide the caller immediate contact with a counselor. Examples of crises that warrant hot line calls include alcoholic, drug, and suicidal crises.

human immunodeficiency virus (HIV) The virulent virus that causes AIDS. It consists of an extremely tiny, double-layered shell, filled with proteins, surrounding a bit of ribonucleic acid (RNA).

hygiene 1. The science dealing with the preservation of health. 2. A condition or practice conducive to health, as cleanliness.

hyperactivity (hyperkinesis) Restless, overactive motor movement and behavior. May be aggressive or destructive. Seen in children with hyperactive conditions or people experiencing a manic episode.

hypervigilance Increased state of guardedness or watchfulness; may be a sign of escalating anxiety or agitation. May involve scanning behaviors as well.

hypoactive sexual desire disorder Persistent or recurrent lack of interest or drive in sexual expression or fantasies.

hypochondriasis Preoccupation with the fear or belief that one has a serious disease, in spite of medical reassurance to the contrary.

hypomania A clinical syndrome in which an individual's predominant mood is elevated, expansive, or irritable, but not as severe as in full-blown manic episodes and without delusions.

hysteria Described in Kaplan and Sadock, as two types: (1) conversion disorder, characterized by bodily symptoms resembling those of physical disease, and (2) dissociative type, manifested by such conditions as somnambulism, various forms of amnesia and fugue states, and multiple personality disorder. Anxiety plays a role in each type.

id In (Freudian) psychoanalytic theory, a construct or concept of the mind that houses all inherited, psychic properties, most notably, the repressed, instinctual drives of sexuality and aggression. Supposedly resides in the unconscious.

identification A defense mechanism that involves the desire or wish to emulate another person and to assume the characteristics of that person. Most notable in adolescence, when identification with peers is an important part of growth and development. It actually begins, however, in early childhood (ages 3 to 6), when identification with the parent of the same sex is a critical developmental task.

identity diffusion The failure to integrate various childhood identifications into a harmonious, adult, psychosocial identity. Also known as *identity confusion* (Erickson).

illogical thinking Thinking that contains erroneous conclusions, irrational ideas, or internal contradictions.

illusions Sensory misperceptions or misinterpretations of actual environmental stimuli. Affects all the senses, but visual and auditory illusions are much more common than tactile, olfactory, and gustatory illusions. May occur as a result of sleep-wake alterations.

immediate memory Memory that includes the last few seconds up to the present time.

imparting information A therapeutic communication skill in which the nurse-therapist makes statements that give the client pertinent information and thus encourages further clarification based on additional input.

inappropriate affect Affect that is incongruent with the content of the client's verbalizations or ideas.

incest Sexual relations between blood relatives or members of the same social unit other than husband or wife.

incoherence The running together of thoughts with no logical connections, resulting in disorganized thought processes.

insertion of thought(s) interruption of stream of thought in which an unwilled thought or idea is introduced into the mind.

insight An understanding of relationships that sheds light on or helps solve a problem; the recognition of sources of emotional difficulty; an understanding of the motivational forces behind one's actions, thoughts, and behaviors; self-knowledge.

institutionalization The process of functional decline characterized by dependency, apathy, resignation, and inability to manage activities of daily life outside an institution and created by an environment that controls decision-making, discourages independence and autonomy, and prevents clients from having relevant interactions with the mainstream community.

intellectualization A defense mechanism that consists of ruminating about philosophic or theoretic data or overusing intellectual or scholarly processes to avoid closeness to one's emotions or expressions. Serves to constrain instinctual drives. Intellectualization constitutes an interruption of the stream of thought.

intelligence The ability to understand, recall, mobilize, and integrate constructively previous learning in meeting new situations.

intoxication Maladaptive behavior associated with alterations of the central nervous system owing to ingestion of a psychoactive substance (substance-specific syndrome).

introjection A defense mechanism that begins in infancy and involves the incorporation of traits, qualities, and characteristics of significant persons. More intense than identification, which is more like imitation.

irrational thinking Thinking that is not based on a universally accepted reality; illogical thinking.

irritable mood A mood in which one is easily annoyed and provoked to anger. Noted in manic episodes.

isolation of affect A defense mechanism by which an individual separates or isolates from his or her thoughts unacceptable or threatening feelings or impulses. Observed in some people during the early stages of grief. May be adaptive as a temporary measure but is maladaptive if the person continues to negate emotions that should be expressed for purposes of overall health and well-being.

judgment The ability or capacity to make a decision based on sound problem solving of a given situation. The exercise or demonstration of objective, wise actions.

-kinesia or -kinesis A combining form used with other terms to mean movement or activity, e.g., dyskinesia, hyperkinesis, hypokinesis.

kleptomania A compulsive disorder that involves the uncontrollable impulse to steal; the objects stolen generally are of no use to the kleptomaniac. Kleptomanic acts may be demonstrated by some people experiencing a manic episode.

knowledge deficit Lack of understanding or awareness regarding all or some aspect of a fact, subject, or concept that may interfere with one's progress toward health or wellness. Used as a nursing diagnosis or etiology.

la belle indifference A condition whose literal definition is "beautiful indifference," characterized by an inappropriate lack of concern about a physical disability or disorder. Seen in clients with conversion disorders. The physical symptom allows the individual to avoid an activity or situation that is perceived as threatening.

labile affect A pattern of observable behaviors that express emotion characterized by repeated, rapid, abrupt shifts.

learned helplessness (excessive dependence) A condition in which a person attempts to establish and maintain contact with another by adopting a helpless, powerless attitude.

lesbianism Sexual activity between females.

lethality assessment A systematic method of assessing a client's suicide risk or potential.

libido In psychoanalytic theory, an individual's sexual drive or energy.

life script Expectations that an individual has for his or her life that have evolved over time, related to the person's life experiences and relationships with significant others. The life script affects many areas of living, including career choices, life partner, and behavior patterns. Used as a concept in transactional analysis theory, which states that one's life script begins as a child and that the adult needs to work on rewriting it to grow and change.

limbic system The part of the brain that is considered the emotional area; includes the hippocampus, lingulate gyrus, isthmus, hippocampal gyrus, and uncus.

limit setting The reasonable setting of boundaries and parameters for client behavior to provide control and safety. Often used with children and adolescents.

linking A therapeutic communication skill in which the nurse responds to the client in a way that ties or links together two or more events, experiences, feelings, or persons; for example, linking together past and present client behaviors to help increase the client's understanding of his or her behavioral patterns.

lithium A basic element or salt used in different forms in the treatment and prevention of manic episodes and other cyclic disorders. (See Appendix M.)

logorrhea (volubility) Copious, coherent, logical speech.

loosening of associations Flow or stream of thought that is characterized by vague, fragmented, unfocused, and illogical speech patterns. Notable in persons with schizophrenia. Listed in Kaplan and Sadock, as a disturbance in structure of associations of thought. Loose associations are generally based on the client's inner repertoire of thought patterns.

magical thinking The belief that one's thoughts, words, or actions will produce an outcome that defies normal laws of cause and effect; the belief that one's words have the power to make things happen. For example, a client may believe his or her thoughts can cause earthquakes. Occurs in schizophrenia.

major depressive episode Depressed mood and/or loss of interest in pleasure in all or almost all activities for a period of at least 2 weeks. (See *mood disorder; depression.*)

malingering Simulation of illness with no evidence of organic pathology.

manic episode Period of behavior characterized by predominantly elevated, expansive mood, either euphoric or irritable, with a duration of at least 1 week. Accompanying behaviors may include increased activity, restlessness, talkativeness, flight of ideas, feeling of racing thoughts, grandiosity, decreased sleep time, short attention span, buying sprees, sexual indiscretion, and inappropriate laughing, joking, or punning.

masochism (sexual masochism) The need to experience emotional or physical pain, in reality or in fantasy, to become sexually aroused.

masturbation Manual stimulation of genitalia or other body parts. The act may be for the purpose of erotic stimulation commonly resulting in orgasm, a conscious expression of hostility toward someone, or an unconscious expression of anxiety.

meditation A method of achieving a state of deep rest and increasing α-wave brain activity that allows the individual to focus on one thing at a time for the purpose of attaining inner peace and emotional harmony.

medulla oblongata The specialized segment of neurologic tissue that attaches the brain to the spinal cord.

mental disorder "A clinically significant behavioral or psychological syndrome or pattern . . . typically associated with painful symptom . . . or impairment, in one or more important areas of functioning" (DSM-III-R, 1987).

mental retardation "Lack of intelligence to a degree in which there is interference with social and vocational performance: Mild (IQ of 52-67), Moderate (IQ of 36-51), Severe (IQ of 20-35), Profound (IQ below 20)" (Kaplan and Sadock, 1988).

mental status examination A record of current findings that includes the description of a client's appearance, behavior, motor activity, speech, alertness, mood, cognition, intelligence, reactions, views, and attitudes.

midlife crisis A period of disequilibrium between ages 35 and 45 years, during which individuals note various signs of aging and experience feelings of boredom, dissatisfaction with life, and uncertainty about the future.

milieu The therapeutic environment; the client's immediate environment.

milieu therapy The purposeful use of people, resources, and events that take place in the client's therapeutic environment (milieu), for the promotion of optimal functioning in activities of daily living, interpersonal interactions, growth and development, and the ability to manage self-care on discharge.

Minnesota Multiphasic Personality Inventory (MMPI) A commonly used complex, lengthy psychologic test with 550 questions that yields a clinical picture of the client's personality style.

mirroring Imitating the client's behavior.

mixed message Communication in which there is incongruence or contradiction between the verbal and nonverbal aspects.

mnemonic disturbances Inability to remember recent events; may extend to global memory loss for both past and recent events.

mood A feeling state or prolonged emotion that influences the whole of one's psychic life.

mood congruence A state in which the mood is congruent or consistent with the person's affect and/or thought processes. For example, a person demonstrates a saddened affect and expresses feelings of sadness appropriate to the mood.

mood disorder A diagnostic category in the DSM-IV that is also referred to as *affective disorder.* Dysfunction or impairment of an individual's mood state either from endogenous or identifiable sources. Endogenous mood disorders are most likely related to a biochemical imbalance of specific neurotransmitters located in areas of the brain that control mood and affect.

mood incongruence A state in which the mood is incongruent or inconsistent with the person's affect or verbal content. For example, a person expresses feelings of happiness yet outwardly manifests a sad affect and verbalizes content that is pessimistic and negative.

mood-congruent delusion A delusion in which the content is appropriate with the mood of the individual. For example, a person expresses feelings of self-importance and elation and states that he or she is the savior of humanity.

mood-incongruent delusion A delusion in which the content is mood-inappropriate. For example, a person expresses elation and exhilaration yet speaks of the world ending.

motor aphasia Disturbance of speech owing to an organic brain disorder in which the ability to speak is lost, although understanding remains intact.

muddled speech A disturbance in the speed of thought associations in which the parts of different thoughts are muddled together.

multiaxial system The five axes used in the DSM-IV to list diagnostic criteria.

multi-infarct dementia Serious cerebrovascular disease resulting in dementia. The person generally experiences a step-wise deterioration with significant episodes, unlike the vague, insidious progression of Alzheimer's disease.

multiple personality disorder A former term for a type of dissociative disorder that is now called *dissociative identity disorder,* in which two or more distinct personalities or personality states exist within one person and recurrently take control of the person's behavior.

mutism An inability to speak owing to a physical defect or refusal to speak as a result of a psychologic or emotional problem.

mutual self-help groups Organized groups that provide support through group interactions between people experiencing the same type of problem, event, or situation, for example, Alcoholics Anonymous.

NANDA Acronym for the North American Nursing Diagnosis Association, an organization made up of nurses who were instrumental in the construction of the NANDA Taxonomy, and who are responsible for reviewing, studying, and accepting specific nursing diagnoses that cover all clinical practice areas.

narcissistic personality disorder A personality disorder in which the essential feature is a pervasive pattern of extreme self-absorption, self-centeredness, grandiosity, and hypersensitivity to the evaluation of others. Individuals seem to lack empathy for others and find it difficult to get in touch with their own feelings and emotions.

negative transference A client's reaction to therapeutic interventions, based on negative feelings such as anger, hate, bitterness, contempt, or envy that have been nurtured from previous unsatisfying relationships.

neologism A newly coined word that generally indicates a formal thought disorder. Neologisms are disturbances in the structure of thought associations in which the client creates new words for psychologic reasons. Noted in clients with schizophrenia who may be experiencing a psychotic episode.

neuroleptic Another term for medications known as *antipsychotics.*

neuroleptic malignant syndrome (NMS) An infrequent yet extremely critical condition in clients who are undergoing neuroleptic drug treatment. Symptoms include diaphoresis, muscle rigidity, and hyperpyrexia and are believed to result from dopamine blockade in the hypothalamus. May be fatal. (See Appendix M.)

neurosis A pre–DSM-III-R category for mental disorders characterized by various anxiety symptoms, thought to be related to unresolved conflicts. No longer a diagnostic category.

neurotransmitter A chemical found in the nervous system (e.g., norepinephrine, serotonin, and dopamine) that facilitates the transmission of nerve impulses across synapses, between neurons. Implicated in affective and schizophrenic disorders.

nihilism The view that existence is senseless and useless.

nihilistic delusion A false feeling that the self, others, or the world is nonexistent.

nonverbal communication The process in which information is passed from one individual to another without speaking but through use of body movements, gestures, posture, and facial expressions. May be conscious or unconscious.

nursing diagnosis A statement that describes a client's health state or response to illness that is treatable by nurses. In NANDA's ninth conference, held in March 1990, *nursing diagnosis* was defined as "a clinical judgment about individual, family, or community responses to actual or potential health problems/life processes. Nursing diagnoses provide the basis for selection of interventions to achieve outcomes for which the nurse is accountable."

nursing process The conscious, systematic set of cognitive and behavioral steps that comprise the clinical acts in nursing practice: assessment, nursing diagnosis, planning, interventions, and evaluation. (See Chapter 1.)

nystagmus Involuntary, rhythmic motion of the eye; may be horizontal, vertical, circular, or mixed.

object permanence The capacity to understand that an absent person or object will return or that something exists even when it is out of one's sight. A function that occurs prior to 2 years of age as the child's memory and cognitive processes develop (Piaget's Sensorimotor Stage, 0 to 2 years).

object relation The emotional attachment one person has for another, as opposed to that person's feelings for himself or herself.

obsession Preoccupation with a thought or idea that is generally upsetting to the individual and that morbidly dominates the mind.

obsessive-compulsive disorder Persistent, recurrent, painful intrusive thoughts, ideas, or urges (obsessions) that are unwilled and cannot be ignored by the individual. Provokes impulsive acts (compulsions) such as hand washing, cleaning, or checking that may be thought of as meaningless and absurd by both client and others but serve to reduce anxiety.

occupational therapy The use of creative techniques and purposeful activities, as well as a therapeutic relationship, to help clients with physical and mental disorders achieve their highest level of functioning. Focus is on activities of daily living and a broad range of vocational skills, including schoolwork and homemaking. Another goal of the occupational therapist is to raise the client's self-esteem and alter the course of illness.

Oedipus complex or Oedipal conflict In psychoanalytic theory, a major process of Freud's phallic stage (3 to 6 years of age), also called the *genital phase,* in which incestuous feelings are attached to the opposite-sex parent and aggressive feelings are directed to the same-sex parent in an attempt to identify with the same-sex parent. Conflicts arise with inappropriate or failed resolution of sex role identity. (Known as the *Oedipus complex* in males and the *Electra complex* in females.)

omnipotence Fantasies of greatness and power beyond capabilities. Can reach delusional proportions. May be noted in psychotic states of mania or in schizophrenia.

one-to-one relationship A mutually acceptable, collaborative, goal-directed relationship, generally between a client and staff member, for the purpose of crisis intervention, counseling, or individual psychotherapy.

open-ended statements Statements that elicit further exploration of the client's problems by encouraging communication. May also be used in the form of a question. Not useful in certain conditions, such as anxiety, confusion, or mania.

oppositional defiant disorder A pattern of negative, hostile, defiant behavior, without violation of others' rights, to a more frequent extent than in others of the same age.

oral stage A theoretic growth and developmental stage conceived by Sigmund Freud, depicting an age of infancy (0 to $1\frac{1}{2}$ years) in which the mouth is the primary source of pleasure. (See Appendix D.)

organic anxiety syndrome Prominent, recurrent panic attacks or generalized anxiety due to a specific organic factor.

organic delusional syndrome Presence of delusions as a result of a specific organic factor.

organic hallucinosis Presence of prominent, persistent, or recurrent hallucinations caused by a specific organic factor.

organic mental disorders A class of disorders characterized by progressive deterioration of the mental processes, caused by permanent brain damage or temporary brain dysfunction. Etiology is known and may be primary (originating in the brain) or secondary to systemic disease. Cognition, memory, emotions, and motivation are affected. Now classified in DSM-IV as delirium, dementia, and amnestic and other cognitive disorders.

organic mental syndromes Cluster of psychologic or behavioral symptoms or abnormalities that tend to occur together; the etiology is unknown.

organic mood syndrome Prominent and persistent depressed, elevated, or expansive mood, owing to a specific organic problem.

organic personality syndrome Persistent personality disturbance as a result of a specific organic factor.

orientation Conscious awareness of person, place, and time.

orientation phase The initial phase of a one-to-one relationship, which is begun by establishing contact with the client.

overactivity A disturbance in behavior characterized by repetitive motor movements and psychomotor agitation, which is often nonproductive and may be in response to inner tension (see *hyperactivity*).

overload In communication theory, sensory input within the client's immediate environment that overwhelms his or her tolerance level or capacity.

overvalued idea A false belief that is maintained without delusional content.

pace To go along with or match the client at whatever rate he or she is moving, talking, or feeling. During hyperventilation in anxiety states, the nurse can pace the client's breathing and promote slower, deeper breaths to eliminate hyperventilation and reduce anxiety.

pacing Rapid, repetitive walking back and forth or around a specific area, generally in an agitated fashion, in response to inner tension. May be a sign of impending aggression or violence.

panic An acute attack or stage of anxiety characterized by personality disorganization that requires immediate intervention. (See Chapter 2 for the stages of anxiety.)

panic disorder with agoraphobia Recurrent panic attacks accompanied by the fear of being in a place or situation in which escape might be difficult or embarrassing, or help may be unavailable.

panic disorder without agoraphobia Recurrent panic attacks without the avoidance behavior that results from agoraphobia.

paranoia Oversuspiciousness. May lead to blaming accusations (projectile behaviors) or persecutory delusions.

paranoid personality disorder A personality disorder with the essential feature being a pervasive and unwarranted tendency to interpret the actions of others as deliberately demeaning or threatening.

paranoid schizophrenia A type of schizophrenia in which the essential feature is preoccupation with one or more systematized delusions or frequent auditory hallucinations related to a single theme. Generally, there is no incoherence, loosening of associations, flat or grossly inappropriate affect, catatonia, or grossly disorganized behavior. Prognosis is often better than in other types of schizophrenia.

paraphilia A sexual disorder in which unusual or bizarre sexual acts are fantasized or enacted in order to achieve sexual excitement.

paraphrasing A therapeutic communication skill in which the nurse restates what she or he has heard the client communicating. It provides an opportunity to test the nurse's understanding of what the client is attempting to communicate and allows the client to hear his or her own words repeated.

parent ego state In transactional analysis theory, the ego state that incorporates the feelings and behaviors learned from parents and/or authority figures. Has been compared to Freud's superego because it deals with right and wrong and other learned values.

parkinsonism An extrapyramidal side effect characterized by motor retardation or akinesia, a masklike facies, rigidity, tremors, "pill-rolling," and salivation. May occur after the first week of psychotropic drug therapy. Thought to result from dopamine blockade.

passive-aggressive behavior Behavior characterized by sarcasm, procrastination, or resistance to requests made by others. A covert use of aggression.

passive-aggressive personality disorder A personality disorder with the essential feature being a pervasive pattern of resistance to demands for adequate performance in social and occupational settings. Resistance may take the form of "forgetfulness," intentional inefficiency, stubbornness, dawdling, or procrastination.

pedophilia The use of prepubertal children to achieve sexual satisfaction.

perception Awareness of objects and relations following peripheral sensory stimulation. A hallucination is an example of a false sensory perception because it is not associated with actual external stimuli.

perseveration Psychopathologic repetition of the same word or idea in response to different questions. Considered a disturbance in the structure of thought associations. Noted in organic mental disorders and schizophrenia.

personality The unique and distinctive human quality that defines and determines the essence of a person's character;

what a person is really like. Comprises deeply ingrained patterns of behavior known as *personality traits.*

personality disorder A nonpsychotic illness characterized by enduring patterns of perceiving, relating to, and thinking about oneself and the environment in ways that are maladaptive. The individual uses inflexible behavior patterns to fulfill own needs and attain self-satisfaction, often at the expense of others and society in general. Results in significant functional impairment and/or subjective distress.

pervasive developmental disorders See *autistic disorder.*

phenothiazines One of the classes of neuroleptic or antipsychotic medications. (See Appendix M.)

phobia A persistent, exaggerated, irrational fear of an object, activity, or situation that is out of proportion to the stimulus and results in avoidance of the feared stimulus in an effort to reduce anxiety. Clinical categories of phobias include agoraphobia with or without panic attacks, social phobia, and simple phobia.

pinpointing A therapeutic skill characterized by calling attention to statements; inconsistencies among statements; or similarities or differences in viewpoints, feelings, or actions. Helpful as a tool for nurses and therapists in interactions with patients.

play therapy Therapy used with children generally between the ages of 3 and 12 years. The child reveals problems on a fantasy level through the use of dolls, puppets, clay, and other toys and materials. The child is encouraged, with the help of the therapist, to act out feelings such as anger, fear, hostility, and frustration. The therapist may intervene to explain to the child his or her responses and behaviors in language that the child can comprehend.

polydrug use or abuse The use or abuse of multiple drugs within the same time frame; includes the use of alcohol.

polypharmacy The mixing of multiple medications; noted in the elderly population, who tend to have a wide variety of medical problems.

positive reinforcement In behavioral theory, operant conditioning, and learning theory, an environmental event (such as a reward or praise) that reinforces or increases the probability of a behavioral response. A technique often used with children and adolescents.

positive transference Client reactions in therapeutic work based on positive feelings, such as love, affection, trust, and respect, that are residual feelings from past, satisfying relationships. May be beneficial or require boundary setting (see *transference* and *countertransference).*

posttraumatic stress disorder Reexperiencing a psychologically terrifying or distressing event that is outside the usual range of human experience (such as rape, war, or a hostage situation) resulting in intense fear, terror, and helplessness.

posture Body stance, position of the limbs, or carriage of the body as a whole. In the mental health assessment, the client's posture is an important indicator of general well-being.

poverty of content of speech Speech that offers little information because of vagueness, vacuous repetitions, or obscure phrases. Considered a disturbance in thought content.

poverty or paucity of speech Restriction in the amount of speech used by an individual. Considered a disturbance in the speed of thought associations.

power rape Rape distinguished by the rapist's intent to command and master another person sexually, not to injure the victim.

primary data source The client as the provider of assessment information.

primary degenerative dementia, Alzheimer's type See *Alzheimer's disease.*

primary gain Obtaining relief from anxiety by the use of a defense mechanism to keep an internal need or conflict out of conscious awareness.

primary idealization The assignment of unrealistic powers to an individual on whom one is dependent.

problem solving A specific form of intellectual activity that involves critical thinking to help an individual deal with a complex situation he or she may not be able to handle with past learned skills. Problem-solving strategies consist of the following sequential steps: observation, definition, preparation, analysis, ideation, incubation, synthesis, evaluation, and development. The nursing process is an example of a systematic set of complex cognitive and behavioral steps in which problem-solving methods are applied.

processing A complex and sophisticated communication skill in which direct attention is focused on the interpersonal dynamics of the nurse-client or nurse-group relationship. Process comments are directed toward content (what is said), feelings, and behavior experienced within the nurse-client or nurse-group relationship.

progressive relaxation A method of deep muscle relaxation based on the premise that muscle tension is the body's physiologic response to anxiety and stress-producing stimuli and that relaxation methods reduce or block anxiety. One relaxation strategy calls for the client to tense and then relax all muscle groups, beginning with the toes and progressing toward the head (unless this type of activity is contraindicated for medical reasons).

projection A defense mechanism in which an individual projects onto others unwanted or undesirable characteristics of self. (See Appendix I.)

projective identification The placement of one's aggressive feelings onto another, thereby justifying one's expressions of anger and self-protection.

pseudodementia Clinical features resembling a dementia not due to organic brain pathology but most often to depression.

psychalgia A psychogenic pain disorder in which the person experiences severe and prolonged pain because of psychologic factors.

psyche The mental or psychosocial structure of a person, as in the internal motivational forces.

psychiatric history A set of interview questions oriented to the medical model, designed to elicit information about an individual's past and current psychiatric experiences. Data may be collected from client or qualified family members and friends, which results in a variety of perceptions.

psychiatric nurse The American Nurses' Association defines a *psychiatric nurse* as a registered nurse who possesses a minimum of a bachelor's degree in nursing.

psychiatric nursing A specialty within the nursing profession in which the focus of the nurse is directed toward the promotion of mental health, the prevention of mental distress, early identification of and intervention in emotional problems that can lead to dysfunctional behaviors and mental disorders, and follow-up care to minimize long-term effects of mental illness.

psychiatry The practice and science of diagnosing and treating mental disorders.

psychoanalysis A type of therapy developed by Sigmund Freud and his followers that deals with repressed, intrapsychic conflicts that are produced through interactions among three theoretic constructs of the mind: the id, ego, and superego. Psychoanalysis employs insight-oriented techniques (e.g., free association and dream analysis) to explore the dynamic, psychogenic, and transference aspects of a client's personality.

psychoanalytic Referring to the constructs of the mind that Freud described as the id (unconscious storehouse of primitive materials), ego (problem solver or mediator, lies mostly in the conscious), superego (conscience or moral system), and the intrapsychic behavior that is produced by interactions among them.

psychoanalytic model of psychiatry An approach founded by Sigmund Freud subscribing to the belief that all psychologic and emotional events are understandable. The meanings behind behaviors are explored through childhood experiences believed to be at the root of adult neuroses. Therapy emanating from this model consists of clarifying the psychologic meaning of events, feelings, and behavior to gain intellectual insight into why one behaves or feels a certain way.

psychodrama A method of group psychotherapy, developed by Jacob Moreno and his followers, in which participants are assigned various roles in improvisational dramatizations of emotionally charged situations and conflicts. The drama is supervised by a person qualified in psychodrama therapy, who guides the participants throughout the exercise. Generally reserved for high-functioning individuals.

psychodynamics Any type of clinical approach to personality (e.g., Freud's) that views personality as a result of the dynamic interplay between conscious and unconscious factors or the result of motivational forces that determine human behavior.

psychogenic Having origin in the mind or in a mental condition or process, for example, a "psychogenic" disorder.

psychogenic amnesia Sudden inability to recall important personal information that cannot be explained by normal forgetfulness.

psychogenic fugue Sudden, unexpected travel away from home or usual place of business, with the assumption of a new identity and inability to recall one's previous identity.

psychogerontology The study of mental health and mental illness and its effects on later life.

psychology The science of the mind or mental state and processes.

psychomotor Pertaining to a response involving both psychologic and motor components.

psychomotor agitation Agitated motor activity.

psychomotor retardation A generalized slowing of psychologic and physical activity, frequently as a symptom of severe depression.

psychopharmacology The branch of pharmacology that deals with the psychologic effects of drugs.

psychopharmacotherapy The use of psychoactive drugs in the symptomatic treatment and management of psychiatric disorders.

psychosis A state in which a person's capacity for recognizing reality and communicating and interacting with others is impaired, thereby greatly diminishing the person's ability to deal with life demands. May be associated with several mental disorders and include thought disorders (delusion), sensory perceptual alterations (hallucinations, illusions), and extremes of affect.

psychosocial Pertaining to the interaction between psychologic and social factors.

psychosomatic Pertaining to a physical disorder that is notably influenced by or caused by emotional or mental factors; involving the mind and the body.

psychosurgery Treatment of a mental disorder by means of brain surgery, for example, lobotomy.

psychotherapy The treatment of psychologic disorders or dysfunctions via a professional technique such as psychoanalysis, group therapy, or behavioral therapy.

psychotropic drugs Chemicals that alter feelings, emotions, and consciousness in a variety of ways; used in the practice of psychiatry to treat a wide range of mental and emotional illnesses.

questioning A very direct communication skill that may be useful when specific information is needed from the client. *Open-ended questioning* focuses on the topic and allows freedom of response. *Closed-ended questioning* limits the client's responses to yes or no. When used excessively, questioning tends to control the nature and extent of the client's responses.

rape A forced, violent sexual act committed against the will of the individual being raped. Threat may be involved.

rape trauma syndrome A syndrome involving specific responses to the traumatic experience of being raped. Also a nursing diagnosis.

rationalization A defense mechanism in which a person justifies ideas, actions, or feelings with seemingly acceptable explanations or reasons.

reaction formation A defense mechanism in which an individual expresses opposite feelings, attitudes, or behaviors toward another person or situation than what would normally be expressed under the circumstances, while repressing unacceptable feelings.

recidivism A tendency to relapse into a previous mode of behavior. For the client with a mental or emotional disorder, recidivism focuses on exacerbation of symptoms and relapse of illness.

reflecting A communication skill in which the nurse reiterates either the content (words) or intent (feeling tone) of the client's message. Reflecting is especially useful in the early stages of the nurse-client relationship because it allows the nurse to acquire important data necessary for planning interventions.

regression Retreating to past developmental levels of behavior, generally in an attempt to reduce overwhelming anxiety. May be used as a defense mechanism.

repression A defense mechanism in which unacceptable feelings are kept out of conscious awareness. Repression is also an operative force in the use of other defense mechanisms and is necessary for emotional survival of the organism.

resistance Reluctance or opposition by the individual to examine anxiety-producing aspects of self. The person uses automatic defenses (denial, repression) and/or learned techniques (arriving late for appointments; worsening symptoms after admission to avoid exploration in group therapy) to avoid personally unacceptable realizations.

restitution or undoing The negation of a previous, intolerable conscious act or experience in order to relieve or reduce feelings of guilt.

rigidity Inflexible; unyielding. May be attitudinal, in which the individual has a need to be precise and accurate, or refer to motor behavior in which the individual assumes a rigid posture related to an illness or medication.

role playing Reenactment of an experience for the purpose of gaining understanding and alleviating emotional distress. The drama and energy involved in role playing can produce a cathartic effect.

Rorschach test (inkblot test) A personality test in which a person states his or her immediate interpretations of a series of 10 standardized cards with inkblot designs on them. This test is believed to reveal many aspects of a person's personality structure and emotional functioning.

sadism The act of experiencing sexual gratification while inflicting physical or emotional pain on another person.

sadistic rape Rape distinguished by brutality as a necessary feature for the rapist to become sexually excited.

scapegoat The person within a family who is the recipient of the negative emotions experienced by various family members.

schizoaffective disorder A mental disorder that appears to comprise features of both schizophrenia and a mood disorder but fails to meet the DSM-IV criteria for either.

schizoid personality disorder A personality disorder with the essential feature a pattern of indifference to social relationships and a restricted range of affect and emotions.

schizophrenia A serious mental disorder characterized by a loss of contact with reality and the appearance of psychotic symptoms during the active phase of the illness; communication is impaired and previous levels of functioning in work, school, social relations, and self-care deteriorate throughout the course of the illness.

schizophreniform disorder A mental disorder that shares all essential features of schizophrenia except that the duration, including all phases, is less than 6 months.

schizotypal personality disorder A personality disorder with a pervasive pattern of peculiar thoughts and ideas, odd appearance and behavior, and deficits in interpersonal relationships.

seasonal affective disorder A major depressive episode with a seasonal pattern.

secondary gain Any benefit or support that a person obtains from the environment as a result of his or her illness, including use of defense mechanisms. Does not include relief from anxiety, which is a primary gain.

seduction An attempt made by a client to manipulate or relate to a nurse or other staff member in a nontherapeutic way (e.g., flattery or familiarity). It is usually nonsexual.

selective attention/inattention A filtering out of extraneous stimuli during the experience of moderate and severe anxiety.

self-awareness The sense of knowing what one is experiencing; it is a major goal of therapeutic work.

self-concept Composite of ideas, perceptions, and attitudes an individual develops about self based on value systems that develop primarily as a result of responses from significant others.

self-disclosure Sharing personal feelings and experiences with others. The nurse and other professionals need to use judgment as to when and how much to disclose to the client.

self-esteem Feelings of self-worth stemming from the individual's positive or negative beliefs about being valuable and capable.

self-fulfilling prophecy A predetermined idea or expectation one has toward oneself that is acted out, thus "proving" itself.

separation-individuation The process of identifying oneself as different from the primary nurturer while maintaining an emotional attachment to that person. An important task of early growth and development.

"silent rape" syndrome A maladaptive reaction to rape in which the victim fails to disclose information about the rape and is unable to resolve feelings. May lead to increased episodes of anxiety and the development of a phobic reaction.

sleep disorders Chronic disturbance of sleep patterns (dyssomnia; amount, quality or timing of sleep; parasomnia; events occurring during sleep, e.g., nightmares).

somatization The conversion of mental states or experiences into bodily symptoms, associated with anxiety.

somatoform disorder A disorder characterized by physiologic complaints or symptoms that are outside the domain of voluntary control and fail to demonstrate organic findings. May be evidence of associated psychologic factors.

somnambulism (sleepwalking) A sleep disorder characterized by repeated acts of rising from bed during sleep and ambulating for a few minutes to half an hour. Generally occurs in stages 3 and 4 of sleep and in the time phase of 30 to 200 minutes after the onset of sleep.

splitting A defense mechanism that prevents one from integrating the good and the bad aspects of oneself or of one's image of another person. The person thus views self or others as either all good or all bad at any given time and acts accordingly; failing to integrate the positive and negative qualities into a cohesive image.

stereotypy Continuous repetition of speech or physical activity. Noted in persons with organic mental disorders and schizophrenia.

strategic therapy Part of communication theory, based on premise by anthropologist Gregory Bateson that behavior makes sense in the context in which it occurs and is continually being shaped by the person's support system. Bateson and his followers attempted to reduce treatment time by focusing on solutions to problems and how best to promote change in human systems. Brief therapy is one variation of strategic therapy.

stress A broad class of experiences in which a demanding situation taxes a person's physical and emotional resources, resulting in a series of adaptive responses by the organism.

stressor A stimulus perceived by the individual or the organism as challenging, threatening, or damaging.

stupor Decreased responsiveness; partial unconsciousness.

sublimation A defense mechanism that involves rechanneling consciously intolerable or socially unacceptable impulses or behaviors into activities that are personally or socially acceptable. Urges may be of a sexual or aggressive nature.

substitution The act of finding another goal when one is blocked. May be adaptive for clients with a mental disorder.

suicidal gesture A more serious warning than suicidal ideation or threat, it involves an action that suggests the act of suicide may be imminent.

suicidal ideation A verbalized thought or idea that indicates a person's desire toward self-harm or self-destruction. Requires immediate intervention.

suicidal threat A statement of suicidal intent accompanied by behavior changes that reflect suicidal ideation.

suicide attempt A serious suicide try involving definite risk. The outcome often depends on the circumstances and is not within the person's control.

summarizing A communication skill in which main ideas are emphasized and summed up to help the client and nurse review the main themes of the conversation.

superego In psychoanalytic theory, a construct of the mind analogous to conscience development, emerging at approximately 3 years of age; a part of the ego that embodies rules (conscience) and values (ego ideal), resulting from parental influences. Faulty influence can lead to an underdeveloped superego, as seen in the antisocial personality, or an overly harsh, punitive superego, as noted in the rigid, unyielding personality types.

suppression The willful or conscious act of putting a thought, idea, or feeling out of one's mind for a variety of reasons, with the ability to recall the thought, idea, or feeling at will.

suspiciousness A pronounced attitude of doubt regarding the trustworthiness, intent, or motives of others. May include objects or situations as well.

symbolization An object, idea, or act that represents another through some common aspect and carries the emotional feeling that is associated with it. May be used as a defense mechanism.

systematic desensitization A type of behavioral therapy in which a person is exposed in steps to a series of predetermined anxiety-provoking situations, graded from least to most frightening, with the goal of reducing the anxiety that these situations promote. Most often used to treat phobias.

systems theory Proposes that a human being is a unified whole possessing his or her own integrity and manifesting characteristics that are more than and different than the sum of his or her parts. The capacity of humans and their surroundings to engage in a continuous interaction process is based on the fact that both are open systems; thus, communication or information and the energy it emits flow freely from one to the other. Nursing's conceptual system is guided by principles that serve human beings in a holistic context. Nursing views the human life process as a phenomenon of wholeness, continuity, and dynamic and creative change. Nursing acknowledges relationships between events and open boundaries that allow one entity to affect another. This is nursing's basis for ordering knowledge and developing hypothetical generalizations and unifying principles.

tangential communication Expressions or responses that are digressive or irrelevant to the topic at hand. A tangential response to a statement disregards the content of the statement and instead focuses on an incidental aspect of the statement, the type of language used, the emotions of the sender, or another facet of the same topic.

tardive dyskinesia The most frequent serious untoward effect of antipsychotic drug therapy. Usually an irreversible and late-onset complication, it is characterized by the presence of abnormal, stereotyped, rhythmic movements of the limbs and torso; tongue protrusion; and chewing movements. May affect any muscle in the body, including the diaphragm. Can occur after abrupt termination of the drug, after reduction in dosage, or after long-term, high-dose therapy. Incidence may be minimized with judicious dose management, drug holidays, and administration of antiparkinsonian drugs.

termination phase The last phase of a therapeutic one-to-one nurse-client relationship, characterized by termination of contact with the client. Termination should be addressed at the beginning of the relationship and brought up at appropriate intervals throughout, to help the client adjust.

tetrahydroaminoacridine (THA) A potent anticholinesterase drug presently being researched for use in restoring some cognitive function in individuals with Alzheimer's disease.

thematic apperception test (TAT) A projective psychologic test that involves asking the client to describe a series of ambiguous pictures.

therapeutic alliance A conscious relationship between a helping person and a client in which each agrees to work with the other to help the client resolve problems and concerns.

therapeutic community (milieu) The environment in which a hospitalized client works through problems and concerns with the help of therapists in a variety of areas. Traditional hierarchical structure and authority figures are minimized. (Originally attributed to Maxwell Jones.)

therapeutic recreation Age-appropriate recreation used purposefully by the nurse for assessment, intervention, and promotion of normal growth and development.

therapeutic use of self The ability of a nurse or other health professional to use learned theory, clinical experience, and self-awareness to benefit the client and to explore one's personal impact on others.

thinking A process that consists of a goal-directed flow of ideas, symbols, and associations initiated by a problem and leading in a logical fashion toward a reality-based conclusion.

thought blocking The sudden stopping of a thought or idea in midstream; an interruption in the train of thinking, unconscious in origin. A disturbance in speed of associations.

thought broadcasting The belief that one's thoughts, as they occur, are broadcast from one's head to the external world. A disturbance in thought content.

thought disorder Thinking characterized by loosened associations, neologisms, and illogical constructs. Includes disturbances in the form, structure, and content of thought.

thought insertion The belief that thoughts that are not one's own are being inserted into one's mind.

thought withdrawal The belief that thoughts have been removed from one's head.

transactional analysis (TA) A type of therapy developed by Eric Berne that analyzes three ego states (adult, child, and parent) as they relate to the communication process.

transference In psychoanalytic theory, an unconscious phenomenon in which the client projects onto the nurse or therapist attitudes, feelings, and desires originally linked with early significant persons. The nurse or therapist represents these figures in the client's current life.

triangling In family systems theory, the process of forming a dysfunctional triad; a major concept in an approach to family therapy developed by Murray Bowen.

trust A feeling of confidence that another person will behave in ways that are beneficial. A feeling of safety regarding another person's intentions and motives.

ulterior transaction A transaction that occurs on two levels: overt (social) and covert (psychologic). Part of the transactional analysis system.

unconscious In psychoanalytic theory, the part of the mind that is out of awareness and contains repressed materials.

undoing See *restitution.*

validation A communication skill that helps the client confirm or deny the content or intent of his or her statement.

values clarification A widely applicable systematic method of helping learners develop an awareness of their beliefs and values, select among alternatives, and act in accordance with identified beliefs. Useful with all age groups and cultures.

verbigeration (polyphasia) Repetition of meaningless words or phrases. Disturbed motor behavior as it relates to speech.

violence Behavior instituted by an individual that threatens or inflicts harm or injury to persons or property.

volubility See *logorrhea.*

voluntary commitment A legal process by which a client chooses to be admitted to a mental health facility and signs a paper to that effect.

voyeurism The attainment of sexual pleasure by observing unsuspecting persons who are naked, undressing, or engaged in sexual activity.

vulnerable Susceptible to being hurt or wounded, physically or mentally (e.g., psychic vulnerability).

waxy-flexibility A term used to describe a catatonic person who maintains the position in which he or she has been placed. The movement of the limbs has been described by caregivers as feeling "waxlike."

Wernicke-Korsakoff syndrome A disorder of the central nervous system most often associated with alcoholism and characterized by confusion, disorientation, and memory loss with confabulation; related to thiamine deficiency. Named after Karl Wernicke and Sergei Sergeivich Korsakoff.

word salad An incoherent mixture of words and phrases consisting of real and imaginary words, lacking comprehension. Occurs in severe states of schizophrenia.

working phase The middle phase of a therapeutic, one-to-one relationship in which problems are analyzed and discussed.

writ of habeas corpus A means by which a client can challenge the legality of his or her detention in a mental health facility.

xenophobia Dread or fear of strangers.

zoophilia (bestiality) Selection of animals as actual or fantasized sexual partners.

zoophobia Dread or fear of animals.

Bibliography

Current

Aguilera D: *Crisis intervention: theory and methodology,* ed 8, St. Louis, 1998, Mosby.

American Nurses Association: *A statement on psychiatric–mental health clinical nursing practice and standards of psychiatric-mental health clinical nursing practice,* Washington, DC, 1994, The Association.

American Psychiatric Association: *Diagnostic and statistical manual of mental disorders,* ed 4, Washington, DC, 1994, The Association.

Armstrong JG, Loewenstein RJ: Characteristics of patients with multiple personality and dissociative disorders on psychological testing, *J Nerv Ment Dis* 178:448, 1990.

Arnold LE, Jensen PS: *Attention-deficit disorders.* In Kaplan H, Sadock B, editors: *Comprehensive textbook of psychiatry,* New York, 1995, Williams & Wilkins.

Arthur D: Alcohol early intervention: a nursing model for screening and intervention strategies, *Australian and New Zealand Journal of Mental Health Nursing* 6:93, 1997.

Atkinson SD: Grieving and loss in parents with a schizophrenic child, *Am J Psychiatry* 151:1137, 1994.

Awan KJ: A piece of my mind . . . for my father, *JAMA* 271:1386, 1994.

Baker C and others: Connecting conversations of caring: recalling the narrative to clinical practice, *Nurs Outlook* 42:65, 1994.

Baratta S and others: The perception of life events in two different cultural settings, *Affective Disorders* 18:97, 1990.

Barkley RA: *Attention-deficit/hyperactivity disorder: a handbook for diagnosis and treatment,* New York, 1990, Guilford.

Beiser M and others: Biological and psychosocial predictors of job performance following a first episode of psychosis, *Am J Psychiatry* 151:857, 1994.

Bennett DA and others: Alzheimer's disease: a comprehensive approach to patient management, *Geriatrics* 49:20, 1994.

Boomsa J, Dingemans CAJ, Dassen TWN: The nursing process in crisis-oriented psychiatric home care, *Journal of Psychiatric and Mental Health Nursing* 4:295, 1997.

Brashares HJ and others: Mood regulation expectancies, coping responses, depression, and sense of burden in female caregiver of Alzheimer's patients, *J Nerv Ment Dis* 182:437, 1994.

Brasie JR and others: Clomipramine ameliorates adventitious movements and compulsions in prepuberal boys with autistic disorder and severe mental retardation, *Neurology* 44:1309, 1994.

Brawman-Mintzer O and others: Somatic symptoms in generalized anxiety disorder with and without co-morbid psychiatric disorders, *Am J Psychiatry* 151:930, 1994.

Bryvis C and others: Mania induced by citalopram (letter), *Arch Gen Psychiatry* 51:664, 1994.

Bulechek GH and McCloskey JC, editors: *Nursing interventions: essential nursing treatments,* ed 2, Philadelphia, 1992, Saunders.

Bulechek GH and McCloskey JC: Nursing interventions, *Nurs Clin North Am,* 27:289-598, 1992.

Butler RN: ApoE: new risk factor for Alzheimer's (editorial), *Geriatrics* 49:10, 1994.

Campbell SB: *Psychiatric disorder in preschool children,* New York, 1990, Guilford.

Cantwell DP: ADHD treatment with nonstimulants. In *Pediatric psychopharmacology,* Washington, 1994, AACAP Press.

Carpenito LJ: *Nursing diagnosis: application to clinical practice,* ed 5, Philadelphia, 1993, JB Lippincott.

Carrol-Johnson R: *Classification of nursing diagnosis: proceedings of the eighth conference,* Philadelphia, 1989, JB Lippincott.

Carslis PV: Ethical and legal issues in the care of Alzheimer's patients, *Med Clin North Am* 78:877, 1994.

Cassady SL and others: Spontaneous dyskinesia in subjects with schizophrenia spectrum personality, *Am J Psychiatry* 155:70, 1998.

Chernomas WM: Experiencing depression: women's perspectives in recovery, *Journal of Psychiatric and Mental Health Nursing* 4:393, 1997.

Clark JB, Queener SF, Karb VB: *Pharmacological basis of nursing practice,* ed 4, St Louis, 1993, Mosby.

Coccaro EF: Clinical outcome of psychopharmacologic treatment of borderline and schizotypal personality disordered subjects, *J Clin Psychiatry* 59(suppl 1):30, 1998.

Cohen D: A primary care checklist for effective family management, *Med Clin North Am* 78:795, 1994.

Crowe M: An analysis of the sociopolitical context of mental health nursing practice, *Australian and New Zealand Journal of Mental Health Nursing* 6:59, 1997.

Data watch, benchmaking study: Nursing labor costs dipped in FY 1993, *Hosp Health Netw* 68:54, 1994.

Davie JK: The nursing process. In Thelan L and others, editors: *Critical care nursing: diagnosis and management,* St Louis, 1994, Mosby.

Davis PC and others: The brain in older persons with and without dementia: findings on MR, PET and SPECT images, *AJR Am J Roentgenol* 162:1267, 1994.

De Oliveira IR and others: Risperidone versus haloperidol in the treatment of schizophrenia: a meta-analysis comparing their efficacy and safety, *J Clin Pharm Ther* 21:349, 1996.

Donner LL and others: Increasing psychiatric inpatients' community adjustment through therapeutic passes, *Arch Psychiatr Nurs* 4:93, 1990.

Ebersole P, Hess P: *Toward healthy aging: human needs and nursing response,* ed 4, St Louis, 1994, Mosby.

Eisdorfer C: Community resources and the management of dementia patients, *Med Clin North Am* 78:869, 1994.

Eisdorfer C and others: Evaluation of the demented patient, *Med Clin North Am* 78:773, 1994.

Elia J: Drug treatment for hyperactive children: therapeutic guidelines, *Drugs* 46:863, 1993.

Esman AH: Child abuse and multiple personality disorder (letter), *Am J Psychiatry* 151:948, 1994.

Fortinash K: *Assessment of mental status.* In Malasanos L, Barkauskas V, Stoltenberg-Allen K, editors: *Health assessment,* ed 4, St Louis, 1990, Mosby.

Fortinash K: *Sexuality alterations.* In Thelan L and others, editors: *Critical care nursing: diagnosis and management,* St Louis, 1994, Mosby.

Glosser G and others: Cross-cultural cognitive examination performance in patients with Parkinson's disease and Alzheimer's disease, *J Nerv Ment Dis* 182:432, 1994.

Goode H and others: Suicide and the use of antidepressants. Depression may not precede suicide (letter), *BMJ* 308:915, 1994.

Gordon M: *Nursing diagnosis: process and applications,* ed 3, St Louis, 1994, Mosby.

Gournay K and others: Dual diagnosis: severe mental health problems and substance abuse/dependence: a major priority for mental health nursing, *Journal of Psychiatric and Mental Health Nursing* 4:89, 1997.

Grilo CM and others: Personality disorders in adolescents with major depression, substance use disorders, and coexisting major depression and substance use disorders, *J Consult Clin Psychol* 65:328, 1997.

Gugel RN: Behavioral approaches for managing patients with Alzheimer's disease and related disorders, *Med Clin North Am* 78:861, 1994.

Hamerman D: Academic medical centers and nursing home affiliations (letter), *Ann Intern Med* 121:389, 1994.

Heinonen O and others: Beta-amyloid protein immunoreactivity in skin is not a reliable marker of Alzheimer's disease: an autopsy-controlled study, *Arch Neurol* 51:799, 1994.

Hodges JR and others: Remote memory and lexical retrieval in a case of frontal Pick's disease, *Arch Neurol* 51:821, 1994.

Hogarth C: Families and family therapy. In Johnson B, editor: *Psychiatric-mental health nursing: adaption and growth,* ed 3, Philadelphia, 1993, JB Lippincott.

Hogstel MD: *Geropsychiatric nursing,* ed 2, St Louis, 1995, Mosby.

Hudziak JJ, and others: Clinical study of the relation of borderline personality disorder to Briquet's syndrome (hysteria), somatization disorder, antisocial personality disorder, and substance abuse disorders, *Am J Psychiatry* 153:1598, 1996.

Iowa Intervention Project: *Nursing interventions, nursing interventions classification (NIC),* ed 2, St Louis, 1996, Mosby.

Jacobs D and others: Age at onset of Alzheimer's disease: relation to pattern of cognitive dysfunction and rate of decline, *Neurology* 44:1215, 1994.

Johnson B and others: The experience of thought-disordered individuals preceding an aggressive incident, *Journal of Psychiatric and Mental Health Nursing* 4:213, 1997.

Jones BN and others: Depression coexisting with dementia: evaluation and treatment, *Med Clin North Am* 78:823, 1994.

Kallman FJ: The genetic theory of schizophrenia: an analysis of 691 schizophrenic twin index families 1946 (classical article), *Am J Psychiatry* 151(suppl 6):188, 1994.

Kane JM: Risperidone (editorial), *Am J Psychiatry* 151:802, 1994.

Kanwischer RW, Hundley J: Screenings for substance abuse in hospitalized psychiatric patients, *Hosp Community Psychiatry* 41:795, 1990.

Kaplan H: *The comprehensive textbook of psychiatry,* ed 6, Baltimore, 1995, Williams & Wilkins.

Kaplan H, Sadock B: *Synopsis of psychiatry–behavioral science–clinical psychiatry,* ed 7, Baltimore, 1994, Williams & Wilkins.

Kendler KS, Gardner CO: Boundaries of major depression: an evaluation of DSM-IV criteria, *Am J Psychiatry* 155:172, 1998.

Kety SS and others: Cerebral blood flow and metabolism in schizophrenia: the effects of barbiturate semi-narcosis, insulin coma and electro shock 1948 (classical article), *Am J Psychiatry* 151(suppl 6):203, 1994.

Kirkpatric B and others: Depressive symptoms and the deficit syndrome of schizophrenia, *J Nerv Ment Dis* 182:452, 1994.

Klender KS and others: Outcome and family study of the subtypes of schizophrenia in the West of Ireland, *Am J Psychiatry* 151:849, 1994.

Kovacs M and others: A controlled prospective study of DSM-III adjustment disorder in childhood: short-term prognosis and long-term predictive validity, *Arch Gen Psychiatry* 51:535, 1994.

Lepola I, Vanhanen L: The patient's daily activities in acute psychiatric care, *Journal of Psychiatric and Mental Health Nursing* 4:29, 1997.

Levy R: Tacrine and lecithin in Alzheimer's disease: patient heterogeneity explains varied response (letter), *BMJ* 308:1506, 1994.

Liebowitz MR and others: Ataque de nervios and panic disorder, *Am J Psychiatry* 151:871, 1994.

Lindemann E: Symptomatology and management of acute grief 1944 (classical article), *Am J Psychiatry* 151(suppl 6):155, 1994.

Linkowski and others: The 24-hour profiles of cortisol, prolactin, and growth hormone secretion in mania, *Arch Gen Psychiatry* 51:616, 1994.

Lipsitz JD and others: Childhood separation anxiety disorder in patients with adult anxiety disorders, *Am J Psychiatry* 15:927, 1994.

Loebel JP and others: The management of other psychiatric states: hallucinations, delusions and other disturbances, *Med Clin North Am* 78:841, 1994.

Lyness SA and others: Cognitive performance in older and middle-aged depressed outpatients and controls, *J Gerontol* 49:129, 1994.

Marder SR and others: Risperidone in the treatment of schizophrenia, *Am J Psychiatry* 151:825, 1994.

Margraf J and others: Guttman scaling in agoraphobia: cross-cultural replication and prediction of treatment response patterns, *Br J Clin Psychol* 29:37, 1990.

Markowitz JC: Psychotherapy of dysthymia, *Am J Psychiatry* 151:1114, 1994.

Marotta C: Alzheimer's disease: how research is changing primary care management (interview by Mark E. Weksler), *Geriatrics* 49:47, 1994.

Masterson JF: Psychotherapy of borderline and narcissistic disorders: establishing a therapeutic alliance (a developmental, self, and object relations approach), *Personality Disorders* 4:182, 1990.

McCaffrey G: The use of leisure activities in a therapeutic community, *Journal of Psychiatric and Mental Health Nursing* 5:53, 1998.

McCay E and others: Sexual abuse comfort scale: a scale to measure nurses' comfort to respond to sexual abuse in psychiatric populations, *Journal of Psychiatric and Mental Health Nursing* 4:361, 1997.

McCloskey JC and others: Standardizing the language for nursing treatments: an overview of the issues, *Nurs Outlook* 42:56, 1994.

Michaels E: Opinions about dementia being revised, conference informs physicians, *Can Med Assoc J* 151:359, 1994.

Midanik L, Clark W: Drinking-related problems in the United States: description and trends, 1984-1990, *J Stud Alcohol* 56:395, 1995.

Mielke DH: Anticonvulsant therapy for mood disorders, *South Med J* 87:685, 1994.

Mitchell J: *Bulimia nervosa,* Minneapolis, 1990, University of Minnesota Press.

Mitrushina and others: A comparison of cognitive profiles in schizophrenia and other psychiatric disorders, *J Clin Psychol* 52:177, 1996.

Munoz DG: Aluminum and Alzheimer's disease (letter), *Can Med Assoc J* 151:268, 1994.

Nakdimen KA: Multiple personality, *Hosp Community Psychiatry* 41:566, 1990.

Negley EN, Manley JT: Environmental interventions in assaultive behavior, *Gerontological Nursing* 16:29, 1990.

Newcorn J, Strain J: Adjustment disorder in children and adolescents, *Journal of the American Academy of Child and Adolescent Psychiatry* 31:318, 1992.

Neziroglu FA, Yaryura-Tobias JA: A review of cognitive-behavioral and pharmacological treatment of body dysmorphic disorder, *Behav Modif* 21:324, 1997.

Nottelmann ED, Jensen PS: Comorbidity of disorders in children and adolescents: developmental perspectives. In *Advances in clinical child psychology,* vol 17, New York, 1995, Plenum.

O'Brien L, Flote J: Providing nursing care for a patient with borderline personality disorder: a phenomenological study, *Australian and New Zealand Journal of Mental Health Nursing* 6:1997.

Olivera AA, Kiefer MW, Manley NK: Tardive dyskinesia in psychiatric patients with substance use disorders, *Am J Drug Alcohol Abuse* 16:57, 1990.

Oxman TE: Delayed recall: demented, depressed or treated? *Lancet* 344:213, 1994.

Pelham WE: *Attention-deficit/hyperactivity disorder: a clinician's guide,* New York, 1994, Plenum.

Pendlebury WW and others: Tacrine and lecithin in Alzheimer's disease. Tacrine is safe and effective (letter), *BMJ* 308:1506, 1994.

Peterson RC and others: Memory function in very early Alzheimer's disease, *Neurology* 44:867, 1994.

Pine DS and others: Anxiety and congenital central hypoventilation syndrome, *Am J Psychiatry* 151:864, 1994.

Piper WE and others: Patient characteristics and success in day treatment, *J Nerv Ment Dis* 182:381, 1994.

Pope HG, Yurgelun TD: Schizophrenic individuals with bipolar first-degree relatives: analysis of two pedigrees, *J Clin Psychiatry* 51:97, 1990.

Provancha LE, Hurst S: *Home health case management: an old approach to a new system,* NSI Home Health Services newsletter, 1994.

Puskar KR and others: Psychiatric nursing management of medication-free psychotic patients, *Arch Psychiatr Nurs* 4:78, 1990.

Rawlins PR, Williams SR, Beck CM: *Mental health–psychiatric nursing,* ed 3, St Louis, 1993, Mosby.

Rawlins R, Heacock P: *Clinical manual of psychiatric nursing,* St Louis, 1992, Mosby.

Reis S: Rumination in two developmentally normal children: case report and review of the literature, *J Fam Pract* 38:521, 1994.

Richards BS: Alzheimer's disease: a disabling neurophysiological disorder with complex nursing implications, *Arch Psychiatr Nurs* 4:39, 1990.

Riggs JE and others: The association between apolipoprotein E allele epsilon 4 and late-onset Alzheimer disease: pathogenic relationship or differential survival bias (letter), *Arch Neurol* 51:750, 1994.

Roberts C and others: Tacrine and lecithin in Alzheimer's disease: serum tacrine concentrations too low (letter), *BMJ* 308:1506, 1994.

Rocio M and others: Suppression of psychoactive effects of cocaine by active immunization, *Nature* 378:727, 1995.

Ross CA and others: Structured interview data on 102 cases of multiple personality disorder from four centers, *Am J Psychiatry* 147:596, 1990.

Rosse RB and others: Gaze discrimination in patients with schizophrenia: preliminary report, *Am J Psychiatry* 151:919, 1994.

Roy MA and others: Validity of the familial and sporadic subtypes of schizophrenia, *Am J Psychiatry* 151:805, 1994.

Roy-Byrne PP: Generalized anxiety and mixed anxiety-depression: association with disability and health care utilization, *J Clin Psychiatry* 57(Suppl 7):86, 1996.

Ryan JP: Nursing theory in perspective (letter), *Nurs Outlook* 42:93, 1994.

Sadock BJ: Group psychotherapy, combined psychotherapy and psychodrama. In Kaplan HL, Sadock BJ, editors: *Comprehensive textbook of psychiatry,* ed 6, Baltimore, 1985, Williams & Wilkins.

Schneider LS and others: Emerging drugs for Alzheimer's disease. Mechanisms of action and prospects for cognitive enhancing medications, *Med Clin North Am* 78:911, 1994.

Schulz SC and others: Treatment and outcomes in adolescents with schizophrenia, *J Clin Psychiatry* 59(Suppl 1):50, 1998.

Silverman JM and others: The Consortium to Establish a Registry for Alzheimer's Disease (CERAD): part VI, family history assessment: a multicenter study of first-degree relatives of Alzheimer's disease probands and nondemented spouse controls, *Neurology* 44:1253, 1994.

Silverman JM and others: Patterns of risk in first-degree relatives of patients with Alzheimer's disease, *Arch Gen Psychiatry* 51:577, 1994.

Simon GE, VonKorff M: Suicide mortality among patients treated for depression in an insured population, *Am J Epidemiol* 147:155, 1998.

Simon J: Therapeutic humor: who's fooling who? *Journal of Psychosocial Nursing in Mental Health Services* 1988.

Sky AJ and others: The use of psychotropic medications in the management of problem behaviors in the patient with Alzheimer's disease, *Med Clin North Am* 78:811, 1994.

Snaith RP: Depression and impotence (letter), *BMJ* 308:1439, 1994.

Skeketee G and others: The psychosocial treatments interview for anxiety disorders: a method for assessing psychotherapeutic procedures in anxiety disorders, *Journal of Psychotherapeutic Practical Research* 6:194, 1997.

Streim JE and others: Federal regulations and the care of patients with dementia in the nursing home, *Med Clin North Am* 78:895, 1994.

Swanson JM: *Classroom interventions with the ADHD children,* Irvine, Calif, 1993, KC Press.

Swanson JM and others: Effects of stimulant medication on learning in children with ADHD, *Journal of Learning Disabilities* 4:219, 1991.

Talley S and others: Effect of psychiatric liaison nurse specialist consultation on the care of medical-surgical patients with sitters, *Arch Psychiatr Nurs* 4:114, 1990.

Taylor AT and others: Fluoxetive in family practice patients, *J Fam Pract* 39:45, 1994.

Thompson JM and others: *Mosby's clinical nursing,* ed 3, St Louis, 1993, Mosby.

Van Gool WA and others: Diagnosis of Alzheimer's disease by apolipoprotein E genotyping (letter), *Lancet* 23:344, 1994.

Wharton RN and others: The use of lithium in the affective psychoses 1966 (classical article), *Am J Psychiatry* 151(Suppl 6):277, 1994.

Wilcock GK: Tacrine and lecithin in Alzheimer's disease: negative conclusions not justified (letter), *BMJ* 308:1507, 1994.

Wisniewski HM: Aluminum tan protein and Alzheimer's disease (letter), *Lancet* 34:204, 1994.

Wittchen Hu and others: DSM-IIIR generalized anxiety disorder in the National Co-morbidity Survey, *Arch Gen Psychiatry* 51:355, 1994.

Yonge OJ: Nurses and patients' perceptions of constant care in an acute care psychiatric facility: a descriptive qualitative study, *Dissertation Abstracts International* 50(11-B):4990, 1990.

Zemetkin AJ: Brain metabolism in teenagers with attention-deficit/hyperactivity disorder. *Arch Gen Psychiatry* 50:333, 1993.

Classics and Standards

Al-Anon: *The 12 steps and traditions of Al-Anon family groups,* New York, 1973, Al-Anon.

Alberti R, Emmons M: *Your perfect right: a guide to assertive behavior,* ed 2, San Luis Obispo, Calif, 1974, Impact.

American Nurses Association: A social policy statement, Kansas City, Mo, 1980, The Association.

American Psychiatric Association: *A psychiatric glossary,* ed 7, Washington, DC, 1994, The Association.

Arieti S: *Interpretation of schizophrenia,* New York, 1974, Basic Books.

Beck A and others: *Cognitive therapy of depression,* New York, 1976, Guilford.

Benson H: *The relaxation response,* New York, 1975, William Morrow.

Berne E: *Games people play,* New York, 1964, Grove.

Bleuler E: *Dementia praecox or the group of schizophrenias* (Zinkin J, translator), New York, 1950, International Universities Press.

Bolby J: *Attachment and loss: separation, anxiety and anger,* New York, 1973, Basic Books.

Bowen M: *Family therapy in clinical practice,* New York, 1978, Jason Aronson.

Burnside I: Listen to the aged, *Am J Nurs* 1975.

Ellis A: *Reason and emotion in psychotherapy,* New York, 1962, Lyle Stuart.

Ellis A, Harper R: *A new guide to rational living,* Hollywood, Calif, 1976, Wilshire.

Engel G: Grief and grieving, *Am J Nurs* 1964.

Erikson E: *Childhood and society,* New York, 1950, WW Norton.

Erikson EH: *Childhood and society,* revised, New York, 1964, WW Norton.

Erikson EH: *Identity, youth and crisis,* New York, 1968, WW Norton.

Fagan C: Psychotherapeutic nursing. In *Psychiatric–mental health nursing: contemporary readings,* New York, 1978, D Van Nostrand.

Ernest Jones, editor: *Collected papers of Sigmund Freud,* New York, 1959, Basic Books.

Freud S: *New introductory lectures on psychoanalysis,* New York, 1933, WW Norton.

Freud S: *Problem of anxiety,* New York, 1936, Basic Books.

Fromm-Reichmann F: *Principles of intensive psychotherapy,* Chicago, 1960, University of Chicago Press.

Hays JS, Larson KH: *Interacting with patients,* New York, 1963, Macmillan.

Holmes TH, Rahe RH: The social readjustment rating scale, *Journal of Psychosomatic Research* 1967.

Horney K: *New ways in psychoanalysis,* New York, 1939, WW Norton.

Horney K: *Our inner conflicts,* New York, 1945, Norton.

Jacobson E: *Progressive relaxation,* Philadelphia, 1938, JB Lippincott.

Jellinek EM: *The disease concept of alcoholism,* New Haven, 1960, Hills-House Press.

Kanner L: To what extent is early infantile autism determined by constitutional inadequacies? *Proc Assoc Res Nerv Ment Dis* 33:378, 1954.

Klein M: A contribution to the psychogenesis of manic-depressive states. In *Contributions to psychoanalysis,* London, 1934, Hogarth.

Kubler-Ross E: *On death and dying,* New York, 1969, Macmillan.

Kubler-Ross E: What is it like to be dying? *Am J Nurs* 1971.

Lange A, Jakubowski P: *Responsible assertive behavior: cognitive/behavioral procedure for trainers,* Champaign, Ill, 1976, Research Press.

Mace NL, Rabins PV: *The 36 hour day: a family guide to caring for persons with Alzheimer's disease, related dementing illnesses, and memory loss in later life,* Baltimore, 1981, Johns Hopkins University Press.

Maslow AH: *Toward a psychology of being,* New York, 1968, D Van Nostrand.

Maslow AH: *Motivation and personality,* New York, 1970, Harper & Row.

Masters W, Johnson V: *Human sexual response,* Boston, 1966, Little, Brown.

May R: *The meaning of anxiety,* New York, 1950, Ronald Press.

Minuchen S: *Families and family therapy,* Cambridge, Mass, 1976, Harvard University Press.

Minuchen S, Fishman HC: *Family therapy techniques,* Cambridge, Mass, 1981, Harvard University Press.

Peplau HE: *Interpersonal relations in nursing,* New York, 1952, GP Putnam.

Peplau HE: Process and concept of learning. In Burd S, Marshall M, editors: *Clinical approaches to psychiatric nursing,* New York, 1963, Macmillan.

Rogers C: Characteristics of a helping relationship, *Pers Guid J* 1958.

Rogers C: *On becoming a person,* Boston, 1961, Houghton Mifflin.

Selye H: *The stress of life,* New York, 1956, McGraw-Hill.

Selye H: *The stress of life,* revised, New York, 1976, McGraw-Hill.

Selye H: *Stress without distress,* New York, 1974, New American Library.

Sullivan HS: *Conceptions of modern psychiatry,* New York, 1953, WW Norton.

Sullivan HS: *The interpersonal theory of psychiatry,* New York, 1953, WW Norton.

Sullivan HS: *Schizophrenia as a human process,* New York, 1962, WW Norton.

Torrey EF: *Surviving schizophrenia: a family manual,* New York, 1983, Harper & Row.

Wolpe J: *The practice of behavior therapy,* ed 2, New York, 1973, Pergamon.

Yalom ID: *The theory and practice of group psychotherapy,* ed 3, New York, 1985, Basic Books.

Index

B

C

G

J

N

O

Q

R

S

T

W

X

Y

Z